Tumours of the Upper Jaw

For Churchill Livingstone
Publisher: Miranda Bromage
Senior Project Editor: Lucy Gardner
Copy Editors: Jane Ward, Isobel Black
Production Controller: Mark Sanderson
Sales Promotion Executive: Caroline Boyd

Tumours of the Upper Jaw

Sir Donald Harrison MD MS PhD
FRCS FRACS(Hon) FRCSE(Hon) FCM(SA)(Hon)
FACS(Hon) FRCSI(Hon) FRSM(Hon)

Emeritus Professor of Laryngology and Otology,
University of London; Emeritus ENT Consultant,
Moorfields Eye Hospital, London

Valerie J. Lund MS FRCS
Reader in Rhinology, Professorial Unit, Institute
of Laryngology and Otology, University College, London;
Honorary Consultant in Otorhinolaryngology, Royal
National Throat, Nose and Ear Hospital Trust, London
and Moorfields Eye Hospital, London

CHURCHILL LIVINGSTONE
EDINBURGH LONDON MADRID MELBOURNE NEW YORK AND TOKYO 1993

CHURCHIL LIVINGSTONE
Medical Division of Longman Group UK Limited

Distributed in the United States of America by Churchill Livingstone
Inc., 650 Avenue of the Americas, New York, NY 10011, and by
associated companies, branches and representatives throughout the
world.

First published 1993

ISBN 0- 443- 04017-6

British Library Cataloguing in Publication Data
A catalogue record for this book is available from the British Library.

Library of Congress Cataloging in Publication Data
Tumours of the upper jaw/edited by Sir Donald Harrison, Valerie J.
Lund
    p.   cm
    Includes index.
    ISBN 0–443–04017–6
    1. Jaw –Tumors. 2. Jaw–Surgery. I. Harrison, D. F. N. (Donald
Frederick Norris) II. Lund, Valerie J.
    [DNLM: 1. Maxillary Neoplasms–diagnosis. 2. Maxillary
Neoplasms–therapy. WU 280 T9255]
  RC280. J3T85 1993
  616. 99'292–dc20
  DNLM/DLC
  for Library of Congress   92–49458

The
publisher's
policy is to use
**paper manufactured
from sustainable forests**

Contents

Preface

The last decade has seen an acceptance of the specialized head and neck oncologist, and an appreciation of the need for a multidisciplinary approach to the management of tumours developing within this unique region of the body. Although the effect of this change of attitude must be to the benefit of the patient, inevitably the consequence is a lessening in experience for the individual clinician. Previously, most neoplasms of the upper jaw found their way to a variety of specialists including ENT, Oral, Ophthalmic and even the General surgeon, none of whom saw enough patients to acquire expertise. However, a combination of personal interest and unique facilities, allowed the Professorial Unit at the Royal National Throat, Nose and Ear Hospital Trust, London, the opportunity of caring for more than 500 patients with malignant neoplasms of the upper jaw over a period of almost 30 years. This book is a compilation of that experience, written however in the light of today's knowledge. In doing so, it is anticipated that the many problems and fascination aroused by the management of upper jaw tumours will be conveyed to the reader, who may be anybody called upon to play a part in the diagnosis or care of these unfortunate individuals.

No excuse is made for including a few clinical conditions which strictly speaking do not fall specifically within the accepted definition of 'neoplasm'. As with odontogenic lesions, we have been guided in our selection by our experience of the patients seen in the Unit and their problems in diagnosis and management. None of this would have been possible without the unstinting enthusiasm and energy shown by the members of the Unit, from both home and abroad, who have played such an important role over almost three decades. Although invidious to mention specific names, we would be amiss not to acknowledge the contributions made by Tony Cheesman and David Howard who have been responsible for much innovative and 'heroic' surgery in this area. In developing craniofacial resection into a safe and cosmetically acceptable procedure, they have contributed greatly to the effective management of many upper jaw lesions. Indeed, this has been one of the few useful oncologic advances in what still remains, a challenging mission to improve the outcome for these patients.

1993

D.F.N.H.
V.J.L.

Acknowledgements

Figures 2.1–2.4, 2.10 and 2.15–2.17 are reproduced from Maran A G D, Lund V J 1990 Clinical rhinology. Georg Thieme Verlag, Stuttgart.

Figure 2.13 is reproduced from Mackay I S, Bull T R (eds) 1987 Scott Brown's otolaryngology, vol 4, rhinology, 5th edn. Butterworths, London.

Figures 4.1, 4.7, 4.8, 5.4, 5.5, 6.4, 6.9, 7.9, 12.1, 12.2, 13.9, 17.6 and 19.11 are reproduced from Lloyd G A S 1988 Diagnostic imaging of the nose and paranasal sinuses. Springer Verlag, Berlin.

We would like to acknowledge the invaluable contribution made by the Pathology Department of the Zoological Society of London.

Authors and contributors

Sir Donald Harrison MD MS PhD FRCS
FRACS(Hon) FRCSE(Hon) FCM(SA)(Hon)
FACS(Hon) FRCSI(Hon) FRSM(Hon)
Emeritus Professor of Laryngology and
Otology, University of London;
Emeritus ENT Consultant, Moorfields Eye
Hospital, London

Valerie J. Lund MS FRCS
Reader in Rhinology, Professorial Unit,
Institute of Laryngology and Otology,
University College, London;
Honorary Consultant in Otorhinolaryngology,
Royal National Throat, Nose and Ear Hospital
Trust, London and Moorfields Eye Hospital,
London

With contributions from:

David J. Howard FRCS FRCS(Ed)
Senior Lecturer in Laryngology, Professorial Unit,
Institute of Laryngology and Otology, University
College, London;
Honorary Consultant in Otorhinolaryngology, Royal
National Throat, Nose and Ear Hospital Trust,
London

Glyn A.S. Lloyd MA DM FRCR
Formerly Director, Department of Radiology, Royal
National Throat, Nose and Ear Hospital Trust, London;
Consultant Radiologist, Moorfields Eye Hospital,
London

Christine Piff
Founder of 'Let's Face It', Support Network for the
Facially Disfigured, Crowthorne, Berks

Philip M. Stell ChM FRCS
Emeritus Professor of Otorhinolaryngology,
Liverpool University

This book is dedicated to
Manuel (Mannie) Lederman FFR DMRE
Consultant Radiotherapist to the Royal Marsden
Hospital, Royal National Throat, Nose and Ear
Hospital, Moorfields Eye Hospital and the Chelsea
Hospital for Women, London.
A pioneer in head and neck oncology with world-
wide recognition, along with his wife, Vera (née
Dalley), he gave an unrivalled professional service
to our patients. His initiation of new ideas, superb
lectures and thoughtful publications contributed
enormously to our understanding of the natural his-
tory of neoplasia within the head and neck. The
upper jaw was his particular interest and we owe
much to his support and encouragement over many
years. His untimely death in 1984 robbed us of a
unique contributor but hopefully this book will serve
as an epitaph to an exceptional man.

Introduction

Tumours arising within or involving the upper jaw were recognized at the time of Hippocrates, who distinguished between hard and soft lesions but believed that treatment only shortened the patient's life! Many of these were probably nasal polyps and not true neoplasms, for by our present definition a tumour is 'an abnormal mass of tissue, the growth of which exceeds and is uncoordinated with that of normal tissue and persists in the same excessive manner after cessation of the stimulus which evoked the change'.

Tumour Registries pay little attention to benign tumours affecting the nose and paranasal sinuses and malignant lesions make up less than 3% of cancers arising within the upper aero-digestive tract, and in most countries form less than 1% of all malignancies. Consequently, upper jaw tumours of all types are uncommon. However, they do present a unique variety of histological variants and an understanding of their natural history and treatment requires a thorough comprehension of the complex anatomy of this region of the body. The intimate relationship of nasal passages to the paranasal sinuses, orbit and anterior cranial fossa presents formidable problems in both diagnosis and tumour control. Individual clinicians will see only a small number of many of these conditions during their lifetime and much of the literature is therefore based upon minimal experience or collated data from a variety of separate institutions, with all the inherent defects of such statistics.

In compiling this book we have drawn heavily on the more recent literature but have also utilized our considerable personal experience, gained over almost 30 years from working within an academic unit which had recourse to large numbers of patients with upper jaw problems. This type of personal experience has now been supplanted by the multidisciplinary team and improvements in local expertise throughout the world has to some extent reduced the volume of external referral. The field of head and neck oncology is now covered by a variety of experts which includes the surgical and medical oncologists, radiotherapist, histopathologist, epidemiologist and biologist, all hopefully for the benefit of the patient.

Head and neck cancer is one of those malignancies for which there is a proven clear relationship to a number of aetiological factors. Whilst the role of tobacco and alcohol is well established in areas such as the oral cavity, pharynx and larynx, industrial carcinogens have been identified as factors in the production of sinus cancer. Adenocarcinoma of the ethmoids is recognized as an industrial disease within the United Kingdom and in Norway a successful educational programme was instituted in the 1970s within the nickel industry. Based upon the association between nickel refining and upper jaw carcinoma, modifications were accepted in the plants in which workers with high nickel plasma levels were moved to low-risk areas, protective masks were worn and a reduction in airborne contamination evolved. This resulted in a 50% fall in mortality rates for maxillary sinus cancer, something which has not happened for the majority of patients in which no specific avoidable aetiological cause has been identified.

Many of the signs and symptoms and radiological findings of upper jaw tumours whether benign or malignant, only become apparent when the disease is well established. Early diagnosis is bedevilled by limitations in histological identification and the inaccessibility of the region. The development of nasal endoscopy and its sophisticated instrumentation has considerably improved our ability to inspect the nasal passages and the maxillary sinus, with increased expectation of identifying early tissue abnormalities. Supplementation of direct visualization by the use of modern radiological techniques has also revolutionized our diagnostic abilities for many upper jaw tumours. Contrast-enhanced computed tomography (CT) in both direct coronal and axial planes allows excellent visualization of bone. Magnetic Resonance Imaging (MRI) combined with paramagnetic agents such as gadolinium-DTPA, enables tumour to be differentiated from inflammatory changes, fluid, fibrosis and in many instances, normal tissues. The improved contrast resolution plus the availability of coronal, sagittal and axial views enhances the diagnostic possibilities and together CT and MRI provide means of accurately delineating tumour boundaries.

The availability of specialized head and neck histo-pathologists has significantly advanced our understanding of the wide range of pathological conditions which affect the upper jaw. Some do not readily fall within a strict definition of 'tumour' but do enter into differential diagnosis. Odontogenic tumours, whilst normally the province of oral pathologists, are frequently seen by other specialists and may cause difficulties in both terminology and management; some are included in this book. Differential diagnosis has been materially affected by the use of monoclonal antibodies which, although originally envisaged as a means of directly attacking tumour cells, have proven of great value in the identification of single tumour antigens. Within the upper jaw the differentiation of anaplastic tumours has been assisted by the use of immunohistochemistry and the pathologist's armamentarium of suitable probes is growing rapidly. No longer does the identification of tumours such as anaplastic carcinoma, olfactory neuroblastoma or endocrine carcinoma have to rely solely on light microscopy. The result has been an awareness of the varying biological behaviour of many of these lesions and the whole biology of human carcinogenesis is undergoing an expansion of interest and knowledge.

Unfortunately a failure to clinically diagnose the majority of upper jaw tumours at an early stage has resulted in a continuation of the problems of the management of advanced cancers. Intracavitary irradiation has been largely replaced by external megavoltage with fractionation dosage. Although no dramatic improvement in cure rates has occurred, severe complications have largely vanished, in part related to the use of computerization in treatment planning. The combination of radiotherapy with surgical excision has been generally accepted for most sinonasal malignancy although relative timing of these two modalities remains a matter for discussion. The development of craniofacial resection and the re-emergence of midfacial degloving has certainly affected the possibilities of adequately resecting a wide range of pathological conditions in this relatively inaccessible site. Morbidity rates are minimal and cosmetic disability so low that these operation are now standard for many benign conditions. Together with the advances and availability of prosthetic devices, such as the integrated osseous implant, much upper jaw surgery can no longer be described as 'mutilating'.

Some mention must be made of the potential implications of research into molecular biology. Recognition of the importance of cellular DNA, with aneuploid DNA content being possibly a prediction of poor survival, is leading to the evaluation of ploidy differences in different histological patterns. This may be of value in management decisions particularly when considering the advisability to major surgical resections or chemotherapy. Despite decades to effort and many clinical studies, our ability to affect significantly the survival or quality of life of patients with squamous carcinoma of the head and neck has not been materially influenced by modern chemotherapy. Complete remission is rare, whilst partial response in many tumours of the upper jaw can be obtained by minor surgery without toxicity. This failure may be related to the use of much chemotherapy in more advanced lesions and in Japan combined therapy (including cytotoxic drugs) has been used successfully for maxillary sinus cancer. However, the absence of prospective studies in large enough numbers and the anxieties in giving immunosuppressive drugs to patients in whom systemic metastases are relatively uncommon, suggests a note of caution.

This book represents a distillate of three decades of experience, during which time our diagnosis and histological accuracy has improved markedly together with our ability to oncologically excise many extensive benign and malignant tumours. Greater understanding of the biological behaviour of many of these unusual lesions together with an ability to restore the functional and cosmetic appearances of patients following loss of maxilla or palate has been to the patients' benefit. However, it would have been unrealistic to have expected a major improvement in actuarial survival rates for the more common malignant tumours and this must wait for further understanding of human cancer and new means of treatment.

1. History of surgery of the upper jaw

P. M. Stell

An historical introduction to major articles or textbooks has become commonplace. Sadly, most of these historical vignettes are, for various reasons, inaccurate, the commonest reason being that the author failed to read the original articles. For example, it is often stated that Watson did the first laryngectomy for syphilis, in 1865. But, the original paper shows that Watson described the larynx, trachea and bronchi of a patient who had syphilis; the only operation carried out during life was a tracheotomy.[1]

A second source of error is an inability to read languages other than English. It is often said that adenoid cystic carcinoma was first described by Billroth in 1859 by the term 'Zylindrome'.[2] This is untrue: the tumour was first described by two Frenchmen, Robin & Laboulbene, as 'tumeur heteradenique' in 1853.[3]

A third source of error is to ignore the context of the historical events. It is stated repeatedly[4] that cancer of the ear was first discussed about 1775 by Wilde & Schwartze. Apart from the fact that Wilde was born in 1815 and Schwartze in 1837, this statement ignores the fact that in 1775, histopathological diagnosis still lay almost a century ahead, so that no such discussion was possible.

A specific example of historical inaccuracy is the large monograph on malignant tumours of the maxilloethmoidal region written by Oehngren in 1933.[5] His extensive historical introduction is marred by two facts: firstly it is obvious that he did not personally read all the original reports for he misquotes names, e.g. Lizzard for Lizars; secondly, he gives no references to the authors he quotes.

In compiling this account of the development of upper jaw surgery, I have read and searched widely through the available literature, attempting to resolve these writings to the technology and politics of the relevant times. The development of the single lens microscope by Antoni van Leeuwenhoek around 1665 (Fig. 1.1) and the discovery of aniline dyes about 1856 by Perkin, an Englishman working in Germany, eventually made histopathology possible.[6] Normal histology developed mainly in

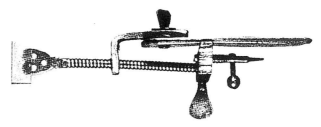

Fig. 1.1 Van Leewenhoek's single lens microscope (circa 1660).

Germany throwing up such well-known names as Schwann and Henle. They were followed by Virchow who laid the foundations of histopathology with his book 'Cellular Pathology'. Virchow was the first to emphasize that classification based on external appearances was arbitrary, rather it should be based on normal cellular structures. He was one of the first to use terms such as epithelioma for squamous carcinoma.[7]

By about 1860 economical and technological advances initiated a German surgical school led by famous men such as Conrad Langenbeck, his nephew Bernard Langenbeck, Billroth, Thiersch, Kocher, Trendelenburg, Czerny, Mululicz, etc. This was the golden age of excisional surgery, and all the first major excisions of the internal organs such as gastrectomy, total laryngectomy, glossectomy, etc. were described at that time in Germany.

Between 1825 and 1875 when maxillectomy was developed, the main contributors came from the French and three British schools: Edinburgh, London and Dublin. The outstanding names were those of Gensoul and Dupuytren in France, Syme, Liston and Lizars of Edinburgh, the English school led by Fergusson, and the Dublin school under Stokes and Butcher. The German schools only contributed towards the end of this period. The school which flourished in Dublin from about 1800–1830, produced such well-known names as Wilde, the father of modern otology (and of Oscar Wilde), Stokes, Adams, Colles, Corrigan, Cheyne, Graves and the now forgotten Butcher, who in his time was preeminent in the field of maxillectomy. Why this school sprang up where and when it did is an historical mystery. Dublin society had been greatly depleted by the departure for London of diplomats and politicians after the Act of Union in 1800. Furthermore Ireland had an entirely agricultural economy, whereas Europe was becoming rapidly industrialized and therefore more prosperous.

SURGICAL PRACTICE IN THE 19TH CENTURY

It is virtually impossible to imagine how primitive were the conditions under which the pioneers of upper jaw surgery worked. Despite the incredible differences in pathology, anaesthesia, instrumentation and, not least, operating facilities, between the early part of the 19th century and today, almost all the fundamental concepts of surgery in this region have developed during a period of 50 years.

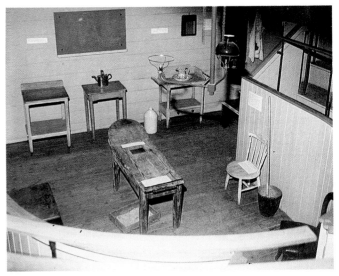

Fig. 1.2 Old St Thomas's operating theatre in use between 1822 and 1861.

Operating conditions

If we could step back in time to 1830, perhaps the first difference that would be apparent would be the surgeon's dress. At that time it was usual to wear an old frock coat which hung on the back of the theatre door: the more encrusted with blood and pus the more honourable it was. Surgical gowns and gloves belong to this century: even after the introduction of asepsis by Lister in 1867 it was usual for surgeons to operate with bare hands until at least 1895.[8]

Resection of the upper jaw was classified as a 'capital operation', so-called because the patient could, and often did, die during or immediately after the operation. It was usual to give notice, not only to the medical profession but also to society in general, of forthcoming operations of this type. Thus the audience included not only medical students but curious bystanders: the famous violinist Paganini carried out a tour of England and Scotland in 1831–1832, and attended a maxillectomy carried out by Earle in 1831. At the end of the operation Earle came forward and was greeted by 'deserved applause'. This operation had to be postponed because the rumour of it had brought together such a multitude that even after an adjournment to the anatomical theatre, it was impracticable to continue with the operation.[9] The operation carried out by Liston in 1835 attracted several hundred spectators. The operating theatre was so-called because the seats were arranged in ascending rows, as in an ordinary theatre, for easier viewing. For similar reasons, it was called an amphitheatre in France (Fig. 1.2).

Pathology

The second enormous difference between the present day and the 50-year period from 1820 to 1870 during which maxillectomy was developed, was in pathological diag-

nosis. Surgeons had no histopathological description of the tumour on which to base their classification until about 1855, and the terms used were merely descriptions of the macroscopical appearance of the tumour. Histopathology was not placed on a firm basis until the publication of Virchow's book in 1856. He was the first to describe tumours on the basis of their cellular appearance.[7] Gross descriptive terms were still being used as late as 1863 when Barton stated that maxillary tumours may be divided into medullary, scirrhous, melanoid or epithelial.[20] Furthermore, even after histopathology became generally available about 1860, histological examination was restricted to postoperative examination.[195] The examination of a biopsy belongs to this century: indeed as late as 1923 Ochsner was vigorously maintaining that preoperative biopsy with a knife led to the setting up of metastases.[10]

A patient described by Dickson in 1840, though not subjected to operation, gives useful insight into the appreciation of gross pathology at that time. The patient was described as having a 'fungus of the antrum with lymphatic contamination, but not visceral taint'. The lymphatic contamination was a lymph node enlarged to the size of an almond in the digastric space. It was clearly appreciated that this was a malignant tumour which had spread to the lymph nodes so that the tumour was therefore incurable. A necropsy was carried out 12 hours after death showing no 'visceral taint', that is no distant metastases.[11]

In 1833 there were three indications for resection of the upper jaw:[12]

1. 'Malignant disease'
2. 'Augmented growth of the bony parts'
3. 'A sort of dropsy'.

The terms used for 'malignant disease' were often so vague that it is now impossible to know what they described. They included tumour, intumescence, malignant disease, medullary disease, sarcoma, etc. The term carcinoma was not used relative to the maxilla until 1878 by a German, Koerte.[13] However, it is clear that the lesions were often carcinoma, and that the terms medullary tumour and sarcoma were squamous carcinomas. The word sarcoma was often used in its literal Greek meaning, that is a 'fleshy tumour'. It did not take on the connotation of a tumour of mesodermal origin until the latter part of the 19th century. Virchow in his classic 'Cellular Pathology' tells us that the term medullary disease arose from the idea that it originated in the nerves and resembled nervous matter. This tumour was originally thought to arise from the body of the sphenoid bone or other bones of the base of the cranium, but Heath showed that it did indeed originate in the maxillary antrum itself.[14] A review of 160 maxillectomies published between 1830 and 1880[11-13, 15-143] shows that about 50 of the 160 were done for carcinoma, although it was said that 'cancer is certainly a very unusual form of growth to occur in the upper jaw'.[69]

'Augmented growth of the bony parts' may refer either to bony tumours or to fibrous dysplasia. 19 of the first 160 cases were described as being bony tumours of some sort, such as exostosis, and many are described as osteosarcoma. Of 14 patients described by Dieffenbach, six were classed as osteosarcoma.[45] This description was not based on histology, and it is unlikely that almost half his patients suffered from so rare a disease. However some of the bony tumours described were clearly osteomas, for example the antral tumour described by Bickersteth in 1857 which could only be examined by sawing it in half.[23] It is interesting to speculate why osteomas (or exostoses) appear to have been so common in the early part of the 19th century.

'A sort of dropsy' was almost certainly expansion of the antrum and erosion of its bony walls by an expanding retention cyst. A patient who had undergone resection of the entire upper jaw for a cyst via a Fergusson type of incision on the face was shown at a meeting of the Medical Society of London in 1874.[68] The surgeon was strongly criticized for carrying out an operation which was more serious than the disease required. Another member pointed out that many of these cysts were of dentigerous origin, and were cured by the removal of the offending teeth, an opinion which would hold good to this day. Another dentigerous cyst of the antrum was described by Bryant who said that doubtless upper jaws had been removed in former times for this affection, its true pathology not having been understood.[144]

Another common diagnosis not included in Guthrie's classification[12] was fibroid tumour or fibroplastic disease. 30 of the first 160 maxillectomies were for such tumours.

From detailed descriptions this tumour had a firm consistency with thin adherent bone, that had been eroded by pressure. Many of these tumours presented with a non-ulcerated swelling of the palate, some later histological studies described fibrous tissue. Many of these tumours are clearly what would now be called angiofibromas, and a series of them is described by the Irish surgeon Butcher.[29-32] However not all these tumours were angiofibromas as they appear to have arisen in both sexes and at all ages. The microscopy of one of these fibrous tumours showed elongated cells forming fibres, calcareous matter deposited along the course of the fibres, and a central hard portion infiltrated by earthy salts converting it into a stony mass.[88] This tumour was almost certainly an ossifying fibroma. A fibrous tumour, described as a fibrosarcoma, was removed from the upper jaw of a man of 58, by the well-known Irish surgeon Stokes in 1873.[145] The histological appearances showed tough fibrous tissue with a few small blood vessels.

At least a dozen maxillectomies were carried out for what was described as necrosis or caries of the upper jaw, due to syphilis,[25,115] typhus,[146] or occupational exposure to phosphorus.[147]

Microscopical examination of tissue removed surgically began in the 1850s: Brainard in 1852 in America was one of the earliest practitioners describing the tumour as presenting no trace of cancerous tissue, and said that no cancer cells were detected under the microscope.[148] This examination was not necessarily based on examination of a section, because Craven in 1863 comments 'under the microscope the juice scraped from the cut surfaces exhibited no fibrous element but simply a confused mass of broken up cells and granular matter'.[37] Thus, in the early stages it appears that some form of cytology was practised on cells scraped from the tumour. Furthermore, examination of sections as we know it, did not develop until the end of the 19th century. Until then specimens for histology were preserved in alcohol[17] and cut by hand, but in about 1866 His made his sliding microtome, which was improved in the following decade. Automatic machines began with Threlfall's, made in 1883. These demanded rigid embedding of the specimen in substances like paraffin wax.[6]

Early histological reports include that by Clark in 1856, who described a tumour 'under the microscope as presenting cells and nuclei of every size and shape. A few commencing characteristics of epithelial cancer were present sufficiently distinctly to show positively that the tumour belonged to that class.'[34] Another tumour[92] was encased in true bone, and histologically showed 'oily globules compressed together but rather more irregular and oval in form, about 1/300th inch in the long diameter. The walls were made of closely packed cellules 1/2000th inch in diameter. No true bony cells could be found. When examined under polarized light at a power of 400 it showed a structure similar to that of horn or ivory.'

Histological descriptions then followed rapidly: of a fibronucleated tumour,[149] 'a section of the mass hardened in spirit showed bundles of fibrous tissue but not arranged so as to form a cancerous stroma; a number of simple round cells and masses of spindle shaped cells';[49] a 'globular epithelioma';[150] a small round cell carcinoma;[151] and a myxosarcoma including a woodcut of the histological appearances.[114] Heiberg in 1861 described an adenoid cystic carcinoma under the then current term of cylindroma; this view was based on histological examination.[152] Other probable adenoid cystic carcinomas were soon described.[47,136] In the latter case histology showed 'an epitheliomatous epulis resembling an adenoma of the breast'.[195] In another case recorded as a cubular epithelioma,[19] histology showed 'the ground work to consist of well-developed fibrous tissue with large groups of cells arranged in some parts like a racemose gland and in other parts like tubular glands. In the centre of most of these groups there was a lumen.' This was probably an adenoid cystic carcinoma, although it might have been an adamantinoma as it was said to resemble identically a 'multilocular epithelioma' previously described in the upper jaw.

Sir William Fergusson must have had an interesting career, spanning as it did the development of both pathology and anaesthesia. The circumstances when he carried out his first operation in 1842[51] must have been very different from those when he removed a maxilla in 1872.[65,153] On the latter occasion histology was available to show that the tumour was composed of fibrous tissue with island-like and spindle-shaped nuclear bodies with a calcareous nodule in its centre, that was probably an ossifying fibroma. He was certainly using chloroform by 1863.[59]

Anaesthesia

In the early days the patient was held or tied down. Nobody records 'dulling the patient with alcohol' but this must surely have been common; laudanum (i.e. morphine) appears to have been given only after the operation. Chloroform was introduced in 1847 and ether in 1842, but chloroform was usually the sole agent used for maxillectomy.

Chloroform was in frequent use by the 1860s, even in the provinces. Unfortunately the patient was often conscious during the greater part of the operation: 'chloroform was administered to its full extent to begin with, but its inhalation was not continued afterwards'.[50] Another report from Australia in 1868 tells us that it 'was tried but abandoned'.[154]

It was often necessary to allow the patient to wake up during the operation if he was bleeding profusely. As late as 1870 it was customary to fix the patient in the armchair as a precaution in case he did wake up.[109] Patients often recovered from the chloroform and 'spat the blood as is often the case on all bystanders'.[155]

Some thought that chloroform was dangerous because 'the irritability of the glottis is weakened if not wholly lost, so that there must be the danger of the trickling of blood from the mouth into the glottis without the excitement of a cough for expelling it from the windpipe'.[74] It was often necessary to suspend the administration of chloroform and allow the patient to recover consciousness because of the 'danger of strangulation from the great amount of blood poured out'. For this reason Rose recommended carrying out the operation with the head hanging.[156] Some surgeons remained unwilling to use chloroform until late in the century.[157]

In the early days chloroform was administered by sprinkling it on a piece of lint,[77] but by 1860 it was being administered by a tube passed through one nostril.[56] Later a special tubular inhaler was developed to be passed through one nostril[43] but this method was rapidly displaced by Trendelenberg's cannula. Trendelenberg had introduced a tracheostomy tube with a cuff in 1870.[158] This cannula had been used for the administration of an anaesthetic through a tracheostomy to the first patient to undergo total laryngectomy by Billroth in 1873,[159] and it was used for a maxillectomy for a cylindroma by Heiberg in Germany in 1872.[152] This method is the obvious way to avoid the dangers of haemorrhage during the administration of chloroform, and had become established by the 1880s: Bellamy in 1883 said 'I was first inclined to do a prophylactic tracheotomy and to use Trendelenberg's tamponade apparatus'.[160]

A further means of preventing pain was to freeze the line of incision with ether.[154]

Instruments

Although surgical instruments of many kinds had been available for centuries there were nonetheless great differences between the early 19th century and the present day. Two examples might suffice to emphasize this: firstly, the only form of illumination was natural daylight. Only one paper in the first 50 years comments on illumination. In Irving's case in 1824 the patient was placed in an armchair opposite a window.[161] The question of illumination is not otherwise discussed; lighting must have been very difficult as efficient illumination, either by gas or electric light, did not come into general use until the 1880s. Secondly, artery forceps for the control of haemorrhage were not invented until the latter part of the century, although ligatures were available for the arteries, and indeed were used by Nivison in 1824.[161] Fergusson's textbook of 1870 shows that the vessel was held by a forceps and the ligature applied.[64]

A common instrument was the cautery, of which there were two types: the actual cautery and the potential cautery. The actual cautery was a hot branding iron, whereas the potential cautery consisted of caustics of different sorts. Division of cautery into these two types was of ancient origin, and their use was described by Parey in the 17th century.[162] The actual cautery was used to deal with carious bone. Parey felt that it was more effective than potential cauteries such as sulphuric acid, scalding oil and molten sulphur, because it could be used more precisely, but that the potential cautery often had to be used because of the pain produced by the actual cautery! In the 19th century discussions as to the relative merits of the two continued: Liston (1821) felt that the actual cautery was preferable in maxillectomy because it was effective and the pain it produced was greater but momentary, whereas the pain of potential cautery persisted for several days.[103]

The term 'actual cautery' continued to be used into this century: Ochsner wrote a paper entitled 'Treatment of cancer of the jaw with the actual cautery' in 1923.[10] The cautery he used was a simple soldering iron heated to red heat in a gas flame. He felt that it was important to hold the iron in place for at least a minute to destroy tissue up to 2 cm away. Also, he thought that the necrotic tissue thus formed stimulated the production of antibodies that attacked the cancer, a concept which re-emerged some 50 years later with the cryosurgical probe. However, by 1926 the diathermy had almost completely replaced the use of soldering irons, as it requires no protection for the surrounding tissues, and may be employed with greater facility.[163] The electrocoagulation was produced by a bipolar high frequency current of the d'Arsonval type.[164] A further extension of the principle of the actual cautery is cryosurgery, which was first used for maxillary carcinoma about 1970.[165]

An interesting illustration of the use of potential cautery is provided by a patient from Wales with a tumour of the palate who was eventually subjected to excision of the jaw in 1843, but who for some time had been under the care first of a wild wart doctor and then a wild wart doctress. These two practitioners had treated the tumour with external applications consisting of a mixture of clay, French brandy and a caustic fluid, probably sulphuric acid.[166] The Welsh wild wart doctors survive to this day and still have a successful practice for the treatment of basal cell carcinomas of the skin using mixtures of this kind.

There was much discussion about the best way of removing the bone, one of the common methods was the use of the lion-jawed forceps designed by Sir William Fergusson (Fig. 1.3).[17] The use of the 'chain saw' (i.e. Giglis' saw) was popularized by Davies in 1858[44] and Heyfelder in 1857.[167] The latter devised a blunt needle passed into the sphenomaxillary fissure to emerge in the

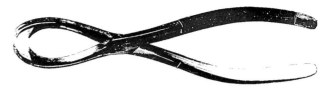

Fig. 1.3 Fergusson's lion forceps.

zygomatic fossa allowing a chain saw to be pulled through for division of the malar bone. He pointed out the advantages of the chain saw over the ordinary saw: the greater ease and rapidity with which the bones can be divided, the avoidance of splintering, the parts are cut from behind forwards avoiding unintentional division by the saw, corners can be rounded, and the division of the bony parts can be effected in a very small space. He strongly criticized Desault's procedure of boring a hole into the antrum with a punch and enlarging it with a short curved knife ('instrument tranchant en forme serpette') because the walls of the antrum in many cases are not thinned. He clearly understood the principle of total excision for cancer when he stated that 'all pathologists and operators on the upper jaw seem with one consent to deprecate the removal of tumours and especially cancerous with a sparing or niggardly hand, their usual counsel in practice being the extirpation of the whole jaw'. Another commonly used means of dividing bone was the Hayes saw.[154]

The speed with which these operations were carried out can but leave us breathless. The length of the operation is only rarely recorded, but Hancock resected the entire upper jaw in 8 min in 1847[76], and Key in 20 min in 1833.[94]

DEVELOPMENT OF SURGERY FOR MAXILLARY CANCER

This surgery developed in three phases: firstly, piecemeal removal of tumours, a phase lasting until 1825; secondly, the establishment of formal excision of the upper jaw beginning about 1825; followed by the development of more refined procedures such as lateral rhinotomy in the latter part of the 19th and early 20th centuries.

The controversy as to who carried out the first maxillectomy was most aptly summed up by Butcher: 'the operations on the upper jaw may, in reality, be classed under two heads, that of exsection and that of disarticulation of the bone'.[29]

Localized removal

The first recorded partial removal of a maxillary tumour was that carried out by Wiseman, surgeon to Charles II, reported in 1676.[168]

A man about twenty-eight years of age came out of the Country recommended to me with a Cancer of his left Cheek, stretching itself from the side of his nose close under the lower Eye-lid to the external Canthus, so making a compass downwards. It was broad in its basis, and rose copped like a Sugarloaf. It gleeted, and was accompanied with Inflammation and much pain. He had also some scirrhous glands under that Jaw. The extirpation of this Cancer had been attempted in the Country; but it growing afterwards bigger and threatening his Eye lately with inflammation, he hastned up, and importuned me to undertake it. I complied with his desire, and four or five days after having prepared all things ready, viz actual Cauteries, Digestives, Defensatives, Bandage, etc. Doctor Walter Needham and my Kinsman Jaques Wiseman being assisting. I pulled the Tumour towards me with one hand, during which I made my Incision close by the Eye-lid, and cut it smooth off as close to the Os jugulare as I could doe it, avoiding the Periosteum. The blood at first spurt out forcibly from many capillaries besides two considerable Arteries: we permitted them to bleed awhile. The lesser Vessels stopped of themselves, and we cauterized the greater afterwards. Then viewing our work, and observing some relique of the Cancer remaining above the external Canthus, we consumed it by actual cautery, and dressed up the Wound with our Digestive, with Embrocations, Desensatives, and moderate bandage to retain them. The third day we took off Dressings, saw it well disposed to digest, and dressed it as before. The second day after, dressing it again, the Cancer appeared rising from the side of the nose and Eye-lid; it also overspread the Cheek-bone. I dressed it as I had done the time before, and the next time came prepared with actual cauteries, and consumed it all, then dressed it up with Lenients. From that time the Ulcer healed daily, and contracted in ten days space to the half; yet since then it begins to bud again here and there, which will put me upon a necessity of using the actual Cautery: and what account to give of it I yet know not.

According to Butcher a part of the upper jaw was removed by Acoluthus, a physician at Breslau in 1693. A woman had a tumour on the jaw after the extraction of a tooth. He enlarged the mouth with a cut, removed part of the swelling, together with four teeth, but was unable at once to get completely round it; 'he attacked it several times at intervals of a few days, sometimes with cutting instruments, and sometimes with the actual cautery, and at last succeeded in curing his patient'.[29] In 1770, White described a tumour of the antrum of two years standing. He removed it by a semicircular incision in the face, scooping away 'matter like rotten cheese and many fragments of rotten bones'; the bony walls of the orbit were already destroyed. He preserved the eye, the optic nerve and part of the alveolus, but stopped at the dura which he could see and feel![169]

Operations for tumours of the upper jaw were thus rarely attempted before 1800, and they are not mentioned at all in the standard 18th century texts such as those by Bell, Heister, Hunter and Pott.[170–173] However, between 1800 and 1820 sporadic attempts were made with increasing frequency at localized excision of diseased tissue.

Localized removal of a tumour after elevating skin flaps, was carried out by Dupuytren in 1818,[174] by Liston in Edinburgh in 1821,[103] by Irving a surgeon in Annan, Scotland on 1 November 1822,[86,161] by Rogers in 1824 in New York,[175] by Ballingal in 1827 in Edinburgh,[18] and by Velpeau of Paris in 1829 and 1830.[176] In all of these cases an incision was made in the face, the soft tissues of the cheek were elevated and a tumour of the antrum was removed by traction on the tumour itself. No deliberate attempt was made to divide the bony attachments of the maxilla and such cases could not really qualify as maxillectomies.

Butcher also tells us that the scooping operation was practiced by Desault, Garengeot, Jourdain, Plaque and others, and has been 'in modern times more especially brought under notice by Dupuytren, in 1820, and since by many surgeons'.[29] Although Dupuytren argued that the greater part of the jaw might be excised he did not do the operation himself.

A similar operation was being carried out as late as 1837 in Germany: Dieffenbach described 17 cases, but only one of these could be classed as a subtotal maxillectomy, the remainder being localized resections of tumours affecting the hard palate or alveolus. The exception was an osteoma probably arising in the ethmoid sinuses which he removed preserving the alveolus and hard palate.[45]

Formal maxillectomy

Guthrie in 1835 said that maxillectomy was one of the great improvements in modern surgery over the previous 16 years for which we were mainly indebted to the French.[12] This statement suggests that the operation began to develop about 1820.

Lizars of Edinburgh, in 1826, proposed the entire removal of the superior maxillary bone, and described the procedure.[106] Speaking of 'polypi, or sarcomatous tumours, which grow in the antrum,' he says:

All the cases which have come within my knowledge (with the exception of one) wherein these sarcomatous tumours have been removed by laying open the antrum, have either returned or terminated fatally. I am, therefore, decidedly of opinion, that unless we remove the whole diseased surface, which can only be done by taking away the entire superior maxillary bone, we merely tamper with the disease, put our patient to excruciating suffering, and ultimately to death. An incision should be made through the cheek, from the angle of the mouth backwards or inwards, to the masseter muscle, carefully avoiding the parotid duct, then to divide the lining membrane of the mouth, and to separate the soft parts from the bone, upwards to the floor of the orbit; secondly, to detach the half of the velum palati from palate bone. Having thus divested the bone to be removed of its soft coverings, the mesial incisive tooth of the affected side is to be removed; then the one superior maxillary bone to be separated from the other, at the mystachial and longitudinal palatine sutures, and also the one palate bone from the other at the same palatine suture, as the latter bone will also require to be removed either by the cutting pliers or a saw; thirdly, the nasal process of the superior maxillary bone should be cut across with the pliers; fourthly, its malar process, where it joins the cheek bone; fifthly the eye, with its muscles and cellular cushion, being carefully held up by a spatula, the floor of the orbit is to be cleared of its soft connections, and the superior maxillary bone separated from the lacrymal and ethmoid bones with a strong scalpel. The only objects now holding the diseased mass are, the pterygoid processes of the sphenoid bone, with the pterygoid muscles. These bony processes will readily yield by depressing or shaking the anterior part of the bone, or they may be divided by the pliers, and the muscles cut with a knife. After the bone with its diseased tumour has been removed, the flap is to be carefully replaced, and the wound in the cheek held together by one or two stitches, adhesive plaster, and bandage. In no other way do I see that this formidable disease can be eradicated.

Lizars attempted the operation in December 1827 'for a medullary sarcomatous tumour of the antrum, from a miner or collier', but had to abandon the operation because of bleeding. He tried again on 1 August 1829 and this time succeeded. He first tied the trunk of the temporal and internal maxillary arteries, and also the external jugular vein which had been divided in the first incision. He cut through the alveolar process and bony plate on the left side of the palatine suture, and completely separated the upper jaw with the saw, Liston's forceps, and strong scissors, but the orbital plate was separated from the eyeball by the handle of the knife. The tumour was medullary sarcomatous, and a portion of it, attached to the pterygoid process of the sphenoid bone, could not be detached, but part of the malar bone involved in the disease was removed. On the 16th day the wound had healed and she left the house on that day. Three days after 'she expired suddenly, but no examination was permitted'. He performed a further successful operation on 10 January 1830.[177]

A very similar procedure was carried out by Syme, also at the Edinburgh Royal Infirmary on 15 May 1829.[129] He made a cruciate incision and, after exposing the tumour, divided the malar bone with a saw and pliers, divided the nasal process of the maxillary bone and cut through the hard palate using cutting pliers after having extracted one of the incisor teeth. He therefore probably did the operation a few weeks before Lizars, although Lizars gave the first description.

The early French literature is reviewed very thoroughly by Gensoul in his monograph of 1833.[179] He describes operations carried out by Garengeot, Desault and Dupuytren up to 1824. He records the great pains he took to find out what operations were actually carried out, both by reading the contemporary accounts and by talking to those present at these operations. His research can be summarized as showing that all the procedures carried out to 1827 consisted of an incision on the face followed by piecemeal removal of diseased tissue; no formal excision had been attempted. Gensoul then described his own patient, a 17-year-old boy with a 2 year history of a swelling in the superior part of the canine

fossa, which he described as a hyperostosis. The tumour measured $7^3/_4 \times 7^1/_2$ inches with a circumference of $16^1/_4$ inches. After much thought and consultation with colleagues he embarked on an operation on 26 May 1827, at the Hotel Dieu in Lyon. After making three incisions in the skin of the face he elevated skin flaps. Then he used a mallet and chisel to divide the lateral wall of the orbit close to the frontozygomatic suture, passed the chisel as far as the pterygomaxillary fissure, and divided the frontal process of the zygoma. Next he applied a very large chisel to the inner canthus and passed it through the lacrimal bone. He divided the ascending process of the nasal bone in a similar manner. He used the knife to divide the soft tissues of the nasal ala from the maxilla, removed the first upper incisor on the left side, and divided the hard palate. Finally, to detach the maxilla from the pterygoid process, he plunged the chisel through the orbit and through the tumour, dividing the superior maxillary nerve, and used the chisel to bevel the specimen into the mouth. Shortly afterwards the patient fainted, but ultimately recovered! This is clearly the first account of a deliberate excision of the upper jaw.

Gensoul also did at least six other similar procedures, some for cancer, one with a 5-year cure. Unusually for that time, he followed his patients for upwards of 5 years, and also recorded the size of his tumours and at one point frankly admits a diagnostic mistake! Even more unusually, he deliberately delayed publication for 6 years to assess the long-term effects. His monograph runs to 77 pages, and in addition describes excision of the lower jaw. Gensoul also acknowledged Lizars' claim to have done the first operation, an apparent reference to Lizars' 'System of Anatomical Plates', published in 1826.

In the early 1850s there was a fairly vicious correspondence under pseudonyms such as 'studens chirugiae' or 'chirurgus',[128, 178] in the medical press about the question of who did the first maxillectomy: Lizars, Syme or Gensoul. Who it was is of little consequence, except perhaps to Lizars, Syme and Gensoul at the time! Such claims for scientific precedence are common: they tell us that the procedure was not a 'maverick' out of its time, but rather that surgery had progressed to the point where the operation was feasible and several surgeons in different countries had decided to try it, indicating that the topic was one of general interest. The main countries contributing to this development were France and Great Britain and, to a lesser extent, Germany. The Surgeon-General's Catalogue tells us that the procedure did not spread to other European countries until the second half of the 19th century.[180] It was first carried out in Belgium in 1845 by Heylen,[182] in Poland in 1852 by Klose,[183] in Italy in 1857 by Gianflone[184] (a previous resection for necrosis had been reported in 1850 by Moretti),[185] in The Netherlands in 1857 by Leonides van Praag,[100] in Austria in 1857 by Dehler,[186] in Portugal in 1862 by Barbosa,[187] in Russia in 1862 by Kade,[93] in Spain in 1864 by Rosa[188] (one case for necrosis had been carried out by Toca in 1858[189]) and in Finland in 1873 by Estlander.[190]

Resection of both upper jaws was first carried out by Heyfelder in Erlangen, Germany in 1844.[82] A report was given in English by his son Oscar in 1857 in the Dublin Journal of Medical Science; Dublin being one of the main centres for this procedure, notably under Butcher, a name now forgotten. The operation was carried out for a large 'pseudo-plasma' arising from the palate, pushing the nose forward. He raised a large bilateral flap up to the inferior orbital margin, and then formally excised both maxillae preserving the nose. No attempt was made to provide a prosthesis. The patient returned to work but died 15 months later of a recurrence in the frontal bone.[167] Oscar Heyfelder stated that the indications for the removal of both upper jaws included the following:

Necrosis and cares

Benign tumours including enchondroma and osteosarcoma

Malignant tumours including epithelial cancer (cancroid of Virchow), cancer gelatiniforme, carcinoma medullare and cystocarcinoma.

Incision

Many incisions have been described for maxillectomy, but they can be divided into two main types. The first is an incision passing from the outer canthus to the angle of the mouth. This was used in the early years – by Ballingal in 1827,[18] Lizars in 1829,[177] Velpeau in 1832,[176] Key in 1834,[94] and Liston in 1835[104] – but appears to have been abandoned by about 1840. The second is an incision passing down the lateral side of the nose. This was first used in 1827 by Gensoul[179] and has become the standard incision. Gensoul brought the incision through the upper lip at the level of the 1st incisor tooth, and Fergusson, in 1842, brought it through the upper lip in the midline.[51] The French school also developed a similar incision without division of the upper lip for partial operations on the upper part of the maxilloethmoidal complex, first described in 1865 by Legouest.[191] A further lateral limb through the lower eyelid was soon added. Farabeuf ascribes to Blandin of Paris an incision running from the inner to the outer canthus at the level of the infraorbital margin,[192] to join the incision running down the side of the nose, but this incision is *not* included in Blandin's original paper of 1834.[24] An incision passing from the inner to the outer canthus within the lower eyelid and through the conjunctiva at the oculo-palpebral fold was described by Michaux in 1854, the purpose being to prevent retraction of the lower eyelid.[193] The incision through the external surface of the lower eyelid just below

the lashes is usually ascribed to Weber. However, the source of this attribution is a mystery: a careful search has failed to reveal any record of a description of this incision by Weber, and the reference to his work[194] relates to fractures of the jaws. The so-called Weber–Fergusson incision would be more accurately termed the Blandin–Gensoul incision. The incision described by Dieffenbach of splitting the patient down the midline did not catch on![45]

Ligation of the carotid arteries

In the earlier operations it was customary to ligate the common or external carotid artery before the operation. For example Earle, in 1831, ligated the common carotid artery on the affected side, apparently with no ill effects[9] whereas Scott in 1830 tied the external carotid artery.[196] Heath in his textbook 'Injuries and Diseases of the Jaws', tells us that this practice had been quite abandoned by the time of writing.[14]

Partial resections

Surgery of the upper jaw continued to be developed for a further century, almost exclusively by the French who introduced the concept of surgery 'à la demande des lesions'.[37]

In 1925 Cornet reviewed this development dividing the upper jaw into three stages: superstructure (the ethmoido-maxillo-orbito-malar complex), a naso-sinus mesostructure, and a palatal infrastructure. He discussed the embryological basis of this division and the main histological tumour types, pointing out that about half are squamous carcinomas. He then discussed the anatomical origin of these tumours – from the ethmoids, the nasal cavity, from the antrum itself and from the hard palate and alveolus – and the route of spread.[197] He carried out experiments with Sebileau on the cadaver, demonstrating that it was impossible to clear the ethmoids via a buccal or transantral approach, and therefore recommended the paralateronasal rhinotomy described by Moure as the operation of choice for tumours of the suprastructure. Sebileau in 1906 described the clinical forms of maxillary cancer (neoplastic, suppurative and putrid) and gave a description of the routes of spread of maxillary cancer into the cheek, nose and mouth, into the nose through the inferior meatus, the canine fossa through the anterior walls, through the socket of an extracted tooth to appear on the upper alveolus, into the orbit through the superior wall, and into the pterygomaxillary or pterygoid fossa through the posterior wall.[197]

Superstructure

In the early years it was thought necessary to resect all the upper jaw, because the methods of investigation had not allowed the exact point of origin and extent of the malignant tumour to be determined. However as early as 1848 Michaux was questioning whether it was necessary to excise the hard palate when it was healthy.[198] He described partial operations for ethmoidal tumours and also preserved the floor of the orbit to maintain the function of the eye.[193] He also stressed the need to exclude extension of the tumour into the cranial cavity. In his monogram of 1854 Michaux described seven different procedures:[193]

1. Ablation of the maxilla and malar bones
2. Ablation of the maxilla alone
3. Removal of the upper portion of the maxilla preserving the hard palate
4. Removal of the inferior portion of the maxilla conserving the floor of the orbit and the ascending process of the maxilla
5. Removal of the palatine arch
6. Resection of the upper alveolus
7. Removal of both maxillae.

In 1865 Legouest made an incision from the inner canthus descending along the nasal ala as far as the centre of the upper lip. He then opened the left nostril widely and retracted the nose towards the healthy side after having divided the articulation of the nasal bone with the ascending ramus. Finally, he turned the internal wall of the maxillary sinus outwards using scissors, after dividing the ascending ramus and the external and inferior part of the anterior opening of the nostril.[191] He did this operation for a boy with a nasopharyngeal polyp; presumably an angiofibroma. Until then these tumours had been treated by total maxillectomy with sacrifice of the orbit, but Legouest made a plea for a more conservative approach.

Cornet tells us that Michel of Nancy in 1869 modified the operations of Michaux and Legouest by omitting the resection of the maxilla itself and by adding an incision perpendicular to the vertical incision to allow partial excision of the orbital rim.[197]

The next development was a lateral rhinotomy described by Moure in 1902 as a radical intervention for malignant tumours arising from the upper part of the nasal fossa or from the ethmoid. He tells us that the orbital route had been previously recommended for approaching tumours of the upper jaw but advocated a different approach as follows. The nose was turned aside after making an incision from the lower part of the frontal bone to the nostril, the nasal bone being exposed using a periosteal elevator. He divided the ascending process of the maxilla and a part of the lacrimal bone after first elevating and retracting the 'membranous nasal canal' so as not to damage it. He then divided the nasal bone within the nose, and finally the nasal spine of the frontal bone. To avoid opening the cranial cavity he passed a gouge

parallel to the cribriform plate as far as the anterior wall of the sphenoid sinus, removing the ethmoids with a large curette working from below upwards. This step was carried out using illumination from a forehead mirror. The operation finished with curettage of diseased areas of the septum, the orbit and sphenoid sinus. He counselled conserving the ridge of the nasal bone to preserve the shape of the nose, and advised packing the postnasal fossa at the start of the operation to prevent inhalation of blood. However, he said that bleeding usually stopped after removal of the tumour, and packing was then no longer necessary. He pointed out that it is possible to reach the sphenoid sinus by this route.[199]

His first patient, a cooper of 55, underwent the operation described above on 9 July 1901. One year later the patient was alive and well with no recurrence. Histology showed an 'epithelioma cylindrique'. Moure did not describe what he meant by this term, but the tumour is described fully in a later French paper by Hautant in 1933. From this description, including the fact that it arises from the olfactory mucosa, and from the accompanying woodcut, it is clear that 'epithelioma cylindrique' would now be called an olfactory neuroblastoma. Indeed this tumour was fully described by the French.[4]

Sebileau further refined this procedure under the name of paralateronasal rhinotomy emphasizing certain technical details, and dividing rhinotomy into high, low or total.[200] Moure's lateral rhinotomy was extended further by Hautant[201] in 1933 using an incision beginning above at the same point as Moure's incision, but then extending laterally beneath the eye. He used chisels to excise all the anterior part of the wall of the maxilla plus the floor of the orbit. This monograph is the first to include a description of the radiological appearances of these tumours.

The French were also the first to point out that sacrifice of the floor of the orbit is excessive if it is not invaded, because the physiological suspension of the eye is lost; 'an eye not lying in its correct place is an eye lost'.

It is interesting that St Clair Thomson said in 1937 that lateral rhinotomy had quite replaced excision of the upper jaw,[202] and yet by 1977 it was described as a neglected operation.[203]

Mesostructure

Cornet in 1925 described unusual tumours which destroy the nasoantral wall and early invade the maxillary antrum.[197] These cases, he says, are suitable for a procedure that preserves both the floor of the orbit and hard palate. He describes a procedure which he terms an extended Caldwell-Luc antrostomy: the initial incision in the gingivobuccal sulcus between the canine and 2nd molar tooth is extended and the entire anterior wall of the sinus is resected. Thereafter, the tumour is removed by careful and meticulous curettage of the antral cavity whose other walls are assessed for erosion.

This was only a minor modification of the operation described by Denker in 1909.[204] After retracting the upper lip, Denker made an incision in the upper buccal sulcus of the affected side, and for 2–3 cm on the opposite side. The soft tissues were then elevated from the face up to the orbital rim. He opened the maxillary antrum through the canine fossa and removed the lateral nasal wall with Luer's forceps and chisel. The lower part of the nasal bone and the nasal process of the maxilla were also resected. If necessary, he cleared the ethmoidal labyrinth and removed the anterior wall of the sphenoid.

Cornet also described a similar procedure[197] for the excision of malignant tumours arising from the inferior part of the nasal fossa (the septum and the inferior turbinate) which he ascribed to Rouge but sadly gives no reference. A careful search has failed to reveal where this procedure is recorded. The steps are as follows:

1. A horizontal sublabial incision extending from one 1st molar to the other in the gingivolabial groove.

2. Exposure of the nose: the curved periosteal elevator is used to denude the bone towards the bony orifice of the nostrils, which it exposes on the lateral part of their circumference, exposing the anterior and inferior nasal spine.

3. Division of the quadrangular cartilage from below upwards using the scissors, and of the nasal spine allowing the superstructure of the nose to be elevated.

4. Pterygomaxillary disarticulation, using a special shears curved on the flat.

5. Extraction of the block held by a Farabeuf's forceps.

Infrastructure

Partial procedures for palatal tumours were described in 1854 by Michaux.[193] He describes resection of the upper alveolus, which he divided above the roots of the teeth with small scissors. He also describes in some detail an operation described by Nelaton of Paris, but unfortunately does not give a reference. Nelaton first elevated the palatal mucosa, providing of course that it was not diseased and next made several holes at the anterior end of the hard palate. He introduced one blade of the scissors through this hole, dividing the hard palate and inferior edge of the septum.

Farabeuf generally made a transverse incision on the face to expose the upper alveolus. He perforated the anterior wall of the antrum to allow scissors to be introduced to cut the attachments of the alveolus.[50] He too ascribes to Nelaton the midline incision in the hard palate, but gives no reference to where Nelaton's work may be found.[192]

Barwell in 1873 removed the hard palate and alveolus from within the mouth, without opening into the nasal cavity.[21] He said that he could find no account of such an operation in any surgical work or journal, completely ignoring the fact that Michaux had given a very full description of this procedure in an extensive monograph 20 years earlier. Barwell's procedure of transoral palatectomy appears to have been empirical, rather than a systematic development based on the study of anatomy and pathology as was the case with the developments described by the French. The final development was that described by Cornet for tumours of the infrastructure. This operation was redescribed in the English literature a quarter of a century later by Wilson, who gave no credit to the French either for describing the operation or for describing the anatomical and pathological principles upon which it is based.[137]

Osteoplastic procedures

The only other contribution from the German school, apart from resection of both maxillae and Denker's sublabial approach, was the development of an osteoplastic approach, originally described by Langenbeck in 1859.[205] His patient was 18 years old, with two fibrous polyps, probably an angiofibroma of the nasopharynx. He first made a skin incision, much like that used for lateral rhinotomy, and divided the nasal cartilages from their attachments. Using a cutting bone forceps he divided the nasal bone close to the septum up to the nasal process of the frontal bone. A second incision divided the bone of the nasal process and continued into the maxillary sinus, ending at the attachment of the nasal process of the maxilla where it forms the lower border of the orbit. He used an elevator to turn the bone back on to the forehead.

In 1863 Voelckers described an osteoplastic flap, pedicled superiorly, of the anterior wall of the antrum for removal of a tumour – again probably an angiofibroma – invading the antrum from the region of the sphenoid sinus.[206]

Combined irradiation

In the early years of the 20th century maxillectomy was also combined with the introduction of radium into the cavity. This method was popular both in England and America.[163, 164, 207, 208] Jacketed tubes, steel points or emanation seeds were used. The radium was applied directly to the tumour using a 50 or 100 mg tube within a silver tube for 15 to 20 hours.[209] An alternative was radium needles contained in a dental plate moulded to fit the cavity.[207]

PROSTHESES

It has been customary since the earliest days to fill the defect left by maxillectomy by some form of dental prosthesis. A prosthesis was made after one of the very first maxillectomies, carried out by Syme in 1835: Nasmyth made an artificial plate and a set of teeth which rendered the patient's appearance, mastication and articulation 'hardly at all defective'.[130] Hart in 1862 tells us of a patient undergoing maxillectomy for scrofula for whom an artificial set of teeth were made by his brother, a dentist.[79] Baker, a surgeon/dentist to Dr Stevens Hospital in Dublin, 'arranged the palate and dental apparatus in a most satisfactory manner so that the patient was enabled to eat with comfort and to articulate with perfect distinctness'.[107]

By the early years of this century the technique of dental restoration was well developed. Woodman describes how a plaster cast must be taken a few days before operation, to allow a temporary denture to be made with a bulbous extension to fit the cavity and prevent prolapse of the cheek. A permanent vulcanite splint, bearing teeth, is made a few months later (Fig. 1.4).[210, 211]

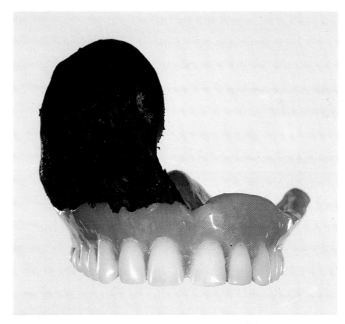

Fig. 1.4 A dental obturator (after Woodman 1923[210]).

SUMMARY

Despite the dramatic technical innovations developed during the last half of the 20th century within the fields of chemotherapy, anaesthesia, illumination and instrumentation, possibly the only new major surgical procedure relevant to upper jaw neoplasia has been the craniofacial resection.

A search through the original European literature has shown that during a period of some 50 years (1825–1875) most of the operations viewed today as standard, were developed without the assistance of adequate illumination, blood replacement, anaesthesia, etc. by a small number of exceptionally gifted and determined surgeons within a small number of European countries. The fact that any patients survived these traumatic experiences is a tribute to these surgeons' skills as well as the patients' own forbearance.

REFERENCES

1. Watson 1865 Ulceration of larynx, tracheotomy, haemoptysis. Edinburgh Medical Journal xi: 78
2. Billroth T 1859 Beobachtungen ueber Geschwuelste der Speicheldrusen. Archiv fur Pathologische Anatomie und Physiologie und fur Klinische Medicin 17: 357–375
3. Robin C, Laboulbene 1853 Trois productions morbides. Compte Rendu de la Societie de Biologie 5: 185–196
4. Berger L Luc, Richard 1924 L'esthesioneuroepitheliome olfactif. Bulletin de l'Association Francaise Pour l'Etude de Cancer 13: 410
5. Oehngren L G 1933 Malignant tumours of the maxillo ethmoidal region. Acta Oto-laryngologia Suppl. xix
6. Pledge H T 1966 Science since 1500. A short history of mathematics, physics, chemistry and biology. Her Majesty's Stationery Office, London, p 166
7. Virchow R 1858 Cellular Pathology as based upon Physiological and Pathological Histology. Churchill, London, pp 464–465
8. Erichsen J E 1895 Diseases of the antrum and upper jaw. In Beck M, Johnson R (eds) The science and art of surgery, 10th edn Vol. II. Longmans, Green, London, pp 627–643
9. Earle 1831–2 Osteo-sarcoma of the antrum, extirpation of the superior maxillary bone. Lancet i: 378–379
10. Ochsner A J 1923 The treatment of cancer of the jaw with the actual cautery. Journal of the American Medical Society 81: 1487–1491
11. Dickson D 1840 Fungus of the antrum: lymphatic contamination: no visceral taint. London Medical Gazette ii (new series): 256–258

12. Guthrie C G 1835–6 Clinical lecture on the removal of the superior maxillary, and other bones of the face. London Medical Gazette xvi: 315–318
13. Koerte W 1880 Resectionen des Oberkiefers. Archiv fur Klinische Chirurgie (Berlin) xxv: 514–516
14. Heath C 1872 In: Injuries and diseases of the jaws, 2nd edn. Churchill, London.
15. Adams 1853 Large fibro-cellular growth in the antrum, removal of the superior maxilla (operation by single incision); recovery. Medical Times and Gazette vii: 89
16. Aikin C A 1839 Excision of the superior maxillary bone. Lancet ii: 217–218
17. Ashurst 1870 Case of fibroid tumour of the upper jaw. American Journal of Medical Science (Philadelphia) lix: 121–123
18. Ballingal 1827 Removal of a sarcomatous tumour from the superior maxillary antrum. Lancet xii: 620
19. Barker A E 1884 Notes of a specimen of tubular epithelioma. Lancet ii: 827
20. Barton J K 1863 Removal of superior maxillary bone, for malignant disease. Dublin Quarterly Journal of Medical Science xxxiv: 32–38
21. Barwell R 1873 Myeloid sarcoma of the upper jaw removed, with nearly all the alveolus of the left side, without opening the cavity of the nose into that of the mouth. Lancet ii: 81
22. Beatson W B 1873 Osseous tumour of the left superior maxilla; removal of the bone. Lancet i: 271
23. Bickersteth E 1857 Excision of the upper jaw. Medical Times and Gazette xiv: 338
24. Blandin E 1834 Case of osteosarcoma of the left upper maxillary bone. Lancet ii: 353–354

25. Braun, H 1875–6 Ueber totale doppelte Oberkieferresectionen. Archiv fur Klinische Chirurgie xix: 728–748
26. Buchanan G 1864 Excision of superior maxillary bone. Edinburgh Medical Journal x: 406
27. Buchanan G 1879 Tumour of antrum: excision of superior maxillary bone: recovery. Glasgow Medical Journal xi: 143–144
28. Burow 1877 Fibroid der Fossa sphenomaxillaris; osteoplastische Oberkieker Resection: Heilung. Berliner Klinische Wochenschrift xiv: 60–63
29. Butcher R G H 1853 On extirpation of the upper jaw. Dublin Quarterly Journal of Medical Science xvi: 18–36
30. Butcher R G H 1860 Excision of nearly the entire left superior maxillary bone. Dublin Quarterly Journal of Medical Science xxix: 259–271
31. Butcher R G H 1861 Successful excision of the entire upper jaw and malar bone, for an enormous tumour involving both, and filling the parotid region. Dublin Quarterly Journal of Medical Science xxxi: 1–12
32. Butcher R G H 1863 Successful excision of the entire upper jaw and palate bone for an enormous fibro-vascular tumour. Dublin Quarterly Journal of Medical Science xxxv: 279–293
33. Canton 1865 Disease of the left upper jaw-bone, originating primarily in a blow from the fist; successful removal of the entire bone. Lancet i: 477–478
34. Clark F Le G 1856 Case of malignant disease of the right upper jaw; excision; recovery. Medical Times and Gazette xiii: 171
35. Collis, Porter 1869 Excision of the upper jaw for malignant tumour of the antrum. British Medical Journal i: 377
36. Coote H 1866 Extirpation of the upper jaw for malignant disease. Lancet ii: 411
37. Craven R 1863 Excision of the superior maxilla and malar bone. Medical Times and Gazette ii: 669–670
38. Craven R 1863 Excision of the superior maxilla for tumour – recovery. Medical Times and Gazette ii: 356–357
39. Craven R 1876 Excision of upper jaw. Medical Times and Gazette ii: 677
40. Crile G W 1906 Excision of cancer of the head and neck. Journal of the American Medical Association 47: 1780–1786
41. Croly H G 1868 Excision of the entire left superior maxilla, by a single incision, for myeloid tumour. Dublin Quarterly Journal of Medical Science xlv: 278–285
42. Crompton 1846 Tumor in the left antrum. London Medical Gazette i (New series): 679–680
43. Cumming A J 1871 Excision of superior maxilla. Lancet i: 231–232
44. Davies R 1858 Encephaloid tumour of antrum. Lancet i: 85–88
45. Dieffenbach 1837-8 On the resection of facial bones. Lancet i: 692–699
46. Dobie W 1853 Fibrous polypus of antrum, etc. evulsion, recovery. Monthly Journal of Medical Science 17: 307–309
47. Dobson N C 1873 Removal of greater part of both superior maxillae simultaneously for malignant disease. British Medical Journal ii: 430–432
48. Dunsmure J 1854 Osteo-sarcoma of upper jaw; excision of superior maxilla; recovery. Edinburgh Medical and Surgical Journal lxxxi: 100–101
49. Erichsen J E 1872 Fibro-plastic tumor of the right upper jaw; excision; recovery. Lancet i: 611–612
50. Fearn S W 1863 Case of fibrous tumour of the antrum, in which the jaw was excised. British Medical Journal ii: 523–524
51. Fergusson W 1841–2 Tumour of the upper jaw – excision of the superior maxillary and malar bone. Lancet i: 710–712
52. Fergusson W 1856 Excisions of the superior maxilla. Medical Times and Gazette xiii: 569
53. Fergusson W 1857 Removal of the upper jaw. Lancet ii: 33–34
54. Fergusson W 1857 Excision of the upper jaw. British Medical Journal ii: 728–729
55. Fergusson W 1860 Vascular fibrous polypus of the antrum extending into the nose - removal. Medical Times and Gazette i: 235
56. Fergusson W 1861 Excision of the superior maxilla – clinical remarks. Medical Times and Gazette i: 550
57. Fergusson W 1861 Fibrous tumour of the antrum extending through the hard palate into the mouth – successful removal. Lancet i: 206–207
58. Fergusson W 1862 Clinical remarks upon a case of removal of the upper jaw, for a tumour extending to the base of the cranium. Lancet ii: 205–206
59. Fergusson W 1863 Extensive tumour of the antrum, involving the floor of the orbit and the soft palate; excision of superior maxilla; recovery. Medical Times and Gazette i: 159–160
60. Fergusson W 1864 Malignant tumour of left antrum, involving left side of hard and the whole of soft palate. Lancet i: 8–9
61. Fergusson W 1865 Removal of a portion of the superior maxilla for a fibrous tumour of the antrum. Medical Times and Gazette i: 600
62. Fergusson W 1868 Case of removal of fibrous polypus attached to base of skull. Medical Times and Gazette i: 211
63. Fergusson W 1870 Two cases of disease of the superior maxillary bone; excision; clinical remarks. Lancet i: 584
64. Fergusson W 1870 Practical surgery, 5th edn. Churchill, London, pp 30–31
65. Fergusson W 1872 Tumour of antrum; removal of greater portion of the superior maxilla. Medical Times and Gazette i: 598
66. Field A G 1858 Resection of the upper jaw. Medical Times and Gazette xvii: 217
67. Fyffe 1853 Encephaloid tumour of the antrum. Dublin Quarterly Journal of Medical Science xv: 470–471
68. Gant 1874 Excision of the antrum of the upper jaw. Lancet i: 164
69. Godlee 1885 Resection of upper jaw for carcinoma, with remarks. Medical Times and Gazette xl: 746
70. Gott W H 1860 Exsection of the right superior maxilla, and a portion of the left for disease of long standing. American Journal of Medical Science (Philadelphia) xxxix: 344–348
71. Gott W A 1871 Encephaloid disease of the right superior maxilla; resection of the bone; recovery. American Journal of Medical Science (Philadelphia) lxii: 289–290
72. Grant J 1843 Tumour of the antrum; removal of the upper jaw-bone. Lancet i: 148–151
73. Greenhow T M 1835–36 Excision of the upper jaw for fungoid disease. Medical Times and Gazette ix: 122
74. Guthrie C G 1850 Removal of the upper jaw. Lancet i: 247–248
75. Hadden 1870 A case of removal of left superior maxilla. Dublin Quarterly Journal of Medical Science 1: 251–254
76. Hancock 1847 Amputation of the upper jaw. Lancet i: 359–360
77. Hancock 1852 Removal of the superior maxilla on the left side, with a large tumour involving that bone. Lancet i: 360
78. Harrison R 1870 Excision of the upper jaw. Liverpool Medical and Surgical Reports iv: 106–107
79. Hart E 1862 Resection of the maxillae, without skin incision. Lancet ii: 59–60
80. Hawkins C 1859 Excision of the upper jaw. British Medical Journal ii: 716–717
81. Hewett P 1859 Removal of the upper jaw for fibro-plastic disease. Lancet i: 537
82. Heyfelder J F M 1844 Totale Resektion beider Oberkiefer. J d. Chir. u. Augenh xxxiii: 633–638
83. Higgens C 1878 Sarcoma of the superior maxilla and orbit; removal; speedy recurrence, and rapid growth. British Medical Journal ii: 722
84. Howse 1850 Removal of the superior maxillary bone. Lancet i: 90–91
85. Hulke 1873 Excision of superior maxilla. British Medical Journal i: 671
86. Irving J 1825 Observations on the case of malignant tumour, successfully removed by operation, from the left antrum maxillare. Edinburgh Medicine and Surgery Journal xxiv: 93–95
87. Jackson A 1877 Myeloid disease of the left superior maxilla; removal of the whole bone without any external incision; recovery. British Medical Journal ii: 478–479
88. Jackson T C 1862 Fibrous tumour of the upper jaw, removed by excision. Transactions of Pathology Society xiv: 236–238
89. Jalland 1885 Tumour of the antrum; excision of the superior maxilla; cure. Lancet ii: 526
90. Johnson H C 1857 Extirpation of the upper jaw for tumour of the antrum. Lancet ii: 602–603
91. Johnson H C 1858 Malignant tumour of the upper jaw, partial excision of that bone. British Medical Journal: 101

92. Johnson Z 1858 Removal of the superior maxilla for disease of that bone. Dublin Quarterly Journal of Medical Science xxvi: 68–86

93. Kade 1862 Totale Resection des rechten Oberkiefers vollstandige Heilung. St Petersburg Medizinische Zeitschrift iii: 157

94. Key C A 1834 Operations – Removal of a great portion of the upper jawbone. Lancet ii: 575–576

95. Key C A 1846 Extirpation of a tumour from the antrum maxillare with removal of the superior maxillary bone, including the palate bone. Dublin Quarterly Journal of Medical Science ii: 552–553

96. Keyworth 1862 Excision of the right superior maxilla on account of fibroid tumour in the antrum. Medical Times and Gazette i: 321–322

97. Lane 1862 Excision of both superior maxillary bones, both palatal bones, both inferior turbinated bones, vomer and part of the ethmoid bones, involved in a tumour; recovery. Lancet i: 96–98

98. Lansdowne 1871 Excision of the superior maxilla for epithelioma of the cheek and hard palate. Lancet ii: 677

99. Leake W J 1860 Exsection of the superior maxillary, together with the malar and palate bones of the right side; recovery. American Journal of Medical Science (Philadelphia) xxxix: 348–351

100. Leonides van Praag J 1857-8 Partielle Resektion des Oberkiefers wegen Epulis. Archiv fur de Hollaender Beitrage Nationale und Heilkunde Utrecht i: 370–398

101. Lewis J S 1979 Tumours of the middle ear cleft and temporal bone. In: Ballantyne, Groves (eds). Scott Brown's Diseases of the ear, nose and throat, Vol. 3 4th edn. Butterworths, London, p 385

102. Lister J 1854 Two cases of tumour of the upper jaw; excision of the superior maxillary bone. London and Edinburgh Monthly Journal of Medical Science xix: 428–433

103. Liston R 1821 Case of Polypus successfully removed by operation from the Antrum Maxillare. Edinburgh Medical and Surgical Journal vii: 397–400

104. Liston R 1835 Osteosarcoma of the jaw; removal of the superior maxillary and malar bones. Lancet i: 917–918

105. Liston R 1841-2 Tumour of the upper jaw-bone; excision and recovery. Lancet i: 67–68

106. Lizars J 1826 The organs of sense. In: A system of anatomical plates. W H Lizars, London, p. 164

107. McDonnell R 1868 Case of excision of a portion of the superior maxilla. British Medical Journal i: 53

108. McFarlane J 1837 Fungus of the antrum. Edinburgh Medical and Surgical Journal xlvii: 25–28

109. Mapother E D 1870 Rhinoplasty and removal of upper jaw. British Medical Journal i: 622

110. Marsden F 1862 Case of excision of the right superior maxilla, and of the palatine process of the left; recovery. Medical Times and Gazette i: 165

111. Marshall H 1865 Case of excision of the upper jaw. British Medical Journal i: 641–642

112. Mash 1865 Fibroplastic tumour of the antrum; excision of the superior maxilla; recovery. Medical Times and Gazette i: 35–36

113. Mueller M 1870 Fall von osteoplastischer Oberkiefer-Resection. Archiv fur Klinische Chirurgie xi: 323–326

114. Neilson J L 1880 Central myxo-sarcoma of the right superior maxilla; removal of entire maxilla and portion of malar bone. American Journal of Medical Science (Philadelphia) lxxix: 437–442

115. Norton A F 1880 Removal of the frontal portion of the frontal bone, the roots of both orbits, the ethmoid bone, parts of both superior maxillae, the vomer, and palate, the left greater wing of the sphenoid bone, and the left eyeball: followed by complete restoration to health. Transactions of Clinical Medicine Society London xiii: 48–51

116. Nunneley 1860 Excision of the superior maxillary bone for a large fibroid tumour attached to its palatal portions, and filling the mouth and fauces. Transactions of Pathology Society London xi: 266

117. Paget 1861 Fibrous tumour of the antrum, successfully removed. Lancet i: 813

118. Paget 1861 Fibrous tumour of the antrum with pulsation – excision – recovery. Medical Times and Gazette ii: 250–251

119. Parkman S 1851 Excision of superior maxillary bone; result unfavourable. American Journal of Medical Science (Philadelphia) xxi: 52–53

120. Peters G A 1885 Excision of the superior maxilla with remarks. New York Medical Journal 41: 57–60

121. Quinton W M 1839 Removal of a tumour from the antrum. Lancet i: 359–360

122. Ransford R 1881 Exostosis of the antrum; removal of superior maxilla; death. Lancet i: 414–415

123. Savory 1871 Removal of the superior maxilla. Lancet ii: 577–578

124. Simon 1858 Excision of the upper jaw on account of fibrous polypus. Medical Times and Gazette xvii: 35

125. Smith H 1852 Tumour of the upper jaw; new operation. Medical Times and Gazette iv: 391–392

126. Smith T 1873 Tumour of the superior maxilla, removal; rapid recovery. Lancet i: 731–732

127. Solly 1869 Myeloid tumour of the upper jaw; excision; recovery. Medical Times and Gazette. i: 464–465

128. Studens Chirurgiae 1854 Excision of the maxillary bone. Medical Times and Gazette viii: 69–70

129. Syme J 1829 Excision of the superior maxillary bone. Edinburgh Medical and Surgical Journal xxxii: 238–239

130. Syme J 1835 Excision of the superior maxillary bone. Edinburgh Medical and Surgical Journal xliv: 1–5

131. Syme J 1843 Peculiar disease of the maxillary antrum, and removal of the bone by a single incision of the cheek. London and Edinburgh Monthly Journal of Medical Science xxx: 495–497

132. Syme J 1852 Excision of the superior maxillary bone. London and Edinburgh Monthly Journal of Medical Science xiv: 530–531

133. Syme J 1862-3 Excision of the greater portion of the upper jaw. Edinburgh Medical Journal viii: 138–139

134. Thorold H 1849 Necrosis of an osseous growth projecting into the antrum of the upper jaw. Medical Times xx: 394–395

135. Trenerry C 1850 Report of a case of extirpation of the superior maxillary bone. Lancet ii: 574–575

136. Wagstaffe W W 1873 Tumour occupying both upper jaws, removed by operation. Transactions of the Pathology Society of London xxiv: 189–191

137. Wilson C P 1955 Growths arising primarily in the antra and anterior ethmoidal regions. Proceedings of the Royal Society of Medicine 48: 72–75

138. Windsor T 1857 Cancer of the upper jaw – removal – death. Medical Times and Gazette xiv: 564–565

139. Stokes W 1868 Excision of the upper jaw. Medical Press and Circular vi: 54–55

140. Stokes W 1872 Excision of the upper jaw, along with an enormous fibro-sarcomatous tumour, which, springing from the base of the skull, passed forwards, causing extensive absorption of the osseous structures surrounding it. Medical Press and Circular xiv: 522–523

141. Tatum T 1858 Fibrous tumour to the base of the skull: resection of the upper jaw bone: removal of the tumour. British Medical Journal lvi: 857–858

142. Thompson H 1870 Removal of the left upper maxilla: recovery. British Medical Journal i: 601

143. Thomson St C S 1916 Malignant disease of the nose and sinuses. Lancet i: 987–991

144. Bryant T 1870 Tumours of the upper and lower jaws: on some cases of cystic disease of the antrum. Guy's Hospital Reports xv (3rd series) 252–255

145. Stokes W 1873 Excision of the upper jaw for the removal of a fibro-sarcomatous tumour growing from the base of the skull. Dublin Journal of Medical Science lvi: 273–287

146. Lawrie J A 1843 Necrosis; removal of the whole of the superior maxilla; division of the masseter; repair of the gap in the cheek; cure. London and Edinburgh Monthly Journal of Medical Science ii: 678–681

147. Ricdinger F 1873 Resection des Oberkiefers mit Erhaltung des mukores-periostealen Ueberzuges des harten Gaumens. Berliner Klinische Wochenschrift. 10: 521–524

148. Brainard D 1852 Case of resection of the superior maxillary and malar bones. American Journal of Medical Science (Philadelphia) xxiv: 131–132

149. Lawson 1872 Extirpation of tumour from the antrum of highmore. Medical Times and Gazette i: 513

150. Lawson 1876 Epithelioma of mucous membrane invading the hard palate; partial excision of superior maxillary bone. Medical Examiner i: 513

151. Walsham W J 1879 Tumour of the antrum; removal of the left superior maxillary bone: from a man aged sixty-seven; recovery. Lancet i: 807

152. Heiberg J 1872 Resection des Oberkiefers wegen Cylindoms, mit vorangeschickter Tracheotomie und Tamponade des Larynx. Heilung. Berliner Klinische Wochenschrift 9: 432–434

153. Fergusson W 1876 Tumour of the antrum. Medical Times and Gazette ii: 439

154. Reid D B 1868 Case of excision of the upper jaw. Lancet ii: 7–8

155. MacLeod G H B 1871-2 Excision of the upper jaw. Glasgow Medical Journal iv: 329

156. Rose E 1874 Vorschlag zur Erleichterung der Operationen am Oberkiefer. Archiv fur Klinische Chirurgie (Berlin) xvii: 454–464

157. Carothers A E 1875 Extirpation of both superior maxillary, left malar, and pterygoid process of left sphenoid bones. American Journal of Medical Science (Philadelphia) lxx: 430–433

158. Trendelenburg 1870 Die Tamponnade der Trachea. Berliner Klinische Wochenscrift 7: 278–281

159. Gussenbauer C 1874 Ueber die erste durch R. Th. Billroth am Menschen ausgefuehrte Kehlkopf Exstirpation und die Anwendung eines Kuenstlichen Kehlkopfes. Archiv fur Klinische Chirurgie 17: 343

160. Bellamy 1883 Removal of the greater portion of both upper jaw bones, without external incision. Medical Times and Gazette ii: 452–453

161. Nivison J F 1825 Case of a malignant tumour successfully removed, by operation, from the left antrum maxillare vel Highmorianum. Edinburgh Medical and Surgical Journal xxiii: 290–293

162. Parey A 1695 The workes of that famous chirurgion Ambrose Parey. Chappell, London, pp 480–481

163. New G B 1926 Malignant tumours of the antrum of Highmore: end results of treatments. Archives of Otolaryngology 4: 201–214

164. Clark W L 1918 Cancer of the oral cavity, jaws and throat. Journal of the American Medical Association 71: 1365–1369

165. Holden H B, McKelvie P 1972 Cryosurgery in the treatment of head and neck neoplasia. British Journal of Surgery 59: 709–712

166. Williams W 1843 Cases of extirpation of the superior maxillary bone. Guy's Hospital Reports i: 462–465

167. Heyfelder O 1857 On the resection of both upper jaw bones. Dublin Quarterly Journal of Medical Science xxiii: 107–119

168. Wiseman R 1676 Observations of a cancer on the left cheek. In: Severall Chirurgicall Treatises. Flesher and Macock, London, p 112

169. White C 1770 An extraordinary tumour on the lower part of the orbit of the eye, thrusting the eye out of its Socket, successfully extirpated. In: Cases in surgery with remarks. Part the First. W Johnston, London, pp 135–139.

170. Bell B 1791 A system of surgery, 5th edn. Bell & Bradfute, Edinburgh

171. Heister L 1759 A general system of surgery, 7th edn. Clarke, Whiston & White, London.

172. Hunter J 1837 The works of John Hunter. Longman, Rees, Orme, Brown, Green and Longman, London

173. Pott P 1779 The chirurgical works of Percival Pott. Lowndes, London

174. Dupuytren M 1839 Lecons Orales de Clinique Chirurgicale. Bailliere, Paris, pp 452–453

175. Rogers D L 1824 Case of osteosarcoma of the superior maxillary bone with the operation for its removal. New York Medical and Physicians Journal iii: 301–303

176. Velpeau A L M 1832 Nouveaux Elements de Medecine Operatoire. Bailliere, Paris, pp 547–552

177. Lizars J 1829-30 Removal of the superior maxillary bone. London Medical Gazette v: 92–93

178. Chirurgus 1853 Letter. Remarks on Mr. Syme being the first to perform the operation of removal of the superior maxillary bone in Europe. Medical Times and Gazette viii: 20–21

179. Gensoul P J 1833 Lettre Chirurgicale sur quelques maladies graves du sinus maxillaire et de l'os maxillaire inferieur. Bailliere, Paris

180. Surgeon-General's Office 1886 Index Catalogue, Vol. VII. Government Printing Office, Washington

181. Stokes W 1883 Fibro-sarcomatous tumour of the superior maxilla, excision of the tumour and greater portion of upper jaw. Dublin Journal of Medical Science xxvi: 348–353

182. Heylen J B 1845 Tumeur cancereuse de l'os maxillaire superieur droit; extirpation; guerison, reflexions; modifications au procede operatoire de Dieffenbach. Annales Societe de Medicine, d'Anvers vi: 409–420

183. Klose C W, Paul J 1852 Krebs des Oberkiefers; Resectio maxillae superioris. Zeitschrift fur Klinische Medicine, Bresle iii: 53

184. Gianflone 1857 Cenno di un fatto di ablazione totale dell'osso mascellare superiore. Morgagni i: 259–261

185. Moretti F 1850 Asportazione quasi totale di ambedue i massilari superiori. Gazz.. med. ital. feder. tosc. Firenze, 2 series i: 89–91

186. Dehler 1857 Partielle Resection des Oberkiefers wegen Necrose. Oesterrische Zeitschrift fur praktical Heilkunde iii: 401–404

187. Barbosa A M 1862 Reseccao de todo o osso maxillar superior do lado direito praticada pela primeira vez em Portugal. Journal Societie de Scientifique de medici de Lisbon, second series xxvi: 441–443

188. Rosa E 1864 Reseccion del maxilar superior, hecha por D.F. Rubio. Siglo Medicina Madrid xi: 406

189. Toca M S 1858 Fungas y caries de la mandibula superior del maxilar: curacion. Cron de l'hospitale, Madrid vi: 469–472

190. Estlander 1873 Resektion af ofverkaken jemte exstirpation af tumor. Finska laksallsk. handl. Helsingfors XV: 271

191. Legouest 1865 Apropos des fibromes nasopharyngiens. Bulletin de le Souciete Imperiale de Chirurgie (2nd series) vi: 523–524

192. Farabeuf 1889 Resections de la Machoire superieure. In: Precis de Manuel Operatoire, 3rd edn. Masson, Paris, pp 870–889

193. Michaux 1854 Resections de la Machoire Superieure. Bulletin de l'Academie Royale de Medecine de Belgique iii: 1–118

194. Weber O 1866 In: Pitha, Billroth (eds) Handbuch der Allgemeinen und Speciellen Chirurgie Vol III. Enke, Stuttgart, pp 232, 247, 283, 285

195. Porter G 1867 Excision of a large portion of the upper-jaw for epuloid disease — recovery. Dublin Medical Science xliii: 106: 257–261

196. Scott 1830–31 Extirpation of the right superior maxillary bone affected with osteosarcoma. Lancet i: 319–320

197. Cornet P 1925 La Chirurgie des Tumeurs malignes du Massif facial superieur 'a la Demande des Lesions'. Annales des Maladies de l'Oreille et du Larynx, xliv: 574–605

198. Michaux 1848–9 Cancer de l'os maxillaire superieur droit penetrant dans la fosse nasale, l'orbite, le sinus frontal, les cellules ethmoidales et le sinus sphenoidal. Extirpation de toute la tumeur par une seule incision pratique sur le ligne mediane de la face, hemorragies consecutives, guerison. Bulletin de l'Acadamie Royale de Medecine de Belgique viii: 1287–1294

199. Moure E J 1902 Traitment des tumeurs malignes primitives de l'ethmoide. Revue Hebdomadaire de Laryngologie, d'Otologie et de Rhinologie 47: 402–412

200. Sebileau I 1906 Les formes cliniques du cancer du sinus maxillaire. Annales des Maladies de l'Oreille et du Larynx xxxii: 430–450

201. Hautant A, Monod O, Klotz A 1933 Les epitheliomas ethmoido-orbitaires: leur traitment par l'association chirurgie-radium: resultats eloignes. Annales d'Oto-Laryngologie: 385–421

202. Thomson St C S, Negus V E 1937 Diseases of the nose and throat, 4th edn. Cassell, London

203. Harrison D F N 1977 Lateral rhinotomy – a neglected operation. Annals of Otology, Rhinology and Laryngology 86: 756–759

204. Denker A 1909 Die operative Behandlung der malignen Tumoren der Nase. Archiv fur Laryngologie und Rhinologie 21: 1–14

205. Langenbeck B 1859 Beitrage zur Osteoplastik. Deutsche Klinik ii: 471–476

206. Voelckers C 1863 Ein Fall von osteoplastischer Resection des Oberkiefers. Archiv fur Klinische Chirurgie iv: 603–607

207. Harmer W D 1935 Treatment of malignant disease in the upper jaw. Lancet i: 129–133

208. Woodman E M 1922 Malignant disease of the nasal accessory sinuses. Journal of Laryngology and Otology 37: 287–295

209. New G B 1918 The use of heat and radium in the treatment of cancer of the jaw and cheeks. Journal of the American Medical Association 71: 1369–1371

210. Woodman E M 1923 Malignant disease of the upper jaw. British Journal of Surgery II: 153–171

211. Woodman E M 1930 Plastic repair after operations on the upper jaw. Proceedings of Royal Society of Medicine 24: 436–439

2. Development and anatomy

DEVELOPMENT OF THE NOSE AND SINUSES[1,2,3a,4]

Growth is an important mechanism for generating changes in form. In general, growth is a moulding process occurring at a later stage of development. Our face and how we look depends upon relative growth of its different parts, which begin from five contiguous facial primordia (Fig. 2.1). These appear around the primitive mouth early in the fourth intrauterine week:

1. The frontonasal process superiorly
2. Paired maxillary processes laterally
3. Paired mandibular processes inferiorly.

Each process has its own characteristic growth pattern and final variations in contour may therefore be the result of quite small differences in individual growth programmes.

By the end of the 4th intrauterine week at 5 mm CR (Crown–Rump) length, bilateral oval-shaped thickenings of the surface ectoderm, the nasal placodes, develop on either side of the frontonasal prominence. With proliferation of the surrounding mesenchyme, the placodes come to lie in depressions termed olfactory pits. As facial development proceeds, the pits deepen into sacs co-incident with enlargement of the surrounding mesenchyme forming medial and lateral nasal prominences (Fig. 2.2). The maxillary processes enlarge, growing towards each other and the medial nasal prominence, but remaining separated from the lateral nasal prominences by the naso-lacrimal groove, which ultimately forms the nasolacrimal duct. Fusion of the medial nasal prominences with each other and the maxillary process produces a central segment from which the philtrum of the upper lip, premaxillary part of the maxilla, associated gingiva and primitive palate derive. From the maxillary processes, the lateral upper lip, remaining maxilla and the secondary palate develop.

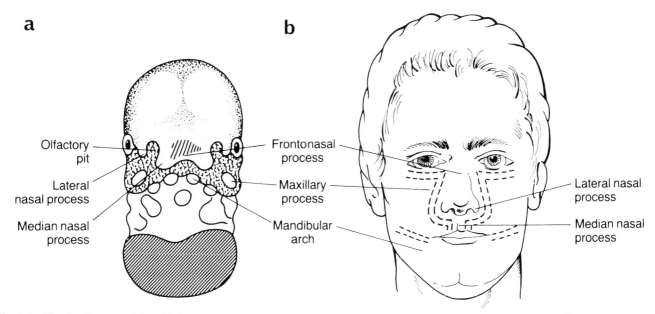

a **b**

Olfactory pit — Frontonasal process

Lateral nasal process — Maxillary process

Median nasal process — Mandibular arch

Lateral nasal process

Median nasal process

Fig. 2.1 The development of the mid-third of the face in (a) a 4 mm CR length embryo; (b) an adult (in Maran + Lund 1990[8]).

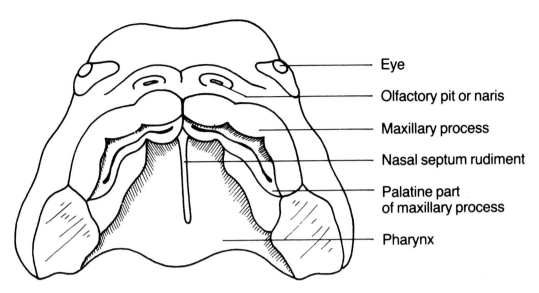

Fig. 2.2 The development of the palate in a 15 mm CR length human embryo (after Hamilton, Boyd & Mossman in Maran & Lund 1990[8]).

Initially the nasal sac is separated from the oral cavity by an oronasal membrane but rupture posterior to the primitive palate produces the primitive choanae, connecting the nasal and oral cavities (15 mm CR length). With secondary palatal development, the choanae become located more posteriorly at the junction between the nasal cavity and pharynx.

Thus the primary palate (median palatine process) develops at the end of the 5th intrauterine week from the merging of the medial nasal prominences and constitutes a wedge of mesoderm which forms the premaxilla. This is the portion of the hard palate anterior to the incisive foramen, containing the incisor teeth and anteriorly forming the anterior nasal spine.

The secondary palate extends posteriorly from the incisive foramen and forms the bulk of the hard and soft palate. Two mesodermal processes, the lateral palatine processes, extend from the inner aspect of the maxillary prominences. Initially the tongue lies between these palatine processes (18–20 mm CR length) but it gradually sinks, allowing the palatine processes to adopt a horizontal position (30–32 mm CR length) (Fig. 2.3). These fuse in the midline with the nasal septum, beginning anteriorly during the 9th intrauterine week and extending

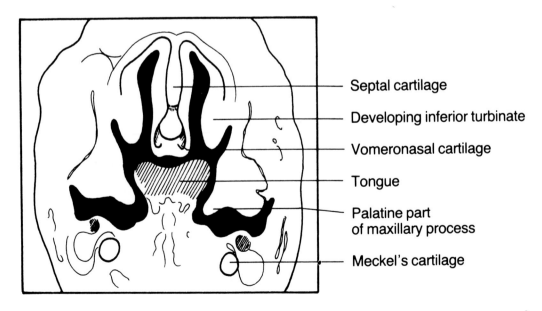

Fig. 2.3 The developing palate of a 20 mm CR length human embryo (after Hamilton, Boyd & Mossman in Maran & Lund 1990[8]).

posteriorly to the uvula by the 12th week (Fig. 2.4).[5] This line of fusion is indicated by the palatine raphe.

The primitive septum, which begins to develop in the 7th to 8th intrauterine week, is entirely cartilaginous initially. The superior part ossifies to form the perpendicular plate, whilst the antero-inferior part persists as the quadrilateral cartilage. The vomer develops from the residual postero-inferior cartilage in the 3rd intrauterine month, ossifying as two bony lamina united inferiorly but diverging in a 'V' shape superiorly, sitting astride the sphenoid rostrum. Antero-inferiorly, the two lamella create a deep groove in which the quadrilateral cartilage lodges. These two bony plates fuse from front to back during the 3rd to 15th years of life,[6] ultimately absorbing the intervening cartilage.

The vomeronasal organs of Jacobson arise as ectodermal invaginations on each side of the nasal septum just superior to the primitive palate in the 8–11 mm CR embryo. They are 4–8 mm long when fully developed at the 6th intrauterine month and are lined by neurosensory epithelium similar to olfactory epithelium (Fig. 2.4). A vomeronasal nerve connects the organ with small accessory olfactory bulbs. In man complete regression usually occurs in late fetal life, leaving only associated vomeronasal cartilages as thin strips between the inferior quadrilateral cartilage in 70% and vomer or a vomeronasal pit in 39%.[7]

On the lateral nasal wall, a series of elevations appear from the 6th intrauterine week which ultimately form the turbinates. The inferior turbinate is the first to develop and is ossified in a 139 mm fetus. Ossification of the middle and superior turbinates occurs in the 5th and 7th months respectively.

The paranasal sinuses arise as evaginations from the nasal cavities. The maxillary sinus is the first to develop (7–10 weeks) and is seen as a shallow groove expanding laterally from the infundibulum in the 4th intrauterine month (Fig. 2.5). This reaches the lateral cartilaginous plate, with subsequent absorption and expansion. At birth a small cavity is present, encroached upon by the upper dentition. It is nevertheless the largest sinus in the neonate ($7 \times 4 \times 4$ mm) and it continues to grow at 2–3 mm a year in conjunction with the development of the mid-third of the face and eruption of the permanent dentition. In old age the sinus may actually enlarge with resorption of the alveolar processes after loss of the teeth.

The maxillary bone has three ossification sites, one for the main mass appearing above the canine fossa in the 6th intrauterine week and two appearing between the 8th and 9th weeks in the anterior premaxillary region. In the 4th intrauterine month the centres fuse to form the alveolar and palatine processes, floor of the orbit, zygomatic process and the frontal process of the maxilla.

The anterior and posterior ethmoid cells develop from furrows on the lateral wall of the nose in the 4th intrauterine month, growing into the lateral ethmoidal mass. Consequently a few cells are present at birth. Ossification of the bone occurs in the cartilaginous nasal capsule from 3 centres, one for the perpendicular plate and one for each labyrinth. At birth the labyrinths are partially ossified, though the rest of the bone is cartilaginous.

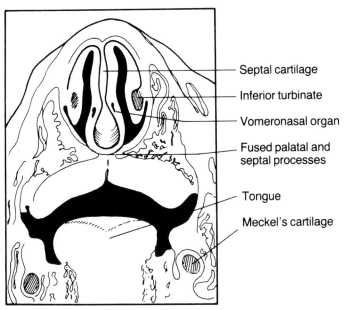

Fig. 2.4 The developing palate of a 48 mm CR length human fetus (after Hamilton, Boyd & Mossman in Maran & Lund 1990[8]).

- Septal cartilage
- Inferior turbinate
- Vomeronasal organ
- Fused palatal and septal processes
- Tongue
- Meckel's cartilage

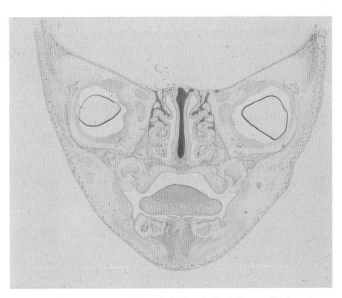

Fig. 2.5 Coronal section through the head of a 150 mm CR length fetus showing turbinate development and early clefts of maxillary and ethmoid sinuses (haematoxylin & eosin).

The sphenoid sinus is recognizable at around the 3rd intrauterine month as an evagination into the sphenoethmoidal recess. At birth it is $0.5 \times 2 \times 2$ mm in size. Expansion continues posteriorly to achieve full size in adolescence, though absorption of bone in old age can lead to further enlargement. The ossification of the sphenoid bone is extremely complex, consisting of at least 14 ossification centres and at birth the bone is in three pieces; a central one consisting of the body and lesser wings, and two lateral parts, each comprising a greater wing and pterygoid process.

The frontal sinus, which is often regarded embryologically as an anterior ethmoid cell, is absent at birth. A sinus cavity is not apparent until 6–12 months and can only be seen on 50% of X-rays at 6–7 years of age. Growth continues into the early twenties.

ANATOMY OF THE UPPER JAW AND ASSOCIATED STRUCTURES

In strict anatomical terms the upper jaw refers to the two maxillary bones, including the upper alveolus, dentition and hard palate. However, given the integrated functional, anatomical and pathological relationships, this term has been extended, for the purposes of this book, to include the nasal cavity and paranasal sinuses. The surgical anatomy of these areas and those important adjacent regions into which disease may readily spread are therefore considered in this chapter.

Nasal cavity[1,3,8]

The nasal cavity is that space between the nasal vestibule and posterior choanae, bounded by the ethmoidal labyrinth and conchae, lacrimal bone, maxilla and inferior turbinate laterally and by the nasal septum medially, dividing it into two. Vertically the nasal cavity extends from the palate to the inferior surface of the cribriform plate.

The bony floor is composed of premaxilla, maxilla and the horizontal plate of the palatine bone. Approximately 12 mm (8–18 mm) behind the anterior end of the floor lies a small pit in the mucous membrane adjacent to the septum. This marks the upper end of the incisive canal containing the terminal branches of the nasopalatine nerve, greater palatine artery and a short mucosal canal (Stenson's organ).

The upper part of the cavity, sometimes referred to as the olfactory cleft, can be divided into a nasal part anteriorly, an ethmoidal section centrally and a sphenoidal portion posteriorly. The nasal spine of the frontal bone and nasal bones form the nasal part, the cribriform plate forms the ethmoidal section and the sphenoethmoidal recess opens into the posterior segment.

The lateral wall is formed by the ethmoid, maxilla, palatine, lacrimal and inferior conchal bones and the medial surface of the medial pterygoid plate. The conchae are a much simplified arrangement of bony baffles which in lower animals are represented by complex ethmoturbinals, maxilloturbinal and nasoturbinal (p. 35). In man an inferior, middle, and superior concha (and in less than 33% of adults a supreme concha) are found. The air spaces lateral to the conchae are termed inferior, middle and superior meatus respectively.

The turbinates are composed of conchal bone, mucoperiosteum, a submucosal cavernous plexus and respiratory mucous membrane. They create turbulence in inspired air and the mucous coating collects particles of dust and bacteria. This is of particular relevance in the middle turbinate where cilial damage and dysplasia can ultimately lead to malignant change (p. 116).

The inferior conchal bone is scroll-shaped and attaches by a downturned maxillary process to the medial wall of the maxilla. The surface of the bone is very irregular, perforated and grooved by many vessels and as a consequence the mucoperiosteum is firmly attached and difficult to dissect. The bone articulates with the lacrimal, ethmoid and palatine bones in addition to the maxilla and it completes the canal for the nasolacrimal duct.

The inferior meatus is the largest meatus and extends almost the entire length of the lateral wall. The attachment of the turbinate renders the meatus highest at the junction of the anterior and middle thirds. The nasolacrimal duct enters at or just anterior to this point. In adults a maximum height of 1.6–2.3 cm (mean 1.92 cm) is found at 1.6 cm along the bony lateral wall.[9] In children the shape is the same though correspondingly smaller. The thickness of the bone of the inferior meatus changes from compact to lamellar, being thinnest under the genu of the turbinate and increasingly thicker as one passes both anteriorly, posteriorly and inferiorly, which is of obvious clinical importance when perforating the bone.

The middle turbinate is an integral part of the ethmoid bone. Its most anterior superior insertion is adjacent to the crista ethmoidalis of the maxilla, forming the agger nasi region which can be pneumatized. The remaining anterior third attaches vertically to the cribriform plate, in a sagittal direction (Fig. 2.6). The middle third attaches laterally to the lamina papyracea by its ground lamella, dividing the ethmoid cells into an anterior and posterior group. In the posterior third, the now almost horizontal ground lamella forms the roof of the most posterior section of the middle meatus and is attached to the lamina papyracea or medial wall of the maxilla (Fig. 2.7). The turbinate is sometimes pneumatized, concha bullosa, occurring in 18% of the normal population (Fig. 2.8) or can be bent paradoxically towards the lateral wall in 17% (Fig. 2.9).

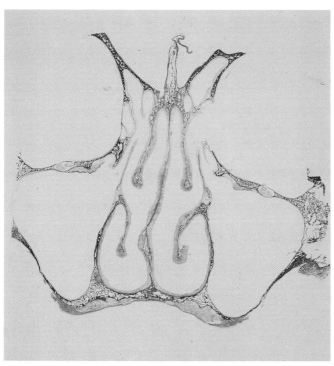

Fig. 2.6 Coronal section through adult mid-facial block through the infundibulum showing vertical superior attachment of the middle turbinate (Van Geison).

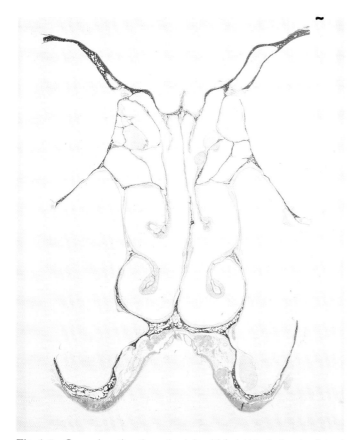

Fig. 2.7 Coronal section through adult mid-facial block showing lateral attachment of ground lamella of the middle turbinate.

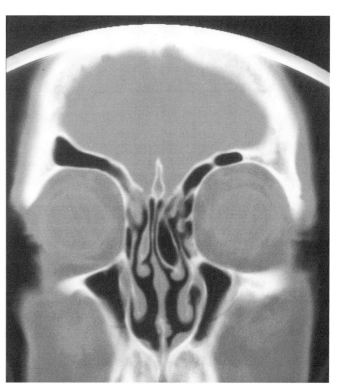

Fig. 2.8 Coronal CT scan showing pneumatized middle turbinate (concha bullosa).

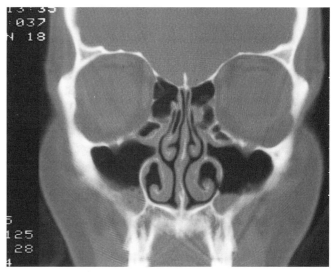

Fig. 2.9 Coronal CT scan showing middle turbinate paradoxically bent towards middle meatus.

The middle meatus is the most complex area of the lateral nasal wall.[10] The bulla occupies the anterior middle meatus, its size dependent upon the degree of pneumatization by the anterior ethmoidal cells. Posteriorly the bulla may fuse with the ground lamella of the middle turbinate but sometimes a cleft exists, the lateral sinus, which can run above the bulla to communicate with the frontal recess. The posterior cells, lying behind the ground lamella, vary in number from one to five. They are intimately related to the optic nerve, and may extend around the nerve and sphenoid sinus (Onodi cells, occurring in 12% of subjects).

Running anterior and inferior to the bulla is a thin curved lamina of bone called the uncinate process of the ethmoid. The attachment of this structure to the lateral wall is variable and in the bony skeleton defects exist between it, the maxilla and inferior turbinate. In life these areas are filled with mucous membrane and connective tissue, to form the fontanelles, lying anterior and posterior to the uncinate process. Accessory ostia are sometimes found in the fontanelles, which are thought to result from sinus infection. Between the concave free posterior margin of the uncinate process and the anterior surface of the ethmoidal bulla is a sickle-shaped two-dimensional cleft, the hiatus semilunaris. This leads anteriorly into the ethmoidal infundibulum which in turn leads into the maxillary ostium (Fig. 2.6).

The ethmoidal infundibulum receives openings from the anterior ethmoidal cells and depending on the configuration of the uncinate process may be joined by the frontal recess into which the frontal sinus opens.

The superior meatus receives the ostia of the posterior ethmoidal cells. A small ridge, the supreme turbinate is sometimes discernible above the superior turbinate. Immediately behind the superior meatus, lies the sphenopalatine foramen. The sphenoethmoidal recess separates the superior concha and anterior face of the sphenoid and receives the opening of the sphenoid sinus.

The nasal septum is composed of a bony and a cartilaginous part. The bony part consists of the perpendicular plate of the ethmoid and the vomer, and two bony crests, of the maxilla and palatine. The cartilaginous part is formed from the quadrilateral cartilage with a contribution from the lower and upper lateral alar cartilages. The perpendicular plate of the ethmoid forms the upper and anterior part of the bony septum and is continuous above with the cribriform plate. The vomer extends from the inferior surface of the body of the sphenoid where its two alae fit either side of the sphenoid rostrum. In so doing it often creates the vomerovaginal canals by approximating with the vaginal processes of the sphenoid, through which pass pharyngeal branches of the maxillary artery. The inferior border articulates with the nasal crest formed by the maxillae and palatine bones. The long anterior border articulates superiorly with the perpendicular plate, a suture line at which deflections often occur and inferiorly with the quadrilateral cartilage. The posterior margin is free, separating the posterior nasal apertures.

The quadrilateral cartilage in addition to joining the ethmoid and vomer often sends a narrow sphenoidal process between these two bones which is most obvious in children and may be the site of spur formation. The upper margin of the septal cartilage is connected to the posterior border of the internasal suture and to the upper lateral cartilages to which it is attached by perichondrium. Inferiorly the septal cartilage sits in the groove of the maxillary crest. Anteriorly it abuts the medial crura of the lower lateral alar cartilages, divided from them by a thin strip of membranous septum.

Histology

A mucosal envelope of mucoperichondrium and mucoperiosteum surrounds the structures of the septum. The septal cartilage is composed of hyaline cartilage and embryologically the cartilage represents the unossified portion of the perpendicular plate of the ethmoid. At birth the mucoperichondrium and mucoperiosteum of these structures are continuous but are separate from the mucoperiosteum covering those other parts of the bony septum arising from separate paired ossification centres, such as vomer, maxillary and palatine nasal crests. This results in the septal cartilage coming to lie in grooves on the vomer and nasal crest which has obvious importance when dissecting in these planes.

The mucous membrane throughout the nasal cavity and paranasal sinuses is principally respiratory with a small area of olfactory epithelium in the superior portion of the nasal cavity adjacent to the cribriform plate. The respiratory epithelium is composed of ciliated pseudostratified columnar cells interspersed with goblet cells. In the submucosa lie seromucinous glands. The mucosa has a prolific vascular structure including cavernous tissue, which is best developed on the turbinates but which is also found on the septum adjacent to the inferior turbinate. Deep to this is a region heavily infiltrated with lymphocytes.

The respiratory epithelium is composed of ciliated and non-ciliated columnar cells, goblet cells and basal cells. The number of ciliated cells increases as one moves posteriorly on the septum. The basal cells are intermediate stem cells capable of differentiation into ciliated columnar or goblet cells. Occasional cuboidal and squamous cells are also found in the epithelium.

The number of cilia on each cell and cilia size varies between different species. In man there are 50–100 per cell though the number varies with age and the position in the nose and they are relatively short at 5 μm. The cilia are composed of the classical multistructural axonema made of nine peripheral doublet and two central single microtubules.

The goblet cells produce mucus, for which they are the main source in the paranasal sinuses. The number of cells varies throughout the nose and sinuses. On the septum there is a gradual increase in numbers passing from anterior to posterior, though the distribution is irregular.

Similarly there is a slight tendency for density to increase from superior to inferior. On the lateral wall, the goblet cell density of the inferior turbinate is higher overall than that on the middle turbinate. The number of glands (about 8/mm^2) is similar on inferior and middle turbinates but decreases as one travels posteriorly.

The seromucinous glands are found in the submucosa of the respiratory epithelium. They are relatively few in number, and show a gradual decrease from anterior to posterior and from superior to inferior so the postero-inferior quadrant has the least concentration but are the main source of mucus production in the nasal cavity.

On each side of the septum is an orifice leading to a blind tubular pouch, 2–6 mm long representing the vomeronasal organ, part of the olfactory system in lower animals (p. 36).

The olfactory epithelium covers a variable area of the septum, dependent on age and extends down from the cribriform plate on to the superior turbinate. This epithelium is composed of receptor cells, supporting cells bearing microvilli, and basal cells which are again stem cells giving the olfactory epithelium the unique property for neural tissue of regeneration. The receptor cells bear olfactory cilia, usually 17 per cell. They differ from respiratory cilia in their radial arrangement, greater length and the poorly developed substructure, preventing beating in a conventional sense. However the sensory endings do terminate in characteristic knob-like vesicular structures and olfactory fibres leave to join the axonal bundle.

Secretion for the olfactory epithelium is provided by the Bowman glands, small, branched, tubular serous structures, found immediately below the epithelium. An abrupt transition zone is found between the respiratory and olfactory epithelium.

Blood supply[11,12]

The nasal cavity is supplied by external and internal carotid arteries. The sphenopalatine branch of the maxillary artery supplies the postero-inferior septum. The greater palatine artery supplies the antero-inferior septum via the incisive canal. The superior labial branch of the facial artery also contributes anteriorly and the internal carotid component derives from anterior and posterior ethmoidal arteries superiorly. All these vessels form a plexiform network in the mucosa and specifically contribute to Keisselbach's plexus localized in Little's area on the anterior septum.

The lateral wall of the nose, like the septum, receives blood from the external and internal carotid systems. The anterior and posterior ethmoidal arteries contribute superiorly, the sphenopalatine supplies the turbinates and meatuses posteriorly and the greater palatine serves the antero-inferior portions.

The cavernous venous system drains posteriorly via the sphenopalatine vessels into the pterygoid plexus and anteriorly into the facial veins. The anterior and posterior ethmoidal veins connect superiorly with the superior ophthalmic system. In addition there can be direct communication with the veins on the orbital surface of the frontal lobes through the cribriform plate and via the foramen caecum into the superior sagittal sinus.

Nerve supply

Ordinary sensation to the septum is mainly supplied by the maxillary division of the trigeminal nerve. The nasopalatine nerve enters via the sphenopalatine foramen and passes medially across the roof of the nose to the upper part of the septum. It then passes forwards and downwards to the incisive canal, through which it passes to supply the hard palate. Thus the postero-inferior septum is supplied, with additional branches from the nerve of the pterygoid canal and the posterior inferior nasal branch of the anterior palatine nerve. The antero-superior part of the septum is supplied by the anterior ethmoidal branch of the nasociliary nerve whilst the antero-inferior portion of the septum receives a branch from the anterior superior alveolar nerve. Accompanying the sensory fibres in these nerves are postganglionic sympathetic fibres to the blood vessels and, with the branches from the pterygopalatine ganglion, postganglionic parasympathetic secretomotor fibres pass to the glands.

The nerve supply of the lateral wall is also similar to that of the septum, with the anterior ethmoidal nerve supplying antero-superiorly and branches of the pterygopalatine ganglion and anterior palatine nerves supplying posteriorly. The sympathetic and parasympathetic supply similarly accompanies the branches of the pterygopalatine ganglion.

Lymphatic drainage

Lymphatics from the anterior septum join those of the external nose running towards the facial vein to the submandibular nodes, potentially bilaterally. In addition drainage from the external nose may be to the parotid lymph nodes. Posteriorly, drainage is along the nasal floor to the upper surface of the soft palate. The lymphatic pathway divides into two on the lateral pharyngeal wall; one of these consists of three or four trunks which run down to join the lymph vessels of the palatine arch and tonsil. The deep cervical chain of lymph nodes lies along this pathway, behind the submandibular gland and the digastric muscles, at the level of the bifurcation of the common carotid artery. The most important node of this group is the jugulofacial lymph node. The other drainage pathway, consisting of two to four vessels, runs directly backwards, closely related to the Eustachian orifice, to the lateral pharyngeal lymph nodes and thence to the deep cervical nodes. Additional connections exist along the olfactory nerves into the subdural and subarachnoid space.

The lateral wall also drains anteriorly with the structures of the external nose to the submandibular nodes and posteriorly to the retropharyngeal and upper deep cervical nodes.

The maxillary bone and sinus[1,3b,8]

Osteology (Fig. 2.10)

The maxilla is the largest facial bone after the mandible, forming most of the roof of the mouth, the floor and lateral wall of the nasal cavity and the floor of the orbit. The body is usually described as a quadrilateral pyramid, and is occupied by the maxillary sinus. The bone has four processes: zygomatic, frontal, palatine and alveolar and articulates with eight bones; its opposite number, the zygoma, frontal, palatine, ethmoid, lacrimal, nasal bone and inferior concha. The anterior surface is directed forwards and slightly laterally, and bears a number of ele-

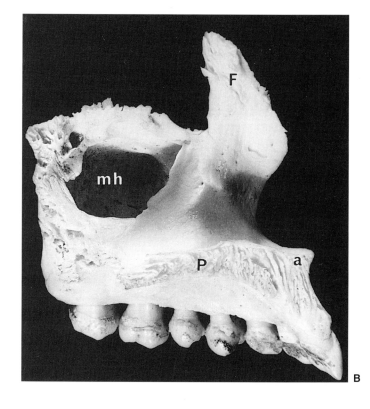

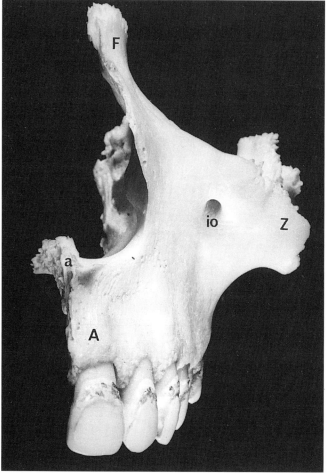

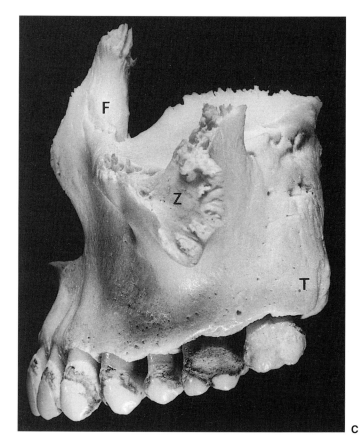

Fig. 2.10   The maxillary bone. **A**, anterior view; **B**, medial view; **C**, lateral view. a, anterior nasal spine; A, alveolar process; F, frontal process; io, infraorbital faramen; mh, maxillary hiatus; P, palatine process; T, tuberosity; z, zygomatic process (Maran & Lund 1990[8]).

vations on the lower surface over the roots of the teeth. Above the elevations are slight depressions, named 'incisive' and 'canine', after the respective teeth. The bone of the canine fossa is relatively thin. Above the canine fossa is the infraorbital foramen, which transmits the infraorbital nerve and vessels. The anterior surface is also characterized by the nasal notch and anterior nasal spine.

The roof of the maxillary sinus forms the majority of the floor of the orbit and is thin and occasionally dehiscent, particularly in the region of the infraorbital groove and canal which run forwards to end as the foramen on the face of the maxilla. Antero-medially lies the lacrimal notch, through which the nasolacrimal duct passes. The posterior edge contributes to the inferior orbital fissure. The posterior infratemporal surface is convex and faces backwards and laterally. Canals for the posterior superior alveolar nerves can be seen on its surface and inferiorly the maxillary tuberosity is found from which the medial pterygoid muscle takes a small attachment.

Inferiorly, the floor of the sinus is thick but is usually encroached upon by the dental roots of the 2nd premolar and three molars which can lead to considerable thinning of bone and dehiscence. This is commonest over the first molar (2.2%). The level of the floor of the sinus relative to the nasal floor changes during life. At birth the cavity is several millimetres higher but by 8 to 9 years the floors are level. With continued development of the middle third of the face as the permanent dentition erupts, the floor of the sinus comes to lie at a lower level than the nasal floor (0.8–10 mm) (Fig. 2.7). The size of the sinus also increases with alveolar absorption following dental extraction in later life.

The medial nasal surface constitutes the floor of the pyramid and contains the maxillary hiatus, a large posterior opening, about 1 cm in diameter, leading into the sinus cavity. This is reduced in size by articulation with a number of other bones; the perpendicular plate of palatine, lacrimal, uncinate process of ethmoid, and inferior concha. The configuration of the hiatus semilunaris, ethmoidal infundibulum and fontanelles has been previously described. The lacrimal canal is created between maxilla, lacrimal bone and inferior concha, through which the nasolacrimal duct passes to the anterior inferior meatus. Posteriorly the greater palatine canal is formed between the perpendicular plate of the palatine and maxilla. Anterior to the nasolacrimal groove is the conchal crest to which the inferior concha attaches, separating the inferior and middle meatuses. The apex of the cavity is directed into the zygomatic process. The average adult Caucasian dimensions of the cavity, giving a mean volume of 14.25 ml, are:

breadth	25–35 mm
height	36–45 mm
length	38–45 mm

The sinus is often incompletely divided by septa and may be encroached upon by posterior ethmoidal cells but in other respects the two maxillary sinuses are relatively symmetrical.

When the two maxillae are articulated, the alveolar processes form an alveolar arch. The frontal process is divided on its lateral surface by the anterior lacrimal crest, to which the medial palpebral ligament is attached. The medial surface articulates with the ethmoid, closing the anterior ethmoidal air cells. Beneath this is an oblique ethmoidal crest, which articulates posteriorly with the middle turbinate and anteriorly underlies the agger nasi. The crest therefore forms the superior limit to the anterior middle meatus.

The palatine process forms a substantial part of the floor of the nasal cavity and roof of mouth, being thicker anteriorly. It articulates with its opposite number in the midline and posteriorly with the palatine bone (Fig. 2.11). The inferior surface is pitted by the attachment of Sharpey's fibres from the palatal periosteum, vascular foramina and depressions from glands. When the two maxillae articulate, the incisive canal, a funnel-shaped hole, is seen behind the incisors. This carries the greater palatine arteries and nasopalatine nerves in separate vascular and neural channels to each side of the nose.

With respect to tumour spread therefore, the maxillary sinus is related superiorly to the orbit and inferiorly to the upper dentition and palate. Posteriorly lies the infratemporal fossa and anteriorly the cheek, with fat and facial musculature.

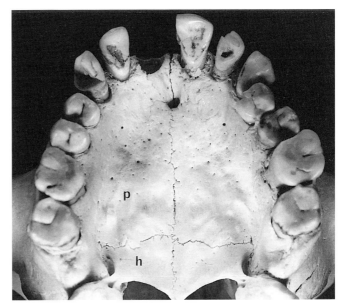

Fig. 2.11 The skull showing inferior view of palate; p, palatine process of maxilla; h, horizontal process of palatine bone (Maran & Lund 1990[8]).

Histology

The maxillary sinus is lined with ciliated columnar respiratory epithelium containing goblet cells and glands. The mucous membrane is relatively thin, less vascular and more loosely adherent to the bony walls than in the nasal cavity. The density of goblet cells in the maxillary sinus is the highest of the paranasal sinuses and similar to that on the inferior turbinate. The seromucinous glands though few in number compared with the goblet cells, are again more numerous in the maxillary sinus compared with the other sinuses and are more concentrated around the ostium.

Blood and nerve supply

The blood supply of the sinus is by small arteries which pierce the bone from the facial, maxillary, infraorbital and greater palatine arteries. Veins accompany these vessels to the anterior facial vein and pterygoid plexus.

The nerve supply is derived from the infraorbital, superior alveolar nerves (anterior, middle and posterior) and greater palatine, all branches of the maxillary division of the trigeminal nerve.[13,14] Near the midpoint of the infraorbital canal, a small branch, the anterior superior alveolar nerve arises and passes in its own canal, the canalis sinusus, to the anterior wall of the maxilla. Reaching the margin of the nasal aperture it passes in front of the anterior end of the inferior concha and reaches the side of the nasal septum in front of the incisive foramen. It supplies the mucous membrane of the anterior wall of the antrum in addition to the pulps of the canines and incisors, the antero-inferior quadrant of the lateral nasal wall, the floor of the nose, and a small portion of anterior septum.

The posterior superior alveolar nerves, usually two in number, arise from the maxillary nerve in the pterygo-palatine fossa and pierce the posterior wall of the maxilla, supplying the mucosa and the molar teeth. The middle superior alveolar nerve, when it is present (in 37% of cases) leaves the infraorbital nerve on the floor of the orbit and runs down in the lateral wall of the antrum to the premolar teeth. Thus one cannot avoid damaging this nerve when it is present during approaches to the anterior antral wall.

The greater palatine supplies the posterior part of the medial wall of the antrum whilst the infraorbital nerve gives perforating branches to the roof of the sinus.

Lymphatic drainage

Anteriorly the lymph drainage is to the submandibular nodes and is relatively poorly developed as evidenced by the rarity of associated lymphadenopathy with infec-tion and malignancy. However, connections have been shown to the Eustachian tube and nasopharynx and thence to the posterior pharyngeal plexus and to the opposite side.

The ethmoid bone and sinuses[1,3,8]

Osteology

This extremely complex bone is situated in the anterior base of the skull, and contributes to the medial wall of the orbits, the nasal septum, roof and lateral walls of the nose. It is approximately $2.5 \times 2.5 \times 2$ cm and weighs around 1g. It is comprised of five parts (Figs 2.7 and 2.12):

> perpendicular plate
> horizontal cribriform plate
> crista galli
> two lateral masses or labyrinths suspended from the horizontal arms in the form of a cross.

The perpendicular plate which forms the central sagittal strut is quadrilateral in shape and forms the upper part of the bony nasal septum. It articulates anteriorly with the nasal spine of the frontal bone and nasal bones, posteriorly with the sphenoidal crest and vomer and inferiorly with the quadrilateral cartilage. Superiorly it attaches to the cribriform plate where it is grooved by olfactory nerve fibres.

The cribriform plate divides the nasal cavity below from the anterior cranial cavity above. It has a triangular projection, the crista galli which is variable in size and pneumatization. Two anterior alae complete the foramen caecum which often transmits an emissary vein to the superior sagittal sinus. The narrow plate on either side is perforated by the many olfactory filaments, processes of dura and ethmoidal vessels and nerves.

The ethmoidal labyrinths consist of a number of thin-walled cells (3–18) and clefts which are divided into anterior and posterior by the ground lamella of the middle turbinate. The lateral walls of the labyrinths constitute the orbital plate or lamina papyracea. The roof of the labyrinths is completed by the frontal bone and similarly the posterior cell is closed by the face of the sphenoid and the orbital process of the palatine bone. Anterior to the orbital plate a few cells are completed by the lacrimal bone and frontal process of the maxilla. These most anterior cells constitute the agger nasi group.

The ethmoid bone has important relationships, dividing as it does the anterior cranial fossa and nasal cavity, with the orbit on either side. The posterior cells are intimately related to the optic canal and may almost ensheath it in some cases (Fig. 2.13). The ethmoid cells can also encroach on the maxilla, can pneumatize the floor of the orbit (Haller cells) (Fig. 2.14), the floor of the frontal sinus and surround the sphenoid.

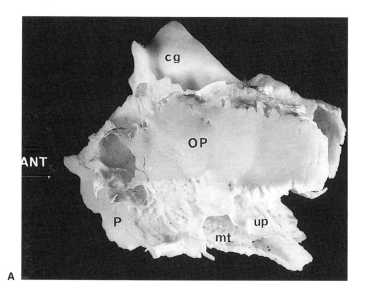

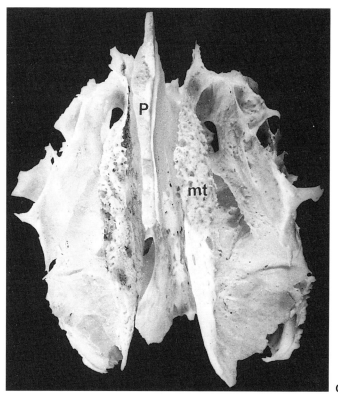

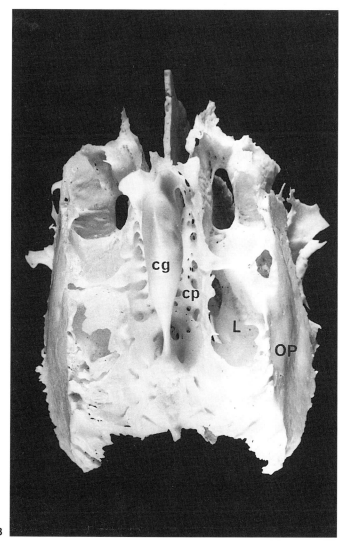

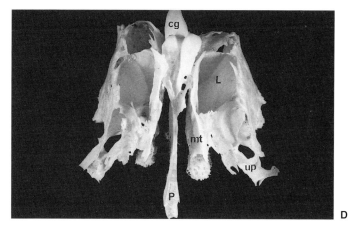

Fig. 2.12 The ethmoid bone. **A**, lateral view; **B**, superior view; **C**, inferior view; **D**, posterior view. cg, crista galli; OP, orbital plate; P, perpendicular plate; mt, middle turbinate; up, uncinate process; cp, cribriform plate; L, labyrinth; ANT, anterior (Maran & Lund 1990[8]).

Histology

The configuration of the ethmoid cells has already been described. They are also lined with ciliated columnar respiratory epithelium, the density of goblet cells being lower than in the maxillary sinus.

Blood and nerve supply

The ethmoidal arteries arise from the ophthalmic artery, a branch of the internal carotid artery. The anterior ethmoidal artery accompanies the nerve and supplies the anterior ethmoidal and frontal sinuses. The vessel travels through the anterior ethmoidal canal in the medial wall of the orbit, on to the superior surface of the cribriform plate, where it gives off an important meningeal branch. The vessel then passes down at the side of the crista galli

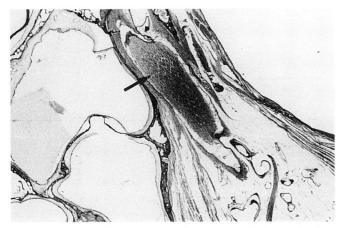

Fig. 2.13 Axial section through an adult midfacial block, showing the intimate relationship between the optic nerve (arrow) and the posterior ethmoidal cells (haematoxylin & eosin) (Lund 1987[15]).

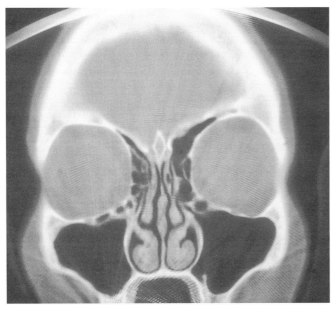

Fig. 2.14 Coronal CT scan showing ethmoidal cells pneumatizing the floor of the orbit (Haller cells).

to the upper nasal septum and lateral wall of the nose, and sends a terminal branch on to the dorsum of the nose between the nasal bone and upper lateral cartilages.

The smaller posterior ethmoidal artery runs through the canal in the medial orbital wall to supply the posterior ethmoidal cells and similarly gives a meningeal branch and terminates in nasal branches to the septum and lateral wall, anastomosing with the sphenopalatine artery. Both vessels, especially the posterior artery are variable and may be absent.

The vascular supply of the ethmoid is derived from the sphenopalatine and ethmoidal (anterior and posterior) arteries and the sinuses are drained by corresponding veins. They are innervated by the anterior and posterior ethmoidal nerves and orbital branches of the pterygopalatine ganglion.

Lymphatic drainage

Lymphatic drainage is to the submandibular nodes anteriorly and retropharyngeal nodes posteriorly.

The sphenoid bone and sinuses [1,3b,8]

The sphenoid is the largest single bone in the skull base, dividing the anterior and middle cranial fossa. It is composed of a body (occupied to a variable degree by two sinuses), two wings (greater and lesser) and two inferior plates (lateral and medial pterygoid plates) (Fig. 2.15).

The jugum on the anterior superior surface of the body articulates with the cribriform plate. This surface bears the chiasmatic sulcus connecting the optic canals, the tuberculum sellae, sella turcica and dorsum sellae with related anterior, middle and posterior clinoid processes. The bone slopes away posteriorly to the dorsum sella towards the clivus. The lateral surface of the body is grooved by the carotid sulcus on each side. The anterior face of the body bears a crest which articulates with the perpendicular plate of the ethmoid. On either side, halfway up the face, lie the openings of the sinuses. These ostia are large on a skull (5–8 mm in diameter) but are partially overlapped and closed by the sphenoidal concha and mucous membrane in life and open into the sphenoethmoidal recess, above the superior concha or turbinate.

The sinus cavities are variable in size and often asymmetric. They measure on average $14 \times 14 \times 12$ mm but pneumatization can extend into the greater wing, pterygoid processes, rostrum and encroach on the basilar part of the occipital bone. Three general types of pneumatization have been described.

1. Conchal pneumatization in which only a rudimentary sinus is present.

2. Pre-sphenoid pneumatization in which the sinus is pneumatized as far as the anterior bony wall of the pituitary fossa. This is found in 40% of the population.

3. Post-sphenoidal and occipital pneumatization in which the pneumatization extends back below the pituitary fossa, occurring in about 60% of people.

The sinuses are divided by a septum which is often paramedian and may have diverticula and other incomplete septa.

The inferior surface of the sphenoid body bears the rostrum which articulates with the vomer. The greater wings contribute to the middle cranial fossa and lateral wall of the orbit. The superior orbital fissure separates it from the lesser wing on each side, the inferior border contributes to the inferior orbital fissure and in addition it is traversed by a number of foramina. The foramen rotundum transmits the maxillary nerve, the foramen ovale transmits the mandibular nerve, accessory meningeal artery and sometimes the lesser petrosal nerve

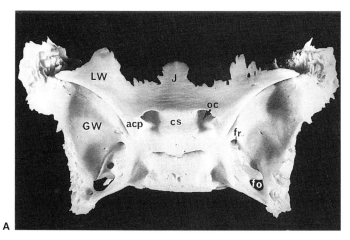

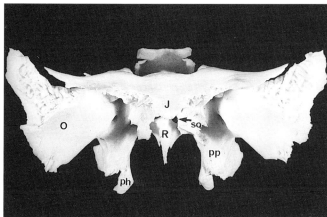

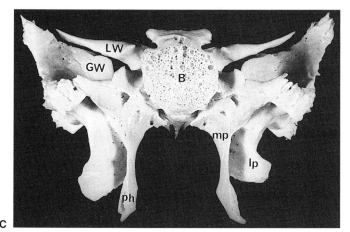

Fig. 2.15 The sphenoid bone, **A**, superior view; **B**, anterior view; **C**, posterior view. J, jugum; oc, optic canal (arrow); fr, foramen rotundum (arrow); cs, chiasmatic sulcus; acp, anterior clinoid process; fo, foramen ovale; GW, greater wing; LW, lesser wing; so, sphenoid ostium (arrow); O, orbital surface; ph, pterygoid hamulus; pp, pterygoid plates; R, rostrum; B, body; mp, medial pterygoid; lp, lateral pterygoid (Maran & Lund 1990[8]).

and through the foramen spinosum the middle meningeal artery passes in company with a meningeal branch of the mandibular nerve. An emissary venous sphenoidal foramen is found related to the foramen ovale in 40% of skulls. The posterior margin of the greater wing contributes to the foramen lacerum.

Each pterygoid process consists of a lateral and medial plate which diverge around the pterygoid fossa and the process is pierced superiorly by the pterygoid canal. The lateral pterygoid muscle arises in part from the lateral surface of the lateral pterygoid plate, the medial pterygoid muscle from its medial surface. The medial pterygoid plate ends in a hamulus around which the tendon of tensor veli palatini passes.

Anteriorly the sphenoid forms the posterior wall of the ethmoid sinuses. The sphenoid sinuses are intimately related to and occasionally ensheath the optic canal. Posteriorly the body articulates with the occipital bone. Laterally lie the cavernous sinuses, extending from the superior orbital fissure to the apex of the petrous temporal bone. They are traversed by the internal carotid artery, with its surrounding sympathetic plexus, the abducent, oculomotor, trochlear nerves and the ophthalmic and maxillary divisions of the trigeminal nerve.

Inferiorly the sphenoid forms the roof of the nasopharynx. The jugum, on the superior surface supports the olfactory tracts. The optic chiasma grooves the surface forming the chiasmatic sulcus and posterior to this and the tuberculum sellae lies the hypophyseal fossa containing the pituitary gland and roofed in by the dural diaphragma sellae. The basilar artery and brain stem are related to the thick posterior basisphenoid.

Blood, nerve and lymphatic supply

The sinuses are supplied by the posterior ethmoidal vessels and nerves plus orbital branches of the pterygopalatine ganglion. Lymphatic drainage is to the retropharyngeal nodes.

The frontal bone and sinuses (Fig. 2.16)[1,3b,8]

The frontal bone forms the forehead and orbital roof. It completes the ethmoid labyrinths and contains the frontal sinuses which form a variable excavation between its inner and outer lamina. The frontal sinuses are as individual as fingerprints. The bone is consequently of varying thickness, being thinnest in the region of the orbital roofs and dehiscences may occur with age.

The frontal sinuses are usually L-shaped, consisting of a vertical and a horizontal compartment; in addition, diverticula, supernumerary sinuses and incomplete septa are described. A complete intersinus septum is usually found but it is often paramedian and may be dehiscent in 9%. The range of variation in size is great:

breadth	28.9 ± 8.6 mm
sagittal length	20.5 ± 7.7 mm

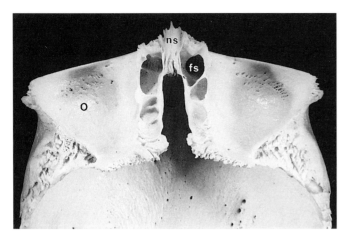

Fig. 2.16   The frontal bone – inferior view. O, orbital roof; fs, frontal sinus; ns, nasal spine.

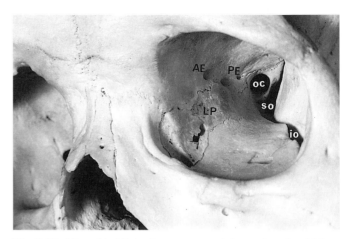

Fig. 2.17   The orbit. LP, lamina papyracea; AE, anterior ethmoidal foramen; PE, posterior ethmoidal foramen; oc, optic canal; so, superior orbital fissure; io, inferior orbital fissure.

However maximum dimensions of 49 mm and 45.5 mm respectively have been reported. 1% of the population have no discernible frontal sinus.

The sinus opens into the anterior extremity of the ethmoidal infundibulum usually directly into the frontal recess forming an 'hour-glass' constriction. However accessory channels are present in 12% of the population with separate ostia draining into the anterior ethmoids in 8% and into the posterior cells in 4%.

The frontal bone articulates with the cribriform plate to form the floor of the anterior cranial fossa (p. 34). The frontal sinus is intimately related to the ethmoid labyrinth from which it derives, and to which the frontal bone forms the roof. Excavation of the bone by the frontal sinus also results in a close relationship to the orbit.

Blood nerve and lymphatic supply

The arterial supply of the sinus is from the supraorbital and anterior ethmoidal arteries. The venous drainage is important clinically as it includes the anastomotic vein in the supraorbital notch connecting supraorbital and superior ophthalmic vessels and also diploic veins draining to the superior sagittal and sphenoparietal sinuses.

The nerve supply is from the supraorbital nerve and the lymphatic drainage is into the submandibular glands.

The orbit[1,3b,8,16]

Osteology (Fig. 2.17)

The orbital cavities are quadrilateral pyramids lying either side of the sagittal plane of the skull between cranium and facial skeleton. The bases of the pyramids are directed forwards, laterally and slightly inferiorly. They each contain the eyeball, extraocular muscles, nerves and vessels and some additional structures traversing the area. There is great variation in dimensions but useful averages are as follows:

depth	40 mm
height of orbital opening	35 mm
width of orbital opening	40 mm
interorbital distance	25 mm
volume	30 ml.

Small increases in volume can lead to considerable proptosis.

Seven bones contribute to the orbit: frontal, zygoma, sphenoid, palatine, ethmoid, lacrimal and maxilla.

The superior wall or roof is vaulted, smooth and triangular in shape. It is composed of the orbital plate of the frontal bone with a posterior contribution from the lesser wing of the sphenoid. At its lateral angle is a fossa for the lacrimal gland, medially is the trochlear fovea. Pneumatization of the roof by the frontal and occasionally ethmoid sinuses is variable. The bone which is thin except in the lesser wing becomes increasingly so with age though dehiscences are comparatively rare. Small veins may perforate the bone particularly in the lacrimal fossa (cribra orbitalia) and lesser wing of sphenoid. The superior margin has two notches or foramina (frontal and supraorbital) which transmit medial and lateral branches of the supraorbital nerves and vessels.

The medial wall is composed of the frontal process of the maxilla, lacrimal bone, orbital plate of the ethmoid (lamina papyracea), and body of the sphenoid. These bones, of which the ethmoid is the largest component, are united by vertical sutures. The wall is roughly oblong, running parallel with the sagittal plane. Anteriorly lies the fossa for the lacrimal sac, limited posteriorly by the posterior lacrimal crest from which the lacrimal part of orbicularis oculi arises.

The medial wall is the thinnest wall (0.2–0.4 mm) and is easily breached by disease. At its junction with the roof is the fronto-ethmoid suture through which pass the anterior and posterior ethmoidal vessels and nerves. The position of these foramina is variable but a rule of 24–12–6 has been suggested, based respectively on the average distance in millimetres from the anterior lacrimal crest to anterior ethmoidal foramen, from anterior to posterior ethmoidal foramina and from posterior ethmoidal foramen to optic foramen.[17] There is, however, considerable variation with the distance between posterior ethmoid and optic canal ranging from 2–9 mm.[18] Furthermore 16% of individuals have no anterior ethmoidal foramen, 30% have multiple foramina and 4.6% have none.

The inferior wall or floor is roughly triangular and slopes slightly downwards from medial to lateral. It is composed of the orbital plate of the maxilla, the orbital surface of the zygoma and the orbital process of the palatine bone. The floor is traversed by the infraorbital sulcus running forwards from the inferior orbital fissure. At a variable point, usually halfway along, it is converted into a canal which emerges on the anterior wall of the maxilla as the infraorbital foramen, 4–7 mm inferior to the orbital margin. This foramen is single in 90% of individuals. It transmits the infraorbital artery and nerve from which the anterior superior alveolar branches are given in most individuals and the middle superior alveolar branch arises in 34% of individuals.

Lateral to the opening of the nasolacrimal canal is a pit marking the origin of the inferior oblique muscle which is the only extrinsic muscle with an extraperiosteal origin. However, this may be intraperiosteal in 9% of cases.[18] The bone of the floor is generally thin (0.5–1 mm) but specific dehiscences in the canal make this area a common site for blow-outs and invasion from the maxilla.

The lateral wall is triangular and makes an angle of 45° with the median plane. It is composed of the orbital surface of the greater wing of the sphenoid, the orbital surface of the zygoma and the zygomatic process of the frontal bone. The sphenoidal part is separated from the roof and floor by superior and inferior orbital fissures respectively. It is the thickest wall of the orbit except posteriorly which represents an area of primitive communication between orbit and temporal fossa.

The superior orbital fissure lies between the greater and lesser wings of the sphenoid. It has a mean length of 20 mm and is widest postero-medially, forming a retort shape. It is divided into three by the common tendinous ring which attaches supero-medially round the margin of the optic canal. The lacrimal, frontal and trochlear nerves pass through it supero-laterally. The superior division of the oculomotor, nasociliary, sympathetic root of ciliary ganglion, inferior division of oculomotor and abducent nerves pass through the ring centrally and a branch of the superior ophthalmic vein usually passes most inferomedially to the ring. The tubercle for the inferior head of lateral rectus is sometimes found on its inferior margin.

The inferior orbital fissure lies between the lateral and inferior walls extending from the root of the greater wing to the zygomatic bone. It is widest antero-laterally and has a mean length of 29 mm. It communicates with the pterygopalatine fossa medially and infratemporal fossa laterally. In life it is filled by membrane through which pass the infraorbital nerves and vessels, zygomatic nerves, and veins draining the orbit into the pterygoid plexus.

The optic foramen or canal lies at the apex of the pyramid between two roots of the lesser wing of the sphenoid connecting orbit with middle cranial fossa. Attached to its margin is the common tendinous ring of Zinn which gives origin to the straight extraocular muscles. It transmits the optic nerve and coverings, ophthalmic artery and sympathetic plexus. It is closely related to the sphenoidal and posterior ethmoidal sinuses.

The orbit has the following relations:

1. Superiorly, the anterior cranial fossa overlies the roof of the orbit but this may be invaded to a variable degree by frontal and ethmoid sinuses. Therefore, above the roof are the meninges, covering the frontal lobes of the brain.

2. Medially, from anterior to posterior, the lateral wall of the nose, infundibulum, ethmoid and sphenoid sinuses. The optic foramen lies most posteriorly.

3. The maxillary sinus is the principle relation inferiorly though occasionally the ethmoid cells can invade the floor.

4. Laterally the orbit is separated anteriorly from the temporal fossa and posteriorly from the middle cranial fossa and temporal lobe of the brain.

Periosteum

The orbital contents are bound and supported by fibrous tissue or orbital fascia which is condensed into four components: periorbita, orbital septum, bulbar sheath and muscular fascia.

The periorbita is the periosteal lining of the body walls to which it is loosely attached. It is firmly adherent to the orbital margins, sutures, foramina, fissures and lacrimal crest, enclosing the fossa and traversing the duct as far as the inferior meatus. It is continuous with the periosteum of the facial bones and posteriorly with the dura surrounding the optic nerve and the structures of the superior orbital fissure and ethmoidal canal.

Special areas of thickening occur in the periorbita round the trochlea and lacrimal sac and from it septa pass into the cavity, separating the lobules of fat. Inferiorly it is thickened to form a definable suspensory ligament, the ligament of Lockwood. It can become ossified, particularly in relation to the inferior orbital canal and has a generous trigeminal nerve supply. Smooth muscle fibres found in the periorbita near to the inferior orbital fissure have been called the muscle of Muller or muscularis orbitalis.

The orbital septum is a fibrous sheet stretching across the entrance to the orbit. It is related to the posterior surface of orbicularis oculi in the lids, attaches to the margin of the orbit and is continuous with the periosteum. It strengthens the lids and contains the fat within the orbital cavity.

The bulbar sheath or Tenon's capsule is a thin fibrous tunic ensheathing all but the corneal part of the eyeball forming a socket. It does not continue posteriorly on to the optic nerve which perforates it as do the ciliary vessels, vorticose veins at the equator and the tendons of the bulbar muscles. Where the bulbar muscles perforate the bulbar sheath, fascial processes pass out on these to the orbital wall. In the region of medial and lateral recti, they are quite well-defined and constitute recognizable check ligaments.

The lower part of the bulbar fascia is thickened to form a supporting sling which has been called the suspensory ligament of Lockwood. This is strengthened by the lateral margins of the sheaths of medial, lateral and inferior recti plus medial and lateral check ligaments. The resulting inferior retinaculum forms a band 15 mm long and 3–4 mm wide and is effective in supporting the globe as evidenced by the maintenance of its position following subtotal maxillectomy.

The palpebral ligaments

The medial and lateral palpebral (canthal) ligaments attach the tarsal plates to the orbital wall. The medial ligament is a strong triangular fibrous band which runs towards the root of the nose and represents a direct continuation of the two tarsal plates. It divides into anterior and posterior limbs which embrace the exposed part of the lacrimal sac and which attach to the anterior and posterior lacrimal crests respectively, thus forming a 'Y' on its side. It has a free lower border while being continuous above with the periosteum of the frontal process of the maxilla and forms a well-marked prominence when the lateral canthus is pulled laterally. The oft-encountered angular vein crosses the ligament usually 8 mm from the medial canthus.

The lateral palpebral ligament attaches to the orbital tubercle on the zygomatic bone approximately 1 cm below the frontozygomatic suture. It is much less defined than its medial counterpart. Its upper border is united with the expansion of levator and the lower border with the inferior oblique and inferior rectus.

The trochlea

The trochlea is a connective tissue sling anchoring the tendinous part of the superior oblique muscle to the orbit. The fovea for the trochlea is a small depression lying close to the fronto-lacrimal suture some 4 mm from the orbital margin and usually 5 mm in diameter. In about 10% of subjects the ligaments which attach the U-shaped cartilage of the pulley to it are ossified. The fovea is then surmounted posteriorly by a spicule or spine of bone. Very occasionally a completely ossified ring is present. Through the pulley, the tendon is enclosed in a synovial sheath beyond which a strong fibrous sheath accompanies the tendon to the eyeball.

The lacrimal apparatus

The lacrimal gland, situated anteriorly in the upper outer quadrant of the orbit, secretes tears which pass into the conjunctival sac and thence to the medial angle. From there tears drain through the lacrimal canaliculi into the lacrimal sac, nasolacrimal duct and thence to the inferior meatus. Under normal circumstances, virtually no tears pass down the duct as just sufficient are produced to lubricate the cornea and conjunctiva.

The gland is composed of two unequal parts, separated to some extent by the levator palpebrae superioris. The larger orbital part is situated in a fossa on the anterior and lateral part of the orbital roof. It is approximately 20×12 mm, almond-shaped and connected by fibrous tissue to the orbital periosteum. It rests in an arch of fascia between the sheaths of the superior and lateral recti. The smaller palpebral portion overlies the lateral third of the upper conjunctival fornix though there are often additional accessory glands present in the fornices and lids (conjunctival glands of Krause).

The gland itself is compound tubuloalveolar in structure and similar to the parotid in appearance. The ducts draining the orbital part are intimately related to the palpebral portion, so removal of the latter effectively abolishes secretion of the entire gland. The gland is supplied by the lacrimal artery (a branch of the ophthalmic) and infraorbital artery (maxillary) and drains into the ophthalmic venous system. Lacrimal nerves derive from the ophthalmic divisions of trigeminal and facial nerves and autonomic supply comes via the greater petrosal and cervical sympathetic trunk.

Blinking distributes the tears, which collect in the medial lacrimal sac. The lacrimal punctum on the papilla lies at the medial end of the lid pointing into the conjunctival sac and receives the tears. This is therefore only visible on everting the lid. A canaliculus (superior and inferior) runs from each punctum. Each is 10 mm long and has a vertical and horizontal portion. They perforate the periorbita and either unite as a common canaliculus or enter separately as small diverticuli of the lacrimal sac – the lacrimal sinus of Maier. The membranous lacrimal sac, lying in the fossa is on average 12 × 4.4 × 2.2 mm in size. It is really a blind-ending tube, opening inferiorly into the nasolacrimal duct. It is covered by orbital periosteum and by the medial palpebral ligament in its upper anterior half but has a loose connective tissue capsule with a venous plexus interposed which can alter flow when engorged.

The naso-lacrimal duct runs as a continuation of the sac in a bony canal down, back and laterally to open in the inferior meatus at or just anterior to the genu of the inferior turbinate. The nasal mucosa is often traversed obliquely producing a small flap or lacrimal plica. There are no true valves in the duct. It is on average 17 mm long with a diameter of 4 mm and is slightly constricted at its junction with the sac. Blockage at any point will result in epiphora.

The teeth[1,3b,8]

Dental anatomy

The functions of the teeth are to facilitate mastication and speech. There are two generations of teeth, a primary deciduous set of 20 and a permanent secondary dentition of 32. Each half set of 16 permanent teeth consists of 4 central incisors, an adjacent canine or cuspid next to which are 2 premolars and 3 molars. Each tooth is composed of two parts, a crown and a root and of three calcified tissues, enamel, cementum and dentine.

The crown is that part of the tooth exposed beyond the gum and is covered with enamel. The root is embedded in the alveolus and is covered with cementum. A neck separates the crown from the root. The crowns of each arch meet at the masticatory or occlusal surface. The crown and root together constitute the tooth body which is composed of dense bone called dentine. The dentine of the crown is covered by enamel which is white, semi-translucent and highly mineralized. As it wears the underlying yellow dentine is exposed.

The dentine of the root is covered by a peridontal membrane which connects the cementum to the bone of the alveolus. Each root has a dental cavity filled with pulp which is a soft fibrous tissue supplied with vessels and nerves entering the root canal via the apical foramen.

The pulp and periodontal membrane have a good blood and nerve supply. The posterior superior dental artery (maxillary) supplies molar and premolar teeth, the anterior superior dental (infraorbital) artery runs to the teeth in the anterior maxillary wall and the middle superior dental (infraorbital) artery, if present, runs in the lateral wall to terminate near the canine and anastomoses with the anterior and posterior branches. A plexus of veins around the apex of each tooth usually join the facial veins or pterygoid plexus posteriorly. Lymphatic drainage from the pulp and periodontal ligament passes either via the palate or submandibular region to the jugulo-digastric group. The nerve supply is predominantly trigeminal via the maxillary division. The anterior, middle and posterior superior alveolar nerves supply the gums, periodontal membrane and pulp cavity of the upper alveolar teeth. The middle nerve is only present in 37% of subjects.

The deciduous dentition by comparison with the permanent teeth are smaller. The crowns are whiter and the enamel softer but thicker. The roots are shorter and the necks more constricted. In form they are generally similar to their permanent counterparts though the molars show greater diversity.

The maxillary alveolar processes extend inferiorly from the bodies of the maxilla and support the teeth within bony sockets, so each maxilla contains a full quadrant of eight permanent or five deciduous teeth. The form of the alveolus is related to the functional demands imposed on the teeth so resorption occurs when these are removed.

The form and depth of each socket depend on the root supported and show considerable variation. Consequently the number of upper teeth whose roots are in direct relation to the maxillary sinus is not constant, but the upper molars are most consistently in close proximity. Assessments of the distance between the root apices of upper teeth and the floor of the antrum have shown that the roots of the 2nd molar are closest to the floor followed, in order of frequency by the 1st molar, 3rd molar, 2nd premolar, 1st premolar and canine.

Dental development

At birth all tooth germs are present except that for the 2nd molar (appearing at 6 weeks) and the 3rd molar (appearing at the 5th year). Calcification begins in the superficial part of the crown and spreads to the root, being complete for deciduous teeth by the 5th intrauterine month. Eruption of the deciduous teeth is variable, beginning at between 6–8 months with the medial incisor and ending at 20–24 months with the 2nd molar. The average time of eruption in years for the upper permanent teeth is as follows:

central incisors	7.0
lateral incisors	8.3
canines	11.2
1st premolars	10.1
2nd premolars	10.7
1st molars	6.2
2nd molars	12.5
3rd molars	17–21

The pterygopalatine fossa[1,3b,8]

This is a small space, the shape of an inverted pyramid, containing the blood and nerve supply of the upper jaw. It is bounded posteriorly by the greater wing of the sphenoid, anteriorly by the posterior wall of the maxilla, superiorly by the inferior surface of the body of the sphenoid, and medially by the perpendicular plate of the palatine. Laterally it opens into the infratemporal fossa via the pterygomaxillary fissure and the apex of the pyramid inferiorly is the pterygopalatine canal.

The space is connected by foramina and canals with five regions of the skull:

1. Anteriorly via the inferior orbital fissure with the orbit, transmitting infraorbital vessels and nerves and ascending branches of pterygopalatine ganglion.
2. Posteriorly via the foramen rotundum with the middle cranial cavity, containing the maxillary nerve and via the pterygoid canal extending to the foramen lacerum.
3. Medially via the sphenopalatine foramen to the nasal cavity.
4. Laterally via the pterygomaxillary fissure to the infratemporal fossa, transmitting maxillary vessels and superior alveolar nerves.
5. Inferiorly via the greater palatine canal to the roof of the mouth, transmitting anterior, middle and posterior palatine nerves and greater and lesser palatine vessels.

The pterygoid or Vidian canal is found below and medial to the foramen rotundum. It transmits the pterygoid nerve (and artery) from the lower part of the anterior wall of the foramen lacerum and thence via the pterygopalatine fossa to join the sphenopalatine ganglion. The pterygoid nerve is composed of the greater and deep petrosal nerves. These respectively carry the preganglionic parasympathetic fibres from the superior salivatory nucleus and the postganglionic sympathetic fibres from the cervical sympathetic chain.

The sphenopalatine foramen is formed superiorly by the body of the sphenoid closing off the sphenopalatine notch of the palatine bone, which is composed anteriorly by the orbital process, posteriorly by the sphenoidal process and inferiorly by the upper border of the perpendicular plate of the palatine. Through it pass the sphenopalatine nerves and vessels to the nasal cavity.

The contents of the pterygopalatine fossa can be divided into a neural compartment of pterygopalatine ganglion and maxillary nerve and a vascular compartment containing the terminal part of the maxillary artery and its respective branches. The maxillary nerve and artery supply the upper teeth, floor of orbit and skin of the face. Branches from the sphenopalatine ganglion travel to the nose and palate. Once tumour has invaded this region, characterized by pain and trismus, the generous vascular and lymphatic drainage compromises virtually all attempts at cure.

The infratemporal fossa[1,3,8]

This irregular space lying beneath the base of the skull between the side wall of the pharynx and the ascending ramus of the mandible is bounded anteriorly by the posterior wall of the maxilla and posteriorly by the styloid apparatus, carotid sheath and prevertebral fascia. From it pathological changes can spread anteriorly into the gingivo-buccal sulcus, superiorly where it is directly continuous with the temporal fossa and inferiorly, through the parapharyngeal space to the superior mediastinum. The roof of the infratemporal fossa is formed by the infratemporal surface of the greater wing of the sphenoid perforated by the foramen ovale and foramen spinosum and a small part of the squamous temporal bone. Medially is the lateral pterygoid plate.

The anterior and medial walls are separated superiorly by the pterygomaxillary fissure through which the infratemporal fossa communicates with the pterygopalatine fossa. The upper end of the pterygomaxillary fossa is continuous with the posterior end of the inferior orbital fissure which is placed between the upper part of the posterior surface of the maxilla and the greater wing of the sphenoid. The fissure connects the infratemporal fossa with the orbit.

Its contents are the medial and lateral pterygoids, the branches of the mandibular nerve, the maxillary artery and the pterygoid venous plexus within the lateral pterygoid muscle. The maxillary artery is divided into three parts in relation to the lateral pterygoid and from each part five branches arise.

The anterior cranial fossa[1,3b,19]

There is considerable morphological variation in this fossa formed by the orbital part of the frontal bone, cribriform plate of the ethmoid, and lesser wings and anterior part of the body of the sphenoid. The anterior fossa supports the olfactory tracts, bulbs and frontal lobes and a number of corresponding grooves and ridges are found on the frontal bone. This area is the thinnest part of the fossa and forms the roof of the orbit. It is only 0.2 mm in the newborn increasing to 1 mm in the adult but thins again with age. The fossa lies at a higher level than the other fossae and has an average length medially (to the optic foramen) of 47.7 mm and laterally of 35 mm (Fig. 2.18).

The frontal bone is split anteriorly by the frontal sinus, and the median plane of the bone is marked by the frontal crest to which the falx cerebri attaches. The jugum of the sphenoid separates the fossa from the sphenoid sinus. Anteriorly the jugum articulates with the cribriform plate and posteriorly it is grooved by the chiasmatic sulcus, connecting the optic canals. The lesser wings curve away laterally and posteriorly, forming a free over-

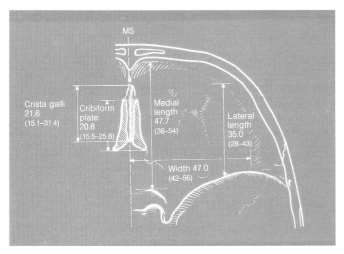

Fig. 2.18 The dimensions of the floor of anterior cranial fossa (after Lang 1983[20]).

hanging border to the middle cranial fossa and bear the anterior clinoid processes. The crista galli lies in the midline. It is variable in shape and size, and is occasionally pneumatized. Anterior to this lies the foramen caecum which often transmits an emissary vein to the superior sagittal sinus. The cribriform plate which divides the nasal and cranial cavities, is so-called because of the foramina transmitting the olfactory nerves. Up to the age of 9 years the plate grows in length, but shortens relatively thereafter due to overgrowth of the planum sphenoidale. The average adult length is 20.8 mm. The anterior ethmoidal canal usually opens between the orbital part of the frontal bone and the cribriform plate and transmits the respective nerve and vessels which run forwards under the dura to gain the nasal cavity by passing down through a slit at the side of the crista. Sometimes these structures can pass through a separate foramen in the frontal bone itself. The posterior ethmoidal canal opens at the posterolateral corner of the plate.

The dura of the anterior cranial fossa is thick, dense and inelastic. Technically it is composed of two layers, meningeal and endosteal, but these are intimately adherent to each other. The falx cerebri, a strong arched process of dura running in the longitudinal fissure between the cerebral hemispheres, attaches to the crista and frontal crest. The free border of the tentorium cerebelli, which covers the cerebellum and supports the occipital lobes, attaches to the anterior clinoid process.

The superior sagittal sinus occupies the attached convex margin of the falx cerebri. It commences at the crista, receiving a vein from the nasal cavity via the foramen caecum. The sinus runs back, grooving the frontal, parietal and squamous parts of the occipital bone. Near the internal occipital protuberance, it deviates to one side (usually to the right) and continues as the trans-

verse sinus. The sinus receives superior cerebral veins and contains the projections of the arachnoid granulations. The sinus communicates with the venous lacunae situated in the dura, a small frontal, and large parietal and occipital lacunae.

COMPARATIVE ANATOMY OF THE UPPER JAW

The comparative anatomy of the mammalian upper jaw and its surrounding structures are worthy of a brief consideration, to highlight not only the interspecies differences but also the similarities which exist in an area which constitutes the first part of the respiratory tract and houses the peripheral olfactory apparatus.[20-28]

The fundamental configuration of the mammalian nasal fossa is remarkably constant. It is divided into two by a midline septum, through it inspired air is moistened, cleansed of particulate matter, subjected to olfactory analysis and, in homiothermic animals, warmed. To this end the mucosal surface area is increased by a series of turbinals, the complexity of which varies between species, generally in relation to olfactory acuity. This and the increased respiratory requirements associated with mammalian metabolism underlie the general alteration in the anterior–posterior dimensions that distinguish the nasal cavity from that of reptiles.

Three sets of turbinals project from the lateral wall and fill the nasal cavity; ethmoturbinals, nasoturbinals and maxilloturbinals. The most complex of these are the ethmoturbinals which are usually arranged in two rows, the ectoturbinals which lie most laterally and the endoturbinals lying medially (Fig. 2.19). These are conventionally denoted by arabic and roman numerals respectively. The ectoturbinals can be very numerous, 31 are found in the horse, and may encroach on the maxil-

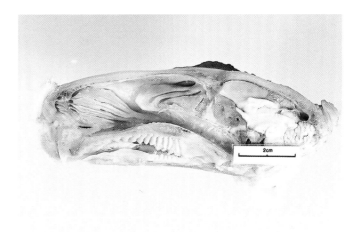

Fig. 2.19 Midline sagittal section through guinea-pig head, showing lateral wall of nose with complex arrangement of ethmoturbinals and maxilloturbinals.

lary sinus cavity whilst the number of endoturbinals are generally in single figures. In many macrosmatic species the nose is effectively divided by a transverse plate into an upper olfactory recess housing the ethmoturbinals above the main respiratory currents and a lower respiratory compartment. This may prolong retention of olfactory substances once sniffed in. The nasoturbinal is usually included with the ethmoturbinals for anatomical and functional consideration but the general development of the nasal cavity has resulted in the maxilloturbinal being completely in the respiratory part of the nose and although often scrolled it never achieves the complexity of the ethmoturbinal (Fig. 2.20).

In the anthropoid nose, there is further reduction in the anterior–posterior length resulting in a short relatively high-roofed cavity. The turbinals are reduced in size, number and degree of branching, resulting in a decreased olfactory surface area consistent with the dominance of vision over olfaction. The olfactory to respiratory mucous membrane surface area ratio of 1 in the cat can be compared with 0.3 in man.[29] Indeed the enlarged orbits obliterate the superior nasal cavity in certain species, and are divided only by an interorbital septum in some or soft tissue alone in others (Fig. 2.21).

In all anthropoids, the ectoturbinals disappear during fetal development and the endoturbinals are reduced to three in number with corresponding reduction in olfactory epithelium. Thus the middle, superior and supreme turbinates correspond to endoturbinals II, III and IV. The nasoturbinal (endoturbinal I) forms the agger nasi region and uncinate process and the maxilloturbinal is equivalent to the inferior turbinate with a separate ossification centre.

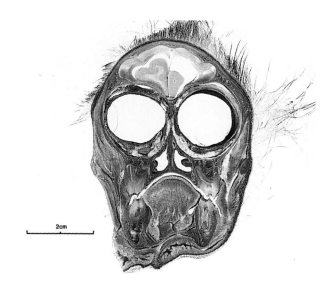

Fig. 2.21 Coronal section through head of *Cercopithecus aethiops* (vervet monkey), showing the orbits separated by an interorbital septum.

The vomeronasal organ constitutes a secondary olfactory organ, lying either side of the base of the nasal septum and having a role in feeding and reproductive behaviour.[30] There is considerable interspecies variation in its degree of development, being prominent in rodents, lagomorphs, ungulates and carnivores but rudimentary in aquatic mammals and man (Fig. 2.22). In rodents, lagomorphs, bats and some ungulates the orifice of the organ

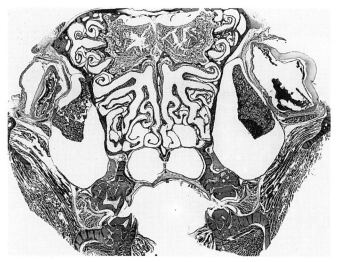

Fig. 2.20 Coronal section through nasal cavity of (Perodicticus Potto) pottoroo showing convoluted ethmoturbinals.

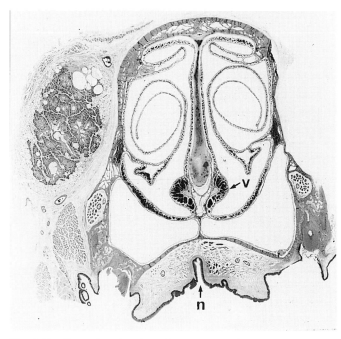

Fig. 2.22 Coronal section through nasal cavity of *Antilope cericapra* (blackbuck) showing the vomeronasal organ (v) surrounded by cartilage and receiving its nerve supply via the nasopalatine canal (n).

opens directly into the nasal cavity. In other species, such as carnivores, it opens via a nasopalatine canal while in the larger ungulates, hippopotamus and duck-billed platypus direct communication occurs with the oral cavity. These differences may not however, be of any functional significance. The organ extends as a pair of blind-ending tubes in the anterior ventral nasal septum usually contained within protective cartilages which have a very variable morphology. The sensory epithelium resembles olfactory epithelium but lacks cilia and pigment in the Bowman's glands.

The paranasal sinuses are a characteristic feature of all terrestial placental mammals, being absent in monotremes, marsupials and aquatic mammals. Whilst the nasal cavity exhibits a similar pattern amongst mammals, the sinuses show considerable variation and despite much complex theorizing, no convincing explanation of their function has emerged.

The maxillary sinus is the most constant feature but may only be an excavation or lateral recess in the maxillary bone rather than an independent cavity. The sinus may be encroached upon by the orbit and dentition in smaller animals but can achieve extensive pneumatization in some species, extending into surrounding bones; nasal, frontal, lacrimal, palatine and nasoturbinal. This is particularly so in carnivores such as the bear and ungulates such as the horse and the elephant. The size of the maxillary sinus does not necessarily correlate with total body size though personal studies of New and Old World monkeys and higher primates demonstrate that the size of the maxillary sinus increases with the size of the skull and orbit.[31]

In the 'dog-faced' monkeys (mandrillus, papio, thercopithecus), the whole lateral wall of the maxilla carrying the maxilloturbinal is displaced inwards resulting in depression of the cheek and a modified lateral recess (Figs 2.23 and 2.24). Although the 'hominoid' monkeys (pan, gorilla, pongo) are also quite prognathic with a protuberant upper alveolus, the occipito–nasion/occipito-alveolar ratio increases proportional to the increase in maxillary sinus dimensions which may reflect the relatively reduced turbinal structure (Fig. 2.25).

Distinction can be made between those monkeys in which a sinus cavity can be demonstrated and those in whom the potential space is occupied by teeth, encroached upon by the orbit and composed of spongiform bone so that no true functional cavity can be determined (Fig. 2.26). Indeed in some, the premolar and molar roots are related directly to the orbit floor. However, it is not possible to demonstrate any statistically significant difference between these two groups. Whilst skull dimensions are on average larger in those with a functional sinus, a number of small monkeys (aotus, callicebus, cebus, pithecus) have a well-developed maxillary sinus (Fig. 2.27, Table 2.1).

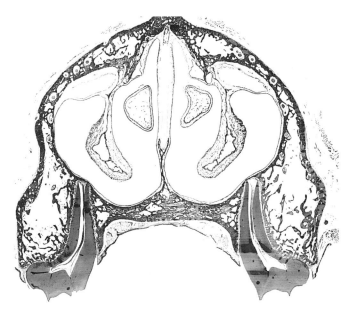

Fig. 2.23 Coronal section through nasal cavity of *Mandrillus sphinx* (mandrill) showing reduced turbinate structure and lateral recess rather than a true maxillary sinus.

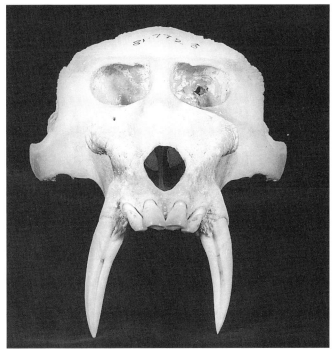

Fig. 2.24 Skull of *Mandrillus sphinx* (mandrill) showing morphology of anterior facial skeleton.

When other parameters are examined, it is still not possible to distinguish the monkeys which possess a functional maxillary sinus as a separate group. The diet of most primates is very varied and whilst one food type may predominate, opportunism often extends the range of food considerably. When the diet of monkeys with lateral

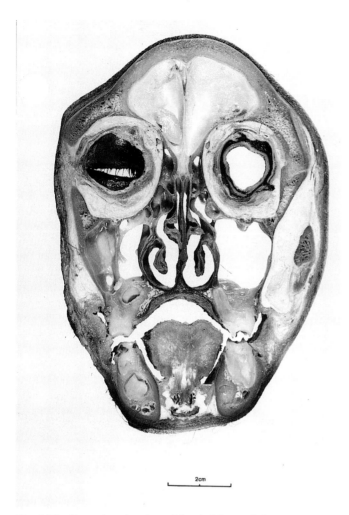

2cm

Fig. 2.25 Coronal section through head of *Pan troglodytes* (chimpanzee) showing well-developed maxillary sinus and reduced turbinal structure.

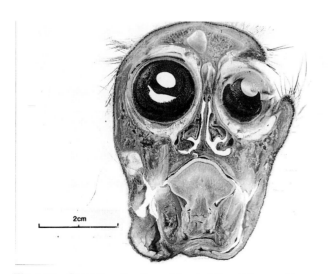

2cm

Fig. 2.26 Coronal section through head of *Cercopithecus aethiops* (vervet monkey) showing potential maxillary sinus region composed of spongioform bone and encroached upon by teeth and orbit.

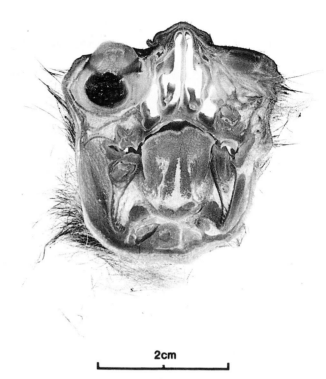

2cm

Fig. 2.27 Coronal section through head of *Aotus trivirgatus* (night monkey), showing well-developed maxillary sinus with teeth lying laterally.

recesses or no functional maxillary sinuses is examined, there is no prediliction for a particular food type and whilst some are vegetarian, others are omnivorous. Similarly, no common pattern emerges amongst monkeys with sinuses, with fruit, vegetable matter, insects and small birds, mammals and eggs being eaten. Even the large apes, whilst predominantly vegetarian, occasionally eat animal material.[32]

The vast majority of Anthropoidae (excluding man) are arboreal, although some like the gorilla and chimpanzee spend part of the day on the ground so there does not appear to be any difference in habitat between the two groups. Similarly the geographical distribution of the monkeys does not relate to the presence of a maxillary sinus, and a mixture of New and Old World monkeys occurs in each group.

When examined by zoological classification in families, the Pongoidae, Hylobatidae and Hominidae (man) have maxillary sinuses but there is great divergence in the Callitrichidae, Cebidae and Cercopithecidae (Table 2.1). Some distinction can be made between the dentition of New and Old World and Anthropoid apes,[33] but this cannot be related satisfactorily to the presence or absence of a maxillary sinus. It is clear that in the smaller monkeys the potential space of the sinus is occupied by teeth roots, e.g. Colobus, Cercopithecus, Erythrocebus (Fig. 2.21). However, in the small monkeys which do have sinuses, e.g. Aotus or Cebus, coronal sections demonstrate the teeth lying lateral to the sinus cavity (Fig. 2.27).

Table 2.1 Presence of maxillary sinus in primate sub-order Anthropoidae (haplorhini)

Family	Species	Common name	Functional maxillary sinus
Callitrichidae	*Callithrix humeralifer*	Marmoset	None
	Leontideus rosalisa	Golden lion tamarin	Present
	Saguinus fuscicollus Weddelli	Tamarin	None
Cebidae	*Aotus trivirgatus*	Night monkey	Present
	Callicebus personatus	Titi monkey	Present
	Cebus capucinus	Capuchin monkey	None
	Saimiri sciureus	Squirrel monkey	None
	Chiropotes satanas	Bearded saki	None
	Cacajao calvus	Bald uakari	None
	Alouatta palliata	Howler monkey	Present
	Ateles paniscus	Black spider monkey	None
	Brachyteles arachnoides	Woolly spider monkey	Present
	Lagothrix lagothricha	Woolly monkey	Present
Cercopithecidae	*Miopithecus talapoin*	Dwarf gueron	None
	Cercopithecus aethiops	Velvet monkey	None
	Cercocebus torquatus torquatus	Mangabey	Lateral recess
	Erythrocebus patas patas	Patas monkey	None
	Papio cynocephalus kindae	Baboon	Lateral recess
	Mandrillus sphinx	Mandrill	Lateral recess
	Thercopithecus gelada	Gelada	Lateral recess
	Macaca mulatta	Rhesus monkey	Present
	Colobus polykomos	Colobus monkey	None
	Presbitis aygula	Langur	None
	Nasalis larvatus	Proboscis monkey	Lateral recess
	Rhinopithecus avunculus	Langur	None
	Pygathrix nigripes	Langur	None
Hylobatidae	*Hylobates syndactylus*	Siamung gibbon	Present
Pongidae	*Gorilla gorilla gorilla*	Gorilla	Present
	Pongo pygmaeus pygmaeus	Orang-utan	Present
Hominidae	*Homo sapiens*	Man	Present

Amongst the great apes, the maxillary sinus and nasal configuration of the gorilla and chimpanzee are very similar to that of man with the natural ostium opening in the same morphological relationship to the middle meatus. The sinus is large in all three species but extends into the hard palate in the chimpanzee whilst in the gorilla there may be extension into the zygoma and invasion of the ethmoid, frontal and sphenoid bones (Fig. 2.28). Similar extensive invasion is seen in the orang-utan, including the palatine and lacrimal bones, which is at the expense of both ethmoid and frontal sinuses but here the sinus opens directly into the nasal cavity.

Most mammals have additional pneumatized chambers communicating with the olfactory region and opening between the lamellae of the ethmoturbinals. The olfactory epithelium may extend into these cavities which are termed 'frontal' or 'sphenoid'. However, they do not necessarily correspond to the same structures in the higher primates where the true frontal sinus consistently opens into the antero-superior part of the middle meatus and developmentally represents an ethmoidal cell. Indeed in some instances these cavities may simply be an extension of the maxillary sinus. The number and extent of these frontal and sphenoid sinuses vary between species, between members of the same species and even between the right and left sides, as a result of changes occurring during the later stages of growth.

No additional pneumatizing chambers are found in the insectivores or aquatic mammals but significant aeration is found in the frontal region of most carnivores, extending even into the parietal region in lions and hyenas. The majority of rodents and lagomorphs, e.g. the rabbit lack extra pneumatization but some, such as the porcupine have frontal development. The big ungulates and elephants have considerable excavation with multiple partitions and supra-cranial extension. The domesticated pig has up to 13 additional sinuses, even more are present in cattle, camels and the horse. In the horse, where a substantial fossil record is available, it appears that frontal pneumatization is directly related to evolutionary changes in cranial proportions.

In small prosimians such as the slender loris and in the majority of the New and Old World monkeys sinus development is confined to the maxilla. Some frontal pneumatization is found in the larger lemurs, in Aotus (Night monkey) and in Cebus (Capuchin monkey) combined

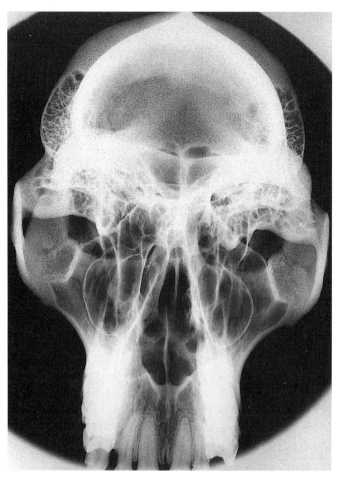

Fig. 2.28 Antero-posterior radiograph of skull of Gorilla gorilla showing extensive paranasal sinus pneumatization.

with some excavation of the presphenoid region. Neither the gibbon nor orang have true frontal sinus development but a small sphenoid cavity is present in the orang and sphenoid pneumatization may extend into the frontal region in the gibbon. Thus the orang and gibbon present the more primitive arrangement when compared with man and the African apes which can be distinguished by the presence of an ethmoid sinus complex in addition to a true frontal and sphenoid sinus. In the chimpanzee and gorilla, pneumatization may involve the orbital roof and the greater wing and pterygoid processes of the sphenoid. The ethmoid cells are few in number in the gorilla (usually three) or can be absent in the chimpanzee compared to the situation in man where the ethmoid, with its many cells and clefts, is most developed.

Examination of these patterns of mammalian sinus pneumatization and the lack of fossil evidence do not allow definitive phylogenetic conclusions to be drawn and fail to clarify their functional significance. Olfaction, humidification, resonance, heat conservation and regulation and respiratory exchange of air have been largely dismissed in the past.[25,26] Pauli emphasized the close correlation between extent of pneumatization and body size but this correlation is less close than originally supposed and does not lend unequivocal support to the 'weight-saving' theory of sinus function.[28]

Consequently we are left with Proetz's statement,[34]

In consideration of the arrangement of the face structures it becomes apparent that the formation of sinuses is necessary for a readjustment to the surrounding parts, and we are not called upon to attribute to these cavities any functional activity. The sinuses, which after all, are nothing but unoccupied spaces, result incidentally.

At present we are not in a position to contradict this view.

REFERENCES

1. Warwick R, Williams P I (eds) 1973 Gray's anatomy, 35th edn, Longman, London, pp 116–120
2. Hamilton W J, Mossman H W (eds) 1972 Human embryology. Heffer, Cambridge, pp 154–158
3. Lang J 1989 Clinical anatomy of the nose, nasal cavity and paranasal sinuses. Georg Thieme Verlag, Stuttgart a: pp 1–5, 31–35, 48–50; b: pp 106–110
4. Moore K L 1982 The developing human. W B Saunders, Philadelphia, pp 197–206
5. Diewert V M 1980 The role of craniofacial growth in palatal shelf elevation. In: Pratt R M, Christiansen R (eds) Current research trends in prenatal craniofacial development. Elsevier North-Holland, New York, pp 165–186
6. Gilbert J G, Heights R, Segal S 1958 Growth of the nose and septorhinoplastic problems in youth. Archives of Otolaryngology 68: 673–682
7. Johnson A, Josephson R, Hawke M 1985 Clinical and histological evidence for the presence of the vomeronasal organ in adult humans. Journal of Otolaryngology 14: 71–79
8. Maran A G D, Lund V J 1990 Clinical rhinology. Georg Thieme Verlag, Stuttgart, pp 5–32
9. Lund V J 1988 Inferior meatal antrostomy. Fundamental considerations of design and function. Journal of Laryngology and Otology (Suppl. 15), pp 3–4

10. Stammberger H 1991 Functional endoscopic sinus surgery. The Messerklinger technique. B C Dekker, Philadelphia, pp 49–88
11. Djindjian R, Merland J J 1978 Superselective arteriography of the external carotid artery. Springer Verlag, Berlin
12. Lasjaunias P L 1981 Craniofacial and upper cervical arteries. Williams and Wilkins, Baltimore
13. Heasman P 1984 Clinical anatomy of the superior alveolar nerves. British Journal of Oral and Maxillo-Facial Surgery 6: 439–447
14. Wood Jones F 1939 The anterior superior alveolar nerve and vessels. Journal of Anatomy 73: 583–591
15. Lund V 1987 In: Mackay I S, Bull T R (eds) Scott Brown's otolaryngology. Vol. 4: Rhinology, 5th edn. Butterworths, London
16. Warwick R 1976 Wolf's anatomy of the eye and orbit, 7th edn revised. H K Lewis, London, pp 1–20
17. Rontal E, Rontal M, Guilford F T 1979 Surgical anatomy of the orbit. Annals of Otology, Rhinology and Laryngology 88: 382–386
18. Harrison D F N 1981 Surgical approach to the medial orbital wall. Annals of Otology, Rhinology and Laryngology 90: 415–419
19. Lang J 1983 Clinical anatomy of the head. Springer-Verlag, Berlin, pp 70
20. Bourne G H 1972 The chimpanzee. Karger, Basel, pp 153–192
21. Cave A J E 1949 Notes on the nasal fossa of a young chimpanzee. Proceedings of the Zoological Society of London 119: 61–63

22. Cave A J E 1973 The primate nasal fossa. Journal of the Linnean Society 5: 377–387
23. Cave A J E, Wheeler Haines R 1939 The paranasal sinuses of the anthropoid ape. Journal of Anatomy 74: 493–523
24. Herschkovitz P 1977 Living New World Monkeys (Platyrrhini) VI. University of Chicago Press pp. 137–151, 317–321
25. Moore W J 1981 The mammalian skull. Cambridge University Press pp. 240–279
26. Negus V 1958 The comparative anatomy and physiology of the nose and paranasal sinuses. E & S Livingstone, Edinburgh, pp 286–327
27. Osman Hill W C 1970 Primates; comparative anatomy and taxonomy. Edinburgh University Press, Vols. I–VIII
28. Paulli S 1900 Uber die Pneumatictat des Schadels bei den Saugethieren. Morphologisches Jahnsuch 28: 147–564
29. Dieulafe L 1906 Morphology and embryology of the nasal fossae of vertebrates (translated by H W Loeb). Annals of Otology, Rhinology and Laryngology 15: 1–60, 267–349, 513–584
30. Harrison D F N 1987 Preliminary thoughts on the incidence, structure and function of the mammalian vomeronasal organ. Acta Otolaryngologica (Stockholm) 103: 489–495
31. Lund V J 1988 The maxillary sinus in the higher primates. Acta Otolaryngologica (Stockholm) 105: 163–171
32. Napier J R, Napier P H 1967 Handbook of living primates. Academic Press, London
33. Berkovitz B K B, Holland G R, Moxham B J 1978 Oral anatomy. Wolfe Medical, Smeets-Weert, Holland
34. Proetz A W 1922 Observations upon the formation and function of the accessory sinuses and mastoid cells. Annals of Otology, Rhinology and Laryngology 31: 1083–1092

3. Diagnostic imaging of the upper jaw and paranasal sinuses

G. A. S. Lloyd

The imaging techniques used for the investigation of the upper jaw have undergone profound changes in the past two decades. Plain radiography, once the only method used, remains as a screening procedure to identify normal sinuses and those with simple allergic or inflammatory disease. High resolution computerized tomography (CT) has replaced pluridirectional tomography for assessing the nose and sinuses prior to endoscopic surgery and to show bone destruction in patients with tumours; whilst gadolinium-enhanced Magnetic Resonance (GdMR) is now the optimum method for the demonstration of the full extent of tumour spread prior to treatment. Angiography has an ancillary role: it is not used diagnostically but is an essential part of embolization procedures. The use of diagnostic ultrasound is limited to the detection of fluid in the frontal sinus and maxillary antrum and has no serious role in the demonstration of upper jaw neoplasia.

PLAIN X-RAY TECHNIQUE

Several technical factors are essential for good radiography of the sinuses. These include accurate coning of the incident beam, a fine focal spot X-ray tube and a Potter-Bucky or fine grid to obtain maximum contrast. The standard projections which may be employed are:

1. Occipito-mental projection (Fig. 3.1)

The subject sits facing the film and the radiographic base line is tilted to 45°. The incident beam is horizontal and is centred on the occipital bone, 3 cm above the external occipital protruberance. This view shows the maxillary antra free of overlap of the petrous bones and, if the mouth is kept open during the examination, the sphenoid sinuses and nasopharynx can be seen through the open mouth.

2. Occipito-frontal projection (Fig. 3.2)

The subject sits facing the film with the orbito-meatal line raised 20°, the incident beam horizontal and the tube

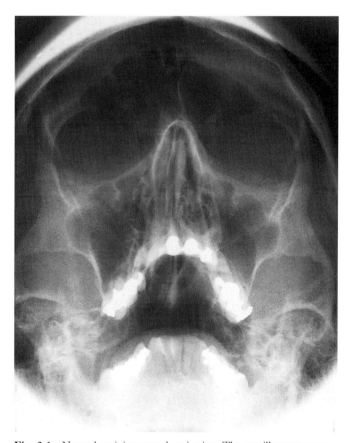

Fig. 3.1 Normal occipito-mental projection. The maxillary antra are shown free of any overlap of the petrous bones.

centred to the nasion. This projection demonstrates the fine detail of the frontal sinuses. The lateral walls of the antra are also seen, although the overlapping petrous bones largely obscure the antra.

3. Lateral projection (Fig. 3.3)

The subject sits with the radiographic baseline horizontal and the sagittal plane parallel to the film. The incident beam is centred through the antrum. The superimposi-

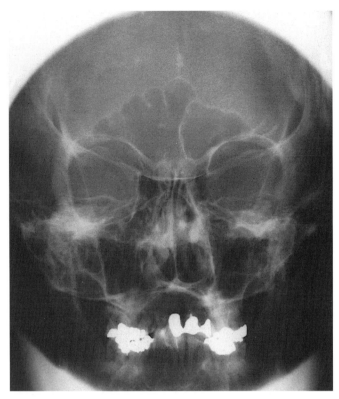

Fig. 3.2   Normal occipito-frontal view of the sinuses.

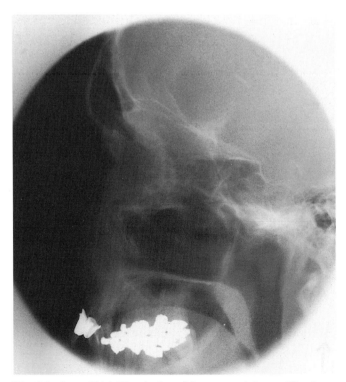

Fig. 3.3   Lateral high kilovolt view of the paranasal sinuses. The air spaces in the nose, sinuses and nasopharynx are better demonstrated by partial elimination of the bone structures.

tion of the frontal sinuses and also of both maxillary antra detracts somewhat from the value of this projection. An alternative version of the lateral projection, which better demonstrates the sinus and nasopharyngeal air spaces, is a high kilovolt lateral film using 150 kV or above and 3 mm of brass filtration.

4. Submento-vertical projection

The head is extended so that the vertex rests against the table top and the incident beam is centred between the angles of the jaw, so that it is at right angles to the baseline. This projection demonstrates the sphenoid sinuses and also the maxillary antra and orbital walls.

5. Oblique projection

Rotation of the sagittal plane of the skull through an angle of 39° will enable the posterior ethmoid cells to be projected through the orbit and will show these cells largely clear of overlap shadows. The optic foramen is seen end-on in this projection.

Sinus examination

Examination of the sinuses should always be made in the erect position with a horizontal X-ray beam to allow the demonstration of fluid levels within the sinus. Fluid in the sinus may be pus or mucopus occurring as a sequel to infection or allergy but may be due to blood after trauma.

The initial radiological investigation of the sinuses is by the plain X-ray technique described above. If the appearances on plain radiography are consistent with allergic or inflammatory disease and there is good correlation with the clinical findings no further investigation is usually necessary. If however, the evidence from plain radiography indicates an expanding or destructive lesion of the sinus walls or a tumour mass, and the clinical findings suggest a less benign process (e.g. pain and paraesthesia, epistaxis, facial swelling, nasal mass or orbital involvement), tomographic investigation is indicated. There are now three tomographic techniques available.

CONVENTIONAL TOMOGRAPHY

Conventional tomography has been almost completely superseded by high-resolution computerized tomography (CT) and now plays only a minor role in the investigation of paranasal sinus disease. It has been reduced to functioning as a simple adjunct to plain radiography at initial examination. For example it is useful in showing whether there is a nasal mass present in association with an opaque sinus, particularly if the maxillary antrum is involved. Small nasal masses often go undetected on plain radiographs, and patients who are found to have unilateral total opacity of the antrum should have immediate tomography as a screening procedure.

Ideally conventional tomography should be performed using a machine capable of complex motion tomography rather than a simple linear movement. A full series of paranasal sinus tomograms consists of:

1. *Coronal projections.* These use an undertilted occipito-mental position of the skull angled 30–35° cranially, or a projection corresponding to the occipito-frontal view with the forehead placed in contact with the table top and the orbito-meatal line at right angles to it (Fig. 3.2).

2. *Lateral tomograms.*

3. *Axial tomography.* For these films a specially designed wooden platform is placed on the table top so that the head may be hyperextended into the sub-mento vertical position.[1]

COMPUTERIZED TOMOGRAPHY

CT scanning has provided an important addition to the radiographic investigation of the paranasal sinuses, and has virtually replaced conventional tomography as a means of assessing tumours, mucocoeles and other expanding lesions in the sinuses. CT has the advantage of showing both bone destruction and the soft tissue extent of disease. In malignant disease it provides an accurate method of staging a tumour prior to radiotherapy or surgery and is important postoperatively to show recurrence of tumour. In addition it has extended the possibilities of differential diagnosis of sinus pathology, not only by showing the soft tissue pattern of disease, but also by a more sensitive demonstration of calcification in a tumour, which in some instances may be characteristic. Occasionally CT may allow the radiologist to make the primary diagnosis of sinus malignancy prior to the clinician, and to indicate the best area for confirmatory biopsy.

Technique

Routine axial and coronal sections should be obtained on all patients. Direct coronal scanning is necessary for adequate demonstration of sinus disease. Reformatted views should be reserved for sagittal sections which are not directly obtainable with most scanner designs. They should only be used to provide coronal scans when direct scanning is for any reason impossible, e.g. if a patient cannot extend the head or cervical spine.

Axial scans (Fig. 3.4)

Axial scans of the sinuses should be orientated in the same plane as those used for CT of the orbit.[2] The posi-

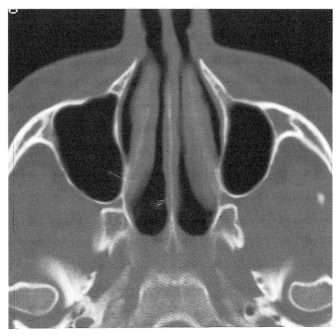

A

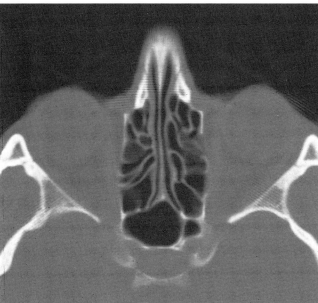

B

Fig. 3.4 Normal axial CT section made (**A**) through the maxillary antra and (**B**) at the level of the ethmoid labyrinth and orbits.

tion of the patient's head is adjusted so that the scanning plane forms an angle of 16° caudally from the orbito-meatal line: in this way the plane of section will conform to the length of the optic nerve, and will also provide axial views of the optic canals and the adjacent posterior ethmoid cells and sphenoid sinuses.

Coronal scans (Fig. 3.5)

Coronal scans are performed by hyperextension of the patient's head and angulation of the gantry with the

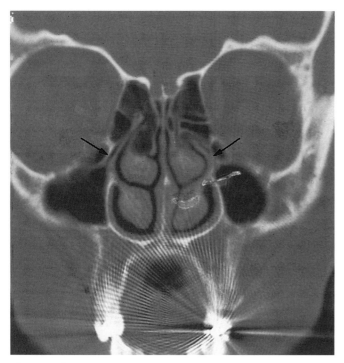

Fig. 3.5 Coronal CT section showing antra, middle meatus and infundibula (arrows).

patient either prone or in the supine position. In some patients it may be impossible to obtain true coronal scans, either because the patient cannot achieve sufficient extension of the neck, or because the angulation may need to be adjusted out of the coronal plane to avoid the effect of metallic dental fillings. These will degrade the image unless suitable computer software modification is available to overcome the problem.

For imaging of the sinuses 5 mm sections in both planes are generally adequate, with contiguous slices through the lesion. Imaging should include both wide window settings for bone detail and narrower window widths for good soft tissue contrast: generally the window settings should be within the range 200–3000 Hounsfield units.

Contrast medium

The CT attenuation values of both normal and abnormal tissues generally show an increase after the administration of intravenous contrast medium. In sinus neoplasia the degree of enhancement varies with tumours of different histology and there is also a considerable variation within the same histological type. Enhancement usually correlates closely with the vascularity of the tissue concerned so that strong enhancement is to be expected for inflammatory tissue while retained secretion and uninfected mucocoeles should not enhance. By utilizing any differential contrast enhancement a distinction can sometimes be made between tumour and adjacent normal or inflammatory tissue. In practice these differences are often unclear, largely because of the wide range of tumour enhancement encountered. This method of assessing tumour extent and recurrence has been largely superseded by magnetic resonance using the contrast agent gadolinium DTPA. In these circumstances, in which CT is used primarily to show bone changes rather than soft tissues, little added information is provided by giving contrast medium prior to CT when magnetic resonance studies are available. In general intravenous contrast should be reserved for the following categories of patient:

1. Patients with vascular tumours such as angiofibroma. In these a bolus injection or drip infusion should be employed, scanning taking place during the actual administration of the contrast to catch the vascular phase of tumour enhancement.

2. Patients with suspected tumour spread into the anterior or middle cranial fossa, i.e. when the blood–brain barrier is involved. The tumour is then outlined against the non-enhancing brain tissue.

3. Patients with sinus infection in whom abscess formation is suspected either in the anterior fossa or in the orbit, when there is an associated orbital cellulitis. This also applies to pyocoeles, which may show typical ring enhancement after contrast.

MAGNETIC RESONANCE IMAGING

Atomic nuclei with an odd number of protons or neutrons possess a magnetic moment and behave like spinning magnets. Hydrogen has such a nucleus and, because of its wide distribution in the body, it is the element most commonly used for magnetic resonance imaging. When placed in a static magnetic field the hydrogen nuclei align their magnetic axes parallel to the field. The sum of these nuclear magnets gives rise to a weak magnetization in the direction of the field, because slightly more of these nuclear magnets align with the field than against it.

Application of an oscillating radio-frequency pulse of a specific frequency introduces energy into the patient and can cause the magnetization to rotate into the transverse plane when a 90° pulse is used. Alternatively the magnetization vector can be completely reversed in direction by a 180° pulse. When the pulse is discontinued the nuclei tend to return to their original orientation in the static magnetic field, while emitting the absorbed energy. When at 90° to the field the transverse nuclear magnetization will cut the receiver coils and induce a resonant signal voltage in the coil. The return to equilibrium for the component in the direction of the static magnetic field is exponential and is described by the time constant T1.

The intensity of the signal is related to the proton density, which refers to the distribution of resonating hydrogen nuclei within the patient. It must be emphasized however, that not all protons give a magnetic resonance signal. The protons in macromolecules such as proteins and DNA and solid structures such as bone and calcification do not usually contribute to the NMR signal, so that bone and calcification are represented as signal voids on magnetic resonance scans. The distribution of the resonating protons is fairly uniform in the soft tissues and differences in density therefore are slight. Contrast between areas of differing proton density can be enhanced if the scan is biased towards T1 or T2 relaxation characteristics. In practice therefore the resultant image is affected by the proton density and by one or other or both of these components.

Pulse sequences

The following pulse sequences are commonly used in magnetic resonance studies:

1. *Saturation recovery.* This is the simplest pulse sequence. 90° radio-frequency pulses are repeatedly applied to the patient and the nuclear magnetic resonance signal is measured after each pulse. Provided the repetition time is short in relation to the T1 relaxation time of the tissue concerned, a proton density image with some T1 weighting will be produced.

2. *Inversion recovery.* This sequence produces images which contain a greater amount of T1 information than is provided by saturation recovery, although the principle is very similar. In inversion recovery the nuclei are caused to resonate by 180° pulse prior to the 90° pulse, so that the nuclei are not at equilibrium when the 90° pulse is applied. The resulting image contains approximately twice the amount of T1 information compared with the saturation recovery mode and is therefore to be preferred when T1 spin characteristics are to be evaluated.

3. *Spin echo.* The spin echo pulse sequence produces a signal to which both T1 and T2 contribute. The pulse sequence is the reverse of inversion recovery in that a 90° pulse is followed by a 180° pulse. The time between the initial 90° pulse and the signal is known as the time to echo; the larger this value the greater the T2 contribution to the signal.

Paramagnetic contrast agents and proton relaxation

The T1 and T2 relaxation times can be affected by the presence of paramagnetic substances. Paramagnetic ions have magnetic moments that are of the order of 1000 times as large as that of protons. These produce large local magnetic fields and can enhance the relaxation rates of water molecules in their immediate vicinity. It is found that the increase in the relaxation rate is directly proportional to the concentration of the paramagnetic agent and to the square of its magnetic moment.

The first paramagnetic agent to be introduced into clinical practice as a magnetic resonance contrast medium was the substance gadolinium DTPA. Gadolinium is a very effective paramagnetic agent but as a free ion it is toxic to liver, spleen and bone marrow. However when chelated to diethylenetriamine penta-acetic acid (DTPA) its toxicity is reduced, permitting it to be used as a safe relaxation enhancing agent. In the soft tissues it is distributed mainly in the extracellular space and to date no serious toxic effects have been recorded with its use.

Technique and application

Multi-slice facility

An advantage of magnetic resonance tomography over other methods is the multi-slice facility which is standard on most current machines. This allows multiple sections to be obtained simultaneously using either 1 cm or 0.5 cm contiguous slices to a depth of up to 12 cm. Coupled with the use of a head coil and three-plane imaging this provides total coverage of the head and neck and allows identification of associated disease away from the primary site in the sinuses, e.g. neck malignancy. This is of obvious importance to the oncologist in treatment planning and represents a major advance over CT scanning.

Slice thickness

Thin slices are advantageous in magnetic resonance tomography when trying to visualize small areas. Definition is improved because the amount of overlap between structures lying obliquely through the slice is reduced and their edges become more distinct. However thin sections suffer from an important disadvantage: the thinner the slice the greater the amount of 'noise' on the scan, increasing the 'noise' to signal ratio and degrading the final image. This effect on the image is less obvious at high static field strengths because the machines with the more powerful magnets possess a higher inherent spatial resolution than the low field strength systems.

Choice of pulse sequences

For optimum tissue characterization T1 and T2 weighted sequences are required. Spin echo sequences using a long time to echo will give maximum T2 weighting and signal differentiation between tissues, depending upon the relaxation times of the tissues concerned. T1 weighting can be achieved using saturation recovery or a spin echo sequence with a short repetition time, producing images of good anatomical detail and containing some T2 information. Greater T1 weighting is produced by the inversion recovery technique. T1 weighting is especially important when a paramagnetic contrast agent is employed.

Tissue characteristics

In general malignant tumours of naso-sinus origin, whether epithelial or mesenchymal, produce signals of medium intensity on T1 weighted spin echo sequences and a medium to strong signal on T2 images. In contrast, retained secretion produces high signal on T2 weighted sequences, the retained secretion always giving a higher signal than tumour. An additional feature is the heterogeneous signal of tumour in comparison with that shown by retained secretion, which is usually homogeneous. The vascularity of the tumour contributes to the lack of homogeneous signal seen in juvenile angiofibroma. In these tumours large vessels can be identified both in the tumour and in the adjacent musculature. They are shown as negative areas of signal or signal void, and when present are diagnostic.

Magnetic resonance scanning can show simple inflammatory or allergic changes in the sinuses. It is possible to demonstrate single or multiple polyps, thickened mucosa, or fluid levels in the presence of infection. In most instances the need to recognize them is simply to be able to distinguish their features from more serious disease. One of the advantages of magnetic resonance over CT is the strong signal which is received on T2 images from retained mucus or mucopus in the sinuses. This enables an important distinction to be made between tumour and secondary mucocoele formation, even within the same sinus cavity. In the same way primary mucocoeles or pyocoeles are optimally demonstrated by this technique. The very vascular nasal mucosa gives a high intensity signal on T2 weighted sequences, which may allow discrimination between nasal mucosa and the less intense signal from tumour. On the other hand when T1 weighted sequences are used the intensities are very similar, and tumour differentiation difficult. Inflamed or oedematous sinus mucosa also produces a signal of high intensity on T2 weighted sequences and may be distinguished from tumour in a like manner. The distinction is especially apparent on heavily weighted T2 images, using a long time to echo and repetition time.

In summary it can be said that mucocoeles, retained secretion and inflamed mucosa give a stronger signal on T2 weighted spin echo sequences than do tumours. In addition examples of dense fibrous tissue in association with paranasal sinus disease may show entirely different magnetic resonance features, characterized by low signal on T2 weighted sequences.

Effects of gadolinium DTPA

Intravenous injection of the paramagnetic contrast agent gadolinium DTPA has effects on the magnetic resonance characteristics of both tumours and normal or inflammatory tissue in the nose and sinuses. As described above, the majority of tumours show high or moderately high signal on T2 weighted sequences. Without the use of contrast, tumours are best shown by this technique and best differentiated from retained secretion or inflamed mucosa. After intravenous gadolinium, naso-sinus tumours show signal enhancement depending upon their vascularity and this may vary from zero to high intensity. Post-contrast T1 weighted series, especially the inversion recovery mode, have been shown to be the best method of tumour demonstration, and are superior to pre-contrast T2 weighted sequences in differentiating tumour from retained secretion and from inflammatory mucosal thickening. Retained secretion does not enhance after contrast, which helps to make differentiation between tumour and fluid in the sinuses more obvious than it is on pre-contrast scans. This also applies to secondary mucocoele formation and to sinuses in which there is inflammatory mucosal thickening and fluid. The high intensity enhancement of the nasal and sinus mucosa is clearly outlined against the non-enhancing fluid.

Gadolinium DTPA pools in the highly vascular capillary bed of the nasal mucosa. This produces a high intensity signal on magnetic resonance scans, and needs to be distinguished from enhancing tumour, which can be difficult if signal intensities are similar. However non-enhancing tumours may be outlined against high signal from the nasal mucosa and from inflammatory mucosal thickening in the sinuses (Fig. 3.6). A totally opaque sinus may be revealed as containing thickened mucosa and fluid rather than tumour. Alternatively all three may be demonstrated in the same sinus cavity.

In the nose and sinuses, tumour tissue can be recognized by its heterogeneous signal; thickened mucosa, polyps and retained secretion present homogeneous signal with or without contrast enhancement. Tumours normally have some degree of signal heterogeneity and this is increased after intravenous gadolinium DTPA, especially on T1 inversion recovery sequences which are most affected by the contrast agent. Differential enhancement of tumour signal is a feature of the post-contrast scans and probably results from areas of varying vascularity in the neoplasm.

Fat suppression and subtraction studies
(Figs 3.7 and 3.8)

The effect of gadolinium is to decrease the T1 and T2 relaxation times of water protons, producing high signal on T1 weighted images and converting the MR signal

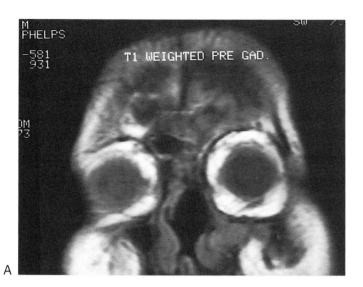

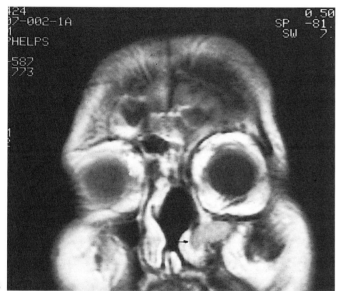

Fig. 3.6   T1 weighted spin echo MR scan showing, **A**, no discrimination between tumour (inverted papilloma) and the mucosa of the inferior meatus (left). **B**, same sequence after intravenous gadolinium to allow discrimination between strong enhancement of nasal mucosa and less strong enhancement of tumour (arrow).

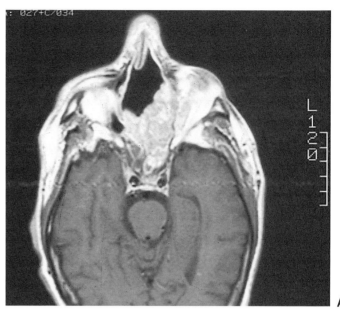

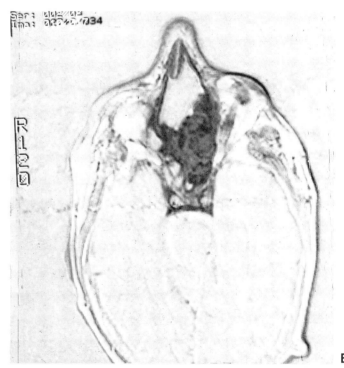

Fig. 3.7   Post-gadolinium section, **A**, pre-subtraction axial MR section showing a recurrent squamous cell carcinoma after cranio-facial surgery. **B**, same section after subtraction: the recurrent sinus tumour is invading the cavernous sinus, which also enhances with the gadolinium.

characteristics of vascular tissue into those closely resembling normal fat. On post gadolinium scans it may then become difficult to dissociate tumour from adjacent fat. Various fat suppression methods have been devised to overcome this problem. A partial solution has been to use STIR (Short Tau Inversion Recovery) sequences which do not record a fat signal. One drawback of this method is that these sequences also suppress signal from gadolinium-enhanced tissue resulting in diminished image contrast. Other methods of fat suppression include chemical shift imaging and a pre-saturation technique. However subtraction is the simplest method. It can be

applied to any MR scanner and does not require any additional sequences to those normally used.

Subtraction GdMR

In this technique the subtraction method used in angiography is applied to magnetic resonance imaging.

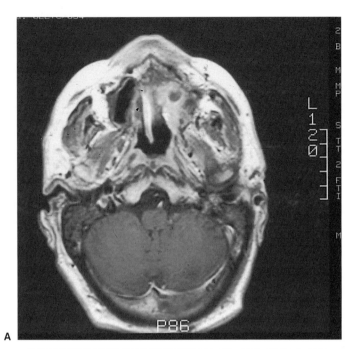

A

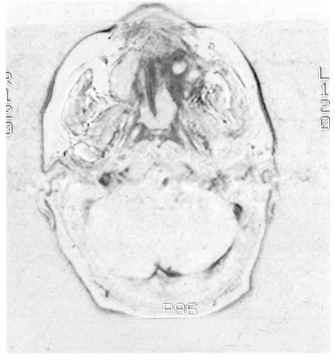

B

Fig. 3.8 Sections from the same patient as Figure 3.7. **A**, post-gadolinium axial section showing skull base. **B**, subtraction made from the section shown in Figure 3.8A demonstrates tumour in the nasopharynx which is invading the Eustachian tube on both sides (arrows). This was not recognized on the unsubtracted images. Biopsy of tissue from the middle ear on both sides was shown to be positive for squamous cell carcinoma.

Essentially pre-contrast T1 weighted images are subtracted from identical scans made after the injection of gadolinium DTPA. In this process the NMR signal is completely removed from the final image so that the den-

sities recorded are dependent only on the vascularity of the tissue concerned. Since adipose tissue has a low vascularity, the fat signal is effectively suppressed in addition to all other non-enhancing structures displayed on the control image. Subtraction has been found most advantageous in situations where the anatomy is complex as at the skull base or in tumour recurrence where normal structures are distorted by previous surgery. It provides a more accurate record of tumour extent than that shown on unsubtracted GdMR scans.

ULTRASOUND

The diagnostic use of ultrasound in the paranasal sinuses has been limited to the detection of fluid in the frontal sinus and maxillary antrum. The first clinical series on the reliability of ultrasonography in the diagnosis of maxillary sinusitis, confirmed by puncture and irrigation, was published by Mann et al,[3] and in 1980 Revonta published an extensive account of the use of ultrasound in the detection of retained secretion in both the maxillary, antra and frontal sinuses.[4] This author's series indicated that ultrasound was in many instances superior to simple radiography in the detection of fluid in these sinuses. Most authors have used the A-scan mode for sinus diagnosis or a modification of this.[5] The A-scan is produced by generating an ultrasonic impulse which is channelled via a transducer through the skin overlying the frontal or maxillary sinus. Air in the sinus reflects the high frequency ultrasound totally and only echoes from the anterior wall are recorded. If secretion is present, ultrasound is transmitted to the posterior bony wall and reflected to the probe, producing a back wall echo after an echo-free zone. These are the signs of retained secretion.

The technique is used on an out-patient basis for screening for the presence of retained secretion: it has little or no application for the demonstration of neoplasia in the upper jaw.

ANGIOGRAPHY AND EMBOLIZATION TECHNIQUES

With the introduction of CT and magnetic resonance imaging angiography is no longer needed diagnostically for tumours of the upper jaw. Its principal use is to monitor embolization procedures, designed to render abnormal tissue ischaemic while maintaining the blood supply to normal structures. It may also be required to deliver chemotherapeutic agents or radioactive microspheres to tumour tissue. For successful embolization the best angiographic facilities are essential with good image intensification and two-plane screening. Digital vascular imaging is an advantage because of the immediate availability of subtraction techniques.

Indications

Embolization may be used as the treatment for selected arteriovenous fistulae, aneurysms and angiomatous malformations, and as an adjunct to surgery for the same conditions. It is also used prior to surgery to reduce the vascularity of hypervascular tumours such as juvenile angiofibroma or meningioma. Other indications include angiomas involving superficial tissues, in which the cosmetic effects of surgery are unlikely to be satisfactory; the palliation of tumours which are inoperable because of their position or nature; and intractable epistaxis.

The initial use of autologous materials such as blood clot, muscle or fat for embolization has been superseded by the injection of foreign substances. These should be non-toxic, non-antigenic and capable of being delivered through a percutaneous catheter. They are divided into solids and liquids. Solids may be injected as particles, coils or as balloons and used to control large arteriovenous fistulae. The first group includes some materials which are relatively quickly absorbed, such as haemostatic gelatin foam. The thrombus induced is associated with little damage to the arterial walls so that this material is excellent for the treatment of haemorrhage in which temporary thrombosis can be life-saving. Some other materials cause more permanent occlusion such as lyophilized dura or polyvinyl alcohol sponge (Ivalon). These substances remain indefinitely within the tissue and produce endothelial damage and thrombosis, which becomes organized and fibrosed. This results in prolonged occlusion of the lumen of the vessels containing emboli.

Liquid embolic materials which solidify on exposure to blood or electrolyte solutions are either silicones, which are used to maintain distension of detachable balloons, or acrylics. The latter have the advantage of potential penetration throughout the abnormal vasculature, causing immediate thrombosis and intimal necrosis followed by organization and fibrosis and a granulomatous arteritis, resulting in permanent occlusion.

Complications of embolization include all the dangers of selective angiography plus those specific to embolization. Aberrant embolization is particularly dangerous when it involves brain tissue and can be caused by reflux of emboli into a cerebral vessel or through an anastomosis between a vessel to the brain and one being embolized. Paralysis of cranial nerves may occur in external carotid embolization especially when acrylic is used, and ischaemia of normal tissues may cause swelling, trismus due to emboli in the muscles of mastication, facial atrophy and tissue necrosis; the last is particularly likely to occur in the tip of the tongue in bilateral lingual embolization and in the ear from emboli in the anterior auricular artery.

Diagnostic approach

The radiological investigation of the upper jaw and paranasal sinuses begins with plain X-ray films. In the first instance these will serve to confirm or eliminate simple allergic or inflammatory disease as the cause of the patient's symptoms; and if the appearances are consistent with this no further investigation is usually necessary. If on the other hand the evidence of plain X-rays indicates an expanding or destructive lesion of the sinus walls or a tumour mass and the clinical findings support the diagnosis of tumour, a more sophisticated technique of investigation is indicated, such as CT or MR. Plain X-rays should never be neglected since both the presence of a lesion and its likely nature are diagnosable in the majority of patients by this simple and inexpensive method. In a series of patients reviewed by Lloyd with upper jaw and sinus pathology, 94% were correctly diagnosed by straight films aided where necessary by conventional tomography.[6] A further advantage of plain radiography is the negligible radiation dose incurred in comparison with two plane CT imaging.

At this stage, in most cases, biopsy will confirm the type of lesion present and establish the histology. The role of CT and MR is then to determine the exact extent and distribution of the neoplasm prior to treatment by surgery or radiotherapy. There are several advantages of MR over CT. The three plane multislice facility using a head coil gives total coverage of the head and neck so that both the primary tumour and any direct or metastatic cervical involvement may be recognized. MR is also superior in terms of tissue recognition. Where CT simply computes voxel attenuation as Hounsfield numbers, several parameters are available by MR: these include proton density imaging, T1 and T2 weighted images and flow studies using the field even echo rephasing technique (FEER) to outline the vasculature. The most important recent advance has been the introduction of the paramagnetic contrast medium, gadolinium DTPA which provides the best means of identifying tumour from inflammatory changes in the upper jaw and sinuses, as well as distinguishing tumour from oedema when the anterior or middle cranial fossa is invaded. Subtraction studies are of most use for showing tumour recurrence especially when the skull base is involved.

Due to the presence of a strong static magnetic field, MR scanning is contraindicated in the presence of metal cardiac pacemakers, aneurysm clips or cochlear implants. Claustrophobia is also a bigger problem in MR than CT; and in a series recorded by Lloyd et al. this accounted for a 4% failure rate.[7] This problem is likely to be overcome in the future by improved technology and design. Faster data acquisition times will also largely obviate motion artefacts resulting from the long scanning times of the early MR machines.

Absence of NMR signal from dense cortical bone and calcium remains the principal disadvantage of magnetic resonance imaging. For the demonstration of bone destruction in upper jaw lesions, conventional tomography was the method of choice before the introduction of CT. CT has the advantage of showing both bone destruction and the soft tissue extent of the tumour. This is particularly important in certain anatomical situations, e.g. in the pterygopalatine fossa, where knowledge of tumour involvement is crucial in terms of operability and prognosis; or again in the cribriform plate area where early bone erosion is an important indication for craniofacial surgery.

Thus the final evaluation is best provided by a combination of GdMR and high resolution CT.

REFERENCES

1. Lloyd G A S 1975 Radiology of the orbit. WB Saunders, London.
2. Lloyd G A S 1979 CT scanning in the diagnosis of orbital disease. Computerised Tomography 3: 247–259
3. Mann W, Beck C, Apostolidis T 1977 Liability of ultrasound in maxillary sinus disease. Archives of Otorhinolaryngology 215: 67–74
4. Revonta M 1980 Ultrasound in the diagnosis of maxillary and frontal sinusitis. Acta Oto-Laryngologica. (Suppl.) 370: 1–54
5. Revonta M 1982 Diagnosis and follow-up of ultrasonographic sinus changes in children. International Journal of Paediatric Otolaryngology 4: 301–308
6. Lloyd G A S 1970 The radiological investigation of proptosis. British Journal of Radiology 43: 1–21
7. Lloyd G A S, Lund V J, Phelps P D, Howard D J 1987 Magnetic resonance imaging in the evaluation of nose and paranasal sinus disease. British Journal of Radiology 60: 957–968

4. Conditions simulating neoplasia

A number of benign conditions which may be mistaken for neoplasia can affect the nose and paranasal sinuses. Some such as mucocoeles and nasal polyps can co-exist with genuine tumours, which may in fact have contributed to their development by obstructing a sinus or producing oedematous change in the adjacent mucous membrane. Because of this, and the range of presentation of neoplasia in this region, we should never be complacent about such apparently benign conditions, until they have been fully investigated. The benign conditions considered are:

1. Cholesterol granuloma
2. Mucocoeles
3. Nasal polyps
4. Fungal infections.

CHOLESTEROL GRANULOMA

Definition and aetiology

This condition is characterized by a foreign body reaction to the presence of cholesterol. Cholesterol is a component of bile acids and steroid hormones. It is found in cell membranes, including erythrocytes, in human high density lipoprotein and also in free form. It is relatively insoluble and can be precipitated in crystalline form when it provokes a significant foreign body reaction. Three main conditions seem necessary for the formation of a cholesterol granuloma: disturbed ventilation, impaired drainage and haemorrhage.[1] Thus trauma or haemorrhage associated with inflammation within a closed cavity which has poor lymphatics provides such conditions.

A number of workers have attempted to induce the condition experimentally.[2-5] Hiraide et al[4] produced extensive subepithelial haemorrhages in the middle ear of monkeys by prolonged obstruction of the Eustachian tube. However, transudate, degenerating tissue or cell breakdown, and even in situ synthesis have also been suggested as possible sources of the cholesterol.[3,5-9]

Incidence

Given the above, it is surprising that this condition is not more common in the middle ear and paranasal sinuses. However, it is relatively rare, with less than 20 cases affecting the sinuses being reported in the literature.[1,10-15]

Age, sex variation

In our own nine cases, the ages ranged from 27–56 years, mean 38 years and there was a male preponderance of 7:2.

Site

In the head and neck, cholesterol granuloma is more commonly encountered in the middle ear and mastoid[6,9,16,17] than in the paranasal sinuses. The maxillary antrum is the sinus most often affected though occasionally the frontal sinus and ethmoids are the primary site or are encroached upon by a lesion arising in the orbit. This is in contradistinction to the distribution of mucocoeles (p. 54).

Clinical features

The patient may present with the usual symptoms of chronic rhinosinusitis, with nasal obstruction, postnasal discharge and facial pain. An expansive mass in the sinus will cause cosmetic deformity and may displace the globe, raising the suspicion of neoplasia. Duration of symptoms may vary from 3 months to 10 years, with a mean of 2.75 years in our series. In five of the nine cases, a history of previous sinus surgery was elicited.

Radiology

Radiologically the appearance fall into two main groups. The first is that of a non-specific inflammatory sinusitis, the second more characteristic finding is of a cyst-like expansion with thinning or complete erosion of the sinus walls.[18] On CT the opacification is of the same density as brain and does not enhance with contrast.[19-21] However on MRI the lesion is characterized by a very high signal on all sequences, T1 spin echo and inversion recovery and T2 spin echo (Fig. 4.1).[22a]

Macroscopic and microscopic appearance

The lesion produces a 'blue' mass lying submucosally which is composed of granulation tissue containing haemosiderin and a marked foreign body reaction. The typical morphological picture shows giant cells arranged around clefts created by the cholesterol crystals which after fixation appear as empty needle-shaped spaces.

Differential diagnosis

The lesion on presentation may have many of the features of neoplasia. In addition it must be distinguished from the variety of cysts (dental, mucous-retention, etc.) which occur in this region and from a mucocoele.

Treatment and prognosis

The need to exclude malignancy often results in biopsy though modern imaging will frequently indicate the diagnosis. Similarly the finding of shimmering amber fluid on antral washout should alert the clinician to this diagnosis. Removal of the diseased mucosa has usually been effected via a Caldwell–Luc approach to the antrum or via an external approach to the fronto-ethmoidal region and normally results in cure.

MUCOCOELES

Definition and aetiology

A mucocoele is an epithelial-lined, mucus-containing sac completely filling the sinus and capable of expansion.[23] This is in contradistinction to a sinus cavity which simply contains mucus. In the fronto-ethmoidal region it may be exclusively confined to either the frontal sinus or a single ethmoidal cell but often involves the horizontal compartment of the frontal sinus which developmentally originates from the anterior ethmoids. Rarely mucocoeles occur in the maxillary or sphenoid sinus.

Historical aspects

It has been suggested that the first description of a pyocoele dates from 1524 and relates to Francis I, King of France.[24] In the medical literature, Lagenbeck described a 'hydatid' affecting the sinuses in 1819[25] and the term 'mucocoele' was coined by Rollet in 1896.[26] In 1907 Turner distinguished frontal and ethmoidal lesions

and discussed possible aetiology.[27] Howarth gave the first comprehensive description of the condition in his Hunterian lecture of 1921[28] and the first report of radiological features came in 1926.[29]

Incidence

Mucocoeles are uncommon as judged by available series (Table 4.1).[23,30-36] A series of 118 cases have been treated at the Royal National Throat, Nose and Ear Hospital

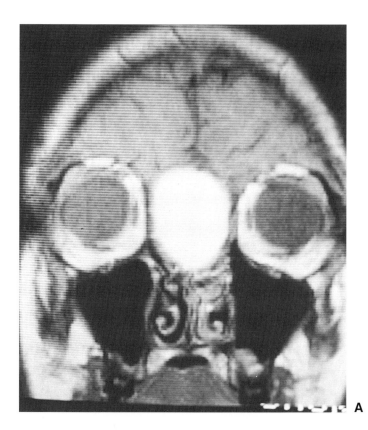

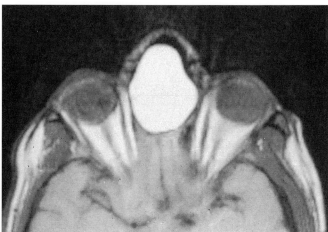

Fig. 4.1 Cholesterol granuloma. **A**, coronal and **B**, axial T1 weighted MR scans showing high signal from large central cystic lesion (Lloyd 1988[22]).

Table 4.1 Mucocoeles: review of major series

Author	No.	Patients Male	Female	Age Range	Fronto–Ethmoid	Ethmoid	Site (%) Maxilla	Sphenoid	Treatment (No.)	Follow-up	Recurrence (%)
Zizmour & Noyek 1968[36]	100	–	–	–	64	30	5	1	–	–	–
Bordley & Bosley 1973[30]	56	32	24	14–68	100	–	–	–	Drainage (1) Lynch–Howarth (6) Osteoplastic flap (28) Radical sinusectomy (21)	– –	30: Lynch–Howarth 21: Osteoplastic flap
Canalis et al 1978[31]	20	11	9	9–74	–	100	–	–	Lynch–Howarth (20)	2–7 yr mean 3.3 yr	20
Natvig & Larsen 1978[23]	112	55	57	10–70	91	6	3	–	Lynch–Howarth (60)	3–29 yr mean 11 yr	18
Hu & Lin 1982[34]	77	41	36	9–72	100	–	–	–	Lynch–Howarth Endonasal	–	–
Kennedy et al 1989[76]	18	10	8	10–76	61	28	11		Endoscopic marsupialization	2–42 mth mean 18 mth	0
Harrison & Lund	118	74	44	10–87 mean 53 yr	92	6	1	1	Lynch–Howarth (118)	mean 3.3 yr	7

during the last 27 years, the majority referred by Moorfields Eye Hospital.

Age, sex and ethnic variation (Table 4.1)

The majority of mucocoeles occur between 40 and 70 years but they have been reported from 23 months to 79 years.[37] There is a slight male preponderance overall. Wolfowitz & Solomon[35] have suggested that the condition is more common in the black population of South Africa but this is based on only 12 cases and no other ethnic differentiation is present in the literature. The Japanese have an apparently high incidence of postoperative maxillary mucocoeles though it is difficult to be sure that these constitute the same lesion as that encountered elsewhere.[38]

Site (Table 4.1)

The vast majority of cases occur in the fronto-ethmoidal complex with a smaller number exclusively affecting the ethmoidal region. The anterior ethmoid cells are most frequently affected (5:1),[22b] mirroring the distribution of chronic inflammation in this region.[39] The maxillary sinus is rarely affected and the sphenoid even less so though reports of these cases more often appear in the neurosurgical literature.[40–43]

The right and left sides are equally affected but the incidence of bilateral mucocoeles is less than 4% in our series (Fig. 4.2).

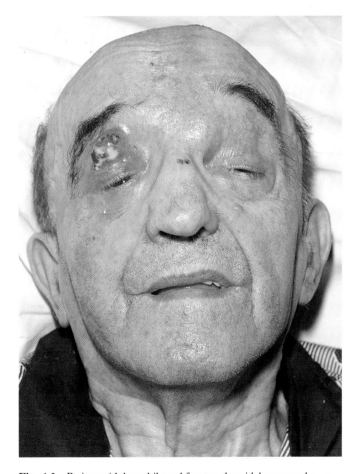

Fig. 4.2 Patient with large bilateral fronto-ethmoidal mucocoeles, an associated discharging fistula and Paget's disease of the skull.

Aetiology

The surgical anatomy of this area, and in particular the fronto-ethmoidal region is one of considerable variation (p. 21–22, 26–28, 29–30) which is reflected in the relative frequency with which mucocoeles are encountered in the different paranasal sinuses. Although alternative drainage pathways from the frontal sinus exist in some patients[44] they may be of little significance if normal mucociliary patterns are in operation.

The formation of a mucocoele has been attributed in the past to a combination of obstruction of sinus drainage, i.e. into the frontonasal recess, and inflammation. It is probable that many patients develop a mucus-filled sinus associated with obstruction but only a small number go on to develop a true mucocoele characterized by expansion and remodelling of the sinus. Experimental studies using animal models have been largely inconclusive. Schenck et al[45] were unable to produce a mucocoele by simple obstruction of the frontonasal duct in dogs but found a mucus-containing cyst partially filling the sinus when mucoperiosteum was stripped in addition to obstruction though they did not believe that this constituted a true mucocoele.

When aetiological factors have been considered in the literature, polyps, trauma, surgery and tumours comprise the obstructive group, infection, increased mucus secretion, cystic degeneration and allergy the inflammatory group.[28,30,31,46–52] However, a paucity of numbers has prevented any close analysis of these factors and if no aetiological factor is obvious, this is usually ignored. In addition one must consider why every patient who experiences midfacial trauma, has nasal polyps, sinus surgery or chronic sinusitis does not develop a mucocoele and why, despite conditions which often affect more than one sinus, patients rarely develop bilateral mucocoeles.

Our own series of 118 patients with fronto-ethmoidal mucocoeles were examined for relevant aetiological factors and to determine the time intervals between these factors and presentation with the mucocoele (Table 4.2). These factors included direct serious trauma involving fracture of facial bones, nasal polyps untreated or removed surgically, frontal sinusitis treated medically or surgically, a miscellaneous group which included benign tumours such as osteomas, schwannomas, inverted papilloma, Paget's disease (Fig. 4.3) and a further group in whom no aetiological factor could be determined.[44] The polyps had been removed intranasally whereas surgical treatment of frontal sinusitis was in all cases by external fronto-ethmoidectomy.

Whilst aetiological factors could be defined in 64%, the largest single group (36%) had no known cause, co-incident with the findings of other authors.[23] When the time interval between the aetiological factor and clinical presentation was considered, it was significantly longer in

Table 4.2 Fronto-ethmoidal mucocoeles: aetiological factors

	None	Trauma	POLYPS No surgery	POLYPS Surgery	INFECTION Antibiotics	INFECTION Surgery	OTHER
Number	45	13	12	14	9	16	9
%	36	11	10	11	8	14	8
Male (%)	60	54	66	71	55	50	55
Female (%)	40	46	34	29	45	50	45
Age range	10–87	20–68	37–70	46–70	18–63	24–80	27–83
Average age	56	47	52	50	42	60	54
Time interval (yr)	–	8–48	–	0.25–30	0.17–8	10–60	3–15
Average time (yr)	–	21	–	11.8	1.8	28	10

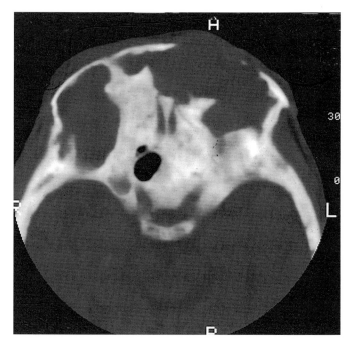

Fig. 4.3   Axial CT scan of patient in Figure 4.2 showing bilateral mucocoeles and Paget's disease.

those in whom trauma or surgery for infection or polyps occurred when compared with the group in whom infection had been treated conservatively with antibiotics (p<0.001 in all cases). This suggests that the latter represents a sterile pyocoele. If no aetiological factor can be defined, it is likely that one is dealing with a vulnerable population in whom there is a degree of narrowing in the sinus outflow, with total obstruction produced by minor sub-clinical change.

Development of the mucocoele appears dependent upon the degree and duration of obstruction and the absence of alternative drainage routes but bone resorption and expansion requires superadded inflammation probably initiated by infection. Histological examination (p. 60) confirms the presence of chronic inflammation, fibrosis and suggests a dynamic balance at the muco-coele/bone interface where osteoclast and osteoblast activity results in osteolysis, new bone formation and sclerosis. In the case of the mucocoele this balance is just tipped in favour of expansion.

This local bone destruction, remodelling and expansion is similar to that observed in odontogenic cysts[53] where previous work[54,55] suggests that most of the bone-resorbing activity is accounted for by prostaglandins, the major one being PGE_2. Work on odontogenic cysts did not allow any comparison with normal tissue but it has been possible to compare fronto-ethmoidal mucocoele lining with that of 'normal' frontal sinuses encountered during craniotomy procedures for non-infective conditions.

These studies show that the lining of the mucocoele is capable of producing bone-resorbing factors, most notably PGE_2 and collagenase,[56] in significantly higher amounts than those present in normal frontal sinus mucosa. Culture of the fronto-ethmoidal mucosa and lining fibroblasts synthesizes PGE_2 so it appears likely that fibroblasts are the primary source of prostaglandins. The products of peripheral blood mononuclear leucocytes can affect the growth and behaviour of fibroblasts. Fibroblasts derived from rheumatoid synovial membrane[57] and from inflamed human gingiva[58] are stimulated to synthesize large quantities of prostaglandins, mainly PGE_2, and collagenase by mononuclear cell factor (MCF) which is probably identical to lymphocyte-activating factor (interleukin 1).[59] Fibroblasts derived from the lining mucosa in these experiments were responsive to mononuclear cell products. The production of this factor by unstimulated mononuclear cell cultures and its enhancement by addition of the mitogen PHA indicate that it may be MCF to which the lining fibroblasts responded.

On the basis of these results and by analogy with the behaviour of connective tissue cells in dental cysts, a sequence of events in the pathogenesis of the fronto-ethmoidal mucocoele may be postulated. Following obstruction of the frontonasal recess by overt or covert causes and in the absence of alternative pathways, a superadded infection leads to chronic inflammation mediated by bacterial antigens. Continued stimulation of lymphocytes and monocytes leads to the production of soluble factors inducing cytokines (such as interleukin 1) which enhance prostaglandin and collagenase synthesis by fibroblasts in the lining mucosa. These bone-resorbing factors in turn stimulate osteoclast and monocyte-mediated bone resorption and so accommodate mucocoele expansion. Studies are underway to elucidate this process further and compare it with the situation in acute and chronic sinusitis but it is interesting to note that positive microbiology can be obtained from ostensibly 'sterile' mucocoeles. Preliminary studies confirm high levels of IL1 and TNF (tumour necrosis factor) in mucocoele lining compared with chronically inflamed mucosa.

A large number of maxillary sinus mucocoeles have been reported in Japan associated almost exclusively with previous radical sinus surgery (Caldwell–Luc) performed for chronic sinus problems 16–19 years previously.[38] The antrostomy was blocked in all cases but the authors also concluded that other factors contributed to the pathogenesis of the mucocoele and it would appear that some cases are simple retention cysts. Som & Shugar[60] suggested that postoperative adhesions were responsible and this was supported by the lateral position of the antral mucocoeles reported in their series, but again it does not explain the continued expansion of the lesion.

Clinical features

Expansion of a fronto-ethmoidal mucocoele occurs in the direction of least resistance through the floor of the orbit and lamina papyracea so that the majority of patients present initially to an ophthalmic surgeon as the condition is one of the most common causes of unilateral proptosis.[61] The majority of patients (91%) exhibit some degree of proptosis though this can range from 1–17 mm (Fig. 4.4). 55% also demonstrate a degree of lateral displacement (2–13 mm, mean 6 mm) and 59% inferior displacement (1–10 mm, mean 4 mm) though this is obviously dependent on the relative frontal and ethmoidal involvement.[62]

95% experience diplopia though this is often minimal in a condition which is slowly progressive. The diplopia is vertical in nature and principally presents in upward gaze and at the extremes of lateral gaze. Ocular mobility is limited in 55% in an upward direction by the presence of the sac which can often be felt in the upper medial quadrant of the orbit, sometimes with a characteristic 'egg-shell' crackling sensation on palpation. An intermittently discharging fistula is sometimes present (4%) (Fig. 4.2). Visual acuity is occasionally reduced and there have been several reports of visual loss in association with infection of the mucocoele.[63,64] The speed of development of all of these symptoms will be significantly increased by additional infection and such pyocoeles will obviously pose a considerable risk to vision.

Mucocoeles confined to the anterior ethmoids usually present with a mass at the medial canthus, producing proptosis and displacement laterally rather than inferiorly. Epiphora can occur if the lacrimal drainage system is compressed.

Due to the proximity of the sphenoid to the optic nerve and cavernous sinus, spheno-ethmoidal mucocoeles present with frontal or retro-orbital headache, facial pain

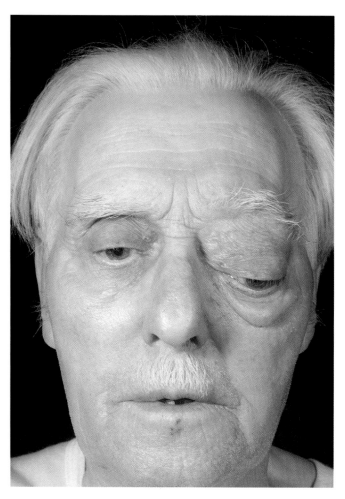

Fig. 4.4 Patient with typical displacement of the globe due to a fronto-ethmoidal mucocoele.

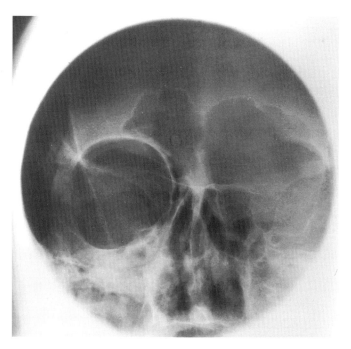

Fig. 4.5 Plain sinus X-ray (occipito-frontal view) of patient in Figure 4.4 showing classical appearances of a fronto-ethmoidal mucocoele; erosion of the supero-medial orbital margin, loss of scalloped frontal sinus margin and sinus opacification.

and orbital symptoms such as diplopia, proptosis, ophthalmoplegia and in more extreme cases visual loss (sphenoid fissure syndrome). Intracranial extension leads to severe complications such as meningitis and raised intracranial pressure.[42,43,52,61,65]

Expansion of a maxillary mucocoele leads to upward displacement of the orbital floor leading to displacement of the globe, diplopia and epiphora, obstruction of the nasal cavity, swelling, numbness of the cheek and dental disturbance.[33] Antral mucocoeles can attain a considerable size if neglected.[66]

Radiology[22b]

In the fronto-ethmoidal region, the classical appearances of an expanded frontal sinus showing loss of the scalloped margin and an overall loss of translucence on the affected side can be seen in the majority of plain sinus X-rays (Fig. 4.5). In addition to osteolysis, a zone of sclerosis at the margin may be seen in some cases[67] and macroscopic

calcification on X-ray has been reported in 5% reflecting the presence of new bone formation.[36]

Other features including depression or erosion of the supra-orbital ridge and extension across the midline to the opposite frontal sinus (shown as a soft tissue bulge) are usually apparent. Loss of the scalloped margin of the sinus walls occurs when the main vertical portion of the frontal sinus is involved, but will not be seen on plain sinus X-ray when only the horizontal part of the fronto-ethmoidal complex is affected. This section of the frontal sinus is either principally or solely affected in 25% of cases. However, computerized tomography is usually employed and more than adequately displays the many possible variations (Fig. 4.6).[68,69] Diagnosis is dependent upon the recognition of the classical findings rather than on the attenuation values of its contents. Although bone erosion may be present, large scale bone destruction is not a feature. CT with intravenous contrast characteristically shows ring enhancement in the presence of a pyocoele.

On magnetic resonance imaging, mucocoeles present a high signal on T2 weighted spin echo sequences and a very low signal on inversion recovery due to a long T1 relaxation time (Fig. 4.7). However, if there has been any haemorrhage, either spontaneous or associated with previous attempts at drainage, a signal of mixed intensity is produced with some loculi producing high signals both on inversion recovery and T1 and T2 weighted spin echo

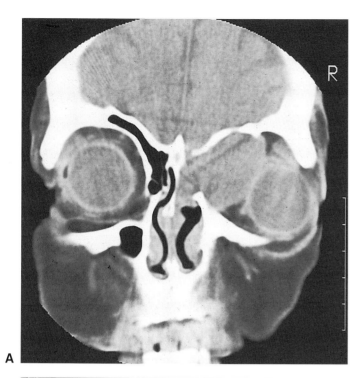

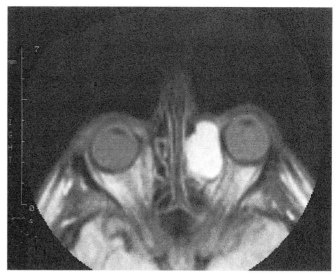

Fig. 4.7 Axial MR scan of anterior ethmoidal mucocoele giving a strong signal on T2 weighted spin echo sequence (Lloyd 1988[22]).

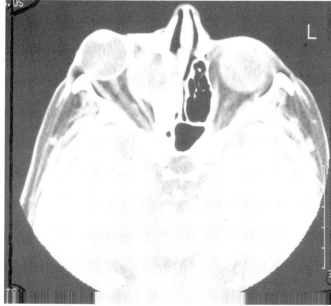

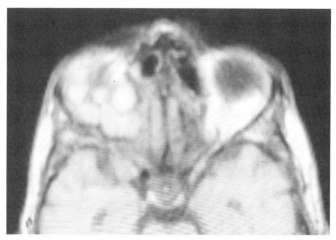

Fig. 4.8 Axial MR scan showing high signal on T1 weighted sequence from loculi of a frontal mucocoele which contained altered blood (Lloyd 1988[22]).

Fig. 4.6 Right fronto-ethmoidal mucocoele. **A**, coronal CT scan; **B**, axial CT scan of same.

sequences. This may be due to the presence of altered blood products such as methaemoglobin which act as paramagnetic agents (Fig. 4.8).[70] Shortening of the T1 relaxation time is due to water absorption in more mature mucocoeles.[71]

Radiologically, ethmoidal mucocoeles are often quite difficult to diagnose on plain X-rays. Occasionally a dacrocystogram shows compression of the nasolacrimal region but ordinarily CT or axial MRI demonstrate the lesion optimally.[72]

In the sphenoid region, initial opacification is followed by expansion of the cavity with elevation or erosion of the floor of the pituitary fossa. This may be seen on lateral plain sinus X-ray and may disappear following drainage of the mucocoele. The sphenoid mucocoele frequently spreads into the posterior ethmoidal cells with erosion of the medial wall of the optic canal. CT scanning is usually employed and may show a diagnostic feature of multiple cyst-like expansions.[73]

In the maxilla an opaque and expanded sinus encroaches on the ethmoids and nasal cavity.[60] An intact bony rim suggests a benign lesion which must be distinguished from slow-growing neoplasms (Fig. 4.9).

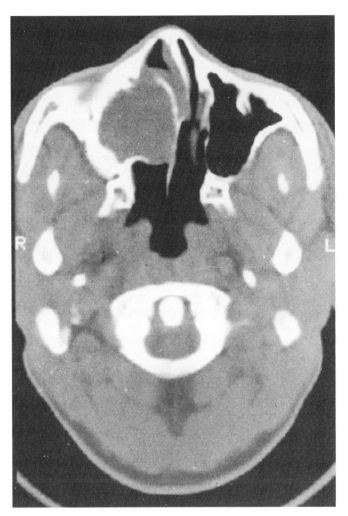

Fig. 4.9 Axial CT scan showing a maxillary mucocoele.

Macroscopic and microscopic appearance

A recent detailed histological analysis showed that all fronto-ethmoidal mucocoeles are lined with pseudo-stratified columnar epithelium though a proportion (37.5%) show additional squamous metaplasia.[74] Goblet cells are present in two-thirds of specimens, frequently showing hyperplasia though there is no increase in the number of seromucinous glands. A degree of chronic inflammation is present in all specimens though this varies in degree and the number of neutrophils is significantly increased if the patient presents with an acute episode. Fibroblast numbers are also increased, irrespective of duration of symptoms as is the vascularity of the submucosa. Woven and lamellar bone is frequently seen as are osteoblasts and osteoclasts; evidence of the dynamic process of erosion, expansion and remodelling that occurs at the muco-coele/bone interface.

These findings are completely at variance with the proposed theory of pressure erosion, which would result in an atrophic lining, and further support a dynamic concept of pathogenesis. Furthermore there is no evidence to support an origin from cystic degeneration of a seromucinous gland. Retention cysts are commonest in the maxilla[75] where mucocoeles are least often found and in none of our cases has a cyst been found almost filling the sinus or a double epithelial lining seen histologically. The sinus mucoperiosteum always appears to constitute the muco-coele lining.

Differential diagnosis

Any condition causing opacification and expansion of the sinuses may be confused with a mucocoele and may also occur synchronously with the condition. Thus acute and chronic infection, polyps including antro-choanal, dental cysts, dermoids, and cholesterol granuloma should be considered. Small mucous retention cysts and pseudo-cysts are frequently found in the floor of the maxillary sinus.[75] They are asymptomatic and do not evolve into true mucocoeles. Osteomyelitis can produce some of the radiological features of mucocoeles though it is not associated with expansion. However, some benign and slow-growing malignant neoplasms (osteoma, schwannoma, inverted papilloma and transitional cell carcinoma) may simulate such change and can also occur concomitantly. This is in contradistinction to the fluid which is often found in sinuses blocked by tumour.

In the sphenoid region any other space-occupying mass must be distinguished, such as pituitary and nasopharyngeal tumours.

Treatment and prognosis

The majority of patients in our series have undergone a modified Lynch–Howarth approach and radical fronto-ethmoidectomy. In the past all the lining mucosa was removed except where erosion of bone has exposed dura and the intersinus septum was widely opened to confirm the presence of a normal contralateral sinus and provide an alternative drainage channel, albeit by gravity.

92% had a large fenestrated (1 cm diameter) silastic tube inserted from the frontal sinus to the nasal cavity. The size is such that it remains wedged in position until removed at a later date in the outpatient department. The tube can occasionally cause some discomfort necessitating early removal but the majority of patients tolerated it for an average of 5 months.

In the immediate postoperative period, it can be anticipated that many patients will experience an increase in diplopia associated with the sudden decompression but this usually settles within a few days or weeks. Disturbance of the trochlea can lead to persistent diplopia due to superior oblique underaction so care should be taken in reattaching the orbital periosteum in this region with a permanent suture.[62] Persistent displacement of the globe presages residual or recurrent problems.

Other postoperative complications are few, including wound infection (1%), CSF leak (1%), frontal sinusitis managed conservatively by antibiotics (11%) and mucocoele recurrence requiring surgery in 7%. 83% have been cured with no further problems. Cosmetic results from the operation were good. Only 4% were troubled by the appearance of the scar and one patient (1%) developed a transitory fistula in the scar associated with infection. When the 11 patients (11%) who did not have a silastic tube inserted are examined, it is apparent that the majority of the recurrences occurred within this group. However, there was not a significantly increased incidence of infection or other postoperative complications.

Nevertheless, the opening created by such a tube is not a 'physiological' one and other means of maintaining the patency of the frontonasal recess may be considered. An endoscopic approach to the problem has been enthusiastically supported[76] but as yet the numbers and length of follow-up are limited (Table 4.3). The frontonasal recess can be a particularly difficult area to visualize and operate in, and not all cases will be amenable to this technique. Furthermore the cosmetic problems of globe displacement may take longer to resolve whilst remodelling of bone occurs though conversely diplopia is less likely to be exacerbated. If regular long-term follow-up is possible, it is worth employing an endoscopic approach which is certainly of value in ethmoidal, sphenoidal and most maxillary mucocoeles. An alternative compromise would be to combine external and endoscopic surgery for fronto-ethmoidal lesions, thus avoiding the silastic tube, and checking long-term patency of the frontonasal recess by regular endoscopic examination.

The Lynch–Howarth fronto-ethmoidectomy can be compared with the alternative operation of osteoplastic flap which has been advocated particularly in the United States. Proponents of each operation cite similar surgical results and postoperative complications as reasons for supporting their respective operations.[23,30,77,78] When the two operations are compared (Table 4.4) both may be associated with cerebrospinal fluid leak and wound infections, though it should be remembered that where fat is used in obliterative procedures, a second wound site for potential infection exists and there is increased risk of fat infection within the frontal sinus. Few patients undergoing a Lynch–Howarth approach are concerned by postoperative cosmetic problems[79] which by careful positioning of the wound, close to the eyebrow and equidistant from medial canthus to nasion, avoids webbing and produces an excellent scar (Fig. 4.10). This must be compared with the linear scar and bony depression that can occur with an osteoplastic flap even with the most careful repair.[78,80] Frontal bossing may also be a problem with the flap, and though the best scar may be unobtrusive in women or men with no tendency to balding, it should be noted that it is just such middle-aged men who form a large proportion of the patients. In

Table 4.3 Surgical treatment of fronto-ethmoidal mucocoeles

Series	Method	No. of cases	Recurrence (%)	Follow-up
Kennedy et al 1989[76]	Endoscopic, fronto-ethmoidectomy	15	0	2–42 mth
Lund	External, fronto-ethmoidectomy	100	4	3–27 yr
Hardy & Montgomery 1976[81]	Osteoplastic flap	116	6	3–19 yr

Table 4.4 Surgical treatment of mucocoeles: complications reported in the literature

Complication	Reference	Patients (No.)	(%)
Osteoplastic flap			
Cosmesis, frontal bossing, depression of bone	Sessions et al 1972[78]	–	–
	Ward & Bauknight 1973[80]	3	–
	Schenck 1975[82]	–	–
	Hardy & Montgomery 1976[81]	13/250	5.2
CSF leak	Hardy & Montgomery 1976[81]	7/250	2.8
Infection:			
Primary operation site	Hardy & Montgomery 1976[81]	14/250	5.6
Fat	Sessions et al 1972[78]	–	–
	Schenck 1975[82]	–	–
	Sessions et al 1972[78]	–	–
Abdominal wound	Schenck 1975[82]	–	–
	Hardy & Montgomery 1976[81]	13/250	5.2
Laceration of dura	Schenck 1975[82]	–	–
	Hardy & Montgomery 1976[81]	7/250	2.8
Nasal skin necrosis	Hardy & Montgomery 1976[81]	2/250	0.8
Fronto-ethmoidectomy			
Infection:			
Primary operation site	Canalis et al 1978[31]	1/112	0.9
	Natvig & Larsen 1978[23]	2/20	10.0
CSF leak	Canalis et al 1978[31]	1/20	5.0

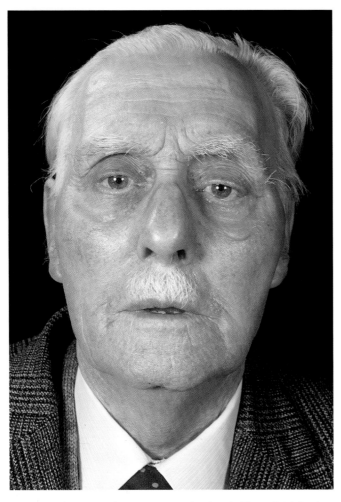

Fig. 4.10 Post-operative appearance of patient in Figure 4.4 following external fronto-ethmoidectomy.

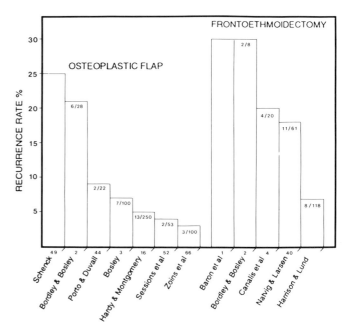

Fig. 4.11 Operative failure due to recurrence of disease for osteoplastic flap and external fronto-ethmoidectomy operations as reported in the literature.

Hardy & Montgomery's series,[81] 5% of patients required further cosmetic surgery including cranioplasty and bone grafting following osteoplastic flaps.

Recurrence of the mucocoele can occur with either operation and even protagonists of the osteoplastic flap such as Schenck[45] have quoted a 25% failure though it would appear that recurrence following external fronto-ethmoidectomy have been overestimated (Fig. 4.11).

In the case of sphenoidal mucocoeles, marsupialization may be sufficient to decompress the area which can be achieved endoscopically or by any number of other approaches to the sphenoid.[83] However, a formal neuro-surgical approach may be indicated for extensive lesions. In the antrum marsupialization may not immediately overcome the visual and cosmetic problems and a Caldwell–Luc, lateral rhinotomy or midfacial degloving approach may be more appropriate depending upon the size of the lesion.

NASAL POLYPS

Definition

The word 'polypus' is latinized Greek, meaning 'many footed' and theoretically can be applied to any pedunculated structure. However, in the nose and antrochoanal area the term refers to specific entities which must be distinguished from genuine neoplasia. Furthermore a considerable spectrum of disease may be encountered from multiple pedicled lesions hanging in the nasal cavity to a generalized polypoid change throughout the sinonasal mucous membrane, with varying aetiology and behaviour.

Historical aspects

The condition was probably first described in India where curettes were used to remove them from before 1000 BC.[88] The term 'polyp' and a method for their removal from the nose was described by Hippocrates[89] and similar illustrations can be seen in Medieval literature. Their inflammatory nature was recognized by Zuckerkandl.[89]

Incidence

This condition is common when compared with neoplasia in the nose and sinuses and has been estimated to affect 4.2% of the adult population.[90] This increases to 6.7% in asthmatics and to between 6–25% of cystic fibrosis patients. Antrochoanal polyps constitute 3.5–6.5% of all polyps in this area.[91]

Age, sex, ethnic variation

The condition is extremely rare under 5 years of age and indeed if polyps are encountered during childhood, the possibility of cystic fibrosis must be excluded. From 20 years onwards, equal numbers are affected in each decade up to 60 years of age after which the incidence decreases. Antrochoanal polyps are more frequent in children and young adults.

Generally the condition is at least twice as common in men and the same male preponderance exists in children with cystic fibrosis. In asthmatics, however, the male to female ratio is equal and in patients with associated aspirin hypersensitivity females predominate (2:1).

The condition is rare in other animals though primates such as the chimpanzee can be affected and recently an experimental model in rabbits has been developed in response to infection (Strajne P., personal communication).

Site

Originally 'nasal' polyps were thought to arise within the ethmoids and prolapse into the nasal cavity and certainly the majority originate in the anterior ethmoidal region though in the clefts as well as within the cells themselves.[92] It has recently been suggested that other areas of the middle meatus may also be affected, wherever there is mucosal juxtaposition such as contact between the uncinate process and middle turbinate. The condition is generally bilateral though one side may be more obviously affected and with the exception of an antrochoanal polyp, the lesions are multiple. Isolated polyps from the posterior ethmoid region or sphenoid sinus are rare.

More sessile polypoid change can also be found throughout the nasal cavity and within the other sinuses, in particular the maxillary antrum. The site of origin of the antrochoanal polyp within the maxilla is debated, the floor or postero-lateral wall being favoured and endoscopic studies suggests that the polyp prolapses out of the sinus through an accessory ostium in the posterior fontanelle rather than through the natural ostium.

Aetiology

The aetiology of this condition is unknown though a number of theories have been fashionable and as indicated it may be incorrect to consider 'nasal polyps' as one pathological entity. In the past, polyps were generally divided into 'allergic' and 'infective' and indeed sinusitis commonly accompanies polyps but it is difficult to determine whether this is a primary or secondary phenomenon. *Haemophilus influenzae* is the commonest

infecting organism[93] as in other cases of bacterial sinusitis. A more likely explanation is a hypersensitivity reaction, mediated by mast cell degranulation. There is certainly no evidence for an allergic aetiology as positive skin prick tests are as common in polyp patients as in the normal population.[89,94,95]

Over one-third of polyp patients also develop intrinsic asthma though the interval may be as long as 20 years[96] and the asthma more commonly precedes the polyps. A further association with intolerance to acetylsalicylic acid has been recognized since 1911 in a small number of patients with polyps and asthma. This ASA triad results from an abnormality of arachidonic acid metabolism which leads to either an increase in leukotrienes[97] or a decrease in prostaglandins.[98]

A number of other conditions can affect the upper respiratory tract mucosa and produce polyps: cystic fibrosis,[99–101] primary ciliary dyskinesia, Young's syndrome and allergic fungal rhinosinusitis (p. 67).[102–104]

Clinical features

Bilateral nasal obstruction, often with a 'valve-like' sensation is present and associated hyposmia which responds capriciously to treatment. Discharge may be clear or mucopurulent dependent on the number of eosinophils or neutrophils present. Epistaxis and pain are not usually features and suggest a more sinister aetiology. Indeed it is remarkable how often patients' symptoms are disproportionately mild in cases of extensive polyposis.

In patients who develop their polyps under 30 years of age, there is often widening of the nasal bridge and a variable degree of hypertelorism (Figs 4.12 and 4.13). This is more a consequence of the age at which the polyps began (i.e. in relation to midfacial skeletal development) than of the length of history.[48]

The actual appearance of the polyps is variable though classically they appear as pale grey–pink translucent 'grapes' hanging in clusters in the upper nasal cavity. They may acquire a more fleshy aspect with time due to squamous metaplasia. Endoscopic examination of the nose will often reveal tiny polyps within the middle meatus which may be the progenitors of the larger lesions and the condition is almost always bilateral even if one side is more obviously affected (Fig. 4.14). The polyps are generally insensitive to touch in contradistinction to polypoid change on the middle turbinate.

Unilateral obstruction of the posterior choanae is produced by an antrochoanal polyp which is usually visible in the postnasal space.

Radiology

On plain sinus X-rays there is a generalized loss of translucence throughout the nasal cavity and sinuses. In

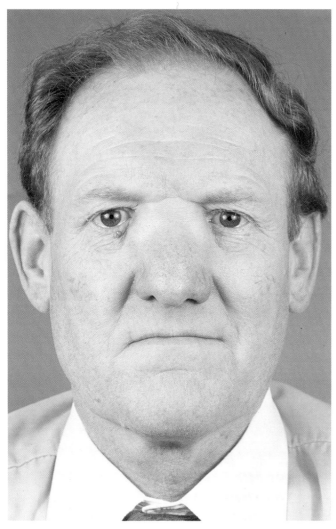

Fig. 4.12 Expansion of the nasal bridge associated with polyps.

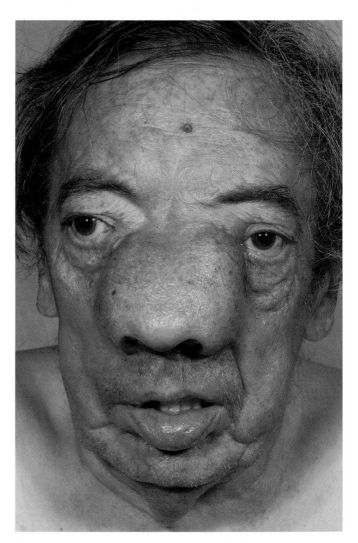

Fig. 4.13 Massive hyperteliorism in a case of long-standing nasal polyps.[48]

20% of cases evidence of ethmoidal expansion can be found,[48] in some cases associated with decalcification and loss of bony septa. However these changes are always bilateral and significant bone erosion especially if unilateral must be regarded as sinister. The degree of expansion is related to the age at which patients first develop the condition (under 30 years) rather than length of history per se.

CT scans also demonstrate the generalized opacification obscuring bony landmarks (Fig. 4.15). A strong signal is seen on T2 weighted MRI which renders the polyps difficult to distinguish from fluid. In fact it is not possible to distinguish polypoid change from the viscous accompanying secretions radiologically.

Mucocoeles may occur in a small percentage of polyp patients producing characteristic radiological features (p. 58–59).

An antrochoanal polyp can be demonstrated on a plain lateral sinus X-ray as a mass in the postnasal space with

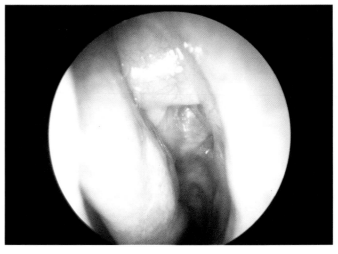

Fig. 4.14 Endoscopic photograph, showing small polyps in the middle meatus.

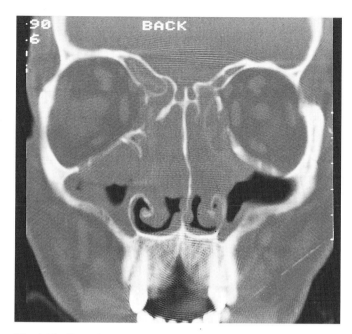

Fig. 4.15 Extensive nasal polyposis. Coronal CT scan showing generalized loss of translucence, expansion of the ethmoidal labyrinth and erosion of ethmoidal septa.

an associated unilaterally opaque maxillary sinus. These findings can be confirmed on CT and T2 weighted MRI which again show a high signal in the antrum and nasopharynx.

Macroscopic and microscopic appearance

Classically multiple pedunculated grey–pink translucent grape-like lesions are seen hanging down from the middle meatus though they may become more fleshy with time due to squamous metaplasia. An antrochoanal polyp by contrast usually presents as a multilobulated structure with a nasal, nasopharyngeal and antral component.

Whatever the aetiology, the primary phase of polypoid formation is increased exudation from the vessels, oedema of the lamina propria and bulging of the respiratory mucosa.[105] Thus the polyp usually consists of oedematous connective tissue, a myxoid stroma and fibroblasts covered by respiratory epithelium. Goblet cell hyperplasia, plasma cell and eosinophilic infiltration are variable. The presence of the latter and degranulated mast cells led to the otherwise unsupported suggestion of an allergic aetiology. Squamous metaplasia and amyloid may occur with time.

Attempts have been made to divide polyps into eosinophilic and neutrophilic or into allergic, chronic inflammatory, those with hyperplasia of glands and those with stromal atypia[106a] which may be helpful histologically but has little clinical relevance. Polyp fluid has been the subject of study and not surprisingly contains all the immunoglobulins, histamine, prostaglandins and leukotrienes amongst others.

The antrochoanal polyp has many of the above features with a pronounced chronic inflammatory infiltrate.

Natural history and prognosis

There is no evidence that simple nasal polyps undergo malignant transformation but it is mandatory to establish their provenance at an early stage in treatment. Whilst they are entirely benign, they have a propensity to recur irrespective of treatment strategies in a most unpredictable and occasionally aggressive fashion. Uncontrolled growth in the young results in marked hypertelorism and the history may be punctuated by superadded infection and mucocoele formation. 21% of our fronto-ethmoidal mucocoele patients had had nasal polyps treated medically or surgically. However, what is more surprising is the rarity of associated mucocoeles given the frequency of polyps and the even less common finding of bilateral mucocoeles under these circumstances.

In ASA-related polyposis, removal of the polyps frequently leads to an improvement in the asthma.[107]

Differential diagnosis

It is mandatory to obtain histology on all nasal polyps prior to medical treatment as a considerable range of conditions, benign and malignant, can present in this way. However in very young children the possibility of an encephalocoele must be considered and appropriately investigated prior to any surgical interference.[108] Other non-neoplastic conditions include inspissated mucus and sarcoid. It should also be remembered that polyps can occur concomitantly with neoplasia so all tissue from both sides of the nose should be examined.

Inverted papilloma and haemangioma may be mistaken clinically and an angiofibroma may resemble an antrochoanal polyp. Modern radiology will allow this condition to be diagnosed without resort to biopsy. Mucinous adenocarcinoma, olfactory neuroblastoma and malignant melanoma have all presented as 'simple' polyps.

Treatment and prognosis

The management of nasal polyps relies upon a combination of medical and surgical strategies dictated by their behaviour in each individual.[109] Steroids given topically,[110] orally or indirectly via intramuscular tetracosactrin are used initially and for maintenance if there are no medical contraindications. Surgery ranges from simple polypectomy using snares, to all forms of ethmoidectomy (endoscopic, intranasal, transantral and external). Personal enthusiasm and expertise will determine which of these is employed. A variety of clinical success rates for each procedure is found in the literature from 75% for intranasal ethmoidectomy[111] to 82% for endoscopic ethmoidectomy.[112] However, it is doubtful whether patients are genuinely 'cured' by surgery and therefore, precise conservative procedures are preferable to radical abalative external operations.

The antrochoanal polyp was traditionally removed using a snare after first performing an antral puncture from which straw-coloured fluid is obtained. Unless the point of origin is adequately extracted, recurrence can be anticipated and in the past a Caldwell–Luc procedure was often advocated. However, endoscopic surgery can often obviate this and is the preferred option ab initio.

FUNGAL INFECTIONS

A number of mycotic agents are capable of infecting the nose and paranasal sinuses producing a variety of lesions, some of which may simulate neoplasia. Fungal infections appear to be increasing in frequency, probably due to a combination of international travel, the rising incidence of immunosuppressed individuals and a greater awareness of the condition. A low threshold of suspicion is required to expedite the diagnosis of fungal infections. To this end, any tissue must be stained specifically for fungus (e.g. using Gomori methenamine-silver or Grocott stains) in addition to culture as this may be more successful and quicker in demonstrating the causative agent.

Considerable geographical differences still exist in the distribution of such diseases. Mycotic infections are still relatively uncommon in the United Kingdom, whereas the Sudan can boast the largest number of cases affecting the upper jaw. In general aspergillosis, zygomycosis, rhinosporidiosis and candidiasis are common in the nose and sinuses, actinomycosis, blastomycosis, sporotrichosis and coccidioidomycosis are moderately common whereas chromomycosis and infection due to Curvularia and Alternaria spp. are exceptionally rare.[106b]

Aspergillosis

The most important and commonest mycosis in the upper jaw is caused by *Aspergillus* spp.[113] Seven pathogenic species have been described. Of these, *A. fumigatus* accounts for 90%, followed by *A. niger* and *A. flavus*. The first reported case of aspergillus maxillary sinusitis was in 1891[114] and whilst it commonly occurs in the Sudan and Saudi Arabia where it is endemic,[115–117] it can occur anywhere and at any age. It has been suggested that it is the arid dry climate which converts this common saprophyte into a pathogen. The maxillary antrum is the most frequently affected[118] followed by the ethmoids though

frontal and sphenoid sinus involvement is less common.[115,117] A number of clinical forms are seen.

In its mildest form a 'fungus-ball' or aspergilloma can fill the maxillary sinus producing minimal symptoms. The 'ball' may be mobile, which can be demonstrated radiologically[119] and is composed of a tangled mass of mycelia covered with giant cells and other inflammatory tissue.

Another non-invasive form occurs, similar to a chronic bacterial sinusitis with rhinorrhoea and nasal obstruction. Indeed it should be suspected in any case of refractory chronic sinusitis where fungal infections can co-exist with secondary bacterial infections such as *Staphylococcus aureus* which may obscure diagnosis. The most characteristic feature is the green–brown sludge which is found filling the sinus cavity, usually the maxilla. A characteristic heterogeneous opacification is seen on CT due to diffuse calcification (Fig. 4.16). Dense nodular areas are sometimes found which can bear some similarity to inverting papilloma or chondrosarcoma. Stammberger et al[120] reported the presence of calcification in 27 out of 59 patients, due to deposition of calcium phosphate combined with traces of heavy metals (silver, lead, copper, cadmium and mercury). This chemical content in part explains the low signal which may be seen on MRI.[22c]

The next stage is that of invasion and it may be the health of the individual which determines this transition from non-invasion though it can occur without obvious immune deficiency. The disease spreads to adjacent structures such as the soft tissues of the cheek and orbit.[121] Evidence of bone destruction may be seen radiologically and serology and skin tests for aspergillus precipitins can be positive but are unreliable. The lesion is composed of giant cells, histiocytes, neutrophils and sometimes microabscesses which may contain hyphae.

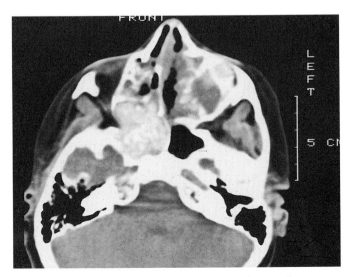

Fig. 4.16 Axial CT scan showing soft tissue mass in posterior ethmoids and right sphenoid with areas of high density typical of fungal sinusitis.

Sometimes a progressive fibrotic or sclerosing form of the condition can occur which may represent the end-stage of the invasive form and which can be readily confused with neoplasia. Large space-occupying lesions can form which threaten vision and invade the anterior and middle cranial fossae. The fungal hyphae are particularly difficult to find amongst the fibrous tissue.

The most serious form is the fulminant which occurs in patients who are immunodeficient.[122-124] Uncontrolled diabetes, systemic steroids, immunosuppressant drugs, aplastic anaemia and malignancy such as leukaemia and lymphoma render the patients vulnerable and it is estimated that 2–7% of deaths in such cases are due to fungal infection.[125-127] Intracranial extension either directly or blood-borne is fatal in a fifth of patients even with treatment. The condition may be mistaken histologically for mucormycosis.

A fourth, 'allergic', form of aspergillosis has recently been recognized.[102-104] It often occurs in young adults with a history of asthma and/or polyps, and produces a pan-sinusitis but without soft tissue or bone invasion. Thick inspissated mucus is found in the sinus and the lining shows a marked eosinophilic reaction with Charcot–Leyden crystals (Fig. 4.17). Fungal hyphae are very scanty and must be carefully sought in the mucus. The condition is similar to allergic broncho-pulmonary aspergillosis.

In all forms, diagnosis using fresh nasal scrapings, mucus and biopsies of the sinus mucosa is important. Surgical drainage and aeration of the area by intranasal procedures (endoscopic or conventional) is often sufficient in the non-invasive and allergic forms, sometimes combined paradoxically with topical or even systemic steroids. Invasive and fulminant forms require more radical therapy, both surgical and medical. Exenteration of the affected area which can even include craniofacial resection and orbital clearance may be necessary, combined with a systemic antifungal agent. Amphotericin B, the mainstay of such treatment must be given parenterally and is associated with significant hepatic toxicity. Newer oral agents such as itraconazole and ketaconazole are less toxic and are likely to supersede amphotericin in the future.

A 49-year-old Nigerian brewery controller was referred from Nigeria with a 3 month history of pronounced right proptosis, periorbital swelling and nasal obstruction. He had lost 16 kg in weight over the preceding 6 months and had periods of

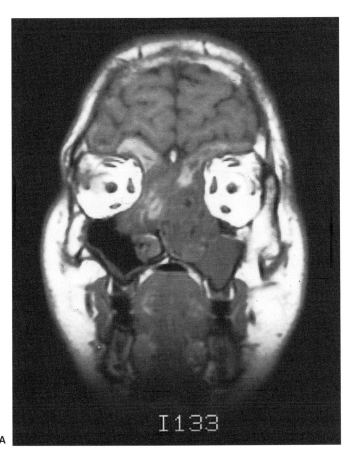
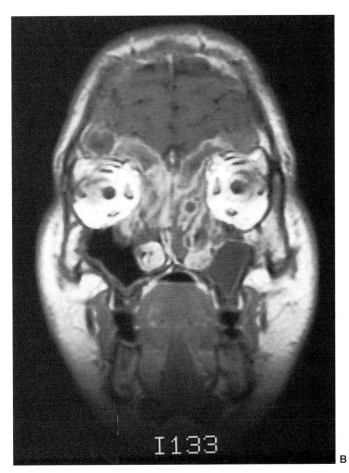

Fig. 4.17 Extensive allergic aspergillus sinusitis. **A**, coronal MR scan, T1 weighted sequence. **B**, same sequence, post-gadolinium showing high signal from inflamed mucosa and polyps compared with inspissated fungal secretions.

confusion and unsteadiness. He was a non-insulin-dependent diabetic well-controlled on chlorpropramide. He had hepatomegaly and abnormal liver function tests consistent with a previous liver biopsy showing cirrhosis. Serology for HIV and hepatitis B were negative, Mantoux tests at 1/10 000 and 1/1000 were negative though a chest X-ray showed bilateral apical shadowing. CT scans showed a large antro-ethmoidal mass with extension into the orbit and through the cribriform plate.

An irregular friable mass was visible in the nose and biopsied. This showed nasal mucosa heavily infiltrated with aspergillus hyphae and culture confirmed *Aspergillus fumigatus*. Despite intensive treatment with amphotericin B combined with surgical debulking of large amounts of necrotic material the patient succumbed a week later. Post-mortem examination revealed an extensive necrotic mass involving all sinuses on the right, the orbit and the anterior cranial fossa. The Aspergillus was present as both a fungal 'ball' and with evidence of infiltration though without any associated granulomatous reaction. Several teeth were found to be missing and Aspergillus was found in the socket of one of these. In addition active cavitating pulmonary tuberculosis was confirmed.

The exact immune status of this patient was uncertain. He had a normal granulomatous reaction to tuberculosis but a negative Mantoux and no granulomatous reaction to the aspergillus hyphae. Although no immune function tests were performed there was indirect evidence of decreased cell-mediated immunity possibly related to the cirrhosis, diabetes and tuberculosis combined with a possible dental source of fungal infection.

Zygomycosis or phycomycosis

This disease is produced by members of the group of zygomycoses or phycomycoses which consists of two orders of fungi: Mucorales and Entomophthorales. *Conidiobolus (Entomophthora) coronatus* belongs to the latter and produces a slowly-progressive subcutaneous infection with considerable fibrosis. There are prominent nasal 'polyps' or granulomas often on the inferior turbinate but spreading into any of the sinuses and subcutaneous tissues. Symptoms are, therefore, obstruction, swelling, discharge and a secondary sinusitis. Biopsy shows multinucleated cells with fungal hyphae. The condition is said to be more common in young men (though not immunosuppressed) and occurs in Central Africa, India and South America.

A rhinocerebral zygomycosis or mucormycosis is caused by *Rhizopus oryzae*. This fungus is found on decaying fruit and bread and is only a threat to the debilitated such as poorly-controlled diabetics and terminal cancer patients.[128] Thus any age and either sex may be affected. The infection which starts in the nose, spreads to the ethmoids.[129,130] It produces arterial thrombosis and necrosis and pursues a rapidly fulminant course with death due to intracranial complications often within days.[129,130] The patient may present with nasal discharge, paraesthesia of the cheek, proptosis, visual loss and severe headaches. X-rays show opacification and bone destruction predominantly in the ethmoid region mimicking a malignant neoplasm though the other sinuses may be affected.[131] CT shows soft tissue invasion and may confirm abscess formation in the frontal lobes.[128]

Rhinosporidiosis

Rhinosporidiosis is a chronic granulomatous zygomycosis caused by *Rhinosporidium seeberi*[132] which is regarded as a fungus though it cannot successfully be grown in culture or transmitted to laboratory animals. The exact mode of transmission is unknown though it is thought to be contracted from horses or cattle dung or by contact with stagnant water contaminated by infected animals.[133] It is found in India, Sri Lanka and Africa from where large series have been reported[134,135] and is again more common in young men. A bleeding polyp studded by sporangia which gives the appearance of a raspberry is found in the vestibule, arising from the anterior septum though the disease can affect any mucosal surface in the respiratory tract, eye or genitalia.[136] The polyps can attain a considerable size and the sporangia have a characteristic histological appearance. At present surgical excision is the mainstay of treatment in the absence of a specific therapeutic agent.

Blastomycosis and histoplasmosis

Three forms of blastomycosis are encountered: South American, North American and European. Of these the South American form is commonest in the upper jaw secondary to pulmonary involvement, producing chronic ulcerative lesions. The causative agent is *Paracoccidiodes brasiliensis* and the condition may be fatal. The lungs are also the primary site for the North American *Blastomyces dermatidis*, a yeast-like fungus which occasionally produces abcesses in the nose and for the European *Cryptococcus neoformans*.

There are morphological similarities between some forms of the blastomycoses and the lesions caused by *Histoplasmosis capsulatum*, another American fungus affecting the reticulo-endothelial system. The pulmonary infection can spread to any organ, including the nose where nodular lesions occur. This must also be distinguished from *Leishmania* and *Toxoplasma* spp. by fungal stains.

Sporotrichosis and coccidioidomycosis

Sporotrichosis (*Sporothrix schenckii*) usually produces lesions in the skin, subcutaneous tissues and lymph nodes but can also occasionally produce nasal nodules as can *Coccidioides immitis*.

Candidosis

Candida albicans is a common nasal mycosis, often

accompanying oral thrush. It usually presents as an acute infection which may be life-threatening in severely debilitated patients such as AIDS sufferers. Occasionally a chronic form of Candida can produce a granuloma. A case occurring in the frontal sinus of a Sikh previously treated for tuberculosis was reported by Osborn in 1963.[137]

Actinomycetes

These organisms are now considered to be bacteria though for many years they were regarded as intermediate between fungus and bacteria, hence their inclusion here.

Actinomycosis (*Actinomyces israeli*) has been occasionally reported in the nose and maxillary sinus[138] though it is more commonly found as a harmless parasite in the mouth. Foul pus may be irrigated from the sinus and there may be associated bone erosion and brawny swelling of the soft tissues with fistulae. The 'characteristic' sulphur granules can also be found with some other bacterial agents such as *Streptococcus* spp. so demonstration of Gram-positive filaments is necessary for diagnosis.

Nocardiosis is caused by some aerobic varieties of Actinomyces (*Nocardia asteroides*) and is even more rare in the upper jaw. One case in an 80-year-old woman presenting with epistaxis is reported by Friedmann.[12b]

REFERENCES

1. Graham J, Michaels L 1978 Cholesterol granuloma of the maxillary antrum. Clinical Otolaryngology 3: 155–160
2. Dota T, Nakamura K, Saheki M, Sasaki Y 1963 Cholesterol granuloma: Experimental observations. Annals of Otology, Rhinology and Laryngology 72: 346–356
3. Friedmann I 1959 Epidermoid cholesteatoma and cholesterol granuloma: experimental and human. Annals of Otology, Rhinology and Laryngology 68: 57–79
4. Hiraide F, Inouye T, Miyakagowa N 1982 Experimental cholesterol granuloma. Histopathological and histochemical studies. Journal of Laryngology and Otology 96: 491–501
5. Main T S, Shimada T, Lim D J 1970 Experimental cholesterol granuloma. Archives of Otolaryngology 91: 356–359
6. Altes A J K 1966 Cholesterol granuloma in the tympanic cavity. Journal of Laryngology and Otology 80: 691–698
7. Beaumont G D 1966 The effects of exclusion of air from pneumatised bones. Journal of Laryngology and Otology 80: 236–249
8. Ojala L 1957 Pneumatization of the bone and environmental factors. Experimental studies in chick humerus. Acta Otolaryngologica Suppl. 133: 1–28
9. Wyler A R, Leech R W, Reynolds A F, Ojemann G A, Mead C 1974 Cholesterol granuloma of the petrous apex: a case report. Journal of Neurosurgery (Baltimore) 41: 765–768
10. Aker Gunes H, Almac A, Canbay E 1988 Cholesterol granuloma of the maxillary antrum. Journal of Laryngology and Otology 102: 630–632
11. Butler S, Grossenbacher R 1989 Cholesterol granuloma of the paranasal sinuses. Journal of Laryngology and Otology 103: 776–779
12. Friedmann I, Osborn D A 1982 Pathology of granulomas and neoplasms of the nose and paranasal sinuses. Churchill Livingstone, Edinburgh a: p 26; b: pp 70–81
13. Hellquist H, Lundgren J, Olofsson J 1984 Cholesterol granuloma of the maxillary and frontal sinuses. Otology, Rhinology and Laryngology 46: 153–158
14. Milton C M, Bickerton R C 1986 A review of maxillary sinus cholesterol granuloma. British Journal of Oral and Maxillofacial Surgery 24: 293–299
15. Niho M 1986 Cholesterol crystals in the temporal bone and paranasal sinuses. International Journal of Pediatric Otorhinolaryngology 11: 79–95
16. Nager G T, Vanderveen T S 1976 Cholesterol granuloma involving the temporal bone. Annals of Otology, Rhinology and Laryngology 85: 204–209
17. Sade J, Teitz A 1982 Cholesterol in cholesteatoma and in otitis media syndrome. American Journal of Otology 3: 203–208
18. Lloyd G A S 1986 Cholesterol granuloma of the facial skeleton. British Journal of Radiology 59: 481–485
19. Bilaniuk L T, Zimmerman R A 1982 Computed tomography in evaluation of the paranasal sinuses. Radiologic Clinics of North America 20: 51–66
20. Griffin C, De La Paz R, Enzmann D 1987 MR and CT correlation of cholesterol cysts of the petrous bone. American Journal of Neuroradiology 8: 825–829
21. Latack J T, Graham M D, Kemink J L, Knake J E 1985 Giant cholesterol cysts of the petrous apex. Radiologic features. American Journal of Neuroradiology 6: 409–413
22. Lloyd G A S 1988 Diagnostic imaging of the nose and paranasal sinuses. Springer Verlag, Berlin a: pp 78–80; b: pp 55–66; c: pp 83–88
23. Natvig K, Larsen T E 1978 Mucocele of the paranasal sinuses. Journal of Laryngology and Otology 92: 1075–1082
24. Hackett F 1934 Francis I. Doubleday Doran and Co, New York, pp 313–316
25. Lagenbeck C J M 1819 Neue Bibliothek fur die Chirurgie und Ophthalmologie. Hahn Hanover 2:365
26. Rollet M 1896 Mucocele de l'angle supero-interne des orbites. Lyon Medecine 81: 573–575
27. Turner A L 1907 Mucocele of the nasal accessory sinuses. Edinburgh Medical Journal 22: 396–501
28. Howarth W G 1921 Mucocele and pyocele of the nasal accessory sinuses. Lancet 2: 744–746
29. Herrnheiser G 1926 Der Rontegenbefund bei der Mucocele oder Pyocele der Stirnhohle und der Siebbeinzellen. Zeitschrift Hals, Nasen, Ohren 14: 319–326
30. Bordley J E, Bosley W R 1973 Mucoceles of the frontal sinus: causes and treatment. Annals of Otology, Rhinology and Laryngology 82: 696–702
31. Canalis R F, Zajchuk J T, Jenkins, H A 1978 Ethmoidal mucoceles. Archives of Otolaryngology, Head and Neck Surgery 104: 286–291
32. De Wilde R, Fossion E, Raas P, Ostyn F 1984 Mucoceles of the paranasal sinuses. Acta Stomatologica Belgica 81: 91–106
33. East D 1985 Mucocoeles of the maxillary antrum. Journal of Laryngology and Otology 99: 49–56
34. Hu X H, Lin D Z 1982 Mucocele des sinus. Revue de Laryngologie, Otologie et Rhinologie 103: 199–201
35. Wolfowitz B L, Solomon A 1972 Mucocoeles of the frontal and ethmoid sinuses. Journal of Laryngology and Otology 86: 79–82
36. Zizmour J, Noyek A M 1968 Cysts and benign tumours of the paranasal sinuses. Seminars in Roentgenology 3: 172–185
37. Timon C I, O'Dwyer T P 1989 Ethmoidal mucocoeles in children. Journal of Laryngology and Otology 103: 284–286
38. Hasegawa M, Saito Y, Watnabe I, Eugene B 1979 Post-operative mucocoeles in the maxillary sinus. Rhinology 17: 253–256
39. Lloyd G A S, Lund V J, Scadding G K 1991 Computerised tomography in the pre-operative evaluation of functional endoscopic sinus surgery. Journal of Laryngology and Otology 105: 181–185
40. Close L G, O'Conner W E 1983 Sphenoethmoidal mucocoeles with intracranial extension. Otolaryngology, Head and Neck Surgery 91: 350–357
41. Diaz F, Fatchow R, Duvall A J, Quick C A, Erickson D L 1978 Mucoceles with intracranial and extracranial extensions. Journal of Neurosurgery 48: 284–288

42. Lundgren A, Olin T 1961 Muco-pyocele of sphenoidal sinus or posterior ethmoidal cells with special reference to apex orbitae syndrome. Acta Otolaryngologica 53: 61–79

43. Nugent G R, Sprinkle P, Bloor B M 1970 Sphenoid sinus mucoceles. Journal of Neurosurgery 32: 443–451

44. Lund V J 1987 Anatomical considerations in the aetiology of fronto-ethmoidal mucoceles. Rhinology 25: 83–88

45. Schenck N L, Rauchbach E, Ogura J H 1974 Frontal sinus disease. II. Development of the frontal sinus model: occlusion of the nasofrontal duct. Laryngoscope 84: 1233–1247

46. Finn D G, Hudson W R, Baylin G 1981 Unilateral polyposis and mucoceles in children. Laryngoscope 91: 1444–1449

47. Kastenbauer E 1967 Uber die Muco- und Pyocelen der Sternoho. Hals, Nasen, Ohren 15: 277–281

48. Lund V J, Lloyd G A S 1983 Radiological changes associated with benign nasal polyps. Journal of Laryngology and Otology 97: 503–510

49. Mendelsohn R S, Cohen B M 1964 Otorhinologic aspects of cystic fibrosis. Archives of Otolaryngology 79: 312–317

50. Palubinskas A J, Davies H 1959 Roentgen features of nasal accessory sinus mucoceles. Radiology 72: 576–584

51. Schuknecht H F, Lindsay J R 1949 Benign cysts of the paranasal sinuses. Archives of Otolaryngology 49: 609–630

52. Sellars S L, De Villiers J C 1981 The sphenoid sinus mucocoele. Journal of Laryngology and Otology 95: 493–502

53. Harris M 1978 Odontogenic cyst growth and prostaglandin-induced bone resorption. Archives of the Royal College of Surgeons 60: 85–91

54. Harris M, Jenkins M V, Bennett A, Wills, M R 1973 Prostaglandin production and bone resorption by dental cysts. Nature 245: 213–215

55. Harvey W, Guat-Chen F, Gordon D, Meghji S, Evans A, Harris M 1984 Evidence for fibroblasts as the major source of prostacyclin synthesis in dental cysts in man. Archives of Oral Biology 29: 223–229

56. Lund V J, Harvey W, Meghji S, Harris M 1988 Prostaglandin synthesis in the pathogenesis of fronto-ethmoidal mucoceles. Acta Otolaryngologica 106:145–151

57. Dayer J M, Robinson D R, Krane S M 1977 Prostaglandin production by rheumatoid synovial cells: stimulation by a factor from human mononuclear cells. Journal of Experimental Medicine 145: 1399–1404

58. Englis D J, D'Souza S M, Meats J E, Wright J, McGuire M B, Russell R G G 1980 Stimulation of prostaglandin biosynthesis induced by mononuclear cell factor added to cells from human gingiva, cartilage, synovium and endometrium. Advances in Prostaglandin, Thromboxane and Leukotrienes Research 8: 1709–1711

59. Mirzel S B, Dayer J M, Krane S M, Mergenhagen S E 1981 Stimulation of rheumatoid synovial cell collagenase and prostaglandin production by partially purified lymphocyte-activating factor (interleukin 1). Proceedings of the National Academy of Science of the USA 78: 2474–2477

60. Som P M, Shugar J M A 1980 Antral mucoceles. A new look. Journal of Computer Assisted Tomography 4: 484–488

61. Wurster C, Levine T, Sisson G 1986 Mucocele of the sphenoid sinus causing sudden onset of blindness. Otolaryngology, Head and Neck Surgery 94: 257–259

62. Lund V J, Rolfe M E 1989 Ophthalmic considerations in fronto-ethmoidal mucocoeles. Journal of Laryngology and Otology 103: 667–669

63. Fujitani T, Takahashi T, Asai T 1984 Optic nerve disturbance caused by frontal and fronto-ethmoidal mucopyoceles. Archives of Otolaryngology 110: 267–269

64. Larson C H, Adkins W Y, Osguthorpe J D 1983 Post-traumatic frontal and frontoethmoid mucoceles causing reversible visual loss. Otolaryngology, Head and Neck Surgery 91: 691–694

65. Weaver R G, Gates G A 1979 Mucoceles of the sphenoid sinus. Otolaryngology, Head and Neck Surgery 87: 168–173

66. Mendelsohn D B, Glass R B J, Hertzanu Y 1984 Giant maxillary antral mucocele. Journal of Laryngology and Otology 98: 305–310

67. Wigh R 1950 Mucoceles of the fronto-ethmoidal sinuses. Radiology 54: 579–590

68. Hesselink J R, Weber A L, New P F, Davis K R, Roberson G H, Taveras J M 1979 Evaluation of mucoceles of the paranasal sinuses with computed tomography. Radiology 133: 397–400

69. Price H I, Danziger A 1980 Computerised tomographic findings in mucocoeles of the frontal and ethmoid sinuses. Clinical Radiology 31: 169–174

70. Gomori J M, Grossman R I, Goldberg H I, Zimmerman R A, Bilaniuk L T 1985 Intracranial hematomas: imaging by high-field MR. Radiology 157: 87–93

71. Som P M, Dillon W P, Fullerton G D, Zimmerman R A, Rajagopalan B, Marom Z 1989 Radiology 172: 515–520

72. Som P M, Shugar J M A 1980 The CT classification of ethmoidal mucoceles. Journal of Computer Assisted Tomography 4: 199–203

73. Takahashi M, Jingu K, Makayama T 1973 Roentgenologic appearances of spheno-ethmoidal mucocoele. Neuroradiology 6: 45–53

74. Lund V J, Milroy C M 1991 Fronto-ethmoidal mucocoeles. A histopathological analysis. Journal of Otology and Laryngology 105: 921–923

75. Paparella M M 1963 Mucosal cyst of the maxillary sinus. Archives of Otolaryngology 77: 96–103

76. Kennedy D W, Josephson J S, Zinreich J, Mattox D E, Goldsmith M M 1989 Endoscopic sinus surgery for mucoceles. Laryngoscope 99: 885–895

77. Goodale R L, Montgomery W W 1961 Anterior osteoplastic frontal sinus operation. Annals of Otology, Rhinology and Laryngology 70: 860–880

78. Sessions R B, Alford B R, Stratton C, et al 1972 Current concepts of frontal sinus surgery: an appraisal of the osteoplastic flap-fat obliteration operation. Laryngoscope 82: 918–930

79. Rubin J S, Lund V J, Salmon B S 1986 Frontoethmoidectomy in the treatment of mucoceles. Archives of Otolaryngology, Head and Neck Surgery 112: 434–436

80. Ward P H, Bauknight S 1973 A serious cosmetic complication of the osteoplastic frontal flap. Archives of Otolaryngology, Head and Neck Surgery 98: 389–390

81. Hardy J M, Montgomery W W 1976 Osteoplastic frontal sinusotomy. Annals of Otology, Rhinology and Laryngology 85: 523–532

82. Schenck N L 1975 Frontal sinus disease: III, Experimental and clinical factors in failure of the frontal osteoplastic operation. Laryngoscope 85: 76–92

83. Stankiewicz J A 1989 Sphenoid sinus mucocoeles. Archives of Otolaryngology, Head And Neck Surgery 115: 735–740

84. Zonis R D, Montgomery W W, Goodale R L 1966 Frontal sinus disease: one hundred cases treated by osteoplastic operation. Laryngoscope 76: 1816–1825

85. Bosley W R 1972 Osteoplastic obliteration of the frontal sinuses. Laryngoscope 82: 1463–1476

86. Baron S H, Dedo H H, Henry C R 1973 The mucoperiosteal flap in frontal sinus surgery. Laryngoscope 83: 1266–1280

87. Porto D P, Duvall A J 1986 Long-term results with nasofrontal duct reconstruction. Laryngoscope 96: 858–862

88. Vancil M E 1969 A historical survey of treatment for nasalpolyposis. Laryngoscope79: 435–445

89. Drake-Lee A B 1987 Nasal polyps. In: Mackay I S, Bull T R (eds) Scott-Browns' Otolaryngology, Vol. 4, Rhinology, 5th edn. Butterworths, London, pp 142–153

90. Settipane G A, Chafee F H 1977 Nasal polyps in asthma and rhinitis. Journal of Allergy and Clinical Immunology 58: 17–21

91. Batsakis J G 1980 Tumors of the head and neck. Williams and Wilkins, Baltimore, pp 139–142

92. Stammberger H 1991 Functional endoscopic sinus surgery. BC Decker, Philadelphia, pp 216–238

93. Majumder B, Bull P D 1982 The incidence of maxillary sinusitis in nasal polyposis. Journal of Laryngology and Otology 96: 937–941

94. Jamal A, Maran A G D 1987 Atopy and nasal polyposis. Journal of Laryngology and Otology 101: 355–358

95. Mygind N, Pedersen C B, Prytz S, Sorensen H 1975 Treatment of nasal polyps with intransal beclomethasone diproprionate aerosol. Clinical Allergy 5: 159–164
96. Maran A G D, Lund V J 1990 Clinical rhinology. Thieme Verlag, Stuttgart, pp 94–99
97. Maloney J 1977 Nasal polyps, nasal polypectomy, asthma and aspirin sensitivity. Journal of Laryngology and Otology 91: 837–846
98. Schwachman H, Kulczychi I L, Mueller H L, Flake C G 1962 Nasal polyposis in patients with cystic fibrosis. Paediatrics 30: 389–401
99. Fonsman J 1970 Mucoviscidosis and nasal polyposis. Acta Otolaryngologica 69: 152–154
100. Sczeklik A, Gryglewski R, Czerniawske-Mysik G 1975 Relationship of inhibition of prostaglandin biosynthesis by analgesics to asthma attacks in aspirin sensitive patients. British Medical Journal 1: 67–69
101. Toma G A, Stein G E 1968 Nasal polyposis in cystic fibrosis. Journal of Laryngology and Otology 82: 265–268
102. Jonathan D, Lund V J, Milroy C 1989 Allergic aspergillus sinusitis: an overlooked diagnosis? Journal of Laryngology and Otology 103: 1181–1186
103. Katzenstein A A, Sale S R, Greenberger P A 1983 Allergic aspergillus sinusitis: a newly recognized form of sinusitis. Journal of Allergy and Clinical Immunology 72: 89–93
104. Waxman J E, Spector J G, Sale S R, Katzenstein A A 1987 Allergic aspergillus sinusitis: concepts in diagnosis and treatment of a new clinical entity. Laryngoscope 97: 261–266
105. Kakoi H, Hiraide F 1987 A histological study of formation and growth of nasal polyps. Acta Otolaryngologica (Stockholm) 103: 137–144
106. Hellquist H B 1990 Pathology of the nose and paranasal sinuses. Butterworths, London a: pp 27–31; b: pp 40–45
107. English G M 1986 Nasal polypectomy and sinus surgery in patients with asthma and aspirin idiosyncrasy. Laryngoscope 96: 374–380
108. Hughes G B, Sharpino G, Hunt W, Tucker H M 1980 Management of congenital midline nasal mass: a review. Head and Neck Surgery 2: 222–233
109. Tos M, Drake-Lee A B, Lund V J, Stammberger H 1989 Treatment of nasal polyps – medication or surgery and which technique. Rhinology (Suppl. 8): 45–49
110. Chalton R, Mackay I S, Wilson R, Cole P 1985 Double-blind placebo controlled trial of betamethasone nasal drops for nasal polyposis. British Medical Journal 281: 788
111. Simonton K 1958 The comprehensive surgical treatment of nasal polyposis. Transactions of the American Academy of Ophthamology and Otolaryngology 65: 75–81
112. Wigand M E, Hosemann W 1989 Microsurgical treatment of recurrent nasal polyposis. Rhinology Suppl. 8: 25–30
113. Levine P A, Yanagisawa E 1977 Pathological quiz case 1. Archives of Otolaryngology 103: 560–562
114. Zarniko C 1891 Aspergillusmykose der Kieferhohle. Deutsche medizinische Wochenschrift 17: 1222
115. Milosev B, Mahgoub S, Abdel A O, El Hassan A M 1969 Aspergilloma of the paranasal sinuses in the Sudan. British Journal of Surgery 56: 132–137
116. Robb P J 1986 Aspergillosis of the paranasal sinuses. Journal of Laryngology and Otology 100: 1071–1077
117. Rudwan M A, Sheikh H A 1976 Aspergilloma of the paranasal sinuses - a common cause of unilateral proptosis in Sudan. Clinical Radiology 27: 497–502
118. Jahrsdorfer R A, Ejercito V S, Johns M M E, Cantrell R W, Sydnor J B 1979 Aspergillosis of the nose and paranasal sinuses. American Journal of Otolaryngology 1: 6–14
119. Beck-Mannagetta J, Necek D 1986 Radiologic findings in aspergillosis of the maxillary sinus. Oral Surgery, Oral Medicine, Oral Pathology 62, 345–349
120. Stammberger H, Jakse R, Beaufort F 1984 Aspergillosis of the paranasal sinuses. X-ray diagnosis, histopathology and clinical aspects. Annals of Otology, Rhinology and Laryngology 93: 251–256
121. Oates J, Clark D R, Chiodini P 1987 Intracranial extension of paranasal sinus aspergillosis. Journal of Laryngology and Otology 101: 188–190
122. Landoy Z, Rotstein C, Shedd D 1985 Aspergillosis of the nose and paranasal sinuses in neutropenic patients at an oncology center. Head and Neck Surgery 8: 83–90
123. Schubert M M, Peterson D E, Meyers J D, Hackman R, Thomas E D 1987 Head and neck aspergillosis in patients undergoing bone marrow transplantation. Cancer 60: 1092–1096
124. Viollier A F, Peterson D E, De Jongh C A, Newman K A, Gray W C, Sutherland J C, Moody M A, Schimpff S C 1986 Aspergillus sinusitis in cancer patients. Cancer 58: 366–371
125. McGill T J, Simpson G, Healy G B 1980 Fulminant aspergillosis of the nose and paranasal sinuses. A new clinical entity. Laryngoscope 90: 748–754
126. Miglets A W, Saunders W H, Ayers L 1978 Aspergillosis of the sphenoid sinus. Archives of Otolaryngology 104: 47–50
127. Milroy C M, Blanshard J D, Lucas S, Michaels L 1989 Aspergillosis of the nose and paranasal sinuses. Journal of Clinical Pathology 42: 123–127
128. Berthier M, Palmieri O, Lylyk P, Leiguarda R 1982 Rhinorbital phycomycosis complicated by cerebral abscess. Neuroradiology 22: 221–224
129. La Touche C J, Sutherland T W, Telling M 1963 Rhinocerebral mucormycosis. Lancet 2: 811–813
130. Yanagisawa E, Friedman S, Kundargi R S, Smith H W 1977 Rhinocerebral phycomycosis. Laryngoscope 87: 1319–1335
131. Becker M H, Ngo N, Berambaum S L 1968 Mycotic infection of the paranasal sinuses. Radiology 90: 49–51
132. Seeber G R 1900 Thesis. Universidad Nacionale, Buenos Aires
133. Michaels L 1987 Ear, nose and throat histopathology. Springer-Verlag, Berlin, pp 145–148
134. Kameswaran S 1966 Surgery in rhinosporidiosis: Experience with 293 cases. International Surgery 46: 602-612
135. Satyanarayana C 1960 Rhinosporidiosis with a record of 255 cases. Acta Otolaryngologica 51: 348–356
136. Subramanyam C S V, Ramano Rao A V 1960 A fatal case of tracheobronchial rhinosporidiosis. British Journal of Surgery 47: 411–413
137. Osborn D A 1963 Mycotic infection of the frontal sinus. Journal of Laryngology and Otology 77: 29–33
138. Stanton M B 1966 Actinomycosis of the maxillary sinus. Journal of Laryngology and Otology 80: 168–174

5. Papillomas of the nasal cavity and paranasal sinuses

Papillomas are benign exophytic neoplasms. They may arise from the skin of the nasal vestibule or from the mucosa of the sinonasal tract.

SQUAMOUS PAPILLOMAS OF THE NASAL VESTIBULE

These lesions are extremely common, and are said to constitute a third of all neoplasms in the nasal cavity. They occur in a wide age range, peaking in middle age and are probably equally common in men and women, though they may present more frequently in women for cosmetic reasons.

A small solitary cauliflower-like pedunculated lesion is seen arising in the vestibule which represents an exophytic squamous proliferation with marked hyperkeratosis (Figs 5.1 and 5.2). They are similar to the verrucous warts found elsewhere in the body and in common with these a viral origin has been proposed in some cases, based on the identification of solitary intranuclear virus-like particles. Like warts, they may also undergo spontaneous regression but can otherwise be removed by local excision

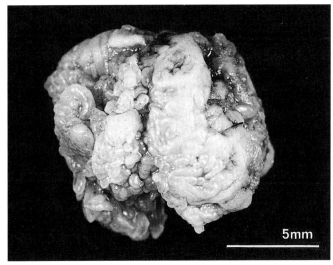

Fig. 5.2 Surgical specimen of squamous papilloma.

and are rarely associated with recurrence and never with malignant change. Occasionally the papillomas may be multifocal when removal can be facilitated with a coagulating laser such as the argon or KTP.

PAPILLOMAS OF THE SINONASAL TRACT

Definition

These lesions arise from the mucosa of the upper respiratory tract and have been described by at least 20 synonyms.

Synonyms

Inverting papilloma, inverted papilloma, Schneiderian papilloma, transitional cell papilloma, cylindric(al) cell papilloma, Ringetz papilloma, papillary adenoma, microcystic papillary adenoma, Ewing's papilloma, papillary sinusitis.

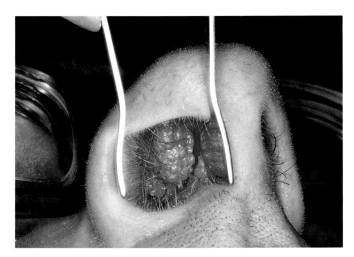

Fig. 5.1 Squamous papilloma arising from the anterior septum.

The origins of the condition serve to explain this plethora of terms.

Historical aspects

In 1847 Kramer[1] used the term 'papillae' to describe a cauliflower-like tumour of the mucous membrane. In 1854, Ward[2] reported a case of nasal papilloma, though Billroth[3] is usually credited with the first description of a true papilloma of the nasal cavity, which he termed a 'villiform cancer'. In 1883 Hoppmann[4] attempted to classify the lesions into hard and soft, though the histological distinction was not clear. Kramer & Som[1] in 1935 reviewed the 81 cases extant in the literature and introduced the term 'true papilloma' and in 1938 Ringetz[5] described the inverting nature of a lesion of cylindrical or transitional cell type. Ringetz used this nomenclature to denote a transition between the squamous and glandular epithelium of the upper respiratory tract. The term was subsequently used by Freidmann[6] but to convey an analogous situation to that of the urogenital tract. Recent authors such as Batsakis[7] have disagreed with this concept and have suggested that the title 'transitional' should be abandoned.

The capacity of the upper respiratory tract to develop such a distinct entity may be explained embryologically. Whereas the majority of the respiratory tract is endodermal in origin, the epithelium of the nasal cavity and sinuses derives from invaginations of the nasal placodes and is therefore ectodermal. This epithelium was described by Victor Conrad Schneider, hence the eponym 'Schneiderian' for both epithelium and tumour.[8]

In 1963 Norris[9] divided these lesions into inverting and exophytic, whilst the term 'inverted' was coined by Lampertico et al in the same year.[10] Both types represent benign neoplastic proliferations arising from the sinonasal mucosa and composed of an epithelial component which may be squamous, respiratory or a combination of both with a mesenchymal stroma.

The inverted tumours arise mainly from the lateral wall of the nasal cavity and sinuses whilst the exophytic or everted lesions occur principally on the septum and have also been termed 'fungiform'. The histological distinction is not completely clear-cut and combinations can occur. Furthermore a subgroup of papillomas composed almost completely of cylindric cells has been described which also tends to occur on the lateral nasal wall.

Papillomas of the sinonasal tract may be classified as:

1. Inverted
2. Everted (fungiform)
3. Cylindric cell.

Incidence

Papillomas are the commonest benign epithelial tumours of the nasal cavity. In the literature, an incidence of between 0.01% and 10% of all neoplasms of the sinonasal tract, both benign and malignant, is quoted.[5,7,11,12]

Age, sex and ethnic variation (Table 5.1)

In the literature the median age varies from 35–60 years, and the age range from 6–85 years. All authors agree that the lesion is rare under 21 years though the fungiform/everted septal lesion affects a younger age group than the inverted or cylindric forms.

Male to female ratios of up to 5:1 have been quoted. Collation of reported cases suggests a male to female ratio of 3.5:1. The male preponderance is more marked in the everted lesion, whereas the cylindric papilloma affects both sexes equally. Caucasians are the commonest ethnic group though the lesion has been reported in Negroes.[9,11,13-17]

Site

Overall about 50% of papillomas, mainly the inverted and cylindric lesions, affect the lateral wall and sinuses whilst the rest, mainly fungiform lesions, arise from the septum. The incidence of inverted papilloma arising on the septum varies from 0–16.7%.[8,9,12,18-24] The middle meatus is the area primarily affected on the lateral wall from whence the tumour can spread into the nasal cavity and maxillary sinus. From here it can also spread inferiorly on to the floor of the nose or up on to the roof. The ethmoids, and less commonly the frontal and sphenoid sinuses, may all be involved. Occasionally the tumour spreads back through the posterior choanae to present in the nasopharynx as an 'antrochoanal polyp' and the palate can also be affected.[37]

The tumour has been described as arising primarily from within the maxillary sinus[38] and more unusually from the posterior pharyngeal wall and nasopharynx where presumably ectopic foci of Schneiderian mucosa can occur.[10,39,40] The lesion is usually unilateral but there are many references to bilateral disease, synchronous and metachronous[11,22,27,33,34,41] suggesting an incidence of around 5%. Similarly while most arise from a single area, a multifocal origin has been described.[11,23]

Aetiology

The aetiology of the lesion is generally regarded as unknown. There is no association with allergy, environmental factors, or smoking.[30] Herrold[42] reported producing papillomas in the anterior nasal cavity of Syrian hamsters using dimethylnitrosamine but the histology of these lesions has been called into question. A 2.7% association has been reported with nasal polyps[7] but these are

Table 5.1 Inverted papilloma: association with carcinoma in major series

	Patients total no.	Male	Female	Age range (yr)	Mean age (yr)	Association with cancer No.	%
Lampertico et al 1963[10]	19	–	–	–	–	3	16
Norris 1963[9]	29	Ratio	3:1	27–76	49	2	7
Brown 1964[18]	30	22	8	–	–	5	12
Oberman 1964[25]	15	12	3	24–72	50	3	20
Skolnik et al 1966[16]	33	26	7	25–72	55	5	15
Fechner & Alford 1968[13]	14	12	2	35–71	57	1	7
Cummings & Goodman 1970[26]	29	18	11	12–71	–	3	10
Osborn 1970[27]	168	140	28	–	50	2	<2
Hyams 1971[11]	149	125	24	11–80	35	19	13
Trible & Lekagul 1971[17]	30	22	8	23–72	49	3	10
Buchanan & Slavin 1972[19]	11	11	0	38–74	53	0	0
Snyder & Perzin 1972[12]	39	30	9	–	–	8	21
Clairmont et al 1975[29]	13	12	1	22–74	49	0	0
Vrabec 1975[22]	24	16	8	35–76	–	3	13
Lasser et al 1976[30]	17	14	3	38–80	60	4	24
Ridolphi et al 1977[8]	30	27	3	13–75	–	1	3
Suh et al 1977[31]	57	47	10	–	–	4	7
Yamaguchi et al 1978[24]	15	–	–	27–62	52	8	53
Calcaterra et al 1980[28]	34	Ratio	3:1	–	47	3	9
Momose et al 1980[32]	115	Ratio	3:1	12–85	–	7	6
Myers et al 1981[33]	19	17	2	25–70	50	6	32
Lawson et al 1983[34]	31	24	7	27–80	56	1	3
Majumdar & Beck 1984[21]	43	32	11	32–76	–	5	12
Woodson et al 1985[35]	90	73	17	–	57	4	4
Segal et al 1986[36]	30	20	10	14–81	51	3	10
Weissler et al 1986[23]	223	159	64	6–87	50	11	5
l 1989[14]	87	71	16	15–80	51	5	6
Myers et al 1990[15]	33	26	7	25–78	66	7	21

regarded as co-incidental rather than precursors of the condition and similarly chronic sinusitis cannot be implicated in its development.

Interest has naturally centred on a possible viral origin for these lesions. Unlike their laryngeal counterparts which occur predominantly in the young, nasal papillomas affect an older age group and no ultrastructural evidence has been found of viral particles[43,44] though Jahnke did find intranuclear particles. However, using the techniques of southern blot molecular hybridization, Respler et al reported the presence of human papilloma virus DNA identical to, or closely related to, human papilloma virus Type II in two cases of nasal inverted papilloma.[45] A recent paper from the MD Anderson reported the presence of human papilloma virus DNA in 76% of 21 patients using in-situ hybridization techniques, with the evidence pointing most strongly to HPV-11.[46]

Clinical features

The clinical manifestations are obviously related to the size and site of the lesion and the length of history can vary from 2 weeks to 20 years. The commonest complaint is unilateral nasal obstruction (75%) though epistaxis frequently occurs from the septal lesions (33%). These are accompanied by rhinorrhoea, mucopurulent postnasal drip and sometimes frontal headache and facial pain. A mass may be seen in the nasal cavity or postnasal space.

Lesions obstructing the frontonasal recess may be associated with a fronto-ethmoidal mucocoele and the more aggressive lesions can produce significant bone destruction and facial deformity with epiphora, proptosis and diplopia resulting from orbital invasion. Indeed, actual transgression of the orbital periosteum has occurred in one of our own patients (Fig. 5.3).

A 55-year-old woman presented with unilateral nasal obstruction. She had a nasal polyp removed 6 years previously but no histology was available. On examination there was a polyp in the right middle meatus and radiological evidence of a fronto-ethmoidal mucocoele. An external fronto-ethmoidectomy was performed via a modified Lynch–Howarth incision and in addition to the mucocoele, a fleshy tumour was found in the middle meatus, extending into the frontonasal recess which was cleared. This proved to be an inverted papilloma. Subsequently, local recurrences occurred after 2, 7 and 10 years, each being removed by local intranasal excision. One year later a lateral rhinotomy was performed which revealed tumour extensively infiltrating adjacent frontal bone with a marked sclerotic reaction, confirming CT scan appearances. A wide clearance was performed and there is no obvious recurrence at 1 year follow-up.

Although the site of the disease is unusual, this case history typifies the frequent local recurrence that occurs in many cases, and which can happen despite reasonable resection once the tumour is established in the more aggressive cases. It is likely that further local recurrence will occur in this patient though there has never been any histological suggestion of malignant transformation.

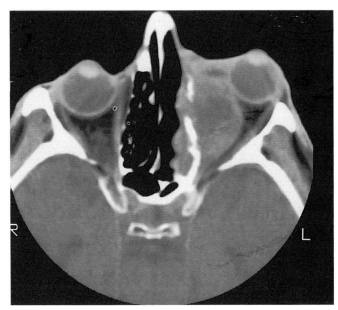

Fig. 5.3   Axial CT scan showing extensive recurrent inverted papilloma which was found to have breached the orbital periosteum.

Radiology (Figs 5.4 and 5.5)

The radiological findings in a personal series of 60 patients[47] confirms those reported by other authors.[17,22,28,32–34,48] On plain sinus X-rays the appearances are often non-specific and may even be apparently normal. There may simply be mucosal thickening of the maxillary antrum (30%), a mass in the nasal cavity (48%) and/or unilateral opacification of the paranasal sinuses.

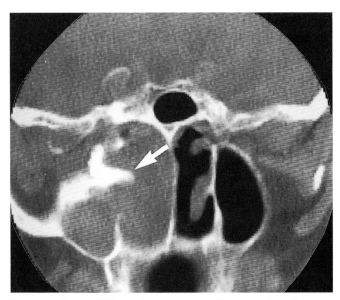

Fig. 5.4   Coronal CT scan showing an extensive inverted papilloma associated with sclerosis and deformation of the posterior maxillary antrum (arrow) (Lloyd 1988[53]).

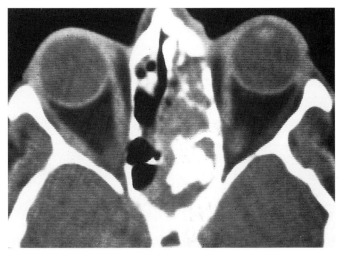

Fig. 5.5   Axial CT scan showing plaques of calcification in an inverted papilloma of the ethmoids (Lloyd 1988[53]).

The maxillary antrum is most commonly affected (53%), though the ethmoids (27%), frontal (10%) and occasionally sphenoid sinuses may also be involved radiologically. The soft tissue mass may be seen in the postnasal space (18%) on lateral views.

The ability of the tumour to destroy bone even in the absence of malignant change and its ability to invaginate between bony trabeculae is best demonstrated on CT scanning. The presence of a mass eroding the middle meatus and invading adjacent sinuses can be seen. The septal skeleton is more usually bowed away from the lesion and may be intact even when the tumour arises primarily from septal mucosa though spread to the opposite nasal cavity by septal destruction has been described.[16,23]

In addition to bone destruction, two features characteristic of this lesion can be seen on CT scanning. Areas of calcification can be seen within the tumour mass and adjacent sinus walls show sclerosis and deformation. The more aggressive lesions have been shown extending into the pterygoid region, infratemporal fossa, orbit and anterior cranial fossa. Although benign papillomas are capable of such behaviour, the possibility of an underlying malignancy in these cases must be suspected and managed appropriately.

Macroscopic and microscopic appearance

The lesions are bulky, polypoid and rubbery. Everted lesions may have a broad base compared with a narrower stalk in the inverted lesion though it is not always possible to define this. The colour varies from grey–pink to fleshy red and the inverted lesions are often quite vascular. It is said that inverted lesions are also more translucent and are frequently mistaken for 'ordinary' polyps either ethmoidal or antrochoanal. Once again this emphasizes the importance of submitting all tissue to histological examination. The association with previous polyps may simply reflect a failure to have diagnosed the condition earlier.[17]

Microscopic appearance

The epithelial component is either squamous or columnar or a combination of both with a variable amount of mucous cells. The mesenchymal stroma can be myxomatous or have a distinctive vascular core which is more often seen in the everted septal lesions. In either case the inflammatory infiltrate is small. The appearances are in keeping with their names. Everted papillomas are exophytic with fronded surface proliferations compared to the characteristic invaginations of inverted papillomas. The invaginations are lined by squamous and ciliated columnar cells, and a high glycogen content may be found in the squamous element. Invaginations of tumour may be found between the trabeculae of bone. Multiple cystic mucus-containing spaces are present and in places intercellular bridges or prickles may be found indicating the epidermoid origins. However, the presence of surface keratin suggests the presence of a concomitant squamous cell carcinoma or a verrucous carcinoma rather than a papilloma.

The cylindric cell subgroup is composed of proliferations of multilayered columnar cells in everted fronds. The cilia are atrophic and both inverted and exophytic components may be seen.

Natural history

Two characteristics of this lesion have been extensively discussed, those of recurrence and malignant transformation.

Recurrence

All three forms of the sinonasal papilloma can recur, though the cylindric cell and everted form have a much reduced tendency to do so (0–20%). Rates of up to 74% have been quoted for inverted papilloma though it has been suggested that 'persistence' would be a better term as this is directly related to the adequacy of surgical excision. A comparison of recurrences rates in series where conservative or radical surgery have been performed confirms this (Table 5.2). The only anomalous results found by Lawson et al[14] and more recently by Myers et al[15] reflect the selection of patients with very localized disease by CT scanning. Multiple recurrences are common, up to seven or more in some series[17] and the time interval of recurrence varies from 10 weeks to 24 years, though most occur within the first 2 years.

The ability of the lesion to spread, the possibility of multicentric origin and the presence of squamous metaplasia in adjacent mucosa all serve to compromise excisional margins. Although specific sites do not seem more prone to recurrence per se, the more inaccessible areas such as frontonasal recess, lacrimal fossa, infraorbital region of the maxilla and horizontal fronto-ethmoidal complex may be less adequately cleared.

Until recently, histological correlation with recurrence had not been found[22] but work on material at the Institute of Laryngology and Otology, London (ILO) suggested a relationship to the presence of mitoses within the tumour, particularly if these were close to the epithe-

Table 5.2 Inverted papilloma: association with recurrence in major series

	Patients total no.	Overall		Recurrence After limited surgery		After radical surgery	
		No.	%	No.	%	No.	%
Lampertico et al 1963[10]	19	9	47				
Norris 1963[9]	29	8	28	8/29	28		
Brown 1964[18]	30	6	46				
Oberman 1964[25]	15	6/13	40				
Fechner & Alford 1968[13]	14	5/10	50	5/10	50		
Cummings & Goodman 1970[26]	29	18	62	16/22	73	1/7	13
Osborn 1970[27]	168	40	24				
Hyams 1971[11]	149	67	45				
Trible & Lekagul 1971[17]	30	19	63	17/24	71	2/6	33
Snyder & Perzin 1972[12]	39	26/35	74	26/35	74		
Lasser et al 1976[30]	17	2	12				
Ridolphi ct al 1977[8]	30	20	67				
Suh et al 1977[31]	57	14/51	27	10/21	45	4/30	13
Calcaterra et al 1980[28]	51	25/51	49	24/32	75	1/19	6
Lawson et al 1983[34]	31	1	3	0/8	0	1/23	4
Scgal et al 1986[36]	30	15	50	14/20	70	1/10	10
Weissler et al 1986[23]	223	103	46	79/112	71	37/126	29
Lawson et al 1989[14]	87	8	9	1/10	10	7/75	9
Myers et al 1990[15]	26	1	4	0/3	0	1/23	4

lial surface.[35] The assessment of histology and recurrence was done independently. Absence of mitoses or rare mitotic figures in each high power field was associated with a 37% recurrence rate, two mitoses per high power field was associated with an 80% recurrence rate and this increased to 87% if there were more than two mitoses in each area examined. This could be utilized when deciding on clinical management.

Malignant transformation

The vexed question of malignant transformation in sinonasal papillomas runs throughout the literature. Neither everted nor cylindric papillomas are usually implicated but the rate for inverted papillomas varies from 0–53% in the literature (Table 5.1) and requires further examination.

Batsakis[7] has defined three circumstances in which this may occur:

1. A carcinoma and a papilloma occur within the same anatomical region but there is no evidence that the papilloma gave origin to the carcinoma
2. A papilloma is found with evidence of in situ or invasive carcinomatous change
3. A papilloma does not recur after treatment but some time later is succeeded by a carcinoma in the same region.

Of these (1) and (3) are considered the most common[6] with true malignant transformation put at less than 2%. In 86 cases at the ILO, no evidence of transformation could be found though four cases of concomitant malignancy occurred.[35] The high figures quoted in some of the earlier series probably reflect problems of initial diagnosis. However, the importance of careful histological examination of all tissue, in particular 'normal' adjacent mucosa should be stressed.

It follows that metastases do not occur, by definition, with benign papillomas.

Differential diagnosis

Clearly frank squamous cell carcinoma and verrucous carcinoma can be mistaken for benign papillomas and may be the cause of confusion in some early series. Squamous metaplasia can occur in ethmoidal polyps but this should never be greater than 12 layers in thickness or there should not be any extensive invagination of the epithelium.

The cylindric cell papilloma variant with many microcysts may be confused with rhinosporidiosis. However, the cysts are always subepithelial in the latter condition compared to the epithelial position of the cysts in the papilloma. More commonly in these circumstances a papillary adenocarcinoma may be misdiagnosed.

Radiologically the changes may suggest the soft tissue mass and opacification of ethmoidal or an antrochoanal polyp, the bone destruction of malignancy, the calcification of chondrosarcoma or fungal sinusitis or the sclerosis of chronic sinusitis.

Treatment (Table 5.2)

All authors are agreed on the role of primary surgery in this condition. The capacity for local aggression, high recurrence rate, multicentricity and suggested association with malignancy, albeit low, would support the most complete surgical excision with the least morbidity. Lesions treated by intranasal excision such as polypectomy, turbinectomy, intranasal and transantral ethmoidectomy have a high incidence of recurrence, around 75%, but these may constitute a group in whom the diagnosis was initially unsuspected. It may be that if subsequent CT scanning demonstrates a limited lesion (Fig. 5.6), or histological assessment of mitoses suggests a less aggressive tumour,[35] a 'wait-and-see' policy may be adopted particularly if supported by other factors such as the age and health of the individual. Such management has been reported by Lawson et al[34] as successful in 8 cases with 6 months to 5 years follow-up and intranasal endoscopic clearance has been advocated for the more limited and accessible lesions. However, most cases are more extensive and aggressive, as confirmed by histology and radiology, and radical surgery is indicated which is best achieved by a midfacial degloving or lateral rhinotomy approach which gives full access to the nasal cavity and paranasal sinuses.[49,50] Recurrence rates of between 0 and 33% have been reported with this technique and it is in many ways superior to conventional Caldwell–Luc and

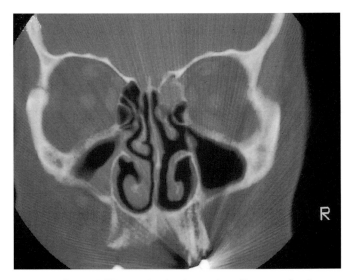

Fig. 5.6 Coronal CT scan showing inverted papilloma confined to a right anterior superior ethmoidal cell.

external fronto-ethmoidectomy procedures where at least 50% recurrence rates may be anticipated.

In the presence of extensive lesions particularly with the suggestion of in situ change, the Weber–Fergusson approach,[37] sub-total maxillectomy and craniofacial resection[51] have been undertaken though a midfacial degloving approach would encompass all but the most extensive antro-ethmoidal lesions.

Radiotherapy is of no value in this benign condition, which is not radiosensitive. Malignant transformation may be induced[52] or osteoradionecrosis produced. Chemotherapy has also been contraindicated though the

recent evidence of a viral origin[46] for the lesions has led to suggestions that interferon may have a role in the most aggressive lesions.

Prognosis

With adequate surgical excision, the prognosis for this condition is excellent but if it is not dealt with adequately, frequent recurrence can be anticipated and once bone infiltration has occurred, eradication can be extremely difficult.

REFERENCES

1. Kramer 1847 Quoted in Kramer R, Som M L 1935 True papillomas of the nasal cavity. Archives of Otolaryngology 22: 22–43
2. Ward N 1854 Follicular tumour involving nasal bones, nasal processes of superior maxillary bone and septum of nose. Removal, death from pneumonia, autopsy. Lancet 2: 460
3. Billroth T 1855 Ueber dem Bau des Schleimpolyp. Reimer, Berlin p 11
4. Hoppmann C M 1883 Die Papillaren Geschwulste der Nasenschleimhaut. Virchows Archiv fur Pathologie und Anatomie 93: 213–258
5. Ringetz N 1938 Pathology of malignant tumours arising in the nasal and paranasal cavities and maxilla. Acta Otolaryngologica Supplement 27: 31–42
6. Friedmann I, Osborn D A 1982 Pathology of granulomas and neoplasms of the nose and paranasal sinuses. Churchill Livingstone, Edinburgh, pp 105–113
7. Batsakis J G 1980 The pathology of head and neck tumors: nasal cavity and paranasal sinuses. Part 5. Head and Neck Surgery 2: 410–419
8. Ridolphi R L, Lieberman P H, Erlandson R A, Moore O S 1977 Schneiderian papillomas: a clinicopathological study of 30 cases. American Journal of Surgical Pathology 1: 43–53
9. Norris H J 1963 Papillary lesions of the nasal cavity and paranasal sinuses. Part II: Inverting papillomas. A study of 29 cases. Laryngoscope 73: 7–17
10. Lampertico P, Russell W O, MacComb W S 1963 Squamous papilloma of upper respiratory epithelium. Acta Pathologica 75: 293–302
11. Hyams V J 1971 Papillomas of the nasal cavity and paranasal sinuses. A clinicopathological study of 315 cases. Annals of Otology, Rhinology and Laryngology 80: 192–206
12. Snyder R N, Perzin K H 1972 Papillomatosis of nasal cavity and paranasal sinuses (inverted papilloma, squamous papilloma). Cancer 30: 668–690
13. Fechner R E, Alford D O 1968 Inverted papilloma and squamous carcinoma. Archives of Otolaryngology 88: 73–78
14. Lawson W, Le Benger J, Som P, Bernard P J, Biller H F 1989 Inverted papilloma: an analysis of 87 cases. Laryngoscope 99: 1117–1124
15. Myers E N, Fernau J L, Johnson J T, Tabet J C, Barnes L 1990 Management of inverted papilloma. Laryngoscope 100: 481–490
16. Skolnik E M, Loewy A, Friedman J E 1966 Inverted papilloma of the nasal cavity. Archives of Otolaryngology 84: 83–89
17. Trible W M, Lekagul S 1971 Inverting papilloma of the nose and paranasal sinuses: report of 30 cases. Laryngoscope 81: 663–668
18. Brown B 1964 The papillomatous tumours of the nose. Journal of Laryngology and Otology 78: 889–905
19. Buchanan G, Slavin G 1972 Tumours of the nose and sinuses. A clinico-pathological study. Journal of Laryngology and Otology 86: 685–696

20. Kelly J H, Joseph M, Carroll E, Goodman M L, Pilch B Z, Levinson R M, Strome M 1980 Inverted papilloma of the nasal septum. Archives of Otolaryngology 106: 767–771
21. Majumdar B, Beck S 1984 Inverted papilloma of the nose. Journal of Laryngology and Otology 98: 467–470
22. Vrabec D P 1975 The inverted Scheiderian papilloma: A clinical and pathological study. Laryngoscope 85: 186–220
23. Weissler M C, Montgomery W W, Turner P A, Montgomery S K, Joseph M P 1986 Inverted papilloma. Annals of Otology, Rhinology and Laryngology 95: 215–221
24. Yamaguchi K T, Shapshay S M, Incze J S, Vaughan C W, Strong M S 1978 Inverted papilloma and squamous cell carcinoma. Journal of Otolaryngology 8: 171–178
25. Oberman H A 1964 Papillomas of the nose and paranasal sinuses. American Journal of Clinical Pathology 42: 245–258
26. Cummings C W, Goodman M L 1970 Inverted papillomas of the nose and paranasal sinuses. Archives of Otolarygology 92: 445–449
27. Osborn D A 1970 Nature and behaviour of transitional tumors in the upper respiratory tract. Cancer 25: 50–60
28. Calcaterra T C, Thompson J W, Paglia D E 1980 Inverting papillomas of the nose and paranasal sinuses. Laryngoscope 90: 53–60
29. Clairmont A A, Wright R E, Rooker D T, Butz W C 1975 Papillomas of the nasal and paranasal cavities. South Medical Journal 68: 41–45
30. Lasser A, Rothfeld P R, Shapiro R S 1976 Epithelial papilloma and squamous cell carcinoma of the nasal cavity and paranasal sinuses. Cancer 38: 2503–2510
31. Suh K W, Facer G W, Devine K D, Weiland L H, Zujko R D 1977 Inverting papilloma of the nose and paranasal sinuses. Laryngoscope 87: 35–46
32. Momose J K, Weber A L, Goodman M, MacMillan A S, Roberson G H 1980 Radiological aspects of inverted papilloma. Radiology 134: 73–79
33. Myers E N, Schramm V L, Barnes E L 1981 Management of inverted papilloma of the nose and paranasal sinuses. Laryngoscope 91: 2071–2084
34. Lawson W, Biller H F, Jacobson A, Som P 1983 The role of conservative surgery in the management of inverted papilloma. Laryngoscope 93:148–155
35. Woodson G E, Robbins T, Michaels L 1985 Inverted papilloma. Considerations in treatment. Archives of Otolaryngology 111: 806–811
36. Segal K, Atar E, Mor C, Har-El G, Sidi J 1986 Inverting papilloma of the nose and paranasal sinuses. Laryngoscope 96: 394–398
37. Ho K H 1988 Inverted papilloma – a modified surgical approach to reconstruction of the palate. British Journal of Oral and Maxillofacial Surgery 26: 115–119
38. Astor F C, Donegan J O, Gluckman J L 1985 Unusual anatomic presentations of inverting papilloma. Head and Neck Surgery 7: 243–245

39. Radcliffe A 1953 Transitional cell papilloma of the posterior pharyngeal wall. Journal of Laryngology and Otology 67: 682
40. Wolff A P, Ossoff R H, Clemis J D 1980 Four unusual neoplasms of the nasopharynx. Otolaryngology, Head and Neck Surgery 88: 753–759
41. Chatterji P, Friedmann I, Soni N K, Solanki R L 1982 Bilateral transitional-type inverted papilloma of the nose and paranasal sinuses. Journal of Laryngology and Otology 96: 281–287
42. Herrold K M 1964 Epithelial papillomas of the nasal cavity. Archives of Pathology 78: 189–195
43. Gaito R A, Gaylord W H, Hilding D A 1965 Ultrastructure of a human nasal papilloma. Laryngoscope 75: 144–152
44. Jahnke V 1971 The fine structure of intranasal papillomas. Annals of Otology, Rhinology and Laryngology 80: 78–81
45. Respler D S, Johm A, Pater A 1987 Isolation and characterisation of papilloma virus DNA from nasal inverting (Schneiderian) papillomas. Annals of Otology, Rhinology and Laryngology 2: 170–173
46. Weber R S, Shillitoe E J, Robbins K T, Luna M A, Batsakis J G, Donovan D T, Adler-Storthz K 1988 Prevalence of human papilloma virus in inverted nasal papillomas. Archives of Otolaryngology, Head and Neck Surgery 114: 23–26
47. Lund V J, Lloyd G 1984 Radiological changes associated with inverted papilloma of the nose and paranasal sinuses. British Journal of Radiology 57: 455–461
48. Rothfeld P, Shapiro R, Lasser A, Kent D 1977 Epithelial (inverted) papilloma – a correlated radiological, histological study. Clinical Radiology 28: 539–544
49. Price J C, Holliday M J, Johns M E 1988 The versatile mid-facial degloving approach. Laryngoscope 98: 291–295
50. Sacks M E, Conley J, Rabuzzi D D 1984 Degloving approach for total excision of inverted papilloma. Laryngoscope 94: 1595–1598
51. Lund V J, Harrison D F N 1988 Craniofacial resection for tumours of the nasal cavity and paranasal sinuses. American Journal of Surgery 156: 187–190
52. Mabery T E, Devine K D, Harrison E G 1965 The problem of malignant transformation in a nasal papilloma. Archives of Otolaryngology 82: 296–300
53. Lloyd G A S 1988 Diagnostic imaging of the nose and paranasal sinuses. Springer Verlag, Berlin

6. Squamous cell carcinoma

The respiratory mucosa of the nasal cavity and paranasal sinuses gives rise to two basic types of epithelial neoplasms, those emanating from metaplastic epithelium (squamous carcinoma) and those originating from mucous glands. The latter comprise only a small percentage of primary tumours in this region and the term 'mucous-gland' tumour is used generically for all non-squamous cell epithelial neoplasms.[1]

The tendency for squamous cell carcinoma formation probably lies in the ultrastructural finding that the basal cells of respiratory mucosa contain more tonofilaments than the remainder of the epithelial cells, and this feature is compatible with the intrinsic potential of these cells to undergo malignant change.[2]

Squamous cell carcinoma within the nose and sinuses shows the same range of histological appearances as elsewhere in the body, being graded according to the degree of differentiation and mitotic activity. This is of little clinical significance since grading is essentially subjective and influenced by variations in sampling. Over 80% are well or moderately well differentiated with occasional verrucous changes.[3a] Very poorly differentiated tumours may occur which present problems in differential diagnosis, particularly with olfactory neuroblastoma or amelanotic melanoma. They carry a poor prognosis although a number of reported cases have been found on immunohistochemistry to have been misdiagnosed.[4]

There are two variants of squamous carcinoma found within the nose and paranasal sinuses which are more commonly seen in other parts of the respiratory tract, particularly the larynx. Verrucous carcinoma is a 'warty' variant being extremely well differentiated with little atypia. Invasion is absent and, although uncommon, this tumour has been reported on the nasal septum and within the maxillary antrum.[5–7] The other variant is the spindle cell carcinoma representing an extreme aspect of differentiation. Histologically, it is bimorphic with one identifiable carcinomatous component and an underlying spindle cell component, which is often pleomorphic resembling a fibrosarcoma. Within the upper jaw they are rare, and Michaels believes that diagnosis is dependent on the presence of invasion or in situ carcinoma as well as the undifferentiated malignant spindle cell tissue.[8]

Aetiology[9]

Although attracting great interest, studies concerning aetiological and epidemiological factors related to nasal and paranasal carcinomata have been bedevilled by difficulties inherent in the analysis of pooled data. Under the International Classification of Disease, Rubric ICD 160 includes not only the nose, nasal cavity and accessory sinuses but also the middle ear.[10] Whilst the last category does not constitute a large number of cases, it does introduce potential errors into subsequent statistics.

In general terms aetiological factors can be considered as environmentally related, occupational or non-occupational, or related to existing pathological changes which may predispose or progress to malignancy. Environmental agents may affect the upper jaw by three routes:

1. Airborne, direct inhalation of particles whose effect depends upon size, density and the host's breathing pattern[11]
2. Absorption, such as the effect of radium adsorbed from the oral mucosa into the facial bones[12]
3. Parental, by experimental administration of toxins such as dioxane, nitrosamines or nickel compounds.[13]

Occupational risks

Changes in working practice and working conditions together with a mobile population make the effects of occupational risks difficult to unravel, particularly when associated with lengthy induction times. The association between adenocarcinoma of the ethmoid and the woodworking trade was unsuspected until 1965 in the United Kingdom,[14,15] whilst the effects of softwood in the development of maxillary sinus cancer was only reported in 1983.[13,16,17] It is surprising that in Japan, where maxillary sinus carcinoma has an unusually high incidence there appears to be little relationship with their traditional wood-working industry.[18]

The leather and shoe industry has also been the subject of extensive epidemiological study in relation to sinonasal squamous cell carcinoma and adenocarcinoma, with some suggestion of an increased incidence amongst its workers. However, three occupations with a proven linkage with carcinoma in the upper jaw are radium dial painting, mustard gas production and nickel refining.[19] The first two are now obsolete but a high relative risk with exposure as short as 6 months has been found in workers in the sintering and roasting processes in the nickel industry although the risk was found to increase with age and duration of exposure.[20,21]

The literature also contains other evidence of occupational risks for nose and sinus malignancy relating to asbestos exposure[22] and the baking industry[23] although the number of substantiated cases remains small.

Non-occupational risks

Some doubt remains as to the role that smoking plays in the production of nasal and paranasal cancer. Within the wood-working industry safety precautions minimize smoking at work but not at home! In 1989 Shimizu et al exonerated both passive and active smoking but a study in The Netherlands suggested a relative risk of 3:1 in the development of sinonasal cancer from this cause.[24,25] Within South Africa the indigenous black population use home-made snuff for their tribal ceremonies and there is evidence that this is associated with their high incidence of advanced antro-ethmoid cancer, possibly due to the additional presence of trace elements such as nickel and chromium together with known carcinogens.[26,27] Acherson et al also associated snuff taking in their classic epidemiological studies of sinonasal cancer in the boot and shoe industry.[28] The direct effect of irradiation in the development of squamous carcinoma has been documented by Roush[23] and until 1954 thorium dioxide (Thorotrast) was used as a radiological contrast agent being injected directly into the maxillary antrum. Peak radioactivity is not achieved with this agent until 15 years and a direct association with subsequent sinus cancer was reported by Rankow et al in 1974.[29]

The relationship between chronic infection and upper jaw malignancy remains uncertain since the former is commonplace and the latter rare. However, in Japan where sinus cancer is more frequent, Shimizu et al have reported a relative risk of 2:3 for squamous cell carcinoma of the maxillary antrum[25] in contradistinction to other reports from the same country.[30] One possible explanation for this disparity may be variations in the use of nasal preparations, for Strader et al in 1988 reported that individuals using nasal drops regularly were 3.5 times more likely to develop upper jaw cancer than non-users.[31]

Except when a confirmed association with an industrial hazard is found aetiological factors are usually difficult to identify for most patients with carcinomas arising within the nasal cavity and paranasal sinuses. Lund carried out a detailed survey of 50 surviving patients from a total cohort of 350 treated in one institution finding evidence of carcinogen contact in more than 20%.[9] However, retrospective studies are reliant upon memory and knowledge, defining 'significant exposure' is fraught with potential errors although it does provide possible avenues for further prospective enquiries.

Incidence

The comprehensive nature of the terms 'nose and paranasal sinuses', which also includes neoplasms of varying biological nature and sites of origin, has led to doubtful validity of much published data relating to tumours in this region. Many papers have been based upon small numbers of patients or collected from numerous institutions taking little note of variations in treatment modalities or policies.

Robin et al[32] have emphasized the importance of accurately studying the natural history of individual neoplasms and published their own data collected from registrations of carcinomata involving the nasal cavity and paranasal sinuses in the Birmingham Regional Cancer Registry from 1957–1972 inclusive. These figures are based on a local population within the United Kingdom of about 5 million with a registration rate of at least 95%. A total of 624 patients were studied and although larger numbers have been recorded by Lewis & Castrol[33] and Lederman,[34] Robin et al suggest that their own data based upon a specific population present a more accurate picture of incidence rates than figures emanating from specialized referral centres.

Distinction must be drawn between true incidence rates and the number of patients being seen since most cases are diagnosed between the ages of 55 and 80 years. More detailed analysis however, shows that this is not a true reflection of the actual incidence rate or 'risk' of the disease. Robin et al tabled the number of patients and incidence rate per 100 000 population for age groups 0–90+ years, and then calculated the incidence rates using the population at risk.[32] Within the younger age groups, cancer was rare but gradually increased until the age of 85 when the rate decreased. Most publications quote the incidence figures for nasal and paranasal cancer as 0.9 (male) and 0.7 (female) per 100 000 population at risk.[35,36] The data published by Robin et al show that after the age of 55 years the rate continues to rise to a peak of 5.85 per 100 000 at the age of 80 years. Though a slightly lower rate follows this peak in males it continues in women possibly because of an increased expectation of life.

Overall, the male to female ratio for squamous cell carcinoma is quoted as 1.5:1 although within the age range of 40 to 90 years of age this ratio is closer to 2:1. There is also a site variation with 'vestibular' carcinoma almost exclusively a male disease. Within the nasal cavity squamous carcinoma is commoner in women as are all anaplastic carcinomas.

Less than 1% of all cancer deaths within the USA between 1950 and 1969 were attributed to sinonasal carcinomata.[37] A similar picture is found within the United Kingdom for the years 1951–1980.[38] Although an incidence figure of about 1 per 100 000 population per year adjusted for age and sex is quoted for many other countries, data from the International Agency for Research shows a considerable ethnic variation. Japan has a figure of 2.6 per 100 000 for men and a similar rate is given for the black population of Nigeria and Jamaica.[36]

Site

The nasal vestibule is defined as the recess immediately within the nostril, bounded by the medial and lateral crura of the alar cartilages, extending to the apex of the nose and limited medially by the nasal septum. The walls are covered by hair-bearing skin and mucous membrane and squamous cell carcinoma located to this area represent about 7% of most sinonasal neoplasms.[39] A further 12% are found on the nasal septum or the remainder of the nasal cavity excluding the lateral nasal wall. Most carcinomata in this region are found within the maxillary sinus (between 60% and 90%) although the advanced stage at diagnosis together with the intimate relationship of the ethmoid and maxillary sinuses, makes accurate delineation of the site of origin, in many cases, difficult to verify.

The degree of lateralization noted in tumours of many bilaterally placed organs, such as the kidney or lung, is usually no greater than 1.2:1. However, a marked left-sided dominance has been found in ethmoidal carcinomata by Robin & Shortridge who attributed this to septal deviation and related deposition of carcinogens on the lateral nasal wall.[40] Morton & Sellars reviewed 330 patients with nasal and paranasal cancer, excluding mesenchymal neoplasms, and confirmed a left-sided dominance for both antral and ethmoidal lesions in their white patients.[41] Lateralization was not present in a much larger group of black patients and the inclusion of maxillary antral tumours was attributed to the difficulty of identifying site of origin in advanced tumours. No data regarding septal deviation was included in this paper and Hopkin et al found no evidence of asymmetry in their review which however, failed to separate tumours by site or histology.[42]

If disturbance of air flow through one side of the nose predisposes the deposition of carcinogenic particles in the region of the ethmoidal sinuses or on the septum, then lateralization might be found in occupations such as the wood-working, leather and boot industries. Identification of high-risk individuals, who could be improved by septal correction, would then be worthwhile.

NASAL VESTIBULAR CARCINOMA

Definition

An area immediately above the nares, bounded laterally by the alar cartilages and medially by the lower part of the nasal septum.[43]

Synonym

Anterior intranasal carcinoma.[39]

Incidence

This is an uncommon, often misdiagnosed malignancy which is frequently reported in the skin literature or amongst neoplasms of the nasal cavity despite its distinct natural history and biological behaviour. Barzan et al[44] whilst reporting 12 cases of their own, tabulated an account of 472 cases taken from the literature between 1967 and 1990, the largest series being that of Vendelbo et al which contained 66 patients.[45] Squamous cell carcinoma is the most frequent neoplasm in this area and must be separated from carcinomas originating in the adjoining nasal mucosa as well as malignant melanoma and basal cell carcinomata. Clear distinction from the commoner nasal lesions is not always possible with extensive tumours although Bodit et al say that carcinomas restricted to the vestibule are far less common than on the nasal septum or nasal floor.[46]

Age, sex, ethnic variation

There is a clear male predominance with 90% occurring in patients over the age of 50 years most of whom are white and smoke.[47] Prolonged exposure to sunlight or dust have been cited as possible aetiological factors in some reports as have enthusiastic smoking and drinking.[44]

Clinical features (Figs 6.1 and 6. 2)

Because of their unique location, vestibular carcinomas present specific problems in diagnosis and treatment. Crusting, painful ulceration with minimal bleeding rarely attracts attention until involvement of the adjoining nasal septum, skin or cartilage occurs. Local invasion of the upper lip allows access to rich lymphatic channels with spread to the facial, submandibular, submental, parotid and cervical lymph nodes. Such metastases can be homo-

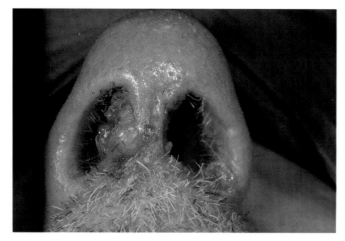

Fig. 6.1 Squamous cell carcinoma affecting the nasal columella.

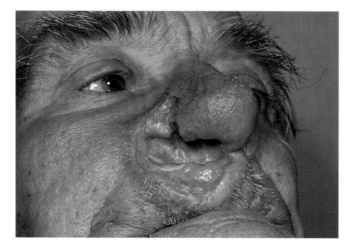

Fig. 6.2 Extensive nasal vestibular squamous cell carcinoma ulcerating into surrounding areas

lateral, contralateral or bilateral although this appears to be unusual at initial presentation.

The actual location is sometimes difficult to specify because the lesion has filled the nasal vestibule making the extent of the tumour within the nasal cavity impossible to determine with accuracy. There is no generally accepted classification of these tumours although some authors divide patients into early lesions, confined to the vestibule, and late lesions with nodes or bone involvement. Wang has proposed a system in which patients are grouped according to the extent of their disease.[47]

T1.   The lesion is limited to the nasal vestibule, is relatively superficial and involves one or more sites within the nasal cavity.

T2.   The lesion has extended to involve the upper lip, nasal skin or nasolabial fold but without fixation to underlying bone.

T3.   Large tumours with extension to the hard palate, most of the upper lip, alveolar, buccal sulcus, turbinates, maxillary sinus or bone involvement.

Lymph node metastases were classified according to accepted International systems.

Vendelbo et al in 1984[45] assessed the prognostic significance of this classification finding it acceptable although admitting that it was often difficult to determine from many of the publications the frequency of the more favourable 'early' lesions. Kagan et al[43] reported 90%, Goepfert et al[48] 80%, Shiffman[39] 75% whilst Barzan et al[44] classified only 50% as T1N0. The last found a delay in diagnosis of 17 months (range 1–24 months) in their 12 patients which probably explained a higher incidence of larger tumours in their series.

Macroscopic and microscopic appearance

The gross appearance is usually an irregular, raised, granular and often ulcerated plaque. Most are well differentiated squamous cell carcinomas although some confusion with dysplastic changes in a benign squamous papilloma must be recognized, irregularity of both rete pegs and papillary formation favouring malignant change. Anaplastic, poorly differentiated squamous cell carcinoma may constitute a diagnostic dilemma and carries an extremely poor prognosis.[49]

Verrucous carcinoma is a 'warty' variant of squamous cell carcinoma characterized by an exophytic growth of extremely well-differentiated squamous epithelium with little cellular atypia. Invasion is not a feature but, if present, the tumour should then be classified as a normal well-differentiated squamous carcinoma.[3b]

The other variant is the spindle cell carcinoma more commonly found in other parts of the upper respiratory tract. This represents the extreme aspect of differentiation with both identifiable carcinoma and an underlying spindle cell component. More usually found within the maxillary antrum producing bone erosion, electron microscopy shows cells of a mesenchymal appearance which may be confused with fibrosarcoma.[8]

Natural history

Although small lesions respond to treatment, extension into surrounding tissue rapidly occurs without necessarily producing excessive symptoms. Many authors report a 10% incidence of multiple malignancies associated with primary vestibular carcinomas, possibly as a result of smoking and drinking.[39,43,50] However, metastasis to the regional lymph nodes remains a major cause of failure to cure and although uncommon at initial presentation, is associated with extension into the lip, septum or floor of the nasal cavity. Incidence rates vary considerably with Wong et al[51] quoting 10%, De Jong et al[52] 23%, Goepfert et al[48] 30% and Kagan et al[43] reporting no instances of nodal disease in their 42 patients, 90% of whom had early lesions.

Differential diagnosis

The only conditions likely to cause difficulties in diagnosis are amelanotic melanoma, basal cell carcinoma, benign squamous papillomata and keratoacanthoma.

Treatment

The small number of patients reported with adequate details of site of origin, e.g. floor, lateral or medial aspect, follow-up and confirmation of clear excisional margins, makes definitive conclusions regarding the best treatment policies unattainable.

Kagan et al[43] summarize the present position when advocating surgical excision or radiotherapy for the early tumours. Surgery consisted of simple excision including margins of surrounding normal tissue or partial rhinotomy in 86% of their patients and 14% needing total rhinectomy. Radiotherapy consisted of 6000 to 7000 rad given over 7–8 weeks by megavoltage. Since 'early' lesions include quite extensive tumours in Wang's classification[47] most oncologists recommend either primary radiotherapy or combination with local excision as shown in Table 6.1, since local recurrence following irradiation can be salvaged by surgery whereas surgical failures do less well with irradiation.[43] Mak et al reported 46 patients treated solely by radiotherapy with 33% developing a local recurrence, possibly because of dosages less than 5400 rad. Eight of these 15 patients (53%) were salvaged by subsequent surgery.[53]

Haynes & Tapley also treated their cases primarily with radiotherapy obtaining 86% control rates with one of their three recurrences salvaged by surgery.[54] It is generally agreed that total rhinectomy is not recommended for early tumours although possibly needed for advanced lesions particularly when the nasal framework is involved (Fig. 6.3).

Barzan et al have used intra-arterial chemotherapy followed by external beam irradiation for large tumours, reporting that 10 of their 12 cases remained free of disease for more than 3 years post-treatment.[44] Cytotoxic drugs were delivered via catheters introduced ipsilaterally or bilaterally through the superficial temporal artery. Methotrexate infusion 20 mg, for 2 days, bleomycin 10 mg for 2 days and vincristine 0.5 mg at days 1 and 3 were followed by a 2 day rest. The cycles were repeated five to eight times and then followed by 4000 to 6000 rad of Cobalt-60 irradiation. All patients achieved complete resolution of their tumour with 10 having more than 3 years' disease-free follow-up.

Goepfert et al advise radical excision with prosthetic replacement for radiation failures of large lesions but, like most others, have had little long-term success especially if nodal metastases are present.[48] It is surprising in view of the propensity of larger lesions to metastasize that few authors recommend prophylactic irradiation to the neck although this might be thought to be an integral part of the initial radiation plan. Wang obtained a 67% 3-year salvage rate in three T3N0 tumours but only 33% in his T3N1 lesions.[47] Radical neck dissection is limited by an inability to remove lymphatic channels between the nose and submandibular lymph nodes although elective neck dissection appears not to be practised even in high risk cases undergoing radical surgery.

5- and 10-year follow-up reveals a late development of second tumours, 11% in Kagan et al's 42 patients[43] and long-term prognosis must be considered as similar to or even worse than that found in other upper aero-digestive tract neoplasms.

Table 6.1 Treatment results for carcinoma of nasal vestibule

Author	No. of patients	Treatment	Results % survival
Goepfert et al 1974[48]	26	Surgery or DXT	78
Haynes & Tapley 1974[54]	22	DXT	86
Shiffman 1979[39]	9	Surgery & DXT	56
Mak et al 1980[53]	47	DXT	85
De Jong et al 1981[52]	22	DXT & surgery	50
Kagan et al 1981[43]	42	Surgery ± DXT	60
Wong et al 1986[51]	56	DXT	87
Chobe et al 1988[50]	32	DXT	87
Vendelbo et al 1990[45]	66	DXT & surgery	78
Barzan et al 1990[44]	12	Surgery, DXT & chemotherapy	100

DXT, radiotherapy

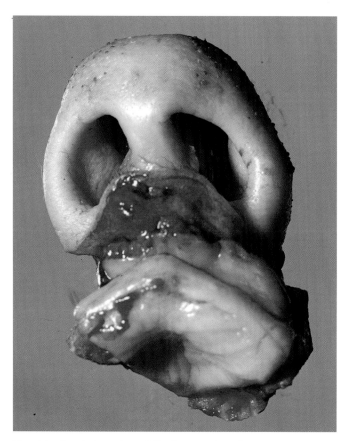

Fig. 6.3 Surgical specimen following resection of nasal vestibular squamous cell carcinoma.

THE NASAL CAVITY

Although Rubric 160 of the International Classification of Diseases of the World Health Organization aggregates neoplasms of the nose, nasal cavities, middle ear and accessory sinuses, subsites exist separating the nose and nasal cavities (ICD 160.0) from the accessory sinuses (ICD 160.2, 160.8, 160.9).

Muir and Nectoux[55] utilized information from cancer registries affiliated to the International Association of Cancer Registries and also data contained in 'Cancer Incidence in Five Continents' to provide detailed ana-tomically-related statistics for the period 1968–1973. A high proportion of the total rubric 160 is constituted by malignant tumours of the paranasal sinuses, largely the maxillary sinus. Considerable variations were however found for both sexes in a number of countries such as Cuba and Israel, possibly because of errors in coding or classification, with some vestibular carcinomata being aligned to the skin. Neoplasms of the nasal cavity how-ever, were found to be rare in countries such as Japan despite their high incidence of maxillary sinus cancer. The deficiencies in extrapolating data such as this in rela-tion to incidence rates has already been considered. Lack of precise anatomical definitions remains a defect when considering sites of origin and this particularly applies to the nasal cavity. Although the nasal vestibule and septum have clear boundaries and configurations, the lateral nasal wall is more complex. At 8 weeks gestation, three soft tissue turbinates are visible and a cartilaginous capsule surrounds the nose. By 9 weeks' flanges of cartilage have invaded the three turbinates and 3 weeks later an 'air space' from which the maxillary sinus develops, becomes visible. The nasal vestibule and lateral wall have an adult configuration by 16 weeks with the ethmoid cells deve-loping from furrows in the lateral wall.[56] For physiological and pathological reasons it would therefore appear logical to include the ethmoid sinuses in discussion of lateral nasal wall carcinomata.

NASAL SEPTAL CARCINOMA

Incidence

A small number of cases were published between 1902 and 1914 by Gibb,[57] Beard[58] and Ridout.[59] By 1969 Yarrington et al had found a total of 50 cases in the litera-ture although they commented that many of these failed to substantiate the diagnosis of a primary squamous cell carcinoma originating in the nasal septum.[60] 10 years later, Young reported 43 patients with malignant septal tumours seen at one institution over a 23-year period,[61] and Weimert et al[62] reviewed 83 cases culled from the literature up to 1978 and adding a further 14 patients of their own. LeLieve et al described the clinical histories of 22 patients seen at the University of Texas, Galveston, 18 of whom had squamous carcinomata.[63] In their paper published in 1988 however, Echeverria-Zumarraga et al said that no more than 300 cases of primary septal carci-noma had been reported in the literature by that date giving an incidence of 9% of all malignant tumours arising within the nasal cavity, which themselves comprise no more than 1% of all malignancies.[64] Most published series have been gathered over many years which itself substantiates the low incidence of this neoplasm.[65,66]

Age, sex and ethnic variation

With such small numbers of patients available for analysis it is difficult to gain more than a general impression of the incidence rate which appears to be between 40 and 80 years with a mean of 60 years. There is a slight male pre-dominance and cases have been recorded from most ethnic groups.

Site and aetiology

With small lesions, where the site of origin is clearly visible, squamous carcinomas usually arise from the ante-rior septum at the muco-cutaneous junction. Despite the known risk of nasal cavity malignancies in certain occupations or industries (p. 81) and the ease with which particulate matter is deposited on the anterior septum, the aetiology of septal cancer remains vague. Both smokers and non-smokers are represented in most series as are the occasional 'nose picker' or snuff user.[63]

The tumour spreads rapidly to involve the nasal vestibule, cavity and nasal framework and, in the absence of a recognized classification system, LeLieve et al have grouped their patients into small, midsized and large tumours. They comment that there is a high correlation between tumours larger than 2 cm and eventual prognosis.[63] They also found synchronous primary tumours in three of their 22 patients (17%) including 'in situ' changes in the floor of the mouth, lip and an adenocarcinoma of the lung. Perhaps of greater importance is the presence of submucosal disease necessitating a wide margin excision rather than merely 'clear' margins.[63]

Clinical features and radiology

Lesions may take a variety of forms ranging from a large fungating friable mass which bleeds readily, to a small flat ulcerated or fissured lesion or even a septal perforation.[64] Anteriorly situated lesions often cause a sore area within the nares with some crusting which is covering superficial ulceration. Persistent crusting, particularly if accompanied by bleeding, when present for several weeks is a significant symptom although diagnosis is usually delayed for 6 months with a range of 1 to 72 months.[67]

The signs and symptoms therefore are similar to those common to many less serious conditions found within the nose and only a high index of suspicion will lead to early diagnosis by biopsy. The extent of the tumour is determined by clinical examination including nasal endoscopy, supplemented by CT and MRI; essential when planning surgical excision. As with vestibular carcinoma, prognosis is related not only to effective local control but also to management of the regional lymph nodes. Cervical metastases occurred in 44% of the patients reported by LeLieve et al[63] which was double that found by Beatty et al[65] and four times the generally quoted rate of 10%.[62] Few patients present with lymph node disease and although their development is reflected in a poor prognosis, and often recurrent local disease, there is little explanation for this variation in incidence rates.

Macroscopic and microscopic appearance

The degree of differentiation varies within these tumours, being in most cases low-grade although Lyons suggests that a further variant may be the degree of cartilaginous invasion, especially in the more active lesions.[66] Deutsch says that a higher recurrence rate is associated with undifferentiated tumours[68] whilst Batsakis et al believe that prognosis is primarily related to site and size rather than the histological grading.[1]

The literature suggests that many septal carcinomas are inadequately treated, possibly because of a failure to appreciate the true extent of the lesion or a desire to avoid severe cosmetic disability. With large tumours, positive margins following excision or local recurrence after radiotherapy, is usually followed by rapid regrowth and a high propensity for lymph node metastases. As with vestibular cancer, these may be homolateral, contralateral or bilateral and indicate a poor outlook with a control rate varying from 0 to 10%.[63]

Differential diagnosis

A wide variety of pathological conditions are found on the nasal septum and must be excluded by histological examination. Amelanotic malignant melanoma, basal cell carcinoma, transitional cell carcinoma, chondrosarcoma, adenoid cystic carcinoma, adenocarcinoma, small cell carcinoma, mucoepidermoid carcinoma and plasmacytoma must all be considered as well as benign lesions such as mycosis, syphilis, tuberculosis, leishmaniasis, leprosy, sarcoid and 'midline granuloma'.

Treatment

Despite variations in treatment strategies, follow-up times and details of tumour extent, there appears to be an agreement that primary septal carcinoma is a serious disease. Although small localized tumours may be completely excised with at least 1 cm margin including the mucoperichondrium and underlying cartilage, most lesions are more extensive when first diagnosed.[69] Larger lesions still confined to the septum can be removed via a sublabial approach or possibly more effectively by a midfacial degloving technique. The success of these limited procedures is not easily evaluated from the literature because of inadequate numbers and data. A variety of modalities have been advocated at one time or another including surgery, radiotherapy or, more popularly, combination therapy. Goepfert et al[48] say that either surgery or radiotherapy are effective or ineffective for survival rates vary from 23%[70] to 100% reported by Whitcomb for his three patients![71] LeLieve et al[63] obtained an absolute 5-year survival rate for their 18 patients of 66% with a median survival time of 45 months, primary control being obtained in 94%. However, seven patients had local excision via a lateral rhinotomy approach, two had radiotherapy alone and the remainder combined therapy. They concluded that although each case must be evaluated individually, septal carcinoma should ideally be treated by wide surgical excision followed by radiation to the primary site and both necks.

Although a lateral rhinotomy approach may be adequate for many tumours, extension to the nasal framework, vestibule or floor may need a total rhinectomy or at least a midfacial degloving procedure (p. 329). Utilizing this rationale, a 5-year survival figure of 60% appears feasible with a better outlook for small lesions. Six of the 13 patients reviewed by Harrison in 1982 were treated by total rhinectomy (Table 6.2). Failure was due to an inability to control disease extending posteriorly despite adjuvant radiotherapy and he suggests that following radiological evaluation, craniofacial resection may be required in addition to total rhinectomy in such cases.[72]

LATERAL NASAL WALL AND ETHMOID SINUS CARCINOMA

Lateral nasal wall tumours are evenly divided between those that are benign and those that are malignant, with inverting papilloma predominating in the former and squamous cell carcinoma the commonest representative of a heterogeneous latter group which originate in the region of the ethmoid labyrinth and middle meatus.

Incidence

The ease with which maxillary sinus cancer invades the ethmoid or enters the nasal cavity, makes assessment of the relative frequency of primary ethmoidal or turbinal carcinoma imprecise. Robin et al in their classic epidemiological study of 624 patients with nasal cavity and paranasal sinus cancer, give a figure of 10% and a male to female ratio of 1:0.6.[32] Hopkin et al analysing 561 patients seen at a single institution over a 15-year period quote an incidence of 19% of all tumours in this region originating within the ethmoid and a male predominance of 3:2.[42] These variations emphasize the problems of site assessment and statistical presentation when unusual

tumours are collated as a single entity. All ethnic groups are represented with considerable variations in age-adjusted incidence rates around the world.[55] Although this may represent artifacts from deficiencies in coding, classification or reporting skills, in some instances it reflects variations in aetiology. This applies particularly to occupationally-induced adenocarcinomata in woodworkers or snuff-induced squamous cell carcinoma of the lateral nasal wall as seen in the South African Bantu.[73,74]

A wide age range is involved varying from 7 to 70 years, the median being around 50 years although Robin et al have shown that incidence rates rise throughout life from about 30 years to 75 years.[32] Jackson et al divided their 115 patients with malignant neoplasms of the nasal cavities and paranasal sinuses into antral and non-antral. 33 were non-antral arising from the nasal septum or lateral nasal wall but they found little variation in the mean age at diagnosis or sex ratio between the two groups.[75] However, in view of Robin & Powell's finding of a 20% error in assessment of malignancies within the ethmoid complex, which exceeded all other sites within the upper jaw, many statistics related to the lateral nasal wall and ethmoid must be viewed with caution.[76]

Aetiology[9]

The close correlation that has been demonstrated between nasal carcinoma and formaldehyde exposure in rats has raised the question of chronic irritation in human sinonasal cancer.[77] In the experimental animal the rate of tumour formation is increased with the level and duration of exposure, although sinonasal cancer was not over-represented in the human mortality study from the National Cancer Institute USA in their study of 26 561 industrial workers exposed to formaldehyde vapour.[78] Discomfort from nasal obstruction and discharge is common amongst wood furniture workers with symptoms

Table 6.2 Nasal septal carcinoma (Harrison & Lund)

Age	Sex	Site	Histology	Treatment	Outcome
61	M	Nasal framework & columella	Poorly differentiated	DXT, rhinectomy	4 yr A&W
63	M	Septum – nares, premaxilla	Well differentiated	DXT, rhinectomy Hard palate resection	10 yr A&W
81	F	Septum – cribriform plate	Moderately differentiated	Rhinectomy – residual disease left	18 mth DOD
54	M	Septum – framework	Moderately differentiated	DXT, rhinectomy Uncontrolled disease posteriorly	3 mth DOD
58	M	Anterior septum, upper lip	Moderately differentiated	Rhinectomy with upper lip	10 mth DOD Lung cancer
71	M	Septum & framework	Well differentiated	Rhinectomy	6 yr A&W

DXT, radiotherapy; A&W alive and well; DOD, dead of disease

apparently related to the concentration of dust particles.[79] Those larger than 5 μm become trapped on the nasal mucosa and histological changes have been observed in the nasal mucosa of workers exposed to wood dust. These show replacement of ciliated columnar epithelium by metaplastic epithelium and goblet cell hypoplasia.[80] Wood dust is now recognized as a carcinogen in man, and responsible for the production of ethmoidal adenocarcinoma. Hardwoods such as beech or oak are more commonly blamed but Voss et al have shown that prolonged exposure to soft wood dust can cause squamous cell carcinoma.[17]

In view of the frequency with which formaldehyde is present in a wide range of occupational environments, such as chemical, furniture, textile and paper industries, Holmstrom & Wihelmsson have studied the pathophysiological effects of combined exposure to these two irritants.[81] Their investigations were complex with data not easily interpreted although histological changes, such as loss of cilia and metaplasia, were found in all groups of workers without evidence of a correlation between exposure dose and cumulative histological changes. In their research, rats exposed to formaldehyde vapour for 24 months developed nasal squamous metaplasia, and in one animal a squamous cell carcinoma. However, animals exposed to dust alone showed no histological changes nor were changes greater in rats exposed to both dust and formaldehyde.

Harrison in his study on the effects of 'dry' snuff found marked atrophy of the turbinals with profound mucosal metaplasia but nasal discharge is rarely complained of by habitual snuff users. The middle meatus was enlarged with old snuff lying in situ. Although there is no evidence that commercial snuff is an important aetiological factor in the production of sinonasal cancer in the Western world, the indigenous Bantu race of South Africa use homemade snuff containing quantities of hard wood ash and have the highest incidence of advanced sinus cancer in the world.[26]

Clinical features

In those patients where both maxillary antrum and ethmoid have been involved the original site of origin may be difficult to establish. Most authors of large series of sinonasal cancers quote an incidence of a primary ethmoidal origin of between 10% and 20%, with a neoplasm situated solely within a turbinate being extremely rare.[42,82]

In the early course of the disease, symptoms are at first trivial taking the form of nasal obstruction and discharge. Some slight bleeding is common but diagnosis is not usually made until there is a substantial intranasal mass or extension has produced facial swelling, proptosis, epiphora or neurological signs related to the infraorbital nerve. The ethmoid is intimately related to the orbit laterally, anterior cranial fossa superiorly and the nasal cavity medially, and the thin lamina papyracea offers little resistance to orbital invasion although penetration of the orbital periosteum is unlikely, i.e. intraorbital but extraperiosteal invasion. Extension into the maxillary antrum is also common and preoperative assessment may fail to detect what is actually an antroethmoidal tumour.[76] The perpendicular plate of the ethmoid is thin allowing spread to the contralateral side and the 1 mm thick cribriform plate also offers little barrier to intracranial spread of tumour. Such extensions, although not clinically detectable, can be shown radiologically; an investigation of considerable importance in the assessment of lateral wall neoplasms.

An obvious but late sign is proptosis, although penetration of the medial orbital wall precedes this event and may only be seen at exploration. Loss of vision from neoplastic invasion of the optic nerve or canal, particularly via the posterior ethmoid cells, is a late symptom as is regional lymph node metastasis, found in about 10% of patients.[32,42] Most of the more obvious symptoms are secondary to tumour extension and diagnosis is delayed on average by 6 months although less with the more aggressive anaplastic carcinomata.

No system of classification for lateral nasal wall/ ethmoid sinus neoplasms is in constant use, and Harrison has suggested that there is little justification for proposing a complex system based upon clinical suppositions and uncertain assessment.[83] Prognosis largely depends on well recognized areas of dangerous spread, such as the orbital apex–cribriform plate–pterygopalatine fossa or skull base, and these can often only be verified at surgery.

Radiology

Radiological evaluation of these tumours plays an increasingly important role in early diagnosis as well as being essential to planning a rational approach to treatment, whether it be radiotherapy or surgery. Conventional sinus views can play a useful adjunct in the investigation of nasal and sinus disease. The medial antral wall and ethmoidal interface are adequately shown on these conventional views, and loss of bone or changes in configuration may assist by invoking suspicion of neoplasia. In addition, views of the optic foramen are helpful in assessing the ethmoid sinus with its bony partitions, lamina papyracea, optic foramen and superior orbital fissure well shown.[84]

However, if a tumour is suspected on the basis of these films or clinical evidence then CT is imperative, although, as Lloyd has shown, isolated ethmoid clouding can be seen in 15% of normal individuals and when confined to only a few cells is without significance.[85] Using direct axial and coronal views, the latter being preferable to reformation because of superior spatial and contrast resolution, tumour extension outside the lateral nasal wall and ethmoid sinus can be visualized. Orbit, intracranial cavity and pterygoid region are well shown although squamous carcinoma displays insufficient density differences, even with contrast enhancement, to allow histological diagnosis.[82] Erosion of the lamina papyracea does not in itself confirm tumour on the orbital periosteum nor does a radiologically intact cribriform plate preclude the possibility of intracranial disease. Final assessment can only be made with confidence at exploration and although Robin and Powell found a low error of 4% in evaluation of 'lower nasal cavity tumour', their 20% total error for ethmoidal carcinomata confirms the inherent difficulties of accurate appraisal at this site.[76] However MRI now provides additional information regarding soft tissue extensions and is particularly useful in intraorbital or intracranial disease (Fig. 6.4).

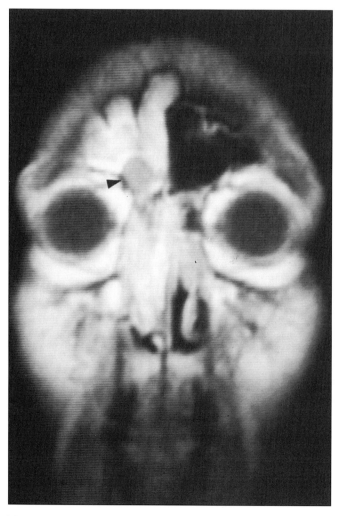

Fig. 6.4 Coronal MR scan, T1 weighted sequence with gadolinium showing extension of squamous cell carcinoma into the frontal sinus (arrow), inflamed mucosa of the frontal sinus and secretion (Lloyd 1988[86]).

The low rate of lymph node involvement confirms that it is an inability to control local disease that is the primary cause of treatment failure. Limitations of surgical excision compounded by an inability to detect microscopical disease is largely responsible for poor cure rates. However, early diagnosis depends largely on radiological detection and both CT and MRI have materially enhanced our prospects of achieving this aim.

Macroscopic and microscopic appearance

With the exception of a very small number of carcinomas thought to have arisen from the inferior turbinate, most lateral wall neoplasms will have come from the maxillary sinus or ethmoidal cells.[1] Friedman & Osborne, pathologists at the Institute of Laryngology and Otology, London found that 37% of all malignant sinus tumours were carcinomas in their evaluation of 1043 nose and paranasal tumours.[87] In smaller series this figure is usually larger, Gadenberg et al in 1984 reporting that half of their 180 malignant sinonasal tumours were squamous cell carcinoma,[88] this disparity probably reflecting the much larger variety of tumours seen in specialized institutions. Most carcinomata in this region are keratinizing, tending to be only moderately well differentiated with a small number of non-keratinizing or anaplastic carcinomas.

The absence of a system of classification for this region, together with the advanced stage at diagnosis and variations in treatment strategies, makes the evaluation of degrees of histological differentiation with prognosis, largely anecdotal. It is tumour extent rather than degree of differentiation that probably influences prognosis, although undifferentiated carcinomas in general do appear to follow a more rapid course. None of the 37 patients with anaplastic carcinomas of the maxillary or ethmoidal sinuses with lymph node metastases reported by Robin and Powell[76] survived more than 3 years.

Areas of carcinoma in situ can be found at the edge of most invasive carcinomas and similar changes have been reported in inverted papillomata, possibly a precursor of subsequent malignant change. However, the development of an epidermal neoplasm in the sinuses is related not only to the tendency for respiratory epithelium to undergo squamous metaplasia but also to a propensity of the undifferentiated basal cells of this epithelium to produce malignant cells, which can then differentiate directly into an epidermoid form. Some of these carcinomas show no differentiation being composed of cells of a primitive appearance. Michaels says that although a carcinoma with a stratified arrangement of well-defined tumour cells but without keratinization or 'prickles' is referred to as non-keratinizing squamous carcinoma, undifferentiated should be reserved for tumour cells with vesicular nuclei and a syncytial appearance.[8]

The designation 'transitional carcinoma' is applied to neoplasms with the features of cylindric cell carcinoma as well as a poorly differentiated, non-keratinizing squamous carcinoma but it is probable that its natural history is similar to that of the commoner squamous cell carcinoma.[75]

Neoplasms with both epithelial and mesenchymal components have been called *keratocarcinosarcoma, spindle-cell carcinoma, pseudosarcomatous squamous cell carcinoma* or *carcinosarcoma*. Batsakis suggests that such lesions should be viewed as a single pathological entity with carcinoma reserved for a true histological malignancy.[89] Shindo et al published a case of carcinosarcoma of the nasal cavity presenting with nasal obstruction and epistaxis of 1 year's duration in a 53-year-old male. CT showed extension into the antroethmoid region and orbit and craniofacial resection produced histologically confirmed clear margins. The patient was given postoperative radiotherapy and remained free from disease 1 year later.[90] However, carcinosarcomata are aggressive neoplasms with a high incidence of local recurrence and a reported mortality of over 80%. Few cases occurring within the sinonasal region have been published and this may reflect some confusion or doubt in histological diagnosis.[91,92]

Natural history

Over 90% of all paranasal sinus cancer will have radiological evidence of invasion of at least one wall at initial diagnosis.[75] Whereas extension of lateral wall tumours into the nasal cavity produces epistaxis and a proliferative mass, orbital invasion threatens vision, producing progressive proptosis. The roof of the ethmoid offers little resistance to intracranial spread nor does the perpendicular plate to contralateral spread. Extension to the maxillary sinus is probably present to some degree in every ethmoidal tumour eventually causing facial swelling, epiphora and ultimately, spread into the pterygopalatine fossa. Untreated and uncontrolled lateral wall carcinoma is progressive and will inevitably produce considerable morbidity before death.

Despite involvement of areas with rich lymphatic drainage, such as the facial skin, regional lymph node metastases are uncommon even with locally advanced tumours originating within the lateral nasal wall. Robin & Powell reported a 12% incidence for ethmoidal carcinoma,[93] whilst other authors combining ethmoid with maxillary sinus give figures ranging from 14% to 20%.[34,42,75] All agree however, that development of metastatic disease carries a uniformly poor prognosis.

Differential diagnosis

Although squamous cell carcinomata are the commonest malignant neoplasms found within the nose and ethmoid sinuses, representing at least half of the total pathology, a wide variety of histological types must be recognized and differentiated. This is of importance not only prognostically but for planning treatment since there is considerable variation in biological behaviour. Biopsy is essential for histological confirmation aided by immuno-histochemistry in many of the anaplastic or untypical lesions.[82]

Treatment

It is a fundamental concept that accurate estimation of the extent of a neoplasm is an essential prerequirement to proper management. Prior to the availability of computered tomography, and later MRI, underestimation led to inadequate surgery or failure to fully irradiate many tumours arising within the lateral nasal wall. Robin & Powell in their evaluation of 282 patients with carcinoma of the nasal cavity and paranasal sinuses found that an error of underestimation was made in 34.7% of the total group, reduced to 20% for the ethmoid complex and 4% for the lower nasal cavity.[76]

Apart from septal carcinomas, excision of the majority of sinonasal neoplasms has been limited by surgical access, although even a radiotherapist as experienced as Lederman admitted that surgical resection was still the mainstay of treatment for upper jaw cancer.[34,94] Ellingwood & Million, discussing 32 patients with sinonasal neoplasms treated solely with radiotherapy between 1964–1975, receiving 6000–8000 rad of Cobalt-60, claimed an unprecedented local control rate of 95% for the nasal cavity and 71% for ethmoidal tumours.[95] Their overall 5-year survival rate of 59% was very different from the 33% determinate 5-year survival rate reported in 1984 by McNicoll et al based upon 105 patients treated by a combination of radiotherapy and surgery.[96] The survival figures of Ellingwood & Million are unusually good since more than half of their patients had extensive disease with orbital or intracranial extension. However, 17 of the 23 surviving patients had radiation complications not found in the report of McNicoll et al although they used a similar irradiation protocol.[91]

Frazell & Lewis[97] published their data concerning 416 patients with nasal and sinus cancer treated between 1935–1954. Following radiotherapy alone, 14% remained free of disease for 5 years or longer (half the cancers were confined to the ethmoid sinus) whereas 35% were 'cured' by surgery alone. Although the statistics are not easy to understand the overall 5-year survival rate appears to be 24.7%, similar to that published by most authors at that time. Despite an acceptance that primary radiotherapy occupies an important role in treatment, an inability to ensure local control or visualize local recurrence, has emphasized the need for post-radiation surgical removal of the area originally involved. Carcinomas situated in the lateral nasal wall can be removed via a lateral rhinotomy approach which although providing excellent visualization of the medial orbital wall and cribriform plate does not permit oncological excision.[98] Harrison has discussed the surgical approaches to the medial wall of the orbit emphasizing the limitations of all extracranial procedures and the need to remove the whole ethmoid block including the cribriform plate.[99]

The management of the orbital contents in both ethmoid and maxillary sinus cancer is discussed separately, but the presence of preformed holes in the cribriform plate ensures that every neoplasm in this region must theoretically be assumed to be intracranial. This area must therefore be resected in all oncological operations designed to radically remove the disease.[100]

Lateral rhinotomy is an incision not an operation, allowing excellent access to the nasal cavity. Varying amounts of the maxilla and ethmoid can be removed safely although the term 'medial maxillectomy' is misleading since rarely is the medial part of the maxilla removed without the adjoining ethmoid. It has attracted some attention because of its value in the management of inverted papilloma but cannot be considered as oncological in ethmoidal neoplasia unless combined with a craniotomy.[101]

Interest has also been shown in a rhinotomy approach to the upper nasal cavity in which the nose is turned inferiorly to provide wide access.[102] This not only gives access to both ethmoids but allows en bloc removal. However, as Biller et al have said, there is also danger to both optic nerves and a risk of nasal deformity and scarring.[103] Mann used this approach on six patients without orbital or dural involvement finding it valuable and producing a 60% 2-year local control.[104]

It has long been apparent, however, that the poor prognosis associated with carcinomas situated within the lateral nasal wall is a consequence of inadequate resection. Harrison in 1973[105] discussing future prospects for improving long-term success, emphasized the need for more radical surgery particularly in relation to the cribriform plate and orbit. This is to some extent now available in the form of craniofacial resection. Originally described by Smith et al in 1954[106] and subsequently improved by Ketcham,[107] this operation has now been developed to become the standard approach to tumours situated in the region of the ethmoid block, whether they be malignant or benign. Cheesman et al have discussed their experience with 60 patients seen over 7 years with a variety of pathologies including seven carcinomas involving the ethmoid. Excellent access together with minimal morbidity allowed removal of lesions beyond the ethmoid, into the anterior cranial cavity and apex of the orbit. In most malignant lesions this was combined with preoperative radiotherapy.[108,109]

Prognosis

The close proximity of the lateral nasal wall and ethmoid sinus to the maxillary antrum, orbit and anterior cranial cavity ensures that most cancers are advanced at initial diagnosis. Although small localized lesions respond to irradiation alone, the difficulty of ensuring local control in these often inaccessible areas suggests that removal of the irradiated tissue by a lateral rhinotomy approach is advisable. For the majority of neoplasms, radiotherapy should be followed by wide field resection using a craniofacial approach. Provisional reports indicate an improvement in local control although data from the larger series, particularly with long-term follow-up, are not yet available. The prognosis for patients with lymph node metastases remains poor although the low incidence has not en-couraged prophylactic irradiation or neck dissection.

CARCINOMA OF THE MAXILLARY SINUS

The commonest neoplasm affecting the upper jaw is found within the maxillary sinus where its intimate relationship to the orbit superiorly, palate and dentition inferiorly, infratemporal fossa posteriorly, face anteriorly and nasal cavity medially, makes early diagnosis and radical excision problematic.

Incidence

It is generally accepted that paranasal sinus malignancies make up less than 1% of all neoplasms and approximately 3% of those originating within the upper aero-digestive system.[110] As with most other tumours, incidence rates vary within differing ethnic populations and, in Japan, paranasal sinus carcinomas comprise more than 1% of the total malignancies and about 25% of all head and neck tumours.[111] Age-adjusted rates of the same order are also found in the African population of Ibadan, Nigeria, in Kingston, Jamaica and in the Bantu people of South Africa. In publishing this geographically distributed morbidity data, Muir & Nectoux emphasize that it depends on accuracy of diagnosis and reporting. In many instances the numbers are small although this does indicate the rarity of malignant sinonasal tumours.[55] Robin et al, in discussing this problem, have also drawn attention to the distinction between true incidence rates and the number of patients actually presenting with the tumour, the latter being a more accurate reflection of the actual rate or 'risk' of the disease.[32] Unfortunately, detailed age-related data are not universally available and incidence rates are possibly best accepted as being about twice the mortality rate.

Age, sex and ethnic variation

Although patients as young as 19 years or as old as 90

years of age have been diagnosed with maxillary sinus cancer, most published cases begin about 35 years with a mean of 60 years.[96,112–115] No specific pattern appears to emerge in relation to age in series where the whole rubric encompassing the nasal cavity and paranasal sinuses, is considered as one. The age-specific incidence curves for Osaka, Japan, an area of high incidence, and for Germany, an area of low incidence, can be taken to represent the age distribution of cancer of the nose and sinuses in general. These curves, illustrated in the paper of Muir & Nectoux, reflect, in fact, the features of any epithelial tumour.[55]

A male predominance of the order 1.7:1 is consistently quoted in the English language publications although ranges of between 1.2:1[55] and 4:1[116] appear in isolated papers. When the sex ratio is determined on the basis of age-adjusted incidence rates it usually shows a two-fold preponderance for males but this is reduced when the maxillary sinus is considered alone rather than encompassing the whole of rubric 160.[55]

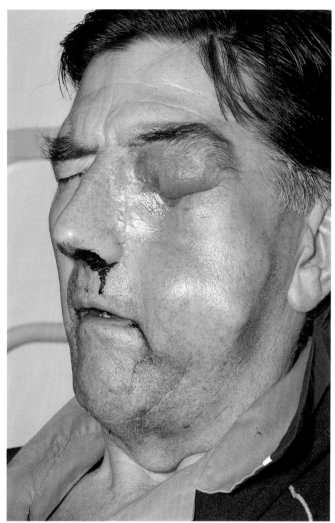

Fig. 6.6 Recurrent squamous cell carcinoma infiltrating soft tissue of cheek.

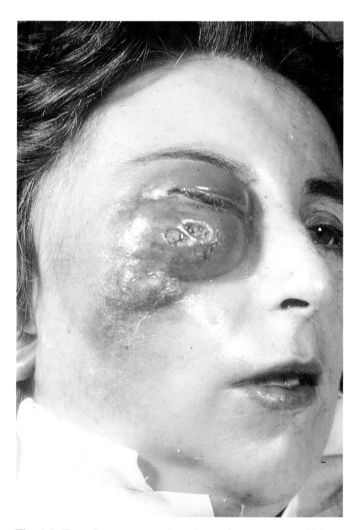

Fig. 6.5 Extensive squamous cell carcinoma from antro-ethmoidal region involving orbit, after injection of disulphine blue.

Site and clinical features (Figs 6.5–6.8)

Carcinomas confined to the maxillary sinus mucosa will only be diagnosed because of an early significant symptom, such as unilateral epiphora or infraorbital neuralgia. Exploration of the sinus for an unrelated cause may very occasionally reveal an unsuspected tumour and with increased use of the endoscope for examination of the sinonasal region, this may occur more frequently.[83] The most frequent symptoms at first onset are cheek swelling (29%), nasal obstruction (28%), and epistaxis (20%), and there is a reported average delay of 3 to 6 months before final diagnosis.[82] At final diagnosis however, 79% have cheek swelling, 70% nasal obstruction or discharge and 52% epistaxis. These figures were published by Miyaguchi et al in their analysis of 845 patients with maxillary sinus carcinoma seen in Japan[117] and show an interesting variation from the data published by Har-El et al based upon their experience of 70 patients seen in

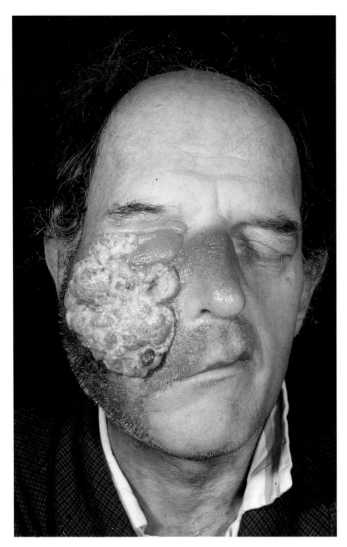

Fig. 6.7 Extensive exophytic squamous cell carcinoma from maxillary sinus.

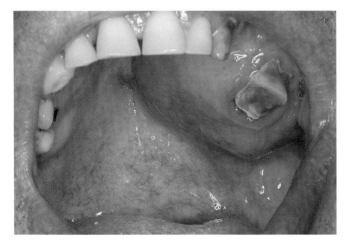

Fig. 6.8 Squamous cell carcinoma from maxillary sinus involving palate and displacing dentition.

Israel. In their study 76% had an intranasal mass, 23% cheek swelling, 14% nasal obstruction or epistaxis and 9% proptosis.[118] Sisson found that 26% of 60 patients presented with facial swellings and 30% with nasal obstruction or epistaxis.[113]

Despite these variations in the frequency of the various initial or presenting symptoms, all are indicative of extra-maxillary disease and convey little of the exact time of onset of the neoplasm. Apart from sensory disturbances involving the infraorbital nerve or occlusion of the naso-lacrimal duct, most symptoms represent invasion or displacement of at least one sinus wall. Ocular signs are less frequent than with ethmoidal neoplasms and, as with trismus, indicate extensive disease. Many of the earlier symptoms are similar to those found in benign sinus disease, hindering the recognition of maxillary sinus cancer at an early stage. This situation may change with the availability of endonasal endoscopic investigatory techniques.

Radiology

Routine films complemented with tomography will show bony destruction, but early diagnosis needs to show firstly the presence of a soft tissue mass. Areas of bony loss or remodelling are secondary changes well evaluated by CT, whilst aggressive destruction implies a rapidly growing tumour leaving little time for new bony growth, a feature of squamous carcinoma. Differential enhancement between inflamed mucosa, non-enhancing secretions and minimal tumour enhancement, provides a means for identifying tumour margins and mapping prior to radio-therapy.[119] However, demineralization of bony walls simulating bone destruction may also occur adjacent to polyps or even in infection, more common in the ethmoid. Accurate assessment therefore depends upon both direct axial and coronal scanning, which allow discrimination of the fascial planes in the infratemporal and pterygopalatine fossae as well as accurately delineating the maxillary sinus walls (Fig. 6.9). CT also demonstrates enlarged lymph nodes in the lateral retropharyngeal space as well as the cervical region.[82,120] Despite the considerable value of CT, small bony dehiscences are not always visible and Robin & Powell estimated that an error of about 4% underestimation will be present in radiological assessment of maxillary sinus carcinomas.[76]

MRI may reduce this figure but since bone erosion alone is significant of serious pathology in most patients, detection of an extramaxillary soft tissue mass may not materially affect future management.

Macroscopic and microscopic appearance

More than 60% of all malignant tumours involving the parasal sinuses are squamous cell carcinomas with at least

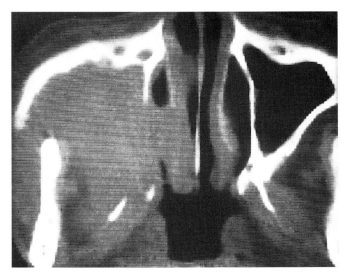

Fig. 6.9 Axial CT scan showing massive invasion of infratemporal fossa by squamous cell carcinoma (Lloyd 1988[86]).

80% arising within the maxillary sinus and in 85% of patients the lesion is keratinized and well differen-tiated. In 1948 Ackerman reported a group of 31 patients with verrucous carcinomas mostly being within the oral cavity.[121] This is a slow-growing squamous cell carcinoma being locally aggressive but rarely metastasizing and was recognized within the maxillary sinus by Elliott et al[6] in 1973, Bacon et al[122] 1989 and Daoud et al[123] in 1991. Histologically, the keratinized squamous epithelium is thick with papillomatosis and a bulbous expanding deep margin. Many of the keratinocytes are 35 μm in diameter with nuclei 12 μm across. Mitotic figures are rare and the reports indicate that this is a slow growing invasive tumour.[124]

Treatment should be by 'adequate' excision as there has been a suggestion, largely unsubstantiated, that radiotherapy may lead to an aggressive change or be ineffective.[125] Radiotherapy however, may be the treatment of choice for recurrence since the biological behaviour of this tumour is insufficiently known to justify very radical surgery.

Spindle cell carcinoma

This is an uncommon, apparently biphasic tumour previously called *pseudosarcoma, pleomorphic carcinoma, epidermoid carcinoma–spindle cell variant* and *pseudosarcomatous squamous cell carcinoma*. Only a small number of cases have been found within the maxillary sinus[126] and although originally regarded as a low-grade, well differentiated squamous carcinoma there is increasing evidence of a more aggressive clinical behaviour pattern. The patient reported by Middlchurst et al[127] had a gingival swelling growing from an antral spindle cell carcinoma excised by partial maxillectomy. 6 months later a soft tissue swelling

developed in the infratemporal fossa with a recurrence in the same maxillary sinus. MRI showed tumour within the nasal cavity, cheek, orbit and pterygopalatine fossa and palliative radiotherapy was given with minimal response. Limited experience suggests that this tumour should be treated in a similar manner to 'normal' squamous cell carcinomata.

Anaplastic carcinoma

The prognosis for anaplastic carcinoma of the paranasal sinuses is said to be worse, site for site, than that for the more common differentiated squamous cell carcinoma. Helliwell et al[49] discussed the biological behaviour of 21 patients with anaplastic carcinoma of the nasal cavity and paranasal sinuses. 14 tumours were within the maxillary sinus and all except two patients were dead within 1 year. Histological diagnosis was confirmed by employing a strict criteria supported by immunohistochemistry, and the average delay between onset of significant symptoms and diagnosis was only 3 months. Orbital involvement was found in half of the antral cases (60% of the total group) and one-third had regional lymph node metastases at presentation. They concluded that anaplastic car-cinoma can be recognized by a combination of light microscopy and immunohistochemistry which differentiates the lesion from lymphoma or malignant melanomata. It is a particularly aggressive tumour and despite combination therapy with both surgery, radiotherapy and chemotherapy, a 5-year survival rate of only 11–15% can be expected. These figures are supported by the publications of Lederman,[128] Robin et al[32] and Kondo et al.[112]

Small cell carcinoma

Baugh et al[129] in 1986 collected details of 33 patients reported as having a small cell carcinoma arising within the nasal cavity or paranasal sinuses. 20 of these cases taken from a paper by Silva et al had been called *neuroendocrine carcinoma,*[130] although Baugh et al believed that they actually represented a variant of small cell carcinoma – differing in clinical behaviour!

Small cell or oat cell carcinoma represents about 10% of all lung neoplasms although small numbers of patients with primary extrapulmonary lesions have been recorded.[131] The first account of a small cell carcinoma arising within the maxillary sinus appeared in 1965 with an unexpected autopsy finding of a lesion within the ethmoid. Koss et al reviewing a series of 14 patients included one patient with an ethmoidal tumour and one in the maxillary antrum.[132] In each instance salivary gland tissue was the presumed site of origin although keratinization was present in each biopsy. Long-term survival is reported for the small number of antral or antro-ethmoidal cases recorded although there appears to be a propensity for local recurrence and invasion has been recognized. Combined therapy is said to be more effective than for squamous carcinoma although it remains unclear from the few available publications whether this is secondary to a better biological behaviour or earlier diagnosis.[133]

Natural history

Squamous carcinoma of the maxillary sinus is a progressive disease making use of areas of natural weakness, such as the inferior orbital fissure or ethmoidal labyrinth, to expand into neighbouring structures. Early diagnosis with tumour still confined within the maxilla is rare and radiological or clinical evidence of penetration of at least one bony wall will be present in a majority of patients at diagnosis. Tumour spread is however, not confined by bony barriers, although both dura and orbital periosteum are relatively resistant to direct penetration. Extension to palate, pterygopalatine fossa, nasal cavity, face and orbit is common as well as to the intracranial cavity and nasopharynx. Regional metastases however, do not correlate with the extent of the primary lesion due to the scanty lymphatics within the sinus mucosa. Spread tends to be related to invasion of areas better provided with lymphatic drainage such as the face, oral cavity or nasopharynx. St Pierre & Baker quote an incidence of 10.6% at initial presentation[113] and Sisson 8.7%.[114] In each series the prognosis for these patients was poor.

Classification

The practice of dividing cancer cases into groups according to 'stages' has arisen because crude survival is higher in patients where the tumour is localized than when it has spread beyond the organ of origin. However, the oncologist is well aware that the stage of the neoplasm at diagnosis is a reflection of rate of growth, histological type, tumour–host relationship and the difficulty of making a definitive diagnosis. Consequently, there is inevitably an inherent weakness in all systems where two dimensional evaluation is used for what is in effect, a three dimensional disease. Variations in biological behaviour are common for most neoplasms but problems in delineation and accessibility are particularly relevant when attempting to classify maxillary sinus carcinomata.

In a supplement of Acta Otolaryngologica (Stockholm) published in 1933, Ohngren presented his personal experience of paranasal sinus cancer. He proposed a classification system based on a hypothetical plane extending from the medial canthus to the angle of the mandible which divided the antrum into an antero-inferior area where tumours had a better prognosis than those situated postero-superiorly. This improvement was primarily due

to better accessibility and relationship to important structures, an observation still true today.[134] He also added another hypothetical line passing vertically through the pupil, producing medial and lateral compartments, the maxilla then being divided into four quadrants. Although this classification has limited clinical application today, it did contribute to the basic concepts upon which other systems have been based, not all as successfully! It is now appreciated that neoplasms do not limit themselves to imaginary lines and the degree of tumour invasion is not covered by this classification although it is relevant to both treatment assessment and prognosis.[118]

Sebileau in 1906 proposed another classification dividing the whole upper jaw into a suprastructure, mesostructure and infrastructure by means of parallel 'imaginary lines' but this system failed to recognize the significance of posterior extension.[135] This defect was recognized, however, by Lederman who modified Sebileau's system by using horizontal planes drawn through the orbital and antral floors together with vertical planes extending down from the medial orbital walls to the nasal floor.[128] This classification had the advantage of including both ethmoidal and nasal cavity lesions although many felt that differences in biological behaviour require that nasal malignancies should be separated from the sinuses.

A contemporary TNM classification was proposed by Sisson et al in 1963 which included some degree of tumour invasion for every T category.[136] Differing localizations of invasion were graded somewhat similarly to Ohngren's regions and its principal advantage lay in its concern for specific invasion of individual sinus walls. However, its complexity with numerous variations made it impractical although the American Joint Committee for Cancer Staging and End-results Reporting (AJC) utilized this system, modified by Rubin[137] in compiling their own proposals (Table 6.3).[138]

In 1967 Sakai & Hamasaki, using their considerable experience of maxillary sinus cancer, proposed a classification system based primarily on the surgical procedures used for each T category.[139] Following some modifications, this is now termed the Japanese Joint Committee (JJC) system using no imaginary planes or compartments (Table 6.4). Other systems are used in Germany and

Table 6.3 Classification of maxillary-sinus cancers (AJC 1977)

T1	Tumour confined to the antral mucosa of the infrastructure with no bone erosion or destruction
T2	Tumour confined to the suprastructural mucosa of the antrum without destruction of the bone or of the antrum's infrastructure and with destruction of medial or inferior bony walls only
T3	Massive tumour with invasion of cribriform plate, posterior ethmoids, sphenoid sinus, nasopharynx, pterygoid plates, or base of skull

Table 6.4 TNM classification of maxillary sinus carcinoma (proposed by the Japanese Joint Committee, 1977)

T	Primary tumour
T1	Tumour confined to the maxillary sinus, with no evidence of bony involvement
T2	Tumour causing destruction of the bony wall, with the external periosteum remaining intact as the capsule and the surrounding tissue not invaded but only compressed
T3	Tumour infiltrated deeply into the surrounding tissue by penetration of the external periosteum, excluding the cases mentioned in T4 category
T4	Tumour extending to the base of the skull, the nasopharynx, the maxilla of the opposite side and/or the facial skin with ulceration
N	Regional lymph nodes, same as UICC classification (1978)

Table 6.5 Classification of maxillary-sinus cancers (according to Harrison[83])

T1	Neoplasm limited to the antral mucosa without evidence of erosion of bone
T2	Erosion of bone without involvement of the facial skin, orbit, ethmoidal labyrinth, or pterygopalatine fossa
T3	Involvement of orbit, ethmoidal labyrinth, or facial skin
T4	Extension of tumour to the nasopharynx, sphenoid sinus, cribriform plate, or pterygopalatine fossa

elsewhere although all suffer from problems of definition and linguistic interpretation, i.e. minimal invasion?

It is obviously difficult to compare treatment results without some conformity of classification, staging being possibly the most important measurable prognostic factor. Harrison in 1978 discussed the deficiencies of existing classification systems particularly in their failure to relate T categories to actual clinical experience. This may be due to these systems being developed by committees rather than experienced oncologists! He concluded that as failure to cure maxillary sinus cancer is primarily due to failure to eradicate the local disease outside the bony walls, these extensions determined prior to treatment, should be the basis for a T classification. Few patients present with metastatic disease, thus accepted nomenclature for N staging could be implemented. Bone erosion within the limits of potential excision, such as the orbital rim or alveolus, are clearly less serious than extension to the pterygopalatine fossa or orbital apex. Although there is no cogent objection to using imaginary planes to divide the upper jaw into regions if it serves a practical purpose, its value in dividing inaccessible mucosal disease, as advocated in the AJC system, appears illogical. Mucosal neoplasia is not confined by hypothetical boundaries and it is impossible to be sure, even on inspection, that disease is not submucosal. Harrison proposed his own classification system for T grouping (Table 6.5) based upon his extensive experience of sinus cancer and its natural behaviour. With more recent experience of craniofacial resection some ethmoidal involvement is accessible to surgical removal and would really fall into T2, otherwise this system reflects those extensions which materially affect ultimate prognosis.

Williatt et al[140] compared the value of six of the currently available classification systems in predicting prognosis in 53 previously untreated squamous cell carcinomas of the maxillary antrum. They used a statistical package to analyse the role of T staging, tumour histology, nodal and systemic spread, patient's age, sex,

treatment, survival and outcome. A table of deviances for a sequence of nested models was built similar to a table of sums of squares used in the analysis of variance. Using these, the significance of prognostic variables, including T staging was assessed. The AJC system and that of Sakai et al failed to stage 47% and 23% of the patients respectively. Of all the systems analysed Harrison's had the most significant correlation with survival (p < 0.01) with T staging proving to be the most important prognostic variable following treatment.

Har-El et al[118] have also analysed staging systems for antral cancer and after recommending a downgrading to T2 for some specific ethmoidal extensions, also concluded that Harrison's system was the most practical means of realistic staging of maxillary sinus carcinomata.

All existing TNM systems are based on factors chosen in part because they can be obtained by clinical or radiological examination. Our inability to quantify the biological behaviour of most neoplasms limits these systems' relationship to prognosis. Eventually technologically based data, such as biological markers and molecular genetics, will have to be incorporated into these systems. Variations also exist in descriptive terminology, limiting the international recognition and application of many classifications and invalidating much statistical information. Classification systems need above all to be both practical and logical if treatment regimes are to receive general understanding; the maxillary sinus is no exception.

Treatment

The treatment of carcinoma of the maxillary sinus has evolved through several stages; at the turn of the century excision with cauterization was the only means of treatment. During subsequent decades, irradiation was favoured although as surgery became safer (and more radical) it gradually replaced radium implants in many cases. Today, most oncologists use a combination of surgery and radiotherapy, although the 'dramatic' improvement in cure rates emanating from Japan following trimodal therapy, is attracting much attention. Unfortunately, comparisons between the end results reported from various institutions cannot be achieved with reasonable accuracy because of variations in classifications and methods used to calculate survival rates. A study of adjusted survival curves indicates that most local recurrences occur within 2 years and over 40% die within the first postoperative year.[114] Consequently, adjusted 5-year actuarial survival rates when compared with 10-year figures give an adequate indication of therapeutic success. Few publications include this data!

Local recurrence is the prime cause of death in maxillary sinus cancer and in an informative paper, Sisson et al[141] have emphasized the need for early diagnosis together with an improvement in initial management. They propose a 'flow chart' covering both diagnostic and therapeutic protocols which exemplifies our present state of knowledge. Patients presenting with chronic nasal or sinus complaints should have an endonasal telescopic examination. Any intranasal lesion should be biopsied and if a suspicion of bone loss is found or there is failure of symptoms to improve with medication, then axial and coronal CT is indicated. They report a reduction in delay between symptoms and diagnosis of 8 to 4 weeks in their patients since utilizing this approach, with 33% of their sinus carcinomas being graded T1 or T2. However, it is doubtful if this is a practical proposition in most centres and patients will continue to present with advanced disease.

Most oncologists recommend a combination of surgery and radiotherapy as providing the best chance of gaining local tumour control although Beale and Garrett found no statistical difference in corrected 5-year survival figures for radiotherapy alone and when combined with surgical excision. Most failures occurred during the first year and the survival of patients with residual disease in the surgical specimen was only 29%, compared with the radiation 'cured' surgical specimen figure of 76%.[142] These conclusions were based upon 112 patients and they emphasized that the irradiated volume was large and included the affected maxilla, ethmoid complex, orbit, frontal and sphenoid sinus, nasal cavity, nasopharynx and pterygoid region. The dose used was 5000 cGy in 4 weeks and the neck was included if nodes were present. Both the radiotherapy and combined groups included between 10 and 20 T4 lesions and the 5-year actuarial survival rate for radiotherapy alone of 42% is remarkable, particularly as 13 of these patients had nodal metastases. However, 13 patients subsequently developed radiation-induced cataracts, six with keratosis or retinal changes and five required enucleation.

Boone and Harle have discussed the complications of radiotherapy used for primary cure of maxillary sinus cancer finding an incidence of 27%.[143] Tsujii et al in their own series of 208 patients given 6000 rad in 4 weeks had brain necrosis or blindness in 21% which they attributed to lack of a CT for treatment planning.[144] Apart from the inoperable, most advanced T4 lesions, radiotherapy is usually combined with surgical excision, being given either pre- or postoperatively depending on treatment protocols. Severe complications are no longer expected or acceptable.

Diagnostic surgery is primarily related to obtaining a biopsy using endoscopic evaluation or exploratory antrostomy. Therapeutic surgery varies from partial maxillectomy to total maxillectomy with orbital clearance or craniofacial resection. The extent of the surgical resection is dependent upon the degree of involvement of surrounding structures, being frequently determined at the time of exploration. Although rare tumours entirely localized to the infrastructure may be suitable for partial maxillectomy, most will require at least a total maxillectomy with clearance of the homolateral ethmoid. Increasing experience with craniofacial procedures has reduced the limitations of resection and neoplasms extending to the apex of the orbit, frontal lobes, pterygopalatine fossa or nasopharynx may still be resected with prospects of worthwhile palliation.

Orbital clearance has not been associated with improvement in 5-year survival rates in most publications although management of orbital extension remains a matter of concern and disagreement.

Management of the orbit

The close topographical relationship of the paranasal sinuses to the orbit, the thin walls dividing them and the multiple vascular and neurological channels which traverse those walls, are all factors responsible for the early invasion of the orbit in sinus neoplasia. The frequency with which this occurs varies, with different authors quoting 26% (Wustrow[145]), 33% (Henderson[146]), 45% (Conley & Baker[147]), whilst Johnson et al give 59%.[148] These variations are influenced by definitions of invasion and individual experience of advanced neoplasms. Diagnosis presents few problems in most cases when there are ophthalmic symptoms such as proptosis, disorders of ocular movement, chemosis or visual loss. Orbital involvement however, may be asymptomatic presenting problems in surgical assessment. Radiology, especially CT and MRI are helpful although not able to visualize all of the orbital walls. Although gross destruction presents few problems in management, an apparently intact wall does not invalidate the possibility of intraorbital disease. A final decision can only be made at exploration.[149,150] Rochels & Nover have successfully used echography to evaluate orbital invasion in 67 patients with paranasal tumours, claiming an ability to differentiate carcinomas from sarcomas.[151] Despite macroscopical tumour within the orbit, the orbital periosteum invariably remains intact and tumour is only found in the periorbital fat via the inferior conjunctival sac (Fig. 6.10).[152] Radical excision is then impossible whilst the eye remains in situ but this

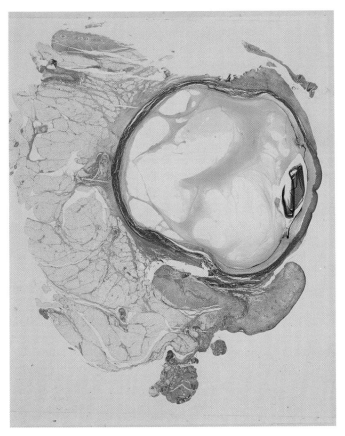

Fig. 6.10 Surgical specimen of orbital clearance with intraconal infiltration by squamous cell carcinoma.

represents an advanced situation with palliation the primary object of treatment. The position is more complex in more favourable cases in which both ocular movement and vision is normal. The concept of preserving orbital contents is supported by many authors[113,145] since clearance frequently represents gross subtotal removal of tumour due to the difficulty of resecting the orbital apex without total orbitotomy. Survival following exenteration varies from 0 to 32%, although these figures ignore the palliative effect of removing a painful, proptosed-ulcerated eye.[152,153] Preservation of the eyelids is possible in most patients, allowing orbital clearance (rather than exenteration) to be succeeded by a skin-lined socket. If bone erosion is limited to the orbital rim or medial wall, an oncological resection is possible and local removal of involved periosteum permits preservation of the orbital contents. The craniofacial approach does provide better access and visualization of the posterior aspect of the medial orbital wall and successful periosteal resection has been reported by Cheesman et al.[154]

A wide variety of changes may be found in the globe following high dose radiotherapy, although Nakissa et al say that if the purpose of treatment is cure then dosage should not be compromised. They treated 30 patients with paranasal sinus cancer with doses varying from 5000

to 7000 rad of Cobalt-60. 17 patients had orbital involvement and all who received more than 6000 rad had posterior ocular problems involving the retina or optic nerve. Five patients were long-term survivors![155]

The majority of patients with ethmoid and maxillary sinus carcinoma are treated with combinations of surgery and radiotherapy and the success of preoperative irradiation can therefore be evaluated at exploration. Som raised a query regarding orbital periosteum without macroscopic tumour but in relation to an area of bone destruction. Should the eye be removed? In practice this is rarely a dilemma, for either disease is left in situ or the periosteum can be resected, the defect being primarily repaired.[156] Where this is not possible, and this applies to many cases where maxillary sinus cancer has entered the posterior part of the orbit via the inferior orbital fissure, preservation of the orbital contents leaves disease at the apex. Subsequent growth soon results in proptosis, chemosis and blindness. Although the inclusion of orbital clearance with total maxillectomy or craniofacial resection does not result in an oncological 'block dissection' nor does it materially effect cure rates, it has a considerable palliative value. Harrison has considered these problems in relation to long-term palliation, emphasizing that with a skin-lined socket, good symptomatic control is possible even with residual disease at the apex.[83] Many of the authors advocating preservation of the eye do not differentiate patients with histologically-confirmed neoplasm on the orbital periosteum from those with bone erosion but 'clear' exposed periosteum. Orbital clearance is clearly not indicated in the absence of proven tumour but palliation is impossible with a painful, proptosed eye.

Table 6.6, a composite analysis of a selection of results taken from papers published within the 1980s when

Table 6.6 Squamous cell carcinoma of maxilla, 5-year survival

Author	No. of patients	5-year survival (%)			
		T2	T3	T4	All
Surgery and DXT					
Weymuller et al 1980[153]	62	–	–	–	35
Lee & Ogura 1981[157]	61	45	28	38	38
St-Pierre & Baker 1983[114]	66	75	28.5	19.4	32.4
McNicoll et al 1984[96]	218	–	–	–	23.3
Linderman et al 1987[162]	55	70	15	25	27
Har-El et al 1988[118]	70	–	–	–	38.6
Sisson et al 1989[141]	60	73	41	15	48
Chemotherapy					
Sakai et al 1983[164]	134	–	–	–	54
Knegt et al 1984[160]	28	–	–	–	52
Tsujii et al 1986[144]	208	100	50	24.4	45.6
LoRusso et al 1987[163]	13	–	36	9.5	?

modern radiotherapeutic and surgical techniques have been used in the treatment of a total of 975 patients with maxillary sinus carcinoma, provides little encouragement. Apart from Japanese data, most have used the AJC classification system and although T2 tumours appear to have a uniformly good 5-year survival rate of 70% (except Lee and Ogura's 45%) variations between T3 and T4 illustrate the difficulties of applying this system in clinical practice. An overall figure of 35% is probably a more realistic reflection of general experience unless an unusually large number of early cases are treated. It is interesting that Lee and Ogura say 'the AJC staging in our group of patients has not been found to correspond well with primary control in combined treatment results, largely due to a failure to recognize the difference between accessible areas of involvement and non-accessible areas following radical resection'. There is little prospect of earlier diagnosis in what is fundamentally an unusual neoplasm and radiotherapy plus surgery has probably reached its zenith. However, provisional results of multimodal therapy, largely carried out in Japan, have produced some remarkable results. Table 6.6 shows the data from four publications and although T staging is not easy to comprehend, an average 5-year survival figure of 45% to 54% for 366 patients is an impressive improvement over past experiences.

Sakai et al[158] first combined cytotoxic therapy (5-fluorouracil with bleomycin) with radiotherapy in 1967–1971, reserving surgery for the 40% failures. From 1972 to 1975 this regime was modified by initially withdrawing the chemotherapy but the incidence of maxillectomy remained at 30% and systemic metastases required the addition of 5-fluorouracil in 68% of these patients. From 1976 to 1992, radiotherapy 5000 rad in 5 weeks together with intra-arterial 5-fluorouracil to a total dose of 2000 mg has been combined with tumour reduction using cryosurgery. The frequency of maxillectomy has been reduced to 22% and the 5-year cumulative survival rate for the 134 patients treated between 1976 and 1979 is 54%. They admit that difficulties with cryosurgery include assessment of tumour infiltration, protection of brain and orbit, together with accurate placement of the probe!

Tsujii et al[144] dispensed with intra-arterial infusion because of the multiplicity of vascular feeders to the maxillary antrum, which includes not only the maxillary artery but the internal carotid and many other branches from the external carotid.[159] Topical 5-fluorouracil ointment is applied following partial maxillectomy and then combined with radiotherapy. Their actuarial survival rate of 45.6% at 5 years dropped to 36.2% at 10 years and 57.8% had persistent disease following one course of treatment. Details of surgical salvage are not given in their paper but they do comment that since 1980 when CT planning was introduced, there has been a reduction in ocular complications and an increase in survival rates.

Knegt et al introduced this approach into The Netherlands in 1976 reporting their results for the period 1976–1981 in 1985.[160] In 60 patients with paranasal sinus carcinoma they obtained a 52% 5-year actuarial survival rate for the 28 patients with maxillary sinus disease. Treatment consisted of 4000 rad preoperative radiotherapy with a 4 Mev linear accelerator followed by partial maxillectomy and curettage of macroscopical tumour. Clearance of the orbit or craniotomy was reserved for those with dural or periosteal disease. 5-Fluorouracil ointment was applied to 'places where the tumour may remain'. Postoperative radiotherapy, 2000 rad in 5 days was started on the 3rd day following surgery. 13 patients (22%) had residual neoplasm which was treated by local removal, more ointment and additional radiotherapy. 12 patients were classified using the AJC system as T3N0, 13 as T4N0 and three of the 28 patients had metastatic disease at diagnosis. Cleaning and packing the antral cavity was described as being painful, requiring morphine analgesia although this subsided unless bone invasion was present. No patients apparently had a maxillectomy.

The search for ways whereby the survival rate for maxillary carcinoma could be improved from its present overall figure of about 35% continues, with the hope that combinations of earlier diagnosis and, in selected cases, more effective surgery may prove of value. Reports of the use of adjuvant chemotherapy to improve survival, and hopefully to reduce the need for maxillectomy, are encouraging but must in part relate to the initial extent of the tumour at diagnosis. A greater awareness of this neoplasm in Japan, combined with the intrinsic deficiencies in classification systems, may be responsible for some of the substantial improvements reported for, in many ways, less radical treatment.

Prognosis

Prospective randomized trials are the best means of identifying prognostic factors. However, the small numbers of available patients with maxillary sinus cancer and the diversity of classification systems and treatment regimes, make these difficult to investigate. Kondo et al[112] carried out a multivariate regression analysis of 95 patients to identify prognostic factors and concluded that T stage was the most significant factor, in terms of both relapse and survival. Since local control is related to these factors, surgical success must also play some role with total maxillectomy preferable to partial procedures. The incidence of cervical lymph node involvement at presentation is variable because of its rarity, with figures varying from 4 to 20%. Salvage rates are low and prophylactic neck dissection is not indicated by any author.[93]

However, this remains an uncommon neoplasm with significant symptoms representing advanced disease. Preoperative staging remains imprecise although improved by the use of CT and MRI, and treatment success isprimarily related to obtaining local control. The presence or development of cervical or systemic metastases carries a

poor prognosis and Shibuya et al[161] found that the risk of another cancer in the unaffected sinus in surviving patients was 67 times greater than that expected by chance!

REFERENCES

1. Batsakis J G, Rice D H, Solomon A R 1980 Pathology of head and neck tumours: squamous and mucous gland carcinoma of the nasal cavity, paranasal sinuses and larynx. Part 6. Head and Neck Surgery 2: 497–508
2. Busutill A, More I A R, McSeveny D 1977 A reappraisal of the ultrastructure of the human respiratory nasal mucosa. Journal of Anatomy 124: 445–458
3. Hellquist H B 1990 Pathology of the nose and paranasal sinuses. Butterworths, London, a: p 88; b: p 1174
4. Frierson H F, Mills S E, Fechner R E 1986 Sinonasal undifferentiated carcinoma, an aggressive neoplasm derived from Schneideran epithelium and distinct from olfactory epithelium. American Journal of Surgical Pathology 10: 771–779
5. Bacon M P, MacLeod T I F 1989 Verrucous carcinoma of the maxillary antrum. Journal of Laryngology and Otology 103: 415–416
6. Elliott G B, MacDougall J A, Elliott J D A 1973 Problems of verrucous carcinoma. Annals of Surgery 177: 21–29
7. Hanna G S, Ali M H 1987 Verrucous carcinoma of the nasal septum. Journal of Laryngology and Otology 101: 184–187
8. Michaels L 1987 Malignant neoplasms of surface epithelium. In: Ear, nose and throat histopathology. Springer-Verlag, Berlin, pp 171–176
9. Lund V J 1991 Malignancy of the nose and sinuses, epidemiological and aetiological considerations. Rhinology 29: 57–68
10. WHO manual of the International Statistical Classification of Diseases, Injuries and Causes of Death. 1967 Vol. 1. World Health Organization, Geneva
11. Anderson H C, Anderson I, Solgaard J 1977 Nasal cancers, symptoms and upper airway functions in woodworkers. British Journal of Industrial Medicine 34: 201–207
12. Rowland R E 1975 The risk of malignancy from internally deposited radioisotopes. In: Radiation research – biomedical, chemical and physical perspectives. Academic Press, New York, pp 146–155
13. Boysen M, Solberg L A, Torjussen W 1984 Histological changes, rhinoscopic findings and nickel concentrations in plasma and urine in retired nickel workers. Archives of Otolaryngology (Stockholm) 97: 105–115
14. Acherson E D, Cowdell R H, Hadfield E 1968 Nasal cancer in woodworkers in the furniture industry. British Medical Journal 2: 587–596
15. Macbeth R G 1965 Malignant disease of the paranasal sinuses. Journal of Laryngology and Otology 79: 592–612
16. Hernberg S, Westerholm P, Schultz L K 1983 Nasal and sinus cancer, connection with occupational exposures in Denmark, Finland and Sweden. Scandinavian Journal of Work and Environmental Health 9: 315–326
17. Voss R, Stenerson T, Oppedal B R 1985 Sinonasal cancer and exposure to softwood. Acta Otolaryngologica (Stockholm) 99: 172–178
18. Takasaka T, Kawamoto K, Nakamura K 1987 A case-control study of nasal cancers. Acta Otolaryngologica (Stockholm) Suppl. 435: 136–142
19. Wada S, Miyanishi P, Nishimoto Y 1968 Mustard gas as a cause of neoplasia in man. Lancet 1: 1161–1163
20. Doll R, Morgan I G, Speizer F E 1970 Cancer of the lung and sinuses in nickel workers. British Journal of Cancer 12: 32–41
21. Pederson E, Hogetueit A C, Anderson A 1973 Cancer of the respiratory tract organs amongst workers in the nickel industry. International Journal of Cancer 12: 32–41
22. Stell P M, McGill T 1977 Asbestos and cancer of the head and neck. Lancet 1: 678

23. Roush G C 1979 Epidemiology of cancer of the nose and paranasal sinuses, current concepts. Head and Neck Surgery 2: 3–11
24. Hayes R B, Kardaun J W, De Bruyn A 1987 Tobacco use and sinonasal cancer. British Journal of Cancer 56: 843–846
25. Shimizu H, Hozawa J, Saito H 1989 Chronic sinusitis and woodworking risk factors in cancer of the maxillary sinus in North East Japan. Laryngoscope 99: 58–61
26. Harrison D F N 1964 Snuff – its use and abuse. British Medical Journal 2: 1649–1652
27. Keen P 1974 Trace elements in plants and soil in relation to cancer. South African Medical Journal 48: 2363–2364
28. Acherson E D, Cowdell R H, Jolles B 1970 British Medical Journal 1: 385–393
29. Rankow R M, Conley J, Fodor P 1974 Carcinoma of the maxillary sinus following thorotrast instillation. Journal of Maxillofacial Surgery 2: 119–126
30. Fukuda K, Motomura M, Yamakawa M 1985 Relationship of occupation with cancer of the maxillary sinus in Hokkaido, Japan. National Cancer Institute Monographs 69: 169–173
31. Strader C H, Vaughan T L, Stergachinis A 1988 Use of nasal preparations and the incidence of sinonasal cancer. Journal of Epidemiology and Community Health 42: 243–248
32. Robin P E, Powell D J, Stansbie J M 1979 Carcinoma of the nasal cavity and paranasal sinuses: incidence and presentation of different histological types. Clinical Otolaryngology 4: 431–456
33. Lewis J S, Castro E B 1972 Cancer of the nasal cavity and paranasal sinuses. Journal of Laryngology and Otology 86: 255–261
34. Lederman M 1970 Tumours of the upper jaw: natural history and treatment. Journal of Laryngology and Otology 84: 369–401
35. Larssen L G, Martensson G 1972 Maxillary antral cancer. Journal of the American Medical Association 219: 342–347
36. Waterhouse J, Muir C S, Correa P, Powell J 1976 Cancer Incidence in Five Continents Vol. III. I.A.R.C. Publications No. 15 International Agency for Research in Cancer, Lyon
37. Mason T J, McKay F W 1974 US Cancer Mortality by County 1950–1969. DHEW Publications, Washington DC No. 74–615
38. Osmond C, Gardner M J, Acheson E D 1983 Trends in cancer mortality, analysis by period of birth and death 1951–1980. H.M.S.O., London
39. Shiffman N S 1979 Anterior intranasal carcinoma. Canadian Journal of Surgery 22: 159–160
40. Robin P E, Shortridge R T J 1979 Lateralization of tumours of the nasal cavity and paranasal sinuses and its relationship to aetiology. Lancet 1: 695–696
41. Morton R P, Sellars S L 1988 Laterality of sinonasal cancer and its aetiological implications. Clinical Otolaryngology 13: 193–196
42. Hopkin N, McNicoll W, Dalley V M 1984 Cancer of the paranasal sinuses and nasal cavities. Journal of Laryngology and Otology 98: 585–595
43. Kagan A R, Nussbaum H, Rao A et al 1981 The management of carcinoma of the nasal vestibule. Head and Neck Surgery 4: 125–128
44. Barzan L, Franchin G, DePaoli A 1990 Carcinoma of the nasal vestibule: a report of 12 cases. Journal of Laryngology and Otology 104: 9–11
45. Vendelbo J L, Franchin G, De Paoli A 1984 Squamous cell carcinoma of the nasal vestibule, treatment results. Acta Radiologica Oncologia 23: 189–192
46. Bodit A O, Kurohara S, Webster J H 1969 Treatment of cancer of the nasal cavity. American Journal of Roentgenology 106: 824–834
47. Wang C C 1975 Treatment of carcinoma of the nasal vestibule by radiation. Cancer 38: 100–106
48. Goepfert H, Guillamondegui O M, Jesse R H 1974 Squamous cell carcinoma of the nasal vestibule. Archives of Laryngology and Otology 100: 8–10

49. Helliwell T R, Yeoh L H, Stell P M 1986 Anaplastic carcinoma of the nose and paranasal sinuses, light microscopy, immunohisto-chemistry and clinical correlation. Cancer 58: 2038–2045

50. Chobe R, McNesse M, Weber R 1988 Radiation therapy for carcinoma of the nasal vestibule. Otolaryngology, Head and Neck Surgery 98: 67–71

51. Wong C S, Cummings B S, Elhakim T 1986 External irradiation of squamous carcinoma of the nasal vestibule. International Journal of Radiation Oncology, Biology and Physics 12: 1943–1946

52. De Jong J M A, Schalekamp W, Nording J 1981 Squamous carcinoma of the nasal vestibule. Clinical Otolaryngology 6: 205–208

53. Mak A C A, van Andel J G, van Woerkom 1980 Radiation therapy for carcinoma of the nasal vestibule. European Journal of Cancer 16: 81–85

54. Haynes W D, Tapley N 1974 Radiation treatment of cancer of the nasal vestibule. American Journal of Roentgenology, Radiation and Therapeutic Medicine 120: 595–612

55. Muir C S, Nectoux J 1980 Descriptive epidemiology of malignant neoplasm of nose, nasal cavity, middle ear and accessory sinuses. Clinical Otolaryngology 5: 195–211

56. Maran A G D, Lund V J 1990 Clinical Rhinology. Thieme Verlag, Berlin, pp 4

57. Gibb J S 1902 Malignant disease of the nose and paranasal sinuses. New York State Journal of Medicine 2: 24–56

58. Beard E A 1905 Malignant disease of the nose and accessory sinuses. New York State Journal of Medicine 10: 57–61

59. Ridout C A S 1914 Carcinoma of the septum nasi – removal of the septum through Olliers incision. British Medical Journal 1: 1017

60. Yarrington C T, Jaquiss G W, Sprinkle P M 1969 Carcinoma of the nose and nasal septum, treatment and reconstruction. Transactions of the American Academy of Ophthalmology and Otolaryngology 73: 1178–1183

61. Young J R 1979 Malignant tumours of the nasal septum. Journal of Laryngology and Otology 93: 817–832

62. Weimert T A, Batsakis J J, Rice D H 1978 Carcinoma of the nasal septum. Journal of Laryngology and Otology 92: 209–213

63. LeLieve W C, Bailey B J, Griffiths C 1984 Carcinoma of the nasal septum. Archives of Otolaryngology 110: 748–751

64. Echeverria-Zumarraga M, Kaiser C, Gavilan C 1988 Nasal septal carcinoma: initial symptoms of nasal sinus perforation. Journal of Laryngology and Otology 102: 834–835

65. Beatty C W, Pearson B W, Kern E B 1982 Carcinoma of the nasal septum, experience of 85 cases. Otolaryngology, Head and Neck Surgery 90: 90–94

66. Lyons G D 1969 Squamous carcinoma of the nasal septum. Archives of Otolaryngology 89: 585–587

67. Ringertz W 1938 Pathology of malignant tumours arising in the nasal cavity, paranasal sinuses and maxilla. Acta Otolaryngologica (Stockholm) Suppl. 27: 1–495

68. Deutsch H J 1966 Carcinoma of the nasal septum, report of a case and review of the literature. Annals of Otology, Rhinology and Laryngology 75: 1049–1057

69. Boulos E J 1984 External rhinoplasty approach for lesions of the nasal vestibule. Laryngoscope 94: 703–704

70. MacComb W S, Martin H E 1942 Cancer of the nasal cavity. American Journal of Radiology 47: 11–23

71. Whitcomb W P 1969 Radiation therapy for carcinoma of the anterior nasal cavity. American Journal of Radiology 105: 550–554

72. Harrison D F N 1982 Total rhinectomy – a worthwhile operation. Journal of Laryngology and Otology 96: 1113–1123

73. Harrison D F N 1967 Snuff – its use and abuse: an essay on nasal physiology. In: Cancer of the nasopharynx. UICC Monograph 1: 119–123

74. Higginson J, Oettle A G 1960 Cancer incidence in the Bantu and 'Cape Coloured' races of South Africa: report of a cancer survey in the Transvaal. 1953–1955. Journal of the National Cancer Institute 24: 589–613

75. Jackson R T, Fitz-Hugh G S, Constable W C 1977 Malignant neoplasms of the nasal cavities and paranasal sinuses. Laryngoscope 87: 726–736

76. Robin P E, Powell D J 1981 Diagnostic errors in cancer of the nasal cavity and paranasal sinuses. Archives of Otolaryngology 107: 138–140

77. Hayes R B, Raatgever J W, Bruyn de A 1986 Cancer of the nasal cavity and paranasal sinuses and formaldehyde exposure. International Journal of Cancer 37: 487–492

78. Blair A, Stewart P, O'Berg M et al 1986 Morbidity amongst industrial workers exposed to formaldehyde. Journal of the National Cancer Institute 76: 1071–1084

79. Wilhelmsson B, Drettner B 1984 Nasal problems in wood furniture workers, a study of symptoms and physiological variables. Acta Otolaryngologica (Stockholm) 98: 321–334

80. Wilhelmsson B, Lundh B 1984 Nasal epithelium in woodworkers in the furniture industry, a histological and cytological study. Acta Otolaryngologica (Stockholm) 98: 548–555

81. Holmstrom M, Wihelmsson B 1988 Respiratory systems and pathophysiological effects of occupational exposure to formaldehyde and wood dust. Scandinavian Journal of Work and Environmental Health 14: 306–311

82. Weber A L, Stanton A C 1984 Malignant tumours of the paranasal sinuses: radiologic, clinical and histopathologic evaluation of 200 cases. Head and Neck Surgery 6: 761–776

83. Harrison D F N 1978 A critical look at the classification of maxillary sinus carcinomata. Annals of Otology, Rhinology and Laryngology 87: 3–9

84. Jing B 1970 Roetgen diagnosis of malignant tumours of the paranasal sinuses and nasal cavity. Annals of Otology, Rhinology and Laryngology 79: 584–592

85. Lloyd G A S 1990 CT of the paranasal sinuses: study of a control series in relation to endoscopic surgery. Journal of Laryngology and Otology 104: 477–481

86. Lloyd G A S 1988 Diagnostic imaging of the nose and paranasal sinuses. Springer Verlag, Berlin

87. Friedman I, Osborne D A 1982 Tumours of the nose and sinuses. In: Pathology of granulomas and neoplasms of the nose and sinuses. Churchill Livingstone, Edinburgh, pp 100–102

88. Gadenberg C C, Hjelm-Hansen M, Sogaard H 1984 Malignant tumours of the paranasal sinuses and nasal cavity – a series of 180 patients. Acta Radiologica and Oncologica 23: 181–187

89. Batsakis J G 1981 'Psuedosarcoma' of the mucous membranes of the head and neck. Journal of Laryngology and Otology 95: 311–316

90. Shindo M L, Stanley R B, Kiyabi M T 1990 Carcinosarcoma of the nasal cavity and paranasal sinuses. Head and Neck Surgery 12: 515–519

91. Feinmesser R, Weisel J, Deutsch E 1982 Carcinosarcoma of the nose and paranasal sinuses – a case report. Rhinology 20: 167–170

92. Hafiz M A, Mira J, Toker C 1989 Post-irradiation carcinosarcoma of the nasal cavity. Otolaryngology, Head and Neck Surgery 97: 319–321

93. Robin P E, Powell D J 1980 Regional node involvement and distant metastases in carcinoma of the nasal cavity and paranasal sinuses. Journal of Laryngology and Otology 94: 301–309

94. Lederman M, Busby E R, Mould R F 1969 The treatment of tumours of the upper jaw. British Journal of Radiology 42: 561–581

95. Ellingwood K E, Million R P 1979 Cancer of the nasal cavity and ethmoid/sphenoid sinuses. Cancer 43: 1517–1526

96. McNicoll W, Hopkin N, Dalley V M 1984 Cancer of the paranasal sinuses and nasal cavities. Part 2 Results of therapy. Journal of Laryngology and Otology 98: 707–718

97. Frazell E L, Lewis J S 1963 Cancer of the nasal cavity and accessory sinuses. Cancer 16: 1293–1301

98. Harrison D F N 1977 Lateral rhinotomy: a neglected operation. Annals of Otology, Rhinology and Laryngology 86: 1–4

99. Harrison D F N 1981 Surgical approach to the medial wall of the orbit. Annals of Otology, Rhinology and Laryngology 90: 415–419

100. Harrison D F N 1984 Surgical pathology of olfactory neuroblastomata. Head and Neck Surgery 7: 751–756

101. Osguthorpe J D, Weisman R A 1991 'Medial maxillectomy' for lateral nasal wall neoplasms. Archives of Otolaryngology 117: 751–756

102. Proust R 1908 La chirurgie de l'hypophyse. Journal de Chirurgie 7: 665–680
103. Biller H F, Slotnik D B, Lawson W 1989 Superior rhinotomy for en bloc resection of bilateral ethmoidal tumours. Archives of Otolaryngology 115: 1463–1466
104. Mann W J 1985 Total rhinotomy for midline lesions of the ethmoids and the nose. Journal of Maxillofacial Surgery 13: 273–276
105. Harrison D F N 1973 The management of malignant tumours affecting the maxillary and ethmoid sinuses. Journal of Laryngology and Otology 87: 749–772
106. Smith R R, Klopp C T, Williams J M 1954 Surgical treatment of cancer of the frontal sinus and adjacent areas. Cancer 7: 991–994
107. Ketcham A S, Chretien P B, Van Buren J M 1973 The ethmoid sinuses: a re-evaluation of surgical resection. American Journal of Surgery 126: 469–473
108. Cheesman A D, Lund V J, Howard D J 1986 Craniofacial resection for tumours of the nasal cavity and paranasal sinuses. Head and Neck Surgery 8: 429–435
109. Jackson I T, Munro I R, Hide T 1984 Treatment of tumours involving the anterior cranial fossa. Head and Neck Surgery 6: 901–913
110. Grant R N, Silverberg E 1970 Cancer Statistics 1970. American Cancer Society, pp 8–14
111. Segi M, Tominaga S, Aoki K 1981 Gann Monograph in Cancer Research No. 26. Japan Scientific Societies Press, Tokyo
112. Kondo M, Ogawa K, Inuyama Y et al 1985 Prognostic factors influencing relapse of squamous carcinoma of the maxillary sinus. Cancer 55: 190–196
113. Sisson G A 1970 Treatment of malignancies of the paranasal sinuses. Laryngoscope 80: 945–953
114. St Pierre S, Baker S R 1983 Squamous cell carcinoma of the maxillary sinus: analysis of 66 cases. Head and Neck Surgery 5: 508–513
115. Bennett M 1970 Paranasal sinus malignancies. Laryngoscope 80: 933–944
116. Baker R, Cherry J, Lott S 1966 Carcinoma of the maxillary sinus. Archives of Otolaryngology 84: 201–204
117. Miyaguchi M, Saki S, Mori N 1990 Symptoms in patients with maxillary sinus carcinoma. Journal of Laryngology and Otology 104: 557–559
118. Har-El G, Hadar T, Krespi Y P 1988 An analysis of staging systems for carcinoma of the maxillary sinus. Ear, Nose and Throat Journal 67: 511–520
119. Som P M 1982 The role of CT in the diagnosis of carcinoma of the paranasal sinuses. Journal of Otolaryngology 11: 340–348
120. Hesselink J R, New P F J, Davis K R 1978 Computed tomography of the paranasal sinuses and face. Journal of Computed Assisted Tomography 2: 568–576
121. Ackerman L 1948 Verrucous carcinoma of the oral cavity. Surgery 23: 670–678
122. Bacon M P, Chevretton E B, Slack R W T 1989 Verrucous carcinoma of the maxillary sinus. Journal of Laryngology and Otology 103: 415–416
123. Daoud A, Lannigan J A, McGlashan A 1991 Verrucous carcinoma of the maxillary sinus. Journal of Laryngology and Otology 105: 696–699
124. Michaels L, Cooper J, Brewer C S 1984 Image analysis in histological diagnosis of verrucous squamous carcinoma of the larynx. Journal of Pathology 143: 329
125. Schwade J G, Wara W M, DeDo H H 1976 Radiotherapy for verrucous carcinoma. Radiology 120: 677–679
126. Ellis G L, Corio R L 1980 Spindle-cell carcinoma of the oral cavity. Oral Surgery, Oral Medicine, Oral Pathology 50: 523–528
127. Middlehurst R S, Blackburn C W, Sloan P 1990 Spindle-cell carcinoma: a case report. British Journal of Oral and Maxillofacial Surgery 28: 114–116
128. Lederman M 1969 Cancer of the upper jaw and nasal chambers. Proceedings of the Royal Society of Medicine 62: 65–72
129. Baugh R F, Wolf G T, McClatchey D 1986 Small cell carcinoma of the head and neck. Head and Neck Surgery 8: 343–354
130. Silva E G, Butler J J, Macckey B, Goepfert H 1982 Neuroblastomas and neuroendocrine carcinoma of the nasal cavity. Cancer 50: 2388–2405
131. Weiss M D, de Fries H O, Taxy J B 1983 Primary small cell carcinoma of the paranasal sinuses. Archives of Otolaryngology 109: 341–343
132. Koss L G, Spiro R H, Hasdu S 1972 Small cell carcinoma of minor salivary gland origin. Cancer 30: 737–741
133. Kimmelman C P, Haller D G 1983 Small cell carcinoma of the head and neck. Otolaryngology, Head and Neck Surgery 91: 708–712
134. Ohngren L G 1933 Malignant tumours of the maxillo-ethmoidal region. Acta Otolaryngologica (Stockholm) 19: 1–476
135. Sebileau P 1906 Les formes cliniques du cancer du sinus maxillaire. Annals malades d'oreille, du larynx, nez et pharynx 32: 430–450
136. Sisson G A, Johnson N E, Amir C S 1963 Cancer of the maxillary sinus: clinical classification and management. Annals of Otology, Rhinology and Laryngology 72: 1050–1059
137. Rubin P 1972 Cancer of the head and neck: nose and paranasal sinuses. Journal of the American Medical Association 219: 336–338
138. Chandler J R, Guillamondegui O M, Sisson G A 1976 Clinical staging of cancer of the head and neck: a new system. American Journal of Surgery 132: 532–538
139. Sakai S, Hamasaki Y 1967 Proposal for the classification of carcinoma of the paranasal sinuses. Acta Otolaryngologica (Stockholm) 63: 42–48
140. Williatt D J, Morton R P, Stell P M 1987 Staging of maxillary sinus cancer – which classification? Annals of Otology, Rhinology and Laryngology 96: 137–141
141. Sisson G A, Toriumi D M, Atiyah R A 1989 Paranasal sinus malignancy: a comprehensive update. Laryngoscope 99: 143–150
142. Beale F A, Garrett P G 1983 Cancer of the paranasal sinuses with particular reference to the maxillary sinus. Laryngoscope 99: 143–150
143. Boone M L M, Harle T H 1968 Malignant disease of the paranasal sinuses and nasal cavity. American Journal of Roentgenology 102: 627–636
144. Tsujii H, Kamada T, Arimoto T et al 1986 Role of rad iotherapy in the management of maxillary sinus cancer. Cancer 57: 2261–2266
145. Wustrow F 1965 Orbital tumours. Saunders, Philadelphia, pp 444–473
146. Henderson J W 1973 Orbital tumours. Saunders, Philadelphia, pp 444–473
147. Conley J, Baker D C 1979 Management of the eye socket in cancer of the paranasal sinuses. Archives of Otolaryngology 105: 702–705
148. Johnson L N, Krohel G B, Yeon E B 1984 Sinus tumours invading the orbit. Ophthalmology 91: 209–217
149. Graamans K, Slootweg P J 1989 Orbital exenteration in surgery of malignant neoplasms of the paranasal sinuses. Archives of Otolaryngology 115: 977–980
150. Harrison D F N 1976 Management of malignant tumours affecting the maxillary and ethmoidal sinuses. Journal of Laryngology and Otology 90: 69–74
151. Rochels R, Nover A 1986 Echography of paranasal tumours invading the orbit. Orbit 6: 123–127
152. Harrison D F N 1980 The ENT surgeon looks at the orbit. Journal of Laryngology and Otology Suppl. 3
153. Weymuller E A, Reardon E J, Nash D 1980 Comparison of treatment modalities in carcinoma of the maxillary sinus. Archives of Otolaryngology 106: 625–629
154. Cheesman A D, Quiney R E, Wright J E 1989 Craniofacial resection for orbital tumours. Annals of the Royal College of Surgeons of England 71: 333–337
155. Nakissa N, Rubin P, Strohl R 1983 Ocular and orbital complications following radiation therapy for paranasal sinus malignancies. Cancer 51: 980–986
156. Som M L 1974 Surgical management of carcinoma of the maxilla. Archives of Otolaryngology 99: 270–273
157. Lee F, Ogura J H 1981 Maxillary sinus carcinoma. Laryngoscope 91: 133–139

158. Sakai S, Honki A, Fuchihata D D, Tanaka Y 1983 Multi-disciplinary treatment of maxillary sinus cancer. Cancer 52: 1360–1364

159. Shibuya H, Suzuki S, Horiuchi J et al 1982 Reappraisal of trimodal combination therapy for maxillary sinus carcinoma. Cancer 50: 2790–2794

160. Knegt P P, Jong P C, Andel J G 1985 Carcinoma of the paranasal sinuses. Cancer 62: 1–5

161. Shibuya H, Amagasa T, Hanai A 1986 Second primary cancer in patients with squamous carcinoma in the maxillary sinus. Cancer 58: 1122–1125

162. Linderman P, Eklund V, Petruson B 1987 Survival after surgical treatment for maxillary neoplasms of epithelial origin. Journal of Laryngology and Otology 101: 564–568

163. LoRusso P, Tapazoglou E, Kish J A 1987 Chemotherapy for paranasal sinus tumours. Cancer 62: 1–5

164. Sakai S, Murata M, Susaki R 1983 Combined therapy for maxillary sinus cancer with special reference to cryosurgery. Rhinology 21: 179–184

7. Nonepidermoid epithelial neoplasms

In comparison with the epidermoid or squamous cell neoplasms which comprise over 80% of tumours in the upper aero-digestive tract, the nonepidermoid epithelial tumours constitute only 4–8%. All the major salivary gland histological types however, are represented though the incidence of malignant tumours in minor salivary glands varies from 13% to 90% depending upon the series.[1] The minor salivary gland tumours account for approximately 18% of all salivary gland neoplasms[2] and the palate is by far the commonest location, accounting for half of these.

A number of classifications have been proposed for the nonepidermoid epithelial tumours, which generally relate to the cell of origin, be it from surface mucosa or sero-mucinous gland (Table 7.1). As the seromucinous glands are derived embryologically from the surface mucosa[3] such distinction may be of academic interest only.

MONOMORPHIC ADENOMAS

As the name implies, these lesions are theoretically composed of one cell type, which lacks the polymorphism of cells and the stroma of the mixed tumour and behaves in a clinically benign fashion.[4] They occasionally occur on

Table 7.1 Nonepidermoid glandular tumours in the upper respiratory tract[6]

| | Origin of tumour | |
	Salivary type	Surface mucosa
Benign	Adenoma – monomorphic – pleomorphic	Papillary adenoma
	Oncocytoma	
Malignant	Adenoid cystic	Adenocarcinoma:
	Mucoepidermoid	papillary
	Acinous	sessile
	Carcinoma ex pleomorphic	neuroendocrine
	Adenocarcinoma	'colonic' type
	Adenosquamous carcinoma	undifferentiated
	Clear cell adenocarcinoma	
	Undifferentiated	

the palate, to one side of the midline and posterior to a line drawn between the first molars but are rather unusual in the upper airway. Despite the lack of a well-defined capsule in this region, the incidence of recurrence is relatively low after local excision.[5,6,7a] As with adenomas from minor salivary glands elsewhere, the cellularity of the tumour does not correlate with the incidence of recurrence which is in agreement with DNA values found in the nuclei of such lesions.[8]

PLEOMORPHIC ADENOMA

Definition

This benign neoplasm is composed of a mixed pattern of epithelial and mesenchymal elements.

Synonyms

Mixed tumour, complex adenoma, pleomorphic sialadenoma.

Historical aspects

Zarniko[9] in his monograph 'Diseases of the Nose and Nasopharynx' presented a case originally described by Eichler[10] in 1898 which may represent the first published adenoma of the nasal septum. Hasslauer[11] in 1900 included 4 adenomas in a group of 160 tumours of the nasal cavity and a further case of a nasal mixed tumour appeared in 1911.[12] However, as with many such early descriptions the criteria for the histological diagnosis are unclear. The epithet 'mixed' was actually introduced by Paget[13] in 1853, but opponents of the dualist theory subsequently adopted the term 'pleomorphic'.

Incidence

The tumour is rare in the nose and sinuses, constituting less than 10% of all glandular tumours in the region.[14a,15,16] It is far more common on the palate where up to 60% of benign pleomorphic tumours arising in the minor salivary glands occur (Table 7.2).

Age, sex and ethnic variation (Table 7.2)

Age ranges of 3 to 82 years appear in the literature[6,17] with a mean in the mid-40s. The male to female ratio is essentially equal compared to the female preponderance which exists for the major salivary gland variety. No ethnic predeliction has been described.

Site

In the nasal cavity the majority occur on the septum, either bony or cartilaginous. Occasionally the lateral wall is affected and rarely the tumour arises in the maxillary antrum.[15,16,22-24]

On the palate, the posterior part is most frequently affected where glandular tissue is more abundant.

Aetiology

No predisposing factors have been demonstrated for this condition. There is certainly no evidence for previous suggestions that the lesions arose from remnants of the vomero-nasal organ.[25] This theory is clearly unnecessary as Tos[26] has demonstrated the distribution of glandular elements throughout the sinonasal tract from which such tumours could readily arise.

Clinical features (Table 7.3)

Such slow-growing lesions present with nasal obstruction and occasionally epistaxis when they arise in the nose, or

Table 7.2 Pleomorphic adenomas of upper jaw: series in literature

Author	Patient total no.	Nose/ sinuses no.	Total no. of minor salivary gland tumours	Age range (yr)	Male:female ratio	Follow-up (yr)	Recurrence
Harrison 1956[18]	12	2	82	40–60	1:1	–	–
Ranger et al 1956[19]	21	4	80	26–80	1:1	–	4/8 after local excision only
Chaudhry et al 1961[17]	27	–	94	17–81	1:1.4	>5 (12) 1–5 (15)	0 1
Bergman 1969[1]	19	1	46	17–86	1:1	–	–
Frable & Elzay 1970[2]	27	–	42	11–83	1:1	2–12	2/27
Hjertman & Eneroth 1970[20]	95	–	170	–	–	–	–
Spiro et al 1973[16]	41	4	492	–	–	–	–
Compagno & Wong 1977[21]	–	40	–	–	–	1–41	3/31
Harrison & Lund	8	4	–	26–66	1:1	2–12	0

Table 7.3 Pleomorphic adenomas of nasal cavity: case reports

Author	Age (yr)	Sex	Symptoms	Duration (yr)	Site	Treatment	Follow-up (mth)
Majed 1971[27]	34	F	Nasal obstruction	Many	Septum	Lateral rhinotomy	5
Worthington 1977[28]	17	M	Swelling of cheek	–	Septum	Lateral rhinotomy	–
Bergstrom & Bjorklund 1981[29]	33	M	Epistaxis	2	Septum	Lateral rhinotomy	50
	32	F	Nasal obstruction	1	Septum	Lateral rhinotomy	20
Baraka et al 1984[30]	18	M	Nasal obstruction and swelling	Many	Inferior turbinate	Lateral rhinotomy	20
Kamal 1984[31]	41	F	Nasal obstruction and epistaxis	1 month	Lateral wall	Lateral rhinotomy	–
Haberman & Stanley 1989[32]	33	M	Nasal obstruction	10	Septum	Lateral rhinotomy	20
Freeman et al 1990[33]	32	F	Nasal obstruction	1	Septum Submandibular lymph node	Septectomy Node excision	12

as a painless mass in the palate which may interfere with a denture (Fig. 7.1). They rarely ulcerate and are consequently often present for many years before medical advice is sought, thereby achieving spectacular proportions (Fig. 7.2).

A 28-year-old woman presented with a palatal swelling which had been present for 18 months. A smooth mass was found on the posterior part of the hard palate adjacent to the tuberosity. Biopsy demonstrated a pleomorphic adenoma following which a partial maxillectomy was performed. With the use of an obturator the patient made a good postoperative recovery and was well with no recurrence after a 4-year follow-up.

A 44-year-old policeman from Ghana was referred by ophthalmic surgeons with a massive tumour involving the right forehead, orbit and maxilla (Fig. 7.2). The lesion had been present for 8 years during which four surgical attempts to remove it had been made and a course of radiotherapy had been given. CT scanning confirmed encroachment into the anterior cranial fossa and a craniofacial resection approach and orbital exenteration was undertaken. The defect was repaired with a temporalis muscle flap in addition to conventional fascia lata and split skin graft. The extent of the lesion makes the exact site of origin difficult to determine and he thus represents an additional extraordinary case to those in Table 7.2. He made an excellent postoperative recovery and has been fitted with a facial prosthesis using osseo-integration techniques.

Radiology

Pleomorphic adenomas in the nose have the non-specific features of any benign unilateral lesion. In the palate, the tumour is not invasive but may cause local excavation of bone, producing a sharply defined interface of cortical bone[34] or localized expansion of the hard palate. It is not possible on present scanty information to extrapolate the complex magnetic resonance appearances of parotid and parapharyngeal pleomorphic tumours to the sinonasal tract.

Macroscopic and microscopic appearance

The tumour is well-demarcated, with a smooth lobulated surface. When cut, the tissue is greyish and homogenous with a degree of translucency dependent upon the myxoid component. Lesions of between 0.7 and 7 cm in diameter have been described.

Microscopic appearance

By definition such tumours have epithelial and mesenchymal elements. The epithelial component is often more prominent than that found in its major salivary counterpart. The mesenchymal element is composed of loosely arranged spindle cells filling the interglandular regions though mucoid, myxoid and chondroid areas may be seen.[7a] A fibrous capsule may be identified or may

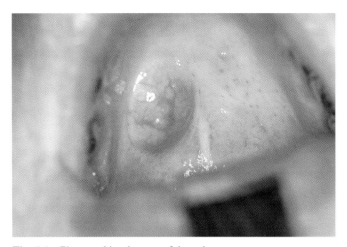

Fig. 7.1 Pleomorphic adenoma of the palate.

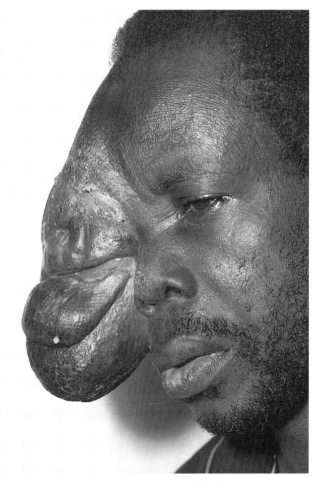

Fig. 7.2 Extensive antro-ethmoidal pleomorphic adenoma (courtesy of D.J. Howard).

result from compression of adjacent tissue. Whilst a rather diffuse infiltrating pattern can be seen in some tumours this does not indicate any clinically malignant potential.[35]

Differential diagnosis

In the absence of a demarcated capsule, it may be necessary to distinguish the tumour from other cellular lesions such as adenocarcinoma, adenoid cystic carcinoma and malignant mixed tumours.

Treatment

The behaviour of these lesions is rarely if ever aggressive and therefore, a wide local excision will suffice in the vast majority of cases. In the nasal cavity a lateral rhinotomy has been used for access (Table 7.3). Some authors have advocated cautery of the area particularly in the palate[2] following surgery but in either case the incidence of recurrence is low (Table 7.2).

Prognosis

The incidence of recurrence in this condition is low. In 31 cases followed for a mean of 7.5 years by Compagno and Wong, three cases recurred and were controlled by further surgery.[21] Similar rates have been described by other authors[2,6,17] though long-term follow-up is required to substantiate such figures. The case reported by Freeman et al[33] is of interest in that the patient had had a benign tumour (histology unknown) removed 17 years earlier. The probable recurrence occurred at the same site and histologically appeared benign but disease was also present in the submandibular lymph node, fulfilling the main criterion of malignancy.

There is little evidence to support the suggestion that stromal composition is related to recurrence.[36]

CARCINOMA EX PLEOMORPHIC ADENOMA AND MALIGNANT MIXED TUMOURS
(Table 7.4)

Two rare malignant forms of pleomorphic tumours in the upper jaw exist. In a carcinoma ex pleomorphic lesion, a malignant epithelial neoplasm arises in a benign pleomorphic adenoma.[37]

In a malignant mixed tumour both epithelial and mesenchymal elements are present and it consequently represents a form of choriocarcinoma.[38] Both are extremely rare and are said to have a greater malignant potential than either adenocarcinoma or adenoid cystic carcinoma.

ONCOCYTOMA

Definition

An oncocytoma is an epithelial tumour composed of large cells containing a granular eosinophilic cytoplasm.

Synonyms

Oxyphil adenoma, oncocytic cell adenoma, eosinophilic or oxyphilic granular cell tumour.

Historical aspects

In 1897 Schaffer[39] described eosinophilic swollen cells in salivary glands, the pharynx, trachea and oesophagus. In 1931 Hamperl[40] used the term 'oncocyte' to describe large cells in major salivary glands filled with acidophilic

Table 7.4 Carcinoma ex pleomorphic and malignant mixed tumours

Author	Site Palate (No.)	Nasal cavity (No.)	Treatment	Outcome	Follow-up (yr)
Carcinoma ex pleomorphic					
Hjertman & Eneroth 1970[20]	3	–	–	–	–
Harrison & Lund	1	–	Wide local excision/radiotherapy	AEW	5
Malignant mixed tumours					
Chaudhry et al 1961[17]	3	–	Wide local excision	1 – recurrence 1 – A&W 1 – DICD	1 1 3
Bergman 1969[1]	1	1	Radical surgery/radiotherapy	2 – AWR	2 (nasal cavity) 7 (palate)
Rafla 1969[12]	–	2	Radiotherapy Radiotherapy/local excision	1 – A&W 1 – AWR	5 5
Frable & Elzay 1970[2]	3	–	1 – Wide local excision 1 – Wide local excision 1 – Wide local excision/radiotherapy	1 – A&W 1 – A&W Dead	4 3 12
Spiro et al 1973[16]	7	1	–	–	–

A&W, alive and well, AWR, alive with recurrent disease, DICD, dead of intercurrent disease granular cytoplasm and in 1936 Gruenfeld & Jorsted[41] reported a lesion in the parotid which they termed an 'oncocytoma'. A similar case had previously appeared in 1927.[42] However, some confusion subsequently ensued in the literature as the term was also used by Jaffe[43] to describe what we now call Warthin's tumour from which it may be clearly distinguished by the lack of lymphoid tissue.

Incidence

Oncocytomas are rare, occurring more often in major rather than minor salivary glands. The incidence in a number of large series varies from 0.1–1% of all salivary gland tumours.[16,44-47] Those affecting the upper jaw are exceptionally rare.

Age, sex and ethnic variation (Table 7.5)

Ages range from 37 to 84 years with no sexual or ethnic preponderance.

Site

Tumours have been described arising in the maxillary sinus, on the palate or in the nasal cavity from whence they may spread to the sinuses.

Aetiology

Oncocytes are found widely distributed in glandular tissue throughout the body, including ovary, adrenal, thyroid, pituitary, liver, pancreas and stomach in addition to major and minor salivary glands.[53] Some discussion has arisen as to whether this lesion represents a true neoplasm or a form of nodular hyperplasia.[54] It was initially thought to be a reaction to trauma or a degenerative process due to ageing but subsequent ultrastructural studies show the cells to be very metabolically active.

Clinical features

Patients present with the usual symptoms of nasal obstruction, rhinorrhoea and epistaxis from nasal lesions; paraesthesia and facial oedema occur with more extensive lesions in the maxilla.

Oncocytomas can exhibit a spectrum of behaviour from benign to malignant.

A 37-year-old female presented with nasal obstruction due to a large left-sided polyp which was subsequently removed. Histology demonstrated an oncocytoma and as CT scanning suggested it was confined to the nasal cavity, clearance via a lateral rhinotomy was undertaken. 6 months later the patient developed epistaxis and noticed a widening of the bridge of the nose. She was referred for craniofacial resection at which a very extensive lesion was found, invading the frontal sinus and anterior cranial fossa and infiltrating the nasal bones which were resected and repaired with iliac crest. A further recurrence was cleared a year later combined with a modified radical neck dissection for nodal disease. The patient died 3 months later.

Considerable discussion surrounded the histology. Examination of the original nasal 'polyp' confirmed oncocytoma but subsequent material was more suggestive of an oncocytic adenocarcinoma which was supported by its natural history.

Radiology

A soft tissue mass with local invasion and bone destruction may be seen, the extent of which will depend upon the aggressiveness of the lesion.

Macroscopic and microscopic appearance

An irregular mass if found, usually lacking the 'capsule' created by compression of surrounding tissue which occurs in the major salivary glands. The benign forms are described as papillary or cystic whereas the more malignant appear solid.

Table 7.5 Oncocytomas of the upper jaw: in world literature

Author	Age (yr)	Sex	Symptoms	Duration	Site	Treatment	Follow-up
Hamperl 1962[49]	55	M	–	–	Nose	–	–
Briggs & Evans 1967[48]	71	F	–	–	Palate	–	2 mth
Cohen & Batsakis 1968[50]	61	M	Obstruction, epistaxis, rhinorrhoea	1 yr	Nose	Caldwell–Luc	8 yr 2 recurrences
Handler & Ward 1979[51]	64	M	Pain, paraesthesia of left cheek	2 yr	Maxilla	Radical maxillectomy	1 yr
Mikhail et al 1988[52]	84	F	Swollen cheek with paraesthesia, diplopia epistaxis	–	Maxilla	Radical maxillectomy	Died 1 yr of intercurrent disease
Harrison & Lund	37	F	Nasal obstruction	3 mth	Nose	Lateral rhinotomy, craniofacial, neck dissection	Died 2 yr of tumour local

Microscopic appearance[55a]

A true oncocyte must:

1. Be present in an organ which is histologically mature
2. Demonstrate high levels of mitochondrial oxidative activity
3. Have large numbers of hypertrophic mitochondria with granular deposits shown on electron microscopy
4. Have no cytoarchitectural features of ductal cells.

Electron microscopy is the best method of demonstration as it can distinguish eosinophilia produced by other organelles such as lysozymes and endoplasmic reticulum. If the above criteria are not fullfilled, the term 'oncocytoid' may be applied.[56]

Differential diagnosis

As oncocytes can occur in association with other definable salivary gland tumours, these lesions must sometimes be distinguished from adenocarcinoma and adenoid cystic carcinoma, as exemplified by the case report (p. 109).

Treatment

Local excision determined by the extent of the tumour is indicated but in the malignant forms, radical neck dissection has sometimes been required for cervical lymphadenopathy. Limited experience precludes any comment on the response of the disease to radiotherapy and chemotherapy.

Prognosis

In common with other histological types, oncocytomas of minor salivary glands are generally more aggressive than their major gland counterparts. The tumour may be locally invasive with bone destruction but can also manifest local lymphatic and distant metastatic spread. Half of the reported cases have behaved in an aggressive fashion and patients may experience frequent recurrence. Prognosis in these circumstances is similar to that for acinic cell or adenocarcinoma so long-term follow-up is required. The location of the primary does not appear to influence subsequent metastasis.[50]

ADENOID CYSTIC CARCINOMA

Definition and aetiology

Adenoid cystic carcinoma is an infiltrating malignant tumour with a characteristic cribriform appearance, deriving from minor seromucinous salivary glands which can occur throughout the mucosa of the upper jaw. No specific aetiologic factors have been determined and there is no association with pleomorphic adenoma.

Synonyms

Cylindroma,[57] adenocystic carcinoma,[58] cribriform adenocarcinoma.[59]

Other terms have included: schleim-cancroid,[60] schlauchknorpelgeschwulst,[61] tubular sarcoma,[62] tubular cancer,[63] cancroid mit hyaliner degeneration,[64] proliferating mucous chondroma,[65] myxosarcoma,[66] proliferating mucous angioma,[67] plexiform angiosarcoma,[68] carcinomatous sarcoma,[69] plexiform sarcoma,[67] alveolar epithelioma with myxomatous invasion,[70] endothelioma interfasciculare,[71] endothelioma hyalinum,[72] angiosarcoma endothelioides,[73] basal cell tumour,[74] basaloma,[75] adenocarcinoma (cylindroma type),[76] adenomyoepithelioma.[77]

Historical aspects

Billroth is frequently credited with the first description of this tumour, occurring in a 22-year-old painter, which he termed 'zylindrome'.[57] In fact the original histological description should be attributed to Robin & Laboulbene[78] who 3 years earlier published an account of three cases of 'heteradenic' tumours in the maxillary antrum, parotid gland and nasal fossa.

A year later they described a further two cases, arising in the lacrimal gland and gum and specifically referred to the presence of perineural spread along adjacent cranial nerves. Billroth's subsequent description, based on three cases of which only one was his own, referred to two types of cylinder, cellular and hyaline.[79] The first he considered glandular canaliculi arising from the lacrimal gland and the second connective tissue deformations in which blood vessels later developed.

Reid is credited with the introduction of 'adenoid cystic',[80] a term used by Foote & Frazell in a fascicle on tumours of the major salivary glands[81] and this term is now widely accepted.

There was considerable confusion initially regarding the malignant potential of the condition. 'Cures' with short-term follow-up were published[82,83] despite a number of reports of cases with distant metastatic spread.[60,72,84–86] Further confusion resulted in 1918 from the classification of adenoid cystic carcinoma with basal cell carcinoma[74] but this was resolved by Speiss in 1930.[87] In 1942 Dockerty & Mayo[76] reported a series of 15 'adenocarcinomas, cylindroma type' with specific malignant properties and capable of perineural spread confirming it as a separate entity.

Incidence

Between 65% and 88% of minor salivary gland tumours in the head and neck are malignant and of these adenoid cystic carcinoma is the commonest form, constituting over one–third of cases.[88–91] However, overall it is said to represent only 1.3% of all tumours of the nose and sinuses[92] so large series with long-term follow-up are rare. It can be found anywhere in the mucous membrane of the upper respiratory tract, and is reported to account for 24% of all palatal tumours[92,109] and 16% of all intraoral minor salivary gland tumours.[17,93]

Age, sex and ethnic variation (Table 7.6)

Our personal series of 49 patients ranges from 23 to 78 years, mean 53 years, with a male to female ratio of 2:1 (Fig. 7.3). A number of other series have reported a similar age range but both a male and female preponderance have been suggested. However, when all published series of adenoid cystic carcinoma affecting the upper jaw are considered the male to female ratio appears equal and the age range of reported cases is from 13 to 84 with the majority of cases occurring in the 4th to 6th decades. No specific ethnic predeliction has been reported.

Site (Table 7.7)

Few large series of adenoid cystic carcinoma of the upper jaw have been published but the maxilla and hard palate appear to be the commonest sites when series are considered individually and overall. The nasal cavity and eth-

Table 7.6 Numbers, sex and age of adenoid cystic carcinoma of the upper jaw in published series

Author	Patient no.	Male	Female	Age range (yr)	Age mean (yr)
Moran et al 1961[94]	10	Ratio 1:1		17–83	48
Tauxe et al 1962[95]	27	16	11	22–63	47
Eby et al 1972[96]	21	Ratio 1:1		16–76	49
Conley & Dingman 1974[88]	35	–	–	40–70	–
Horee 1974[97]	28	12	16	30–77	53
Spiro et al 1974[91]	43	Ratio 1:1		20–84	–
Perzin et al 1978[98]	21	–	–	15–81	–
Marsh & Shannon Allen 1979[99]	7	2	5	39–72	51
Miller & Calcaterra 1980[100]	18	9	9	13–78	46
Chilla et al 1980[92]	11	4	7	50–70	–
Matsuba et al 1984[101]	28	–	–	50–65	–
Dal Maso & Lippi 1985[102]	11	Ratio 1:1.3		51–77	61
Harrison & Lund	49	32	17	23–78	50

Table 7.7 Site of adenoid cystic carcinoma in upper jaw in published series

Author	Patient no.	Maxilla	Nasal cavity	Ethmoid sinus	Sphenoid sinus	Frontal sinus	Hard palate	Superior alveolus
Moran et al 1961[94]	10	–	1	–	–	–	9	–
Tauxe et al 1962[95]	27	19	4	1	1	–	–	2U/K
Eby et al 1972[96]	21	6	1	1	–	1	9	3
Horee 1974[97]	28	12	–	5	–	–	9	2
Spiro et al 1974[91]	43	29	14	–	–	–	–	–
Osborn 1977[90]	23	10	1	1	–	–	11	–
Marsh & Shannon Allen 1979[99]	7	3	2	1	1	–	–	–
Miller & Calceterra 1980[100]	18	7	4	–	–	–	7	–
Szanto et al 1984[106]	32	17	1	–	–	–	14	–
Dal Maso & Lippi 1985[102]	11	4	3	1	–	–	3	–
Harrison & Lund	49	24	6	9	–	1	9	–

U/K, unknown

moid are next in order of frequency and there have been occasional cases reported occurring in the sphenoid and frontal sinus. The antro-ethmoid region may be involved by lesions arising in and around the nasolacrimal duct which inevitably affect the orbit. The orbit is involved in up to two-thirds of cases in some series.[14b] In addition the superior alveolus has been reported as a site in several cases.

Any part of the nasal cavity may be affected and the position on the palate has already been commented on relative to the distribution of minor salivary gland tissue.

Clinical features

Depending upon the site of origin, the common clinical features include nasal obstruction, rhinorrhoea, and epistaxis. Facial pain, tingling and paraesthesia particularly affecting the infraorbital division of the trigeminal nerve have been specifically commented upon by authors cognizant of the potential for perineural infiltration. Conley & Dingman quote an incidence of 18%[88] but this symptom has occurred rarely in our patients or those of others.[96]

Orbital involvement may produce proptosis (40% of our cases) and diplopia, with eventual visual loss though the changes are often gradual due to the protracted course of the condition. Indeed the history may vary between 1 month and 15 years[95,96] with a marked tendency for late presentation. Occasionally patients have presented with a small mass adjacent to the medial canthus associated with the lacrimal sac and have been initially referred to an ophthalmic surgeon.

Palatal lesions present as a firm mass, which is rarely painful or ulcerated and may only be noticed when upper dentures fail to fit (Fig. 7.4). It usually lies to one side of the midline in keeping with the distribution of minor salivary gland tissue. This tissue is rarely found anterior to a line drawn between the first molars, and does not occur in the midline of the hard palate nor in the gingiva.

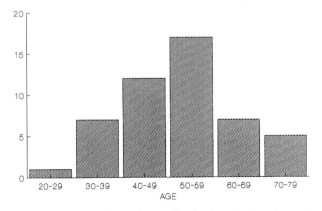

Fig. 7.3 Adenoid cystic carcinoma: distribution of patients by age (in personal series).

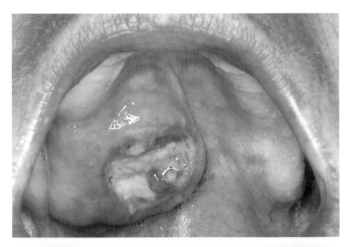

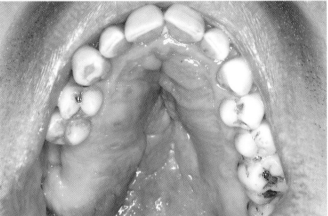

Fig. 7.4 Examples of palatal lesions in adenoid cystic carcinoma.

The incidence of independent glandular aggregates has been quoted as 250 for the hard palate, 100 for the soft palate and 12 for the uvula and this is reflected in the relative distribution of salivary gland tumours in this region.[103]

A 42-year-old accountant had presented at another hospital in 1967 with a small mass on the right palate which had been treated with local excision followed by radiotherapy when histology revealed adenoid cystic carcinoma. He had no problems for 11 years when a local recurrence was found and it was again removed by conservative surgery. A further recurrence 3 years later led to his referral to our care and he underwent a subtotal inferior maxillectomy. Multiple examinations under anaesthesia followed but there was no sign of local disease until 1984, another 3 years later. However, in the meantime a routine chest X-ray revealed a secondary deposit in the left lung field.

A total maxillectomy was performed and this was succeeded by more radical surgery over the next 3 years culminating in an infratemporal fossa and orbital clearance with a pectoralis major myocutaneous flap repair. The pulmonary secondaries continued to increase but the patient underwent a number of anaesthetics without any respiratory problems and was not clinically dyspnoeic (Fig. 7.5). Local disease was periodically debulked by cyrosurgery when the obturator was displaced, until he finally succumbed 23 years after the initial diagnosis.

Radiology

There are few specific radiological features other than those of a malignant tumour on conventional radiology and enhanced computerized tomography, with evidence of a soft tissue mass and bone destruction. The tumour may erode the cribriform plate and roof of ethmoids to enter the anterior cranial fossa and frequently spreads posteriorly into the sphenoid and orbit, thence into the cavernous sinus and middle cranial fossa.

Perineural spread may cause swelling of the nerve and it is occasionally possible to demonstrate enlargement of the foramen ovale and rotundum consequent upon maxillary and mandibular nerve infiltration[104] or similarly expansion of the infra-orbital canal.[105] We have examined 22 patients with MRI/gadolinium DPTA (GdMR) and this particular feature may be elegantly demonstrated by this technique. The deep extension of these tumours into the skull base and middle fossa is now best demonstrated by subtraction GdMR.

The frequency of pulmonary metastases in this condition means that regular chest X-rays should be performed.

Macroscopic and microscopic appearance

There are no specific features to this tumour except that it is a firm mass, which often does not ulcerate and spreads by insidious infiltration through tissue planes. It may be grey–pink in colour but is frequently indistinguishable from normal tissue and this should be borne in mind when taking biopsies.

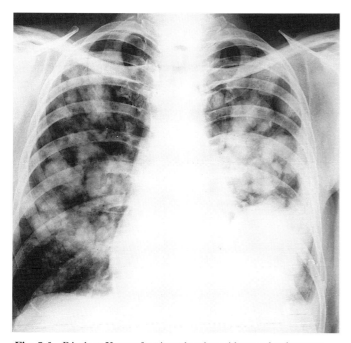

Fig. 7.5 PA chest X-ray of patient showing widespread pulmonary metastases which have been present for 3 years.

Microscopic appearance

Considerable effort has been made to classify this tumour histologically and to use this as a prognostic determinant. The classical appearances are those of a cribriform or lace–like pattern produced by the two component cell types, duct lining cells and myoepithelial cells, arranged around cystic spaces. The holes or 'pseudocysts' contain amorphous material which may be basophilic or eosinophilic and shows some features of connective tissue mucin. Some areas are more solid with no cysts whilst others have elongated tubular structures predominating. Based on these features three histological types have been described: *tubular, cribriform* and *solid*, in order of worsening behaviour and prognosis.

The *solid* type has been suggested as the most aggressive form by a number of authors[92,96,98,107–112] but many others have found no correlation between histology and outcome.[7b,17,55b,81,89–91,95,113] When one considers the small number of cases and the difficulty in defining tumours which are usually mixtures of the different elements, a preoccupation with such classifications would seem unrewarding.

Differential diagnosis

Tumours with a cribriform appearance must be distinguished from ameloblastomas and pleomorphic tumours, whereas the more solid lesions may resemble basal cell tumours. Adenoid cystic carcinoma can also be confused with adenocarcinoma and mucoepidermoid tumours.

Natural history

This tumour has a unique natural history characterized by frequent local recurrence and early spread by perineural infiltration and haematogenous dissemination. In consequence the majority of patients have one or more local recurrences during the course of the disease, usually occurring within the first 5 years following treatment but sometimes reappearing 14 years or more later (Table 7.8).[88,90,91,95,114] Although the usual pattern of the disease is one of insidious growth over many years, some patients manifest a more aggressive course and considerable effort has been made to distinguish predictive factors.

The tumour's particular capacity for perineural spread was noted in some of the earliest descriptions[78] though it was specifically attributed to spread along perineural lymphatic channels by Leroux & Leroux-Robert in 1934.[115] In fact the tumour appears to ensheath the nerve by infiltrating the perineural spaces though the frequency with which this occurs varies between 14% and 40%.[76,116–118] Of even greater therapeutic importance is the possibility of embolization along these spaces which can lead to deposits at some distance from the lesion as demons-

Table 7.8   Percentage incidence of local recurrence and metastatic disease in adenoid cystic carcinoma of the upper jaw in published series

Author	No.	Local recurrence (%)	Metastatic disease (%)
Moran et al 1961[94]	10	70	41
Tauxe et al 1962[95]	27	92	22
Conley & Dingman 1974⋆[88]	78	42	41
Spiro et al 1974[91]	43	67	42
Osborn 1977[90]	23	50	–
Marsh & Shannon Allen 1979[99]	7	71	57
Chilla et al 1980[92]	11	90	18
Matsuba et al 1984[101]	28	N/A	58 (paranasal sinuses) 22 (palate)
Harrison & Lund	49	95	40

⋆All cases of minor salivary gland tumours

trated in a section of optic nerve (Fig. 7.6) showing a distant focus of tumour.

No adequate explanation has been made for the tumour's predilection for blood and perineural spread nor for the relative paucity of lymphatic dissemination. Regional lymph nodes are occasionally involved but principally by direct extension.[92,95,99,119] However, an incidence of between 9% and 16% of cervical lymph node involvement has been noted in some series at presentation and during the disease course.[88,94,119,120]

The true incidence of systemic metastases is always difficult to assess but has been quoted at 20–50% (Table 7.8). The organs affected in order of frequency are lung, brain, bone, and liver and skin nodules can also occur. Although the majority of patients manifest metastatic disease after local recurrence, most do so within the first 5 years and up to 5% of patients have evidence of secondaries at initial presentation.[88] By contrast metastatic spread may manifest itself 15 to 22 years later. As a con-

sequence patients can never be regarded as cured of this particular tumour and 5-year survival figures are rendered meaningless.

However it is important to recognize that the presence of metastases does not necessarily imply a rapid demise and patients may live several years with disseminated disease which has obvious therapeutic implications.

Treatment

Clearly small numbers of a tumour with such unusual biological properties make it difficult to demonstrate that any treatment modality offers statistically significant improvement in long-term survival. However, it is apparent from our own series and those of other authors that whilst radical primary surgery may not be curative nor affect the frequency of metastatic disease, the number and speed of local recurrence is considerably reduced. Bearing in mind the capacity for embolic spread along nerves, one cannot support the suggestion of Conley that all implicated cranial nerves should be extirpated to the skull base. It would appear more rational to offer the most radical operation which also combines an acceptable morbidity. In most cases this would be a craniofacial resection or total maxillectomy with or without orbital clearance or in the case of a localized lesion on the palate, a subtotal maxillectomy preserving the orbital floor. Local recurrence can be dealt with by further debulking procedures, cryosurgery and lasering as appropriate.

The low incidence of cervical node involvement means that neck dissection is rarely indicated and certainly never as a prophylactic measure. However, the frequency of pulmonary metastases which do not in themselves imply rapid deterioration has led to the practice in a number of centres of wedge resection or lobectomy, procedures which conserve functional ventilatory reserve. It is also of interest that patients can withstand general anaesthesia

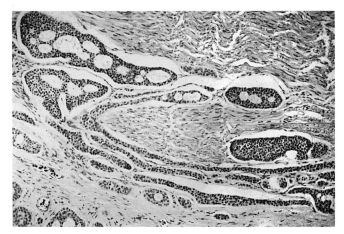

Fig. 7.6   Photomicrograph showing section of optic nerve with distant focus of adenoid cystic carcinoma from ethmoidal tumour (haematoxylin and eosin × 73).[234]

for further surgical procedures even in the presence of widespread lung secondaries.

With regard to radiotherapy, the tumour may be radiosensitive but it is not radiocurable so though this modality may occasionally contribute to control in combination with surgery, it has no effect on 5-year survival. Chemotherapy has no part to play in this condition.

From a practical point of view, carbamazepine can be very successful in the control of pain, particularly as it relates to neuronal involvement.

Prognosis

Such is the natural history of this tumour, that 5-year survival figures are meaningless and large numbers with long-term follow-up are not available. A number of authors have attempted to determine prognostic factors, most notably using a histological classification (p. 113) and more recently DNA flow cytometry has been used in an attempt to predict the more aggressive tumours.[121]

Other factors which have been examined have included size, site, patient age, and symptoms such as pain but once again there is no universal agreement on these points.[91,98,106] Other histological features such as mitoses and perineural invasion do not appear to be relevant though not surprisingly the presence of tumour at resection margins, and involvement of lymph nodes and bone are associated with a poorer outcome.

Based on our own series of 49 patients with up to 24 years' follow-up and the experiences of others, a number of facts emerge. Adenoid cystic carcinoma of minor salivary glands is worse than that affecting major glands and that affecting the nose and sinuses is a more aggressive disease than in other areas of the head and neck. It is doubtful that any patient is actually cured of the condition and apparent cure simply results from death due to some other cause in an ostensibly disease-free interval. The choice between conservative and radical management may not alter prognosis and in view of the tumour's potential for embolic perineural spread, supra-radical surgery is not justified. It is clear however, that the incidence and speed of local recurrence is reduced by radical surgery and as death is usually due to local disease with its attendant miseries, a balance between radical surgery and minimum morbidity should be sought.

In addition a policy of continued local treatment, even in the presence of distant metastases can be advocated in view of the limited morbidity engendered by their presence and their limited effect on prognosis.

Examination of determinant survival for all cases in the upper jaw shows a gradual loss of patients, from around two-thirds at 5 years to 10% or less at 20 years though some authors have suggested a slightly better prognosis for palatal lesions (Table 7.9).

In considering why adenoid cystic carcinoma of the upper jaw does particularly badly when compared with similar pathology in the major salivary glands, examination of our own patients leads one to the conclusion that as is so often the case in this region, the combination of late presentation and close proximity to 'special' anatomical areas inevitably compromises the surgical options. This contention is supported by the somewhat better prognosis of palatal lesions.

ADENOCARCINOMA

Definition

Adenocarcinoma is a malignant epithelial tumour characterized by the presence of glandular structures. It may arise from surface epithelium and minor salivary gland tissue.

Table 7.9 Determinant survival in adenoid cystic carcinoma of the upper jaw in published series

Author	No.	Survival (%) after years				
		3	5	10	15	20
Tauxe et al 1962[95]	22	–	73	41	7	0
Stuteville & Corley 1967[122]	Palate		58		–	–
Adams & Duvall 1971[113]	Palate	30	–	10	–	–
Conley & Dingman 1974[88]	78	–	64	34	23	8
Spiro et al 1974[91]	43					
	All	–	31	18	10	7
	Nose	–	–	7	–	–
	Palate	–	–	16	–	–
Perzin et al 1978[98]	Palate	–	50	–	–	–
Szanto et al 1984[106]	32					
	All	–	60	37	23	–
	Maxilla	–	–	–	8	–
	Palate	–	–	–	38	–
Harrison & Lund	49	–	53	24	18	2

Historical aspects

Reports of this histological type began in the early 1900s.[123,124] In 1935 Ahlbom[125] found five cases out of nine glandular tumours in the nose and sinuses and Ringertz's major review of sinonasal malignancy[126] described ten cases arising in the antro-ethmoidal region.

Incidence

In studies of malignant tumours of the nose and sinuses, adenocarcinoma constitutes between 4 and 9%.[7c,55c,126–128] In our series it constitutes 12% of malignancy of the upper jaw, the higher percentage reflecting referral for craniofacial resection.

Age, sex and ethnic variation (Table 7.10)

Because of the importance of occupational factors in the aetiology of this tumour, it is found predominantly in men. An overall ratio of 4:1 occurs but this may increase to 11:1 in the older age groups reflecting longer carcinogenic exposure. It has been suggested that when the tumour is graded into low- or high-grade malignancy, the male preponderance is confined to the high-grade group, with an equal male to female ratio in the low-grade tumours.[138]

Any age can be affected, from 9–90 years though the average age is usually between 50 and 60, with a tendency for the higher grade tumours to present in the slightly older.[138,139a] The peak incidence appears to occur about 5 years earlier than for squamous cell carcinoma.[127] In women the menopause may be responsible for a temporary downturn in incidence around 50 years which is similar to Clemmesen's hook observed in breast cancer and is most likely to occur in sinonasal malignancy of glandular origin such as adenocarcinoma.[140]

Site (Table 7.11)

The tumour arises high in the nasal cavity and ethmoid region though some of the larger series contain large numbers of antral lesions. This may again be determined by the relative importance of aetiological factors. Lesions on the palate are relatively uncommon.

Aetiology (Table 7.12)

A number of aetiological factors have been found to be associated with adenocarcinoma of the sinuses, the mechanism for which has been the subject of considerable research. The most notable is the association with the wood-working industry. The route by which these environmental agents have their effect is principally airborne, by direct inhalation of particles whose effect will depend upon their size, density and the breathing pattern of the host.[144–146]

Reports on the association between adenocarcinoma of the ethmoid and the wood-working trade, in particular hardwood exposure, began in 1965 in the United Kingdom and have subsequently appeared from many other countries.[147–160] Soft-wood exposure by contrast is implicated in the development of squamous and anaplastic carcinoma.[161–163] It is also noteworthy that Japan, a country where squamous cell carcinoma of the maxilla predominates, has a large traditional wood-working industry and has found no such association.[164]

The increased relative risk is similar to that for carcinoma of the bronchus in smokers with a cumulative lifetime risk of 1 in 120 and a 500–1000 times greater risk than the general population of developing the condition. It became a recognized industrial disease in Great Britain in 1969 and subsequent studies on wood-workers showed dysplasia in adjacent non-neoplastic epithelium and impaired mucociliary function.[165,166] This cuboidal meta-

Table 7.10   Adenocarcinoma of upper jaw: distribution by sex and age

Author	No.	Male:Female	Age range (yr)	Average age (yr)
Ringertz 1938[126]	10	5:5	20–79	54
Wille 1947[129]	10	–	–	–
Larsson & Maartensson 1954[130]	11	–	–	–
Hemenway & Lindsay 1959[131]	13	–	–	–
Chaudhry et al 1961[17]	8	4:2	–	62
Huizing 1962[132]	13	–	–	–
Batsakis et al 1963[133]	9	9:0	41–75	52
Gamez-Araujo et al 1975[134]	18	17:1	25–80	60
Saunders & Ruff 1976[135]	16	13:3	45–85	–
Goepfert et al 1983[136]	30	18:12	–	–
Alessi et al 1988[137]	13	6:7	23–69	50
Harrison & Lund	46	38:8	34–78	58

Table 7.11 Adenocarcinoma of upper jaw: distribution by site

Author	Total	Ethmoid	Maxilla	Antro-ethmoid	Nasal cavity	Sphenoid	Frontal	Palate	Lacrimal
McDonald & Havens 1946[15]	9	–	–	9	–	–	–	–	–
Wille 1947[129]	10	–	–	–	–	–	–	–	–
Larsson & Maartensson 1954[130]	11	–	–	–	–	–	–	–	–
Chaudhry et al 1961[17]	8	–	–	–	–	–	–	8	–
Batsakis et al 1963[133]	9	7	2	–	–	–	–	–	–
Luna et al 1968[35]	2	–	–	–	–	–	–	–	–
Rafla 1969[12]	14	7	5	–	1	1	–	–	–
Lewis & Castro 1972[141]	129	16	74	–	39	–	–	–	–
Spiro et al 1973[16]	40	4	20	–	16	–	–	–	–
Gamez-Araujo et al 1975[134]	18	1	10	–	5	2	–	–	–
Saunders & Ruff 1976[135]	16	14	2	–	–	–	–	–	–
Robin et al 1979[127]	39	21	10	–	–	–	–	–	–
Tran et al 1987[142]	2	–	–	–	–	–	–	2	–
Alessi et al 1988[137]	13	9	2	–	1	1	–	–	–
Kraus et al 1990[143]	9	–	–	9	–	–	–	–	–
Harrison & Lund	46	22	7	7	4	–	–	4	2

Table 7.12 Occupational agents correlated with sinonasal cancer (after Roush 1979[178])

Occupation	Relative risk	Suspected carcinogen	Latent period (yr)	Histology	Other associated cancers
Wood-workers	70	Dust 5 μm diameter Tar Aldehydes Aflatoxins Chromium Tannins	35	Adenocarcinoma (hardwood) Squamous (softwood)	Lung, testis, brain
Leather/Shoe manufacturers	87	Dust Tar Aldehydes Aflatoxins Tannins	55	Adenocarcinoma	Rectum, bladder
Chrome pigment manufacturers	>21	Calcium chromate Zinc potassium chromate	–	Adenocarcinoma	Lung
Isopropyl alcohol manufacturers	>21	Isopropyl oil	<20	Adenocarcinoma	Larynx
Textile and clothing	5–8	Wool dust and dyes	–	Adenocarcinoma Malignant melanoma	Tongue, mouth, pharynx

plasia was found in 19 out of 22 wood-workers with adenocarcinoma though the actual carcinogenic agent has not been defined. Specific jobs are more implicated than others, principally those where large amounts of fine dust are produced such as sanding and turning, at high temperatures which may alter the components in some way. Consequently joiners and cabinet makers are particularly at risk.

The particle size is of importance as only those greater than 5 μm will be deposited on the middle turbinate, smaller ones reaching the lower respiratory tract. Length of exposure is also relevant as in the original reports a mean period of 40 years was cited. However, it is clear that under certain circumstances 9 years or less may be sufficient. The incidence of disease may have reached it

speak in men entering the industry between 1915–24 with no documented deaths before 1950, but it is not possible to predict the effect of improved factory conditions and changes in work practice because of the latent period of 22–70 years. Consequently there is still a need for screening of those workers at risk (Fig. 7.7).

Experimental studies have been performed on wood dust exposure in rats and hamsters using appropriately sized particles, different levels of exposure and in combination with another carcinogen, diethylnitrosamine (DEN). These have produced chronic irritation and dysplasia and with higher exposure levels and DEN, nasal tumours. However, the carcinogenic effect of wood-dust alone appeared to be weak, consistent with the long latent period.[167–169] Adenocarcinoma occurred in 46 patients in

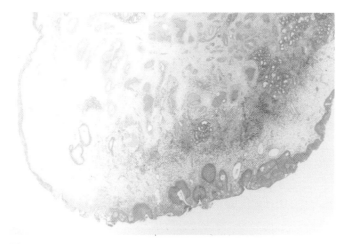

Fig. 7.7   Histology section through middle turbinate of wood-worker showing dysplastic change in mucosa.

our series of 500 malignancies of the upper jaw, only 10 of whom were wood-workers so although it is an important definable factor, the link is not absolute.

The leather and shoe industry has also been the subject of extensive epidemiological study for squamous and adenocarcinoma since Acheson's report in 1975.[170] Other occupations which are associated with an increased risk of adenocarcinoma are the manufacture of chrome pigment,[171–173] isopropyl alcohol,[174–176] and the textile and clothing trade, the last also being associated with malignant melanoma.[177] Adenocarcinoma has also been reported in association with the baking trade[178] and there is one case in the literature of this ethmoidal tumour occurring 30 years after radiotherapy for a bilateral retinoblastoma.[179]

Clinical features

These are initially innocuous such as nasal obstruction and discharge. Persistence of these with additional unilateral epistaxis, pain, epiphora and other orbital symptoms may lead to referral but the lesion has been likened to 'a fire which smoulders unnoticed within the walls of a house'[15] and is usually quite extensive at presentation. The lesion may present with a midline glabellar mass overlying and involving the frontal bones (Fig. 7.8).

A 50-year-old male began working as a machinist with hardwoods, notably oak, mahogany and teak in 1948. He continued in this trade until 1976 though the conditions under which he worked, particularly ventilation of the workshop, varied considerably during this time. He experienced mild nasal obstruction from the early 1970s which his general practitioner treated with nasal sprays. Polyps were removed in 1981 but presumably were not submitted for histology as it was not until a subsequent removal 2 years later that adenocarcinoma of the ethmoid region was diagnosed. He underwent a course of radiotherapy and was then referred from the local hospital for craniofacial surgery. He is alive and well without sign of recurrence 6 years later.

Radiology (Figs 7.9 and 7.10)

In our own series the tumour predominantly occurred in the upper nasal cavity and adjacent ethmoid, in contrast to squamous cell carcinomas which principally affect the antrum. Consequently the orbit and anterior cranial fossa are affected at an early stage, which can be shown by contrast-enhanced computerized tomography. Occasionally small areas of calcification may be seen similar to those found in adenocarcinoma of the gastro-intestinal tract.

Appearances on magnetic resonance are not specific to the histological type, showing a moderately high signal on T2 weighted spin echo sequences which can be readily distinguished from the higher signal from adjacent secretion. A combination of coronal CT and sagittal MRI with contrast enhancement will provide the best information on intracranial and intraorbital extension.

Macroscopic and microscopic appearance

The lesion may be a pale grey friable mass of exophytic papillary appearance or deeply infiltrating and sessile. It is often quite gelatinous.

Microscopic appearance

Adenocarcinoma has been classified in a number of ways and attempts made to relate this to prognosis. Heffner et al[138] divided them into low- and high-grade tumours which related to the degree of differentiation. It was felt that the low-grade lesions with small uniform glands lined by regular columnar cells, rare mitoses and areas of calcification were associated with a better prognosis. This was in contrast to the high-grade tumours with solid sheets of cells, an irregular pattern and many mitoses.

The tumour has also been described as papillary, sessile or alveolar-mucoid. The last includes a 'colloid' or 'colonic' subgroup. Because of the presence of many argentaffin, Paneth and goblet cells several authors have suggested they arise at the junction of endoderm and ectoderm and belie a common gastro-intestinal origin.[128,180–182] Colloid adenocarcinoma was first described by Ringertz[126] in 1938 and although a worse prognosis has been postulated for this type, this may be more related to the site and extent of the lesion than the histological variant.

Electron microscopy demonstrates secretory granules which should be distinguished from those found in acinic cell carcinoma.

Differential diagnosis

The similarity between a mucoid papillary adenocarcinoma and a benign polyp emphasizes the need to send all such material for histological examination. Furthermore a

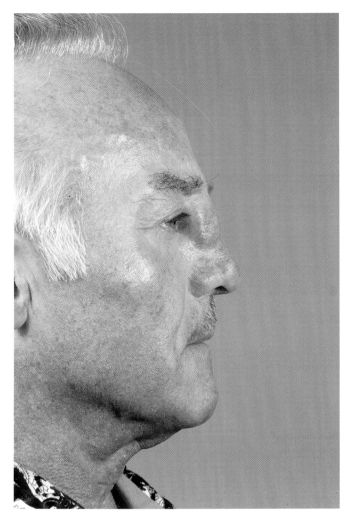

Fig. 7.8 Ethmoidal adenocarcinoma presenting with a glabellar mass.

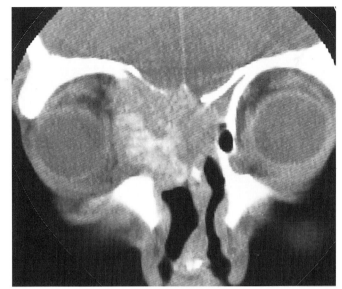

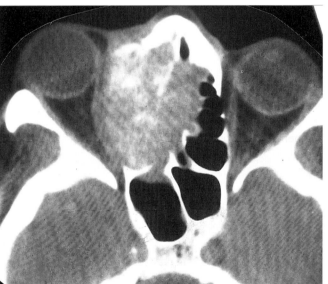

Fig. 7.9 **A**, coronal CT scan showing calcification in ethmoidal adenocarcinoma with erosion of cribriform plate and **B**, axial CT scan of same (Lloyd 1988[105]).

report of a monomorphic adenoma should be questioned as the low-grade lesions may be misdiagnosed in this way.

The presence of microcysts and an abundant myxoid stroma should distinguish cylindric cell papilloma from adenocarcinoma.

Treatment

It is well established that radical surgery is the most effective treatment for this lesion which is relatively resistant to radiotherapy and chemotherapy.[12,138,183,184] In the past the majority of cases were managed by a radical maxillectomy or extended lateral rhinotomy frequently with sacrifice of the eye. The advent of the combined craniofacial approach has enabled an oncologic clearance with access to the anterior cranial fossa and orbit (p.331)[185–188] which is particularly advantageous in ethmoidal adenocarcinoma.[189–191]

In our series of 46 patients (Table 7.13), 28 have undergone craniofacial resection, 24 of whom had already received radiotherapy and/or surgery. In the 18 patients with palatal lesions or antro-ethmoidal disease which predated the craniofacial resection, 13 underwent radical surgery, four received radiotherapy or chemotherapy alone and one patient was not treated. Although the numbers are small, differences in outcome may be assessed below.

Prognosis

The improved prognosis associated with low-grade adenocarcinoma has been supported by Heffner et al[138] and others.[7c,137,139a] For 23 patients with low-grade disease and a median follow-up of 6.3 years, two were dead of disease, 21 alive, three with disease. In the high-grade group of 27 patients, 21 were dead of disease all within 3

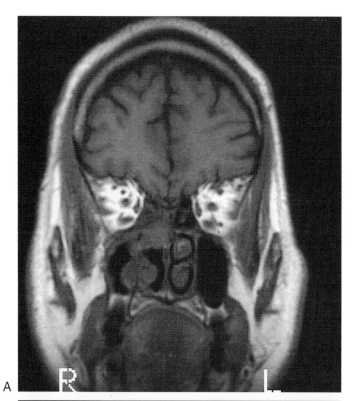

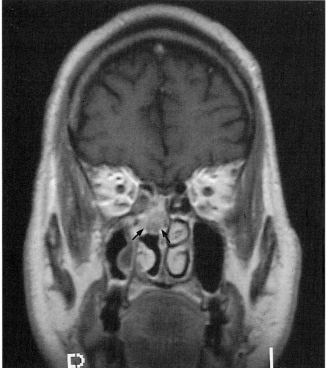

Fig. 7.10 Coronal MR scan, **A**, T1 weighted sequence in wood-worker with adenocarcinoma of right ethmoid. **B**, same sequence with gadolinium showing discrimination of tumour from adjacent mucous membrane.

years, and six were alive, four with tumour. This view of a more benign natural history in low-grade tumours is not supported by Matsuba[192] or Goepfert.[136]

Table 7.13 Adenocarcinoma: personal series

Patients:	
Total	46
Sex (M:F)	38:8
Age range (yr)	34–78
Average age (yr)	58
Wood-workers	10
Site:	
Ethmoid	22
Maxilla	7
Antro-ethmoid	7
Nasal cavity	4
Palate	4
Lacrimal	2
Previous treatment:	
Surgery	7
Radiotherapy	7
Both	11
None	21
Treatment:	
Surgery	40
Craniofacial resection	28
Radical maxillectomy	7
Lateral rhinotomy	5
Radiotherapy	4
Chemotherapy	1
None	1
Additional radiotherapy	7
Additional surgery	4
Outcome:	
Alive and well	17
Alive with disease	3
Dead	23
Lost	12
Survival (12–13 yr)	11
Causes of death:	
Local recurrence	11
Metastases	6
Other	7

Other authors[16,139a,184] have felt that the prognosis worsened as one moved from papillary to sessile and finally alveolar-mucoid. In addition Spiro et al[16] suggested that sex, age, site, size and not surprisingly the presence of cervical metastases at presentation and inadequate surgery also determined prognosis!

Robin et al[127] agreed that women fared better though this has not been our own experience given that they constitute a small proportion of the whole group. It is hardly surprising that site should be important given the proximity of the vital structures and late presentation from the ethmoidal lesions compared to the palate. Indeed three of the four palatal lesions in our series are alive and well with 5-, 10- and 13-year follow-up.

In comparing survival in our 28 patients managed primarily by craniofacial resection with those 14 previously treated by maxillectomy/lateral rhinotomy or other modalities, a 50% crude survival or 62% actuarial survival (which takes into account five deaths from intercurrent disease) emerges for the craniofacial patients. Six of those patients treated prior to craniofacial have unfortunately been lost to follow-up, two are alive and well and six are dead, one of intercurrent disease. The follow-up in the surviving craniofacial group ranges from 11 months to 9 years, mean 55 months and interval from surgery to death ranges from 4 to 92 months, mean 32 months. A similar interval between surgery and death is found in the pre-craniofacial group.

The impact of the craniofacial procedure may therefore be judged by comparison with previously quoted overall 5-year survival of 30%,[12,182,192] 39%[135] and 54%.[184] However, it is clear that 5-year survival figures fail to give the complete picture as at least one of our patients developed recurrence nearly 8 years after surgery.

Cervical metastases probably occur only in 2–3% of cases and in most series the majority of patients succumb to local recurrence, with distant metastases occurring rarely.[113,126,130,137,180,184,193] Certainly 50% of our craniofacial patients died with local disease but a similar number developed distant metastases to lung, bone and brain which may be the result of improved local control afforded by the craniofacial resection. This again emphasizes the necessity for long-term follow-up.

MUCOEPIDERMOID CARCINOMA

Definition

This malignant neoplasm is characterized by the presence of squamous cells, mucus-secreting cells and intermediate cells though whether it originates from epithelium or minor salivary gland ducts is debated.

Synonyms

Adenosquamous carcinoma,[194] mucoepidermoid tumour.

Historical aspects

Mucoepidermoid tumours were first described in relation to the parotid by Masson & Berger in 1924.[195] In 1945 Stewart et al[196] described a series of 45 cases, 4 of which arose in the nose and sinuses.

Incidence

The relative incidence of this tumour reported in the literature is shown in Table 7.14. It is certainly one of the less common tumours affecting this region but is nevertheless the second commonest malignancy of minor salivary glands. Spiro et al[16] found it to constitute 16% of glandular tumours in the sinonasal tract (20/122), compared with 12% in our ILO material rendering it less

than 1% of all sinonasal tumours. When the oral cavity is considered, mucoepidermoid lesions comprise between 11–21%.[17,35,197]

Age, sex and ethnic variation (Table 7.14)

A wide age range is found in the literature, from 10–80 years with no specific predeliction though it is reportedly the most common malignant major salivary gland tumour in children. The sexes appear to be equally affected.

Site

Armed Forces Institute of Pathology data shows the nasal cavity is as commonly affected as the maxillary antrum but a review of other available series suggests that the maxilla is the commoner site.[139b] In the oral cavity approximately half of the cases occur on the palate.

Batsakis et al[201] distinguish a separate subgroup of mucoepidermoid carcinoma which they termed the central mucoepidermoid carcinoma of the jaw. This may arise from ectopic or embryologically trapped salivary gland tissue and affects women in their 4th to 5th decades. The mandible is twice more often the site of this lesion than the maxilla.

Aetiology

No known agent or occupation has been implicated in its genesis.

Clinical features

The usual symptoms of obstruction and epistaxis occur with nasal lesions, a painless mass or occasionally a fistula may develop in the upper jaw, with proptosis and epiphora if the orbit is involved.

Radiology

No specific features are associated with this lesion. However, the central mucoepidermoid lesion of the jaw can produce a radiolucent area which must be distinguished from a dentigerous cyst or ameloblastoma.

Macroscopic and microscopic appearance

A firm mass is usually seen sometimes with obvious cystic areas.

Microscopic appearance

Opinion is divided as to the origin of this tumour which is characterized by mucus-secreting cells, squamous cells

Table 7.14 Mucoepidermoid carcinoma of upper jaw: distribution by age, sex and site in literature

Author	No.	Total no. of tumour cases in series	Minor salivary gland tumours	Male	Female	Age range (yr)	Average age (yr)	Palate	Antrum	Nasal cavity	Ethmoid	Alveolus	Other
Ranger et al 1956[19]	3	80	All	–	–	–	–	3					
Fine et al 1960[93]	19	79	All	7	13	28–63	49	9				10	
Chaudhry et al 1961[17]	10	94	Intra-oral	5	5	16–70	51	5					5
Stuteville & Corley 1967[197]	17	80	Intra-oral	10	7	17–78	44	10					7
Luna et al 1968[35]	9	68	Intra-oral	7	2	24–74	56	5					4
Smith et al 1968[198]	6	22	Upper & lower jaw	3	3	34–63	42	1	5				
Bergman 1969[1]	2	46	All	–	–		–		1				
Rafla 1969[12]	2	37	Nose and sinuses	–	–		–		2		1		
Eneroth 1971[109]	27	170	Palate	–	–		–	27					
Frable & Elzay 1970[2]	11	73	All	5	6	14–70	7th decade	7					4
Healey et al 1970[199]	10	13	All	–	–	15–70	52	2	7	1			
Spiro et al 1973[16]	41	492	All	–	–		–	21	13	7			
Da-Quan & Guang-Yan 1987[200]	10	131	All malignant	–	–		–						
Tran et al 1987[142]	12	38	Palate	–	–		–	12					
Harrison & Lund	4	500	Upper jaw	4	–	26–46	38		3	1			

and intermediate cells forming solid cellular masses and tubulo-cystic structures. Electron microscopy confirms the presence of mucus secretory granules and glycogen particles but it is unclear whether the lesion arises from the mucosa or minor salivary mucoserous glands.[139b]

Differential diagnosis

Difficulties may arise when an unrepresentative biopsy is obtained. If cystic areas predominate the lesion may be erroneously labelled as an adenocarcinoma, if solid, a squamous cell tumour may be diagnosed.

Natural history

Mucoepidermoid tumours can demonstrate a spectrum of activity from well differentiated low-grade to high-grade more aggressive lesions. However, they should never be regarded as entirely benign and have the potential for metastatic spread and frequent recurrence.[201]

Treatment

Because of their unknown potential, mucoepidermoid lesions should be treated definitively with primary surgical excision, i.e. by some form of maxillectomy. This may be combined with radiotherapy but in general these tumours are radioresistant or at best only moderately radiosensitive.

Prognosis

As can be seen in Table 7.15, these small series show a considerable range of survival, consistent with the spectrum of activity. The nasal cavity appears a more favourable site than the maxilla though overall the prognosis appears better than for adenoid cystic carcinoma. Long-term survival can be expected with the low-grade lesions whereas the high-grade tumours are characterized by recurrence and metastases even when survival exceeds 5 years. In the Spiro et al series[16] of 76 cases in minor salivary glands (41 in upper jaw) overall 10-years, determinate cure rate was 69%, ranging from 79–50% depending on the degree of differentiation.

ACINIC CELL CARCINOMA

Definition

This tumour of salivary tissue is rare in minor glands and in the upper jaw in particular. Thus its characteristics have largely been extrapolated from its behaviour in major salivary gland tissue.

Historical aspects

In 1892 Nasse[202] reported an acinic tumour of the parotid. Its occurrence in the major salivary glands subsequently became well established.[81]

Table 7.15 Mucoepidermoid carcinoma of upper jaw: treatment and outcome in literature

| Author | No. | Treatment | | | Outcome | | | | | |
		Surgery	DXT	Surgery + DXT	A&W	AWR	Dead of Disease ICD		Lost	Metastases (%)
Stuteville & Corley 1967[197]	17	13		4	8 (>5 yr)		3		6	
Luna et al 1968[35]	9				4 (>5 yr)		3	1	1	
Smith et al 1968[198]	6	5		1	3 (1–4 yr, 1–14 yr, 1–35 yr)		3			
Bergman 1969[1]	2			2		2				50
Rafla 1969[12]	2						1		1	
Eneroth 1971[109]	27									18
Frable & Elzay 1970[2]	11	11			7 3 (>5 yr)	1			2 1	
Healey et al 1970[199]	10	4		6	2		6 (5/7 maxilla)	2		20 (cervical lymph nodes)
Spiro et al 1973[16]	41									30 (lymph nodes, 10 (distant 2°s)
Tran et al 1987[142]	12	10		2						
Harrison & Lund	4	1	1	2	1 (>13 yr)		2 (<1 yr)		1	

A&W, alive and well; AWR, alive with recurrence; ICD, intercurrent disease; 2°s, secondaries; DXT, radiotherapy

Incidence

In the minor salivary glands, acinic cell carcinoma is rare compared with the parotid where it constitutes 2.5–4% of tumours. It is exceptionally rare in the nose and sinuses and only a few case reports are found in the literature (Table 7.16). Inoue et al[203] found 80 cases affecting minor salivary glands of which the majority arose in the oral cavity.

Age and sex variation

Acinic cell carcinoma can occur at any age, including childhood[204] and in either sex, though women seem to predominate in the few case reports available (Table 7.16).

Site

Lesions on the lateral wall of the nasal cavity, antro-ethmoid region and hard palate have been described.

Aetiology

No predisposing factors are known.

Clinical features and radiology

Epistaxis was the main symptom in three of the cases reported but radiological evidence of bone destruction has not been described.

Macroscopic and microscopic appearance

A circumscribed or polypoid mass is found. In the major glands the lesion can be multifocal and bilateral but has not been reported in the upper jaw.

Microscopic appearance

The lesion is described as arising from two cell sources:

1. Reserve cells of the terminal tubules
2. Intercalated ducts.[201]

In its most differentiated form, the tumour resembles an enlarged normal salivary lobule, when least differentiated it is similar to an early phase of development of the salivary unit.

The growth pattern has been divided into solid, papillary-cystic, follicular and microcystic of which solid is the commonest.[209] Whilst one pattern may predominate, a mixture is often found which may make diagnosis difficult. Consequently attention has been given to ultrastructural morphology,[210] DNA content[211,212] and immunocytochemistry.[213]

Differential diagnosis

A combination of immunohistochemical demonstration of intracellular amylase and electron microscopy will help to distinguish acinic cell lesions from adenocarcinoma.

Natural history and treatment

Batsakis et al[201] take issue with the opinion that acinic cell tumours so rarely become malignant and metastasize that they should not be termed carcinoma[214] believing the patient to be ill-served by regarding it as a benign lesion. Consequently the tumour should be excised widely.

Local recurrence has occurred in several case reports but the incidence of metastases is difficult to assess with such few cases and short follow-up. In the major glands a determinate survival rate of 89% for 5 years, fell to 56% at 20 years.[215] Distant metastases were found in 15% of cases and to lymph nodes in 10%.[216,217]

METASTASES TO THE UPPER JAW

Definition

Metastatic disease to the upper jaw must emanate from a distant site and excludes those tumours that spread from adjacent areas or recur locally in this region. The majority are therefore derived from neoplasms occurring below the clavicle.

Table 7.16 Acinic cell carcinoma of the upper jaw: reports in literature

Author	No.	Sex	Age (yr)	Site	Total no. of minor salivary gland tumours
Chaudhry et al 1961[17]	1	–	–	Palate	1414
Hjertman & Eneroth 1970[20]	1	–	–	Palate	170
Kleinsasser 1970[205]	3	–	–	Nasal cavity	–
Manace & Goldman 1971[206]	1	F	47	Antro-ethmoid	–
Spiro et al 1973[16]	2	–	–	Nasal cavity Gum	492
Perzin et al 1981[207]	1	F	75	Nasal cavity	–
Ordonez & Batsakis 1986[208]	1	F	60	Nasal cavity	–

Historical aspects

The first reference to such a lesion was by Perls[224] in 1872 when a metastasis to the sphenoid from the bronchus was recorded. In 1893 another deposit in the sphenoid was described by Von Eiselberg,[277] deriving from the thyroid and in 1905 the first case of a secondary in the sinuses from a renal tumour was published by Albrecht.[289]

Incidence

Secondary deposits presenting in the head and neck appear to be extremely uncommon but determining an exact incidence is difficult as their true origins may remain undiscovered. Skeletal surveys are not always routine and post-mortem examination may not include a detailed examination of the sinus region.

In a review of metastatic disease in general, Abrams et al[290] found none in the nose and sinuses. It might be expected that those tumours with a propensity for bone secondaries, such as breast, thyroid and prostate, would feature more frequently in this respect but this is not found in practice. It is thought that red marrow is a prerequisite for a deposit to establish itself and proliferate.[291] The relative paucity of active marrow in the upper jaw may be reflected in the rarity of bony metastases.

A population-based study in Minnesota over 50 years demonstrated that 3.6% of all upper aero-digestive tract carcinomas are metastases and that this was the first evidence of malignancy in half of the cases.[280] Of the 11 cases reported, two involved the upper jaw. In a study of 1500 cases of prostatic cancer, 1% were associated with secondaries in the head and neck but these were almost exclusively to cervical lymph nodes.[292]

Metastatic disease in the bones of the jaw usually involves the mandible rather than maxilla. In a series of 115 cases of secondaries in the jaw described by Batsakis & McBurney,[291] 20 cases involved the maxilla alone and two both mandible and maxilla, the rest being mandibular.

In a review of metastases to the ear, nose and throat, Friedmann and Osborn[14c] found that less than 50% involved the nose and sinuses of which 80% derived from the kidney, i.e. four out of five cases. The kidney is by far the commonest source of such secondaries and it has been estimated that 6% of these tumours metastasize to the head and neck,[291] mainly to this area.

We have seen five cases of proven metastatic disease in 500 cases of nose and sinus malignant tumours in a 26-year period, i.e. 1%, consistent with other reports.[280]

Age and sex variation

The age and sex distribution is determined by the source of the tumour and is shown in Table 7.17. In reviewing all published cases of secondary deposits in the nose and sinuses, these have been found in patients with a wide age range, the majority occurring in the 6th and 7th decades. Our five cases are shown separately in Table 7.18.

Site (Table 7.19)

Metastases to this region favour the maxilla, irrespective of the source. Renal secondaries are also found in the ethmoids with relative frequency. Occasionally the

Table 7.17 Metastases to the upper jaw published in literature: incidence and histology

Site of origin	No.	Age range (yr)	Average age (yr)	Male:Female sex ratio	Histology
Kidney[218-253]	44	34–76	59	1.7:1	Hypernephroma
Bronchus[219-221,224,225,254-256,293-296]	14	38–81	57	6:1	Squamous, anaplastic
Breast[218-220,257-263]	10	46–75	63	all female	Adenocarcinoma
Testicle[218,220,264-267]	8	34–69	56	all male	Seminoma
Uterus[14c,268-272]	7	3 mth–58	–	all female	Leiomyosarcoma choriocarcinoma
Thyroid[219,273-277]	6	28–61	–	1:1	Follicular
Colon & rectum[218,221,222,262,278,279]	6	33–78	–	1:1	Adenocarcinoma
Stomach[220,221,280,281]	4	45–67	55	all male	Adenocarcinoma, squamous
Prostate[219,282]	3	57, 61, 77	–	all male	Adenocarcinoma
Skin melanoma[283-285]	3	21, 24, 47	–	2:1	Malignant melanoma
Pancreas[218,281]	2	33, 65	–	Both female	Anaplastic
Adrenal[286,287]	2	17 mth, 5 yr	–	1:1	Neuroblastoma
Bladder[280,288]	2	74, 80	–	1:1	Squamous, transitional

Table 7.18 Metastases to the upper jaw: personal cases

No.	Site of origin	Age	Sex	Site	Histology	Relation of primary to secondary	Treatment of secondaries	Outcome
*1	Kidney	49	M	Ethmoid	Clear cell adeno-carcinoma	Secondary appeared first	External fronto-ethmoidectomy, radiotherapy	Died after 8 yr
2	Pancreas	56	M	Ethmoid	Adeno-carcinoma	Primary appeared 4 mth later	Craniofacial, radiotherapy	Died after 4 mth
3	Pancreas	61	M	Ethmoid	Anaplastic	Primary appeared 8 mth later	Craniofacial, radiotherapy, chemotherapy	Lost to follow-up, presumed dead
4	Malignant melanoma on skin of back	34	M	Nasal cavity	Malignant melanoma	Secondary appeared 2 yr later	Craniofacial, radiotherapy, chemotherapy	Died after 27 mth
5	Malignant melanoma on leg	55	F	Nasal cavity	Malignant melanoma	Secondary appeared 9 yr later	Lateral rhinotomy	Alive and well 6 yr

*Case report

Table 7.19 Metastases to the upper jaw published in literature: distribution by site

Site of origin	No.	Maxilla	Ethmoid	Frontal	Sphenoid	Nasal cavity	Palate	Alveolar ridge
*Kidney[218–253]	44	23	13	9	2	6	1	2
*Bronchus[219–221,224,225,254–256,293–296]	14	5	1	1	2	3	–	5
Breast[218–220,257–263]	10	7	–	–	1	2	–	–
Testicle[218,220,264–267]	8	5	–	–	–	1	–	2
Uterus[14c,268–272]	7	4	–	1	–	–	1	1
Thyroid[219,273–277]	6	2	–	1	2	1	–	–
*Colon & rectum[218,221,222,262,278,279]	6	3	–	–	2	–	1	1
*Stomach[220,221,280,281]	4	3	1	–	–	–	–	1
Prostate[219,282]	3	1	–	–	2	–	–	–
Skin melanoma[283–285]	3	2	–	–	–	1	–	–
*Pancreas[218,281]	2	1	1	–	– female	1	–	–
Adrenal[286,287]	2	1	–	–	–	–	–	1
Bladder[280,288]	2	2	–	–	–	–	–	–

*Multiple sites affected

alveolar ridge and upper gingivae can be the site of a secondary deposit but this is rare in the absence of bone involvement. It is of interest that both the frontal and sphenoid sinuses can be affected when they are so infrequently the site of primary disease. Consequently suspicions should be aroused by such a finding.

Aetiology

The kidney is the commonest source of metastases, followed by bronchus and breast. The urogenital and gastro-intestinal tracts have only occasionally been reported. It has been suggested[259] that embolization occurs via the vertebral venous plexus with increases in intrathoracic or intra-abdominal pressure, to involve the pterygoid venous plexus. The vascularity of the source organs has also been commented on but it is of more interest that metastases to the nose and sinuses occur so infrequently under these circumstances.

Clinical features (Table 7.20)

Lesions in the maxillary bone may present with pain which can precede radiological changes by up to 15 months.[291] There may be swelling of the cheek, nasal obstruction or loosening of the teeth. Orbital involvement may produce diplopia and proptosis and neurological symptoms result from disease in the sphenoid. Secon-

Table 7.20 Metastases to the upper jaw: symptoms at presentation in published series*

Site of origin	No.	Epistaxis	Swelling mass	Pain	Nasal obstruction	Other (ocular/neurolical
Kidney[218-253]	44	28	7	3	9	3
Bronchus[219-221,224,225,254-256,293-296]	14	–	5	3	1	4
Breast[218-220,257-263]	10	–	5	3	–	2
Urogenital	20	–	–	–	–	–
Testicle[218,220,264-267]	8	1	10	1	2	4
Uterus[14c,268-272]	7	–	–	–	–	–
Prostate[219,282]	3	–	–	–	–	–
Bladder[280,288]	2	–	–	–	1	1
Gastro-intestinal	10	–	–	–	–	–
Colon & rectum[218,221,222,262,278,279]	6		3	2	1	1
Stomach[220,221,280,281]	4	–	–	–	–	–
Miscellaneous	13	3	5	1	1	3
Thyroid[219,273-277]	6	–	–	–	–	–
Pancreas[218,281]	2	–	–	–	–	–
Melanoma[283-285]	3	–	–	–	–	–
Adrenal[286,287]	2	–	–	–	–	–

*Multiple symptoms present in some patients

daries of renal origin frequently produce significant epistaxis[220,230,231,234,235,240] which reflects the vascularity of the tumour. These symptoms may occur before those from the primary in over half the cases. Alternatively the secondary can appear some time after the primary has been removed.[226,234] The deposit can occur alone or in association with supraclavicular and superior cervical lymphadenopathy.[245,262] Very rarely the metastases can be bilateral.[245]

It is clearly important to perform a thorough general examination of the patient.

A 49-year-old male presented with a left pleural effusion and a mass in the left fronto-ethmoidal region (Table 7.18). Exploration by an external fronto-ethmoidectomy approach revealed a soft-tissue mass which was biopsied and proved to be a clear-cell carcinoma consistent with a renal origin. An intravenous pyelogram showed a space-occupying lesion in the left kidney which was removed. This case predates the introduction of the craniofacial approach and consequently the sinus lesion was treated with radiotherapy.

2 years later a bone metastasis was discovered in the left 6th rib for which a course of chemotherapy was given. Further rib lesions appeared after 3 years and were treated with radiotherapy. A deposit subsequently appeared in the right maxilla, followed by skin metastases and the patient died later that year when post-mortem confirmed extensive disseminated disease. 8 years had elapsed between the initial diagnosis and death.

Radiology

Deposits in the bone of the upper jaw may appear as osteolytic lesions, often in the molar area associated with the presence of red marrow. Alternatively the features may be non-specific with bone destruction and a soft tissue mass.

The source organ may be demonstrated by an intravenous pyelogram, chest X-ray or barium studies.

Macroscopic and microscopic appearance

Macroscopic appearance is non-specific although tumours of renal origin are often pale yellow in colour.

Microscopic appearance (Table 7.17)

Hypernephroma accounts for 83% of malignant renal tumours[259] and has characteristic histology. The cells are large clear, pale and vacuolated with a high glycogen content. Special stains for lipid and glycogen can be used and electron microscopy demonstrates cytoplasmic inclusions and fine microvilli arising from the tumour cells. The stroma is vascular[7d] hence the frequent presenting of epistaxis.

The other histological types such as anaplastic, other adenocarcinomas, malignant melanoma and neuroblastomas can arise both primarily or as secondary deposits in this area. Electron microscopy and immunocytochemistry may be helpful in their diagnosis.

Differential diagnosis

Clear cell tumours may be confused with acinic cell carcinoma and occasionally the angiomatoid varieties have been diagnosed as haemangiomas.

Natural history

Symptoms from the lesion in the nose and sinuses may precede or succeed those from the primary. When the secondary succeeds the primary, it may do so by anything from 10 months to 13 years so it is important to take a careful history of past medical treatment.[218,234,235,246,252,262] However, the slow growth of hypernephroma confined by its capsule means that up to 60% of patients may present with secondary symptoms[245] and in 38 patients with bony secondaries from renal malignancy, 75% of these became apparent before the primary was recognized. Thus the secondary may symptomatically precede the primary by anything up to 6 years[242] and this has also been our own experience with tumours in the tail of pancreas.

Treatment

The presence of a secondary deposit in this region is rarely an isolated event and usually signifies disseminated disease although solitary metastases are possible from the kidney. Consequently the aim of treatment must be palliative and directed principally at pain relief. However, radical resection of both primary and secondary renal tumours has sometimes produced moderate survival as in two of our cases. In the literature, radiotherapy has often been used either alone or in combination with surgery and occasionally chemotherapy. Three of our cases underwent craniofacial resection, four out of five received radiotherapy in addition to surgery and two also received chemotherapy. It is not always apparent that the lesion represents a metastasis and pancreatic tumours are notoriously difficult to diagnose early. However as the craniofacial procedure offers excellent palliation with minimal morbidity it might still be undertaken even when the situation is recognized.

Prognosis

As it is usually evidence of generalized carcinomatosis, the presence of metastatic disease in the nose and sinuses is inevitably associated with a dismal prognosis. Two-thirds of patients are dead within the year and less than 10% survive 4 years. Although hypernephroma is reputed to produce isolated secondaries,[235] post-mortem examination frequently reveals multi-organ involvement[235,297] so radical treatment can be unrewarding. A review of all cases with secondaries in the antrum, irrespective of histology and treatment, demonstrated an average survival time of 20 months.[242] It is also worth noting that the average length of survival in untreated cases was 33 months.

The rarity of this condition and its potential for symptomatically preceding its progenitor by some years renders generalized screening of all patients with tumours in this area unnecessary. However, a careful history, the presence of isolated involvement of the frontal and sphenoid sinus and certain histologies, may suggest the possibility of an alternative primary source, leading to selective investigation and management based on the concept of genuine palliation.

REFERENCES

1. Bergman F 1969 Tumors of the minor salivary glands. A report of 46 cases. Cancer 23: 538–543
2. Frable W J, Elzay R P 1970 Tumors of minor salivary glands. A report of 73 cases. Cancer 25: 932–941
3. Batsakis J G, Rice D H, Solomon A R 1980 The pathology of head and neck tumors: Squamous and mucous-gland carcinomas of the nasal cavity, paranasal sinuses and larynx. Part 6. Head and Neck Surgery 2: 497–508
4. Batsakis J G, Regezi J A, Bloch D 1979 The pathology of head and neck tumors: Salivary glands. Part 3. Head and Neck Surgery 1: 260–273
5. Eneroth C M, Zetterberg A 1973 Nuclear DNA content as a criterion of malignancy in salivary gland tumours of the oral cavity. Acta Otolaryngologica 75: 296–298
6. Hyams V J, Batsakis J G, Michaels L 1988 Tumors of the upper respiratory tract and ear. Atlas of tumor pathology, 2nd Series, Fascicle 25, Armed Forces Institute of Pathology, Washington DC, pp 85–88
7. Michaels L 1987 Ear, nose and throat histopathology. Springer Verlag, Berlin a: pp 180–181; b: pp 182–185; c: pp 177–180; d: p 235
8. Eneroth C M, Hjertman L, Moberger G 1972 Salivary adenomas of the palate. Acta Otolaryngologica 73: 305–315
9. Zarniko C 1910 Die Krankheilen der Nase und des Nasenrachens, Karger, Berlin, pp 310–322
10. Eichler W 1898 Adenom einen von der Nasenschliemhaut ausgahenden polypen vortauschend. Archives of Laryngology 7: 134
11. Hasslauer G 1900 Tumoren der Nasenscheidewand. Archives of Laryngology 10: 60
12. Rafla S 1969 Mucous gland tumors of paranasal sinuses. Cancer 24: 683–691
13. Paget J 1853 Cartilaginous tumours. Lecture VII in Lectures on Surgical Pathology, Longmans 2: 201–205
14. Friedmann I, Osborn D A 1982 Pathology of granulomas and neoplasms of the nose and paranasal sinuses. Churchill Livingstone, Edinburgh a: pp 150–152; b: pp 152–157; c: p 300
15. McDonald J R, Havens F Z 1948 A study of malignant tumors of glandular nature in the nose, throat and mouth. Surgical Clinics of North America 28: 1087–1106
16. Spiro R H, Koss L G, Hajdu S I, Strong E W 1973 Tumors of minor salivary origin. A clinicopathologic study of 492 cases. Cancer 31: 117–129
17. Chaudhry A P, Vickers R A, Gorlin R J 1961 Intraoral minor salivary gland tumors. An analysis of 1414 cases. Oral Surgery, Oral Medicine, Oral Pathology 14: 1194–1226
18. Harrison K 1956 A study of ectopic mixed salivary tumours. Annals of the Royal College of Surgeons of England 18: 99–122
19. Ranger D, Thackray A C, Lucas R B 1956 Mucous gland tumours. British Journal of Cancer 10: 1–16
20. Hjertman L, Eneroth C M 1970 Tumours of the palate. Acta Otolaryngologica 263: 179–182
21. Compagno J, Wong R T 1977 Intranasal mixed tumours (pleomorphic adenomas). A clinicopathologic study of 40 cases. American Journal of Clinical Pathology 68: 213–218.
22. Martis C S, Karakasis D T 1971 Pleomorphic adenoma arising in the maxillary sinus. Plastic and Reconstructive Surgery 47: 290–292

23. Potdor G G, Paymaster J C 1969 Tumors of minor salivary glands. Oral Surgery, Oral Medicine and Oral Pathology 28: 310–319
24. Russell H 1955 Adenomatous tumours of the anterior foregut region showing the cylindroma pattern. British Journal of Surgery 43: 248–254
25. Stevenson H N 1932 Mixed tumour of the nasal septum. Annals of Otorhinolaryngology 41: 563–570
26. Tos M 1982 Goblet cells and glands in the nose and paranasal sinuses. In: Proctor D F, Andersen I B (eds) The Nose: Upper airway physiology and the atmospheric environment. Elsevier, Amsterdam, pp 99–144
27. Majed M A 1971 Pleomorphic adenoma of the nasal septum. Journal of Laryngology and Otology 85: 975–976
28. Worthington P 1977 Pleomorphic adenoma of the nasal septum. British Journal of Oral Surgery 14: 245–252
29. Bergstrom B, Bjorklund A 1981 Pleomorphic adenoma of the nasal septum. Journal of Laryngology and Otology 95: 179–181
30. Baraka M E, Sadek A A, Salem M H 1984 Pleomorphic adenoma of the inferior turbinate. Journal of Laryngology and Otology 98: 925–928
31. Kamal K A 1984 Pleomorphic adenoma of the nose. Journal of Laryngology and Otology 98: 917–923
32. Haberman R S, Stanley D E 1989 Pleomorphic adenoma of the nasal septum. Otolaryngology, Head and Neck Surgery 100: 610–612
33. Freeman S B, Kennedy K S, Parker G S, Tatum S A 1990 Metastasizing pleomorphic adenoma of the nasal septum. Archives of Otolaryngology, Head and Neck Surgery 116: 1331–1333
34. Weber A L 1981 Pleomorphic adenoma of the hard palate. Annals of Otology, Rhinology and Laryngology 90: 192–193
35. Luna M A, Stimson P G, Bardwil J N 1968 Minor salivary gland tumors of the oral cavity. Oral Surgery 25: 71–86
36. Krolls S O, Boyers R C 1972 Mixed tumours of the salivary glands, long term follow up. Cancer 30: 276–281
37. Thackray A C, Lucas R B 1974 Tumors of the major salivary glands. Atlas of tumor pathology, 2nd Series, Fascicle 10, Armed Forces Institute of Pathology, Washington DC
38. Hellquist H, Michaels L 1986 Malignant mixed tumour. A salivary gland tumour showing carcinomatous and sarcomatous features. Virchows Archives of Pathological Anatomy and Histopathology (Berlin) 409: 93–103
39. Schaffer J 1897 Beitrage zur Histologie menschlicher Organe. IV, Zunge, V, Munde-Schlundkopf, VI. Oesophagus, VII, Cardia. Sitzungsb D K Akad D Mathetiek und Naturwissenschaften berichte der Königliche Akademie der Wissenschaften, Wien, Pt 3 106: 353–455
40. Hamperl H 1931 Beitrage zur normalen und pathologischen Histologie menschlicher Speicheldrusen. Zeitschrift fur mikroskopische und anatomische Forschung 27: 1–55
41. Gruenfeld G E, Jorsted L H 1936 Adenoma of the parotid salivary gland: oncocyte tumor. American Journal of Cancer 26: 571–575
42. McFarland J 1927 Adenoma of the salivary glands with a report of a possible case. American Journal of Medical Science 174: 362–378
43. Jaffe R H 1932 Adenolymphomas (oncocytomas) of parotid gland. American Journal of Cancer 16: 1415–1423
44. Blanck C, Eneroth C M, Jakobsson P 1970 Oncocytoma of the parotid gland: neoplasia or nodular hyperplasia. Cancer 24: 919–925
45. Foote F W, Frazell E L 1954 Tumors of the major salivary glands. Atlas of tumor pathology, Section IV, Fascicle 11. Armed Forces Institute of Pathology, Washington DC, pp 137–144
46. Kirklin J W, McDonald J R, Harrington S W, New G B 1951 Parotid tumors: Histopathology, clinical behaviour and end-results. Surgery, Gynaecology and Obstetrics 97: 721–733
47. Tandler B, Huffer R V P, Erlaredson R A 1970 Ultrastructure of oncocytoma of the parotid gland. Laboratory Investigation 23: 567–580
48. Briggs J, Evans J N G 1967 Malignant oxyphilic granular-cell tumor (oncocytoma) of the palate. Oral Surgery 23: 796–802
49. Hamperl H 1962 Benign and malignant oncocytoma. Cancer 15: 1019–1027
50. Cohen M A, Batsakis J G 1968 Oncocytic tumors (oncocytomas) of minor salivary glands. Archives of Otolaryngology 88: 71–73
51. Handler S D, Ward P H 1979 Oncocytoma of the maxillary sinus. Laryngoscope 89: 372–376
52. Mikhail R A, Reed D N, Bybee D B, Okoye M I, Dodds M E 1988 Malignant oncocytoma of the maxillary sinus – an ultrastructural study. Head and Neck Surgery 10: 427–431
53. Hamperl H 1950 Oncocytes and the so-called Hurthle cell tumor. Archives of Pathology 563–567
54. Johns M E, Regezi J A, Batsakis J G 1977 Oncocytic neoplasms of salivary glands: an ultrastructural study. Laryngoscope 87: 862–871
55. Batsakis J G 1980 Tumors of the head and neck 2nd edn., Williams & Wilkins, Baltimore, a: pp 85-86; b: pp 78–79; c: pp 77–83
56. Johns M E, Batsakis J G, Short C D 1973 Oncocytic and oncocytoid tumors of the salivary glands. Laryngoscope 83: 1940–1952
57. Billroth T 1856 Die Cylindergeschwulst (Cylindroma). In: Untersuchungen uber die Entwicklung der Blutgefasse, nebst Beobachtungen aus der koniglichen chirurgischen. Universtas-Klinik zu Berlin, Reimer, Berlin, pp 55–69
58. Guttman M R 1936 Primary adenocystic carcinoma or cylindroma of trachea. Annals of Otology 45: 894–901
59. Friedmann I, Osborn D A 1966 In: Wright G P, Symmers W St C (eds) Malignant tumours of the nasopharynx in systemic pathology. Longman, London
60. Foerster A 1854–1859 Atlas die mikroskopischen pathologischen Anatomie. Voss, Leipzig, p 78
61. Meckel von Hemsbach H 1856 Uber Knorpel-Wucherung: Mit einem Anhang von T Billroth: Schauch-Knorpel Geschwulst. Annals Charite-Krankenhospital, Berlin 7: 60–115
62. Friedreich N 1863 Zur Casuistik der Neubildungen. Virchow Archiv A. Pathological Anatomy and Histopathology 27: 375–388
63. Tommasi C 1864 Uber die Entstehungsweise des Friedreich'schen Schlauchsarkoms. Archiv fur Pathologischen Anatomie 31: 111–117
64. Koester K 1867 Cancroid mit hyaliner Degeneration (Cylindroma) (Billroth's). Virchow Archiv A. Pathological Anatomy and Histopathology 40: 468–504
65. Boettcher A 1867 Uber Structur und Entwickelung der als 'Schlauchknorpelgeschwulst, Cylindroma' bekannten Neubildung. Archiv fur Pathologischen Anatomie 38: 400–428
66. Czerny V 1869 Plexiformes Myxosarcom aus der Orbita. Archiv Klinischen Chirurgie 11: 234–241
67. von Ewetsky T 1877 Zur Cylindromfrage. Archiv fur Pathologischen Anatomie 69: 36-55
68. Waldeyer W 1872 Die Entwickelung der Carcinome. Virchow Archiv A. Pathological Anatomy and Histopathology 55: 67–159
69. Sattler H 1874 Uber die sogenannten Cylindrome und deren Stellung im onkologischen Systeme. Reimer, Berlin, pp 100
70. Malassez L 1883 Sur le 'Cylindrome' (epitheliome alveolaire avec envahissement myxomateux). Archives de Physiologie Normale et Pathologique 1: 123-129; 186–213
71. Ackermann T 1883 Die Histogenese und Histologie der Sarkoma, Sammlung Klinische Vortsch Chirurgie 54–84: 1971–2040
72. Klebs E 1887 Die allgemeine Pathologie oder die Lehre von den Ursachen und dem Wesen der Krankheitprocesse. Jena, VEB Gustav Fischer Verlag 2: 836
73. Bizzozero G 1911 In: Kaufmann E (ed) Lehrbuch der speziellen pathologischen. I Anatomie fur Studierende und Artze, Reimer, Berlin, p 115
74. Krompecher E 1918 Zur Kenntniss der Basalzellenkrebse der Nase, der Nebenhohlen, der Kehlkopfes und der Trachea. Archiv fur Laryngologie und Rhinologie 31: 443–460
75. Beck J C, Guttman M R 1936 Basaloma or so-called cylindroma of air passages. Annals of Otology 45: 618–631
76. Dockerty M B, Mayo C W 1942 Primary tumors of submaxillary gland with special reference to mixed tumours. Surgery, Gynecology and Obstetrics 74: 1033–1045
77. Bauer W H, Fox R A 1945 Adenomyoepithelioma (Cylindroma) of palatal mucous glands. Archives of Pathology 39: 96–102

78. Robin C, Laboulbene A 1853 Memoire sur trois productions morbides non decrites. Compte Rendu Societe Biologique 5: 185–196

79. Billroth T 1859 Beobachtungen uber Geschwulste der Speicheldrusen. Virchows Archiv A, Pathological Anatomy and Histopathology 17: 357–375

80. Reid J D 1952 Adenoid cystic carcinoma (cylindroma) of the bronchial tree. Cancer 5: 685–694

81. Foote F W, Frazell E L 1953 Tumors of major salivary glands. Cancer 6: 1065–1133

82. Ferreri G 1928 Contribution a l'etude clinique et anatomo-pathologique de cylindrome du maxillaire superieur. Acta Otolaryngologica 12: 411–430

83. Kramer R, Som M L 1939 Cylindroma of the upper air passages: A Cylindromatous type of mixed tumor. Archives of Otolaryngology 29: 356–370

84. Eidesheim G 1909 Ein Beitrag zum vorkommen primarer bosartiger Neubildungen in der Trachea (Cylindrom). Lehmann, Leipzig, pp 25

85 Eigler G 1932 Uber Endotheliome, Peritheliome, Cylindrome und ahnliche Tumoren der oberen Luftwege. Archiv fur Ohren, Nasen und Kehlkopfheilkunde 132: 209–253

86. Nussbaum R 1930 Ein Fall von Zylindrom des Warzenfortsatzes. Archiv fur Ohren, Nasen und Kehlkopfheilkunde 125: 307–309

87. Speis J W 1930 Adenoid cystic carcinoma: generalised metastases in 3 cases of basal cell type. Archives of Surgery 21: 365–404

88. Conley J, Dingman D L 1974 Adenoid cystic carcinoma in the head and neck (cylindroma). Archives of Otolaryngology 100: 81–90

89. Leafstedt S W, Gaeta J F, Sako K, Shedd D P 1971 Adenoid cystic carcinoma of major and minor salivary glands. American Journal of Surgery 122: 756–762

90. Osborn D A 1977 Morphology and the natural history of cribriform adenocarcinoma (adenoid cystic carcinoma). Journal of Clinical Pathology 30: 195–205

91. Spiro R H, Huvos A G, Strong E W 1974 Adenoid cystic carcinoma of salivary origin. American Journal of Surgery 128: 512–520

92. Chilla R, Schroth R, Eysholdt U, Droese M 1980 Adenoid cystic carcinoma of the head and neck. Controllable and uncontrollable factors in treatment and prognosis. Otology, Rhinology and Laryngology 42: 346–367

93. Fine G, Marshall R B, Horn R C 1960 Tumours of minor salivary glands. Cancer 13: 653–669

94. Moran J J, Becker S M, Brady L W, Rambo V B 1961 Adenoid cystic carcinoma. Cancer 14: 1235–1250

95. Tauxe W N, McDonald J R, Devine K D 1962 A century of cylindromas. Archives of Otolaryngology 75: 94–106

96. Eby L S, Johnson D S, Baker H W 1972 Adenoid cystic carcinoma of the head and neck. Cancer 29: 1160–1168

97. Horee W A 1974 Adenoid cystic carcinoma of the maxilla. Archives of Otolaryngology 100: 469–472

98. Perzin K H, Gullane P, Clairmont A C 1978 Adenoid cystic carcinoma arising in salivary glands. Cancer 42: 265–282

99. Marsh W L, Shannon Allen M 1979 Adenoid cystic carcinoma. Cancer 43: 1463–1473

100. Miller R H, Calcaterra T C 1980 Adenoid cystic carcinoma of the nose, paranasal sinuses and palate. Archives of Otolaryngology 106: 424–426

101. Matsuba H M, Thawley S E, Simpson J R, Levine L A, Mauney M 1984 Adenoid cystic carcinoma of major and minor salivary gland origin. Laryngoscope 94: 1316–1318

102. Dal Maso M, Lippi L 1985 Adenoid cystic carcinoma of the head and neck: a clinical study of 37 cases. Laryngoscope 95: 177–181

103. Coates H L C, Devine K D, Desanto L W, Weiland L H 1975 Glandular tumours of the palate. Surgery, Gynecology and Obstetrics 140: 589

104. Dodd G D, Jing B 1972 Radiographic findings in adenoid cystic carcinoma of the head and neck. Annals of Otology, Rhinology and Laryngology 81: 591–598

105. Lloyd G A S 1988 Diagnostic imaging of the nose and paranasal sinuses. Springer Verlag, London

106. Szanto P A, Luna M A, Tortoledo M E, White R A 1984 Histologic grading of adenoid cystic carcinoma of the salivary glands. Cancer 54: 1062–1069

107. Batsakis J G, Luna M A, El-Naggar A 1990 Histopathologic grading of salivary gland neoplasms. III Adenoid Cystic Carcinoma. Annals of Otology, Rhinology and Laryngology 99: 1007–1009

108. Byers R M, Jessee R H, Guillamondegui O M, Luna M A 1973 Malignant tumors of the submaxillary gland. American Journal of Surgery 126: 458–463

109. Eneroth C M 1971 Salivary gland tumors in the parotid gland, submandibular gland and the palate region. Cancer 27: 1415–1418

110. Stewart J 1961 Carcinoma of salivary glands showing the cylindroma pattern. British Journal of Surgery 49: 241–245

111. Tarpley T M, Giansanti J S 1976 Adenoid cystic carcinoma. Analysis of 50 oral cases. Oral Surgery, Oral Medicine and Oral Pathology 41: 484–497

112. Thackray A C, Lucas R B 1960 The histology of cylindromas of mucous gland origin. British Journal of Cancer 14: 612–619

113. Adams A, Duvall A 1971 Adenocarcinomas of the head and neck. Archives of Otolaryngology 93: 261–270

114. Howard D J, Lund V J 1985 Reflections on the management of adenoid cystic carcinoma of the nasal cavity and paranasal sinuses. Otolaryngology, Head and Neck Surgery 93: 338–341

115. Leroux R, Leroux-Robert J 1934 Essai de classification architecturale des tumeurs des glands salivaires. Bulletin de l'Association Francaise pour l'etude du cancer 23: 304–340

116. Belsey R H R, Valentine J C 1951 Cylindromatous mucous-gland tumours of the trachea and bronchi: a report of three cases. Journal of Pathology and Bacteriology 63: 377–387

117. Berdal P, De Besche A, Mylius E 1970 Cylindroma of salivary glands. Acta Otolaryngologica 263: 173–178

118. Smout M S, French A J 1961 Prognosis of pseudo-adenomatous basal cell carcinoma: cylindroma, adenocystic carcinoma. Archives of Pathology 72: 107–112

119. Shannon Allen M, Marsh W L 1976 Lymph node involvement by direct extension in adenoid cystic carcinoma. Cancer 38: 2017–2021

120. Stell P M, Cruickshank A H, Stoney P J, McCormick M S 1985 Lymph node metastases in adenoid cystic carcinoma. American Journal of Otolaryngology 6: 433–436

121. Grace B, Patterson B, Cummings B, Gullane P, Bryce D, Penzarella T DNA flow cytometry is a better prognostic indicator in adenoid cystic carcinoma than histological grading. Otolaryngology Head and Neck Surgery (in press)

122. Stuteville O H, Corley R D 1967 Surgical management of tumors of intraoral minor salivary glands. Cancer 20: 1578–1586

123. Citelli S, Calamida U 1903 Beitrage zu Lehre von dem Epitheliomen der Nasenschleimhaut. Archiv fur Laryngologie 13: 273–287

124. Harma L, Glas E 1907 Die malignen Tumoren der inneren Nase. Deutsche Zeitschrift Chirurgie 89: 433–539

125. Ahlbom H E 1935 Mucous and salivary gland tumours. Acta Radiologica Suppl. 23

126. Ringertz N 1938 Pathology of malignant tumours arising in the nasal and paranasal cavities and maxilla. Acta Otolaryngologica Suppl. 27

127. Robin P E, Powell D J, Stansbie J M 1979 Carcinoma of the nasal cavity and paranasal sinuses: incidence and presentation of different histological types. Clinical Otolaryngology 4: 431–456

128. Worsoe Petersen J 1965 Colloid carcinoma of the nasal cavity and sinuses. Archives of Otolaryngology 82: 181–185

129. Wille C 1947 Malignant tumors in nose and in accessory sinuses. Acta Otolaryngologica Suppl. 65

130. Larsson L G, Maartensson G 1954 Carcinoma of paranasal sinuses and nasal cavities. Acta Radiologica 42: 149–172

131. Hemenway W G, Lindsay J R 1959 Malignancies of paranasal sinuses. Acta Otolaryngologica 70: 71–74

132. Huizing E H 1962 Report of malignant tumors of nose, paranasal sinuses and nasopharynx. Practica Otolaryngologica 24: 127–132

133. Batsakis J G, Holtz F, Sueper R 1963 Adenocarcinoma of nasal and paranasal cavities. Archives of Otolaryngology 77: 625–633

134. Gamez-Araujo J J, Ayala A G, Guillamondegui O 1975 Mucinous adenocarcinoma of nose and paranasal sinuses. Cancer 36: 1100–1105
135. Saunders S H, Ruff T 1976 Adenocarcinoma of the para-nasal sinuses. Journal of Laryngology and Otology 90: 157–166
136. Goepfert H, Luna M A, Lindberg R, White A K 1983 Malignant salivary gland tumors of the paranasal sinuses and nasal cavity. Archives of Otolaryngology 109: 662–668
137. Alessi D M, Trapp T K, Fu Y S, Calcaterrra T C 1988 Non-salivary sinonasal adenocarcinoma. Archives of Otolaryngology, Head and Neck Surgery 114: 996–999
138. Heffner D K, Hyams V J, Hauck K W, Lingeman C 1982 Low-grade adenocarcinoma of the nasal cavity and paranasal sinuses. Cancer 50: 312–322
139. Hyams V J, Batsakis J G, Michaels L 1986 Tumors of the upper respiratory tract and ear. Armed Forces Institute of Pathology a: pp 95–100; b: pp 104–106
140. Roush G C, Schymura M J, Stevenson J M, Holford T R 1987 Time and age trends for sinonasal cancer in Connecticut incidence and US mortality rates. Cancer 60: 422–428
141. Lewis J S, Castro E B 1972 Cancer of the nasal cavity and paranasal sinuses. Journal of Laryngology and Otology 86: 255–262
142. Tran L, Sadeghi A, Hanson D, Ellerbroek N, Calcaterra T C, Parker R G 1987 Salivary gland tumors of the palate. Laryngoscope 97: 1343–1345
143. Kraus D H, Roberts J K, Medendorp S V, Levine H L, Wood B G, Tucker H M, Lavertu P 1990 Nonsquamous cell malignancies of the paranasal sinuses. Annals of Otology, Rhinology and Laryngology 99: 5–11
144. Andersen H C, Andersen I, Solgaard J 1977 Nasal cancers, symptoms and upper airway function in woodworkers. British Journal of Industrial Medicine 34: 201–207
145. Stokinger H E 1977 Routes of entry and modes of action. In: Key M M, Henschel A F, Butler J (eds) Occupational diseases, a guide to their recognition. DHEW, Washington DC, pp 11–21
146. Wilhelmsson B, Drettner B 1984 Nasal problems in wood furniture workers. A study of symptoms and physiological variables. Acta Otolaryngologica 98: 548–555
147. Acheson E D, Cowdell R H, Hadfield E, Macbeth R G 1968 Nasal cancer in woodworkers in the furniture industry. British Medical Journal 2: 587–596
148. Brinton L A, Blot W J, Stone B J, Fraumeni J F 1977 A death certificate of nasal cancer among furniture workers in North Carolina. Cancer Research 37: 3473–3474
149. Cecchi F, Buiatti E, Kriebel D, Nastasi L, Santucci M 1963 Adenocarcinoma of the nose and paranasal sinuses in shoemakers and woodworkers in the province of Florence, Italy (1963–77). British Journal of Industrial Medicine 37: 222–225
150. Debois J M 1969 Tumoren van de neusholte bij houtbewerkers. Tijdschr Geneesk 25: 92–93
151. Delemare J F M, Themans H H 1971 Het adenocarcinoom van de neusholten. Ned Tijdschr Geneesk 115: 688–690
152. Elwood J M 1981 Wood exposure and smoking: association with cancer of the nasal cavity and paranasal sinuses in British Columbia. Canadian Medical Association Journal 124: 1573–1577
153. Engzell U 1978 Occupational etiology and nasal cancer. Acta Otolaryngologica 86 (Suppl. 360): 126–128
154. Gignoux M, Bernard P 1969 Tumeurs malignes de l'ethmoide chez les travailleurs du bois. Journal de Medecine (Lyon) 50: 731–736
155. Hadfield E H 1970 A study of adenocarcinoma of the paranasal sinuses in woodworkers in the furniture industry. Annals of Royal College of Surgeons of England 46: 301–319
156. Hayes R B, Gerin M, Raatgever J W, De Bruyn A 1986 Wood-related occupations, wood dust exposure and sinonasal cancer. American Journal of Epidemiology 124: 569–577
157. Ironside P, Matthews J 1975 Carcinoma of the nose and paranasal sinuses in woodworkers in the state of Victoria, Australia. Cancer 36: 1115–1121
158. Macbeth R G 1965 Malignant disease of the paranasal sinuses. Journal of Laryngology and Otology 79: 592–612
159. Mosbech B J, Acheson E D 1971 Nasal cancer in furniture-makers in Denmark. Danish Medical Bulletin 18: 34–35
160. Tola S, Hernberg S, Collan Y, Linderborg H, Korkala M L 1980 A case-control study of the etiology of nasal cancer in Finland. International Archives of Occupational and Environmental Health 46: 79–85
161. Boysen M, Voss R, Solberg L A 1986 The nasal mucosa in softwood-exposed furniture workers. Acta Otolaryngologica 101: 501–508
162. Hernberg S, Westerholm P, Schultz Larsen K 1983 Nasal and sinonasal cancer. Connection with occupational exposures in Denmark, Finland and Sweden. Scandinavian Journal of Work and Environmental Health 9: 315–326
163. Voss R, Stenersen T, Oppedal B R, Boysen M 1985 Sinonasal cancer and exposure to softwood. Acta Otolaryngologica 99: 172–178
164. Takasaka T, Kawamoto K, Nakamura K 1987 A case-control study of nasal cancers. Acta Otolaryngologica Suppl. 435: 136–142
165. Black A, Evans J C, Hadfield E, Macbeth R G, Morgan A, Walsh M 1974 Impairment of nasal mucociliary clearance in woodworkers in the furniture industry. British Journal of Industrial Medicine 31: 10–17
166. Wilhelmsson B, Hellquist H, Olofsson J, Klintenberg C 1985 Nasal cuboidal metaplasia with dysplasia. Acta Otolaryngologica 99: 641–648
167. Drettner B, Wilhelmsson B, Lundh B 1985 Experimental studies on carcinogenesis in the nasal mucosa. Acta Otolaryngologica 99: 205–207
168. Guney E, Tanyeri Y, Kandemir B, Yalcin S 1987 The effect of wood dust on the nasal cavity and paranasal sinuses. Rhinology 25: 273–277
169. Wilhelmsson B, Lundh B, Drettner B, Stenkvist B 1985 Effects of wood dust exposure and diethylnitrosamine: a pilot study in Syrian golden hamsters. Acta Otolaryngologica (Stockholm) 99: 160–171
170. Acheson E D, Cowdell R H, Jolles B 1975 Nasal cancer in the Northamptonshire boot and shoe industry. British Medical Journal 1: 385–393
171. Enterline P E 1974 Respiratory cancer among chromate workers. Journal of Oral Medicine 16: 523–526
172. Heuper W C 1966 Occupational and environmental cancers of the respiratory system. In: Rentchnick P (ed) Recent results in cancer research, 3. Springer Verlag, New York
173. Levy L S, Verritt S 1975 Carcinogenic and mutagenic activities of chromium-containing materials. British Journal of Cancer 32: 262–263
174. Fraumeni J F Jr 1968 Respiratory carcinogenesis: an epidemiological appraisal. Journal of National Cancer Institute 55: 1039–1044
175. International Agency for Research on Cancer Working Group 1976 Isopropyl alcohol and isopropyl oils. In: Evaluation of carcinogenic risk of chemicals to man. World Health Organization, Geneva, pp 223–243
176. National Institute for Occupational Safety and Health 1976 Criteria for a Recommended Standard Occupational Exposure to Isopropyl Alcohol. DHEW Publication, Washington DC, No. 76–142
177. Acheson E D, Cowdell R H, Rang E 1972 Adenocarcinoma of the nasal cavity and sinuses in England and Wales. British Journal of Industrial Medicine 29: 21–30
178. Roush G C 1979 Epidemiology of cancer of the nose and paranasal sinuses: current concepts. Head and Neck Surgery 2: 3–11
179. Rowe L D, Lane R, Snow J B 1980 Adenocarcinoma of the ethmoid following radiotherapy for bilateral retinoblastoma. Laryngoscope 90: 61–69
180. Jarvi O 1945 Heterotopic tumors with an intestinal mucous membrane structure in the nasal cavity. Acta Otolaryngologica 33: 471–485
181. Raiford T S 1932 Mucoid carcinoma of the gastrointestinal tract. Surgery, Gynecology and Obstetrics 55: 409–417
182. Sanchez-Casis G, Devine K D, Weiland L H 1971 Nasal adenocarcinomas that closely simulate colonic carcinomas. Cancer 28: 714–720

183. Elner A, Koch H 1974 Combined radiological and surgical therapy of cancer of the ethmoid. Acta Otolaryngologica 78: 270–276
184. Klintenberg C, Olofsson J, Hellquist H, Sokjer H 1984 Adenocarcinoma of the ethmoid sinuses. A review of 28 cases with special reference to wood dust exposure. Cancer 54: 482–488
185. Cheesman A D, Lund V J, Howard D J 1986 Craniofacial resection for tumours of the nose and paranasal sinuses. Head and Neck Surgery 8: 429–435
186. Ketcham A S, Wilkins R H, Van Buren J M, Smith R R 1963 A combined intracranial facial approach to the paranasal sinuses. American Journal of Surgery 106: 698–703
187. Lund V J, Harrison D F N 1988 Craniofacial resection for tumors of the nasal cavity and paranasal sinuses. American Journal of Surgery 156: 187–190
188. Smith R R, Klopp C T, Williams J M 1954 Surgical treatment of cancer of the frontal sinus and adjacent areas. Cancer 7: 991–994
189. Bridger G P 1980 Radical surgery for ethmoid cancer. Archives of Otolaryngology 106: 630–634
190. Guggenheim P, Kleitsch W P 1967 Combined craniotomy, rhinotomy for ethmoid cancer. Annals of Otolaryngology 76: 105–117
191. Weaver D F 1961 Cancer of the ethmoid sinuses. Archives of Otolaryngologica 74: 333–339
192. Matsuba H M, Mauney M, Simpson J R, Thawley S E, Pikul F J 1988 Adenocarcinoma of major and minor salivary gland origin. Laryngoscope 98: 784–788
193. Salassa J R, McDonald T J, Weiland L H 1980 'Colonic type' adenocarcinomas of the nasal cavity and paranasal sinuses. Otolaryngology, Head and Neck Surgery 88: 133–135
194. Gerughty R M, Henniger G R, Brown F M 1968 Adenosquamous carcinoma of the nasal, oral and laryngeal cavities. Cancer 22: 1140–1155
195. Masson P, Berger L 1924 Epitheliomes a double metaplasie de la parotide. Bulletin de l'Association Francaise pour l'etude du cancer 13: 366–375
196. Stewart F W, Foote F W, Becker W F 1945 Mucoepidermoid tumours of salivary glands. Annals of Surgery 122: 820–844
197. Stuteville O H, Corley R D 1967 Surgical management of tumours of intraoral minor salivary glands. Cancer 20: 1578–1586
198. Smith R L, Dahlin D C, Waite D E 1968 Mucoepidermoid carcinomas of the jawbones. Journal of Oral Surgery 26: 387–393
199. Healey W V, Perzin K H, Smith L 1970 Mucoepidermoid carcinoma of salivary gland origin. Cancer 26: 368–388
200. Da-Quan M, Guang-Yan Y 1987 Tumours of the minor salivary glands. A clinicopathologic study of 243 cases. Acta Otolaryngologica 103: 325–331
201. Batsakis J G, Chinn E, Regezi J A, Repola D A 1978 The pathology of head and neck tumors: salivary glands, part 2. Head and Neck Surgery 1: 167–180
202. Nasse D 1892 Die Geschwulste der Speicheldrusen und verwandte Tumoren des Kopfes. Archiv Klinische Chirurgie 44: 233–302
203. Inoue T, Shimono M, Yamamura T, Saito I, Watanabe O 1984 Acinic cell carcinoma arising in the glossopalatine glands: a report of two cases with electron microscopic observations. Oral Surgery, Oral Medicine, Oral Pathology 57: 398–407
204. Krolls S O, Trodahl J N, Boyers R C 1972 Salivary gland lesions in children: a survey of 430 cases. Cancer 30: 459–469
205. Kleinsasser O 1970 Acinuszelltumoren der Schleimdrusen. Archiv fur klinische und experimentelle Ohren, Nasen und Kehlkopfheilkunde 195: 345–354
206. Manace E D, Goldman J L 1971 Acinic cell carcinoma of paranasal sinuses. Laryngoscope 81: 1074–1082
207. Perzin K H, Cantor J O, Johannessen J V 1981 Acinic cell carcinoma arising in nasal cavity. Cancer 47: 1818–1822
208. Ordonez N G, Batsakis J G 1986 Acinic cell carcinoma of the nasal cavity: electron-optic and immunohistochemical observations. Journal of Laryngology and Otology 100: 345–349
209. Abrams A M, Cornyn J, Scofield H H, Hanse L S 1965 Acinic cell adenocarcinoma of the major salivary glands. Cancer 18: 1145–1162
210. Dardick I, George D, Diane Jones M T 1987 Ultrastructural morphology and cellular differentiation in acinic cell carcinoma. Oral Surgery, Oral Medicine, Oral Pathology 63: 325–334
211. Eneroth C M, Silfversward C, Zetterberg A 1974 Malignancy of acinic cell tumours elucidated by microspectrophotometric DNA analysis. Acta Otolaryngologica 77: 126–130
212. Gustafsson H, Lindholm C, Carlsoo B 1987 DNA cytophotometry of acinic cell carcinoma and its relation to prognosis. Acta Otolaryngologica 104: 370–376
213. Hellquist H B 1990 Pathology of the nose and paranasal sinuses. Butterworths, London, pp 118
214. Evans R W, Cruickshank A H 1970 Epithelial tumours of the salivary glands. Saunders, Philadelphia, pp 117
215. Eneroth C M, Jakobsson P A, Blanck C 1966 Acinic cell carcinoma of the parotid gland. Cancer 19: 1761–1772
216. Chong G C, Beahrs O H, Woolner L B 1974 Surgical management of acinic cell carcinoma of the parotid gland. Surgery, Gynecology and Obstetrics 138: 65–68
217. Spiro R H, Huvos A G, Strong E W 1975 Cancer of the parotid gland: a clinicopathologic study of 288 primary cases. American Journal of Surgery 130: 452–459
218. Bernstein J M, Montgomery W W, Balogh K 1966 Metastatic tumors to the maxilla, nose and paranasal sinuses. Laryngoscope 76: 621–650
219. Barrs D M, McDonald T J, Whisnant J P 1979 Metastatic tumors to the sphenoid sinus. Laryngoscope 89: 1239–1243
220. Garrett M J 1959 Metastatic tumours of the paranasal sinuses simulating primary growths. Journal of the Faculty of Radiologists (London) 10: 151–155
221. Meyer I, Shuklar G 1965 Malignant tumors metastatic to mouth and jaws. Oral Surgery, Oral Medicine, Oral Pathology 20: 350–362
222. Tolan T L 1939 Report of two cases of carcinoma of sphenoid and ethmoids. Annals of Otology, Rhinology and Laryngology 48: 1069–1072
223. Hamberger C A 1943 Hypernefrommetastas i sin ethmoidale och sphenoidale. Nordsk Medicin 20: 2229–2234
224. Perls M 1872 Beitrage zur Geschwulstlehre. Virchow Archiv A. Pathological Anatomy and Histology (Berlin) 56: 437–444
225. Salman S, Darlington C G 1944 Rare (unusual) malignant tumors of the jaws. American Journal of Orthodontics 30: 725–749
226. Achar M V R 1955 Metastatic hypernephroma occurring in nasal septum. Archives of Otolaryngology 62: 644–648
227. Arrowsmith H 1916 Malignant hypernephroma of the ethmoidal region. Laryngoscope 26: 909–912
228. Atkins R T 1924 Metastatic hypernephroma of the nasal septum and accessory sinuses. Laryngoscope 34: 740–742
229. Barmwater K 1931 Endothelioma cavi nasi. Zentralblatt fur Hals, Nasen und Ohrenheilkunde 17: 42–48
230. Biendara E 1951 Zur Klinik der Hypernephrommetasten im Nasen-nebenhohlengebiet. Zeitschrift fur Laryngologie und Rhinologie 30: 313–317
231. Burns J R, Edwards M H, Essel J F, Cowlbeck D D 1956 Epistaxis resulting from metastatic renal carcinoma. Journal of the American Medical Association 161: 226–227
232. Carnevale-Ricci F 1936 Metastasi nel seno frontale di un ipernefroma latente. Archivo Italiano di Otologica, Rhinologica, Laringologica 48: 73–82
233. Connor C E 1938 Metastatic hypernephroma of right frontal ethmoid and maxillary sinuses. Archives of Otolaryngology 28: 994–998
234. Edwards W G 1964 Epistaxis from metastatic renal carcinoma. Journal of Laryngology and Otology 78: 96–102
235. Eneroth C M, Martensson G, Thulin A 1961 Profuse epistaxis in hypernephroma metastases. Acta Otolaryngologica 53: 546–550
236. Esau D 1925 Fruhzeitige Fernmetastasen bei verborgenem Karzinom. Medizinische Klinische 21: 1086–1094
237. Friedmann I, Osborn D A 1965 Metastatic tumours to the ear, nose and throat region. Journal of Laryngology and Otology 79: 576–587
238. Freiman K A 1961 Prispevek k vyskytu hypernephromu ve vedlejsich nosnich dutirach. Ceskoslovenska Otolaryngologie 10: 362–366

239. Grimaud A P, Wayoff D 1954 Metastase ethmoidale isolee d'un hypernephrome malin opere. Journal Francaise Otologie, Rhinologie et Laryngologie 3: 495–498

240. Harrison M S, Doey W D, Osborn D A 1964 Intra-nasal metastasis from renal carcinoma. Journal of Laryngology and Otology 78: 103–107

241. Hlavacek T 1961 A contribution to the presence of hypernephroma in the paranasal sinuses. Cited by Freiman K in Ceskoslovenska Otolaryngologie 10: 362–366

242. Kent S E, Majumdar B 1985 Metastatic tumours in the maxillary sinus. Journal of Laryngology and Otology 99: 459–463

243. Kretschmer H L 1930 Metastasis from hypernephroma to the nasal sinuses. Massachusetts General Hospital Case Report. New England Journal of Medicine 202: 657–658

244. Kurokawa K 1941 Hypernephroma des linken Oberkiefers. Zentralblatt Hals, Nasen und Ohrenheilkunde 34: 413–421

245. Matsumoto Y, Yanagihara N 1982 Renal clear cell carcinoma metastatic to the nose and paranasal sinuses. Laryngoscope 92: 1190–1193

246. Oppikofer E 1931 Die hypernephrommetasten in der oberen Luftwegen und in Gehororgan. Archiv fur Ohren, Nasen und Kehlkheilkunde 129: 271–292

247. Preysing 1909 Einige Beispiele von diagnostischen Irrtumer und von selteneren Tumoren. Medizinische Klinische 5: 1738–1741

248. Storath E 1913 Ein Full von Hypernephrommeastase in der Nasenhohle nebst Vorschlagen fur operation der malignen Nasentumoren uberhaupt. Zeitschrift Ohrenheilkunde 69: 157–171

249. Van Duyse D, Marbaix 1922 Metastase ethmoido-orbitaire d'hypernephrome latent. Archives Ophthalmologie (Paris) 39: 396–409

250. Heindl A 1930 Uber Geschwulste der sternhohle. Monatsschrift fur Ohrenheilkunde 64: 128–137

251. Scudder C L 1906 Bone metastases of hypernephroma. Annals of Surgery 44: 851–865

252. Sellstrom L G 1962 Hypernephroma metastases in the ear and nose region. Acta Otolaryngologica 55: 545–552

253. Stein G 1929 Hypernephrommetastase als Epulis. Deutschen Zeitschrift fur Chirurgie 219: 318–320

254. Gottlieb M 1937 Metastatic carcinoma of the upper jaw from a primary bronchogenic tumor. Report of a case. Journal of the American Dental Association 24: 1075–1079

255. Kranes A 1950 Unusual metastatic spread of bronchial carcinoma. Massachusetts General Hospital Case Report. New England Journal of Medicine 243: 1043–1077

256. Reuter G 1960 Metastasis to the frame of the nose of a lung tumor. Krebsarzt 15: 61–63

257. Archilei G 1959 Metastasi orbita-paranasale da carcinoma mammario. Bollettino Malattia Orecchio 77: 218–229

258. Blake H, Blake F 1960 Breast carcinoma metastatic to maxilla. Oral Surgery, Oral Medicine, Oral Pathology 13: 1099–1102

259. Nahum A M, Bailey B J 1963 Malignant tumors metastatic to the paranasal sinuses: case report and review of the literature. Laryngoscope 73: 942–953

260. O'Connell D 1958 Metastasis in the nasal bones. Journal of the Faculty of Radiologists 9: 97–98

261. Robin I G 1939 Malignant disease of the maxilla with special reference to carcinoma of the antrum. Guy's Hospital Reports 19: 301–329

262. Robinson D 1973 Antral metastases from carcinoma. Journal of Laryngology and Otology 87: 603–609

263. Ungerecht H 1950 Spatmetastase eines Mamma-Carcinoms. Zentralblatt fur Hals, Nasen und Ohrenheilkunde 40: 130–133

264. Castigliano S G, Rominger C J 1954 Metastatic malignancy of the jaws. American Journal of Surgery 87: 496–507

265. Marx H 1953 Die Nasenheilkunde in Einzeldarstellungen, 6th edn. Gustav Fischer, Jena, pp 17

266. Minnigerode B 1962 Seminommetasen in den Kieferhohlen, HNO 10: 334–336

267. Worgan D 1967 Metastatic maxillary antrum seminoma. Journal of Laryngology and Otology 81: 241–243

268. Cohen J 1931 Metastase eines Uterusscheidenkarzinoma in der Nase. Zeitschrift fur Laryngologie und Otologie 21: 452

269. Mercer R D, Lammert A C, Anderson R, Hazard J B 1958 Choriocarcinoma in mother and infant. Journal of the American Medical Association 166: 482–485

270. Mukherjee D K 1978 Choriocarcinoma of the nose. Annals of Otology, Rhinology and Laryngology 87: 257–259

271. Salimi R 1977 Metastatic choriocarcinoma of the nasal mucosa. Journal of Surgical Oncology 9: 301–305

272. Subramanyam C, Lal M 1970 Unusual presentation of chorion epithelioma malignum. Medical Journal of Malaya 24: 306–307

273. Auriti F 1921 Adenoma a struttura tiroidea del setto nasale. Archivio Italiano di Otologica, Rhinologica, Laringologica 4: 120–127

274. Cinberg J Z, Solomon M P, Ozbardacki G 1980 Thyroid carcinoma and secondary malignancy of the sinonasal tract. Archives of Otolaryngology 106: 239–241

275. De Vincentius I 1959 Sulle metastasi del cancro tiroideo di interesse otorinolaringolatrico. Annali di Laringologica 33: 39–48

276. Renner G J, Davis W E, Templer J W 1984 Metastasis of thyroid carcinoma to the paranasal sinuses. Otolaryngology, Head and Neck Surgery 92: 233–237

277. Von Eiselberg A 1893 Uber Knochen-Metastasen des Schilddrusen Krebses. Verhandlungen der Deutschen Gesellschaft fur Chirurgie 22: 255–259

278. Clausen F, Poulsen H 1963 Metastatic carcinoma to the jaws. Acta Pathologica Scandinavia 57: 361–374

279. Humphrey A A, Amos N H 1936 Metastatic gingival adenocarcinoma from a primary lesion of the colon. American Journal of Cancer 28: 128–130

280. Bouqout J E, Weiland L H, Kurland L T 1989 Metastases to and from the upper aerodigestive tract in the population of Rochester, Minnesota, 1935–1984. Head and Neck Surgery 11: 212–218

281. Hommerich D W 1954 Zur Kenntnis sekundarer Geschwulste der Nasennebenhohlen. Archiv fur Ohren, Nasen, Kehlkopfheilkunde 166: 229–231

282. Har-El G, Avidor I, Weisbord A, Sidi J 1987 Carcinoma of the prostate metastatic to the maxillary antrum. Head and Neck Surgery 10: 55–58

283. Hada B 1914 Zur Kenntnis der Melanome. Virchows Archiv fur Pathologische Anatomie 215: 216–232

284. Phillips C 1928 Cited by Schmittmann M 1935 In: Handbuch der speziellen Pathologischen Anatomie und Histologie, Vol III. Springer, Berlin, pp 246

285. Meyer J E, Rogers W P, Leiter B 1979 Metastatic melanoma involving the left maxillary antrum. Journal of Laryngology and Otology 93: 1011–1013

286. Goldman H M 1960 Cited in Oral Pathology by K H Thomas and H M Goldman, CV Mosby, St Louis, pp 238

287. Young G 1935 Growth of right maxillary neuroblastoma metastasis from suprarenals. Journal of Laryngology and Otology 50: 860–861

288. Kawai N, Asakura K, Sambe S, Kataura A, Enomoto K 1989 Metastatic squamous cell carcinoma of the paranasal sinuses from a primary squamous cell carcinoma of the urinarybladder. Journal of Laryngology and Otology 103: 602–604

289. Albrecht P 1905 Hypernephrom in Siebeingebiet. Archiv fur Klinische Chirurgie 77: 1073

290. Abrams H L, Spiro R, Goldstein N 1950 Metastases in carcinoma. Cancer 3: 74–85

291. Batsakis J G, McBurney T A 1971 Metastatic neoplasm to the head and neck. Surgery, Gynecology and Obstetrics 133: 673–677

292. Flocks R H, Boatman D L 1973 Incidence of head and neck metastases from genito-urinary neoplasms. Laryngoscope 83: 1527–1539

293. Aisenberg M S, Inman C L 1956 Tumors that have metastasized to the jaws. Oral Surgery, Oral Medicine and Oral Pathology 9: 1210–1217

294. Barbey A 1928 Cited by Schmittmann M 1934. In: Handbuch der speziellen Pathologischen Anatomie und Histologie, Vol III, Springer, Berlin, pp 246

295. Carruth J A S 1972 Carcinoma of the bronchus presenting as a malignancy of the maxillary antrum. Journal of Laryngology and Otology 86: 293–296

296. Von Eicken C 1934 Hypernephrom in Siebeingebiet. Zeitschrift fur Laryngologie, Rhinologie und Otologie 25: 52–54

297. Ljunggren E 1960 Synpunkter pa njurtumorer. Schola postgraduate medica. Svenska Lakartiden 39: 2685

8. Mesenchymal malignancy

The tumours included in this section are those non-epithelial tumours of fibrous, adipose and other connective tissue not dealt with in subsequent chapters. Considerable debate is found in the histopathology literature on the classification of lesions derived from fibroblasts. Like the other tumours herein discussed, tumours of fibrous tissue are rare in the sinonasal tract. Thus a simple division into benign fibromatous lesions and malignant fibrosarcoma and fibrous histiocytoma has been made for practical purposes. This chapter covers:

1. Fibroma and fibromatosis
2. Fibrosarcoma
3. Lipoma and liposarcoma
4. Myxoma
5. Malignant fibrous histiocytoma
6. Ewing's sarcoma
7. Alveolar soft part sarcoma

FIBROMA AND FIBROMATOSIS

The existence of the fibroma as a true tumour entity in the sinonasal tract is doubted by many pathologists.[1a,2-4a] Although Fu & Perzin[5] reported four cases in their series of 256 non-epithelial tumours of this region, it is thought that such lesions represent a reactive process of hyperplasia rather than neoplasia and even Fu & Perzin thought some might represent an area of inflammation or a polyp which had been replaced by fibrous tissue. Whatever the circumstances these are rare incidental findings, usually affecting the nasal cavity and composed of mature well-differentiated sparsely cellular fibrous tissue. They should be differentiated from meningioma[4] and are cured by simple excision.

The entity of fibromatosis is recognized in the head and neck. It has been defined as an infiltrating fibroblastic proliferation showing none of the histologic features of an inflammatory response nor features of unequivocal neoplasia.[6] The lesion is generally regarded as a well-differentiated or non-metastasizing fibrosarcoma or is sometimes called a desmoid tumour. The lesion is locally aggressive but incapable of metastasis.

It is also extremely unusual in the upper jaw and in the few cases reported showed a wide age range (2–76)[3a,5] and no predilection for either sex. The distribution appears to be nasal cavity, antrum or both and no known causaive factors are known. Clinical features include nasal obstruction, swelling of the cheek and nose, bleeding, facial pain and an oroantral fistula following dental extraction. Radiology of the two cases seen at the Royal National Throat Nose and Ear Hospital (both aged 2 years) showed a benign expansile lesion.[7]

Histologically the tumour is composed of relatively mature fibrous tissue with abundant collagen. This and the uniform growth pattern, scarcity of mitoses, and absence of abnormal mitoses distinguish it from other fibrosarcomas.

The tumour will recur unless widely excised as evidenced by 6 cases reported by Fu & Perzin.[5] Three recurred between 6 months and 11 years after incomplete excision compared with no recurrence in the other three patients, 3, 8 and 9 years after radical en bloc resection (partial or total maxillectomy). The site and extent of the lesion may obviously compromise surgery but radiotherapy alone or in combination is ineffective. Fibromatosis has occasionally been responsible for death due to local invasion as in one case 18 years after initial treatment.[5]

The differential diagnosis should include fibro-osseous disease, other fibrosarcomas, myxoma, neurofibroma and angiofibroma.

A 2-year-old Polish boy was referred in 1987 with a swelling of the left maxilla (Fig. 8.1). His mother had noticed an asymmetry since 3 months old and when this increased in size, it was biopsied and diagnosed as infantile (desmoid-type) fibromatosis. A rapid acceleration in the tumour's growth prompted referral and when first seen he had a prominent mass arising from the upper alveolus. A partial maxillectomy was performed via a lateral rhinotomy incision. The lesion had expanded into the antral cavity, disrupting dentition and infiltrated the alveolus. Subsequent correspondence suggests

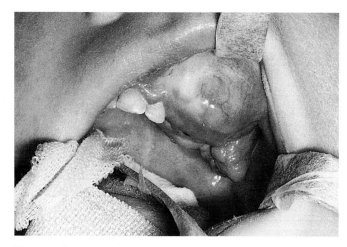

Fig. 8.1 Intraoperative photograph showing benign fibromatosis affecting maxilla of 2-year-old boy.

reasonable development of the residual dentition and some prominent fibrotic scarring in the gingival sulcus has not progressed during the last 4 years.

FIBROSARCOMA

Definition

Fibrosarcoma is a malignant tumour of spindle-shaped cells which produce reticulin and collagen, shows no other evidence of cellular differentiation and is capable of recurrence and metastasis.[8] Furthermore Fu & Perzin[5] emphasized that the diagnosis of fibrosarcoma should only be made when other tumours which demonstrate fibrous tissue and collagen have been ruled out.

Historical aspects

In 1869 Billroth[9] reported a spindle-cell sarcoma of the nasal septum. 71 similar cases were reviewed by Johnston[10] in 1904, some of which were probably fibrosarcomas and a bilateral sinonasal case, who died of meningitis, was reported in 1927.[11]

Incidence

Fibrosarcoma is generally a rare tumour. It has been estimated to constitute 0.5% of all malignancies and 5% of all primary malignant bone tumours.[1b,12] It is particularly rare in the upper jaw with less than 100 cases reported in the last 25 years. In Stout's series of 218 fibrosarcomas,[13] seven occurred in the upper respiratory tract and of Swain's 40 cases of head and neck fibrosarcomas,[14] only 5 affected the sinonasal tract. The maxilla constitutes between 0–6% of all primary fibrosarcomas of bone.[15,16]

Age, sex and ethnic variation

The tumour can affect any age but predominates in the 4th–6th decades. In large series of all fibrosarcomas, a small but definite peak is found in the first years of life when it can be difficult to distinguish from benign fibromatosis. In this age group it is second only to rhabdomyosarcoma as the most common soft tissue sarcoma. There are no major differences in the tumour characteristics in the different age groups except that prognosis may be better in the very young.

In fibrosarcoma as a whole and in those affecting the upper jaw a slight male preponderance is described but this was not the finding in our seven cases (Table 8.1).

Site

In the head and neck region, the soft tissues of the face and neck are most commonly involved followed by the maxillary sinus, the other paranasal sinuses and nasopharynx.[1b]

Fibrosarcoma may derive from soft-tissue (e.g. periosteum) or have an intraosseous (medullary) origin. In the upper jaw it is extremely difficult to distinguish between such origins though the soft tissues are a more likely source. Multiple diffuse fibrosarcomas affecting the skull and facial bones have been reported.[33]

Aetiology

Specific aetiological factors such as trauma have been discounted and the occasional case report implicating radiotherapy[34] has not been supported experimentally.

Clinical features

These are the usual symptoms and signs of malignancy: a mass, pain or swelling of the cheek, nasal obstruction, serosanguinous discharge, ulceration of the palate and loosening of the teeth (Fig. 8.2). There has been one case report of the tumour presenting as a frontal mucocoele.[29]

A 51-year-old woman from Saudi Arabia was referred with residual fibrosarcoma of the right maxillary sinus. She had originally presented with a 4 month history of painful swelling of the right cheek and ulceration of the hard palate. A local removal had been performed 5 months earlier, followed by a full course of radiotherapy during which the tumour had actually enlarged. When seen she had severe facial pain and trismus with an obvious mass affecting the maxillary sinus, orbit, hard palate, soft tissues of the cheek and involvement of the mandible.

Radical surgical excision including orbital clearance, total ethmo-maxillectomy, partial mandibulectomy and pterygoid dissection was performed. Residual disease was left on the base of the skull and the patient returned home where she died 4 months later.

Radiology

Radiological examination, principally by CT scanning, of our cases shows non-specific bone expansion and destruction.

Table 8.1 Fibrosarcoma of the upper jaw: cited in literature

Author	No.	Sex M	Sex F	Age (av. yr)	Age range	Site N	Site M	Site E	Site F	Site Other	Treatment S	S/DXT/C	DXT	None	Prognosis A&W	AWR	DOD	DICD	Lost no FU	METS	Local recurrence
Stratton 1953[17]	1	1		56							1				4 yr						1
Hoggins & Brady 1962[18]	1		1	35			1				1								1		
Karlan & Kunin 1963[19]	1	1		14			1				1				1 yr						
Prasad & Kanjilal 1969[20]	1	1		8								1					6/12				
Richardson & Maguda 1970[21]	2	2		56, 56							2				10/12		4 yr				
Cronin 1973[22]	3	2	1	33, 33, 52			2		1		2	1					54/12		2		1
Swain et al 1974[14]	5					1	4								20% 6 yr						
Fu & Perzin 1976[5]	13	8	5	47	10–77	2	4	4		3 Pan sinus	6 Radical (1wDXT) 5 Local		2		3–14 yr 6 yr	7½ yr	2 yr	7 yr	3	1	1 5
Goepfert et al 1977[23]	2	1	1	44, 36			1			1 Palate	2				6 yr		12 yr				
Shah 1977[24]	1	1		66		1					1				2 yr						
Agarwal et al 1980[25]	1	1											1		3 yr						
Broniatowski & Haria 1981[26]	2	2		47, 68			2				2						3/12	6/12		Lung	1
Kadri & Pratt 1981[27]	1	1		58			1				1				9/12						
Slootweg & Muller 1984[28]	2	1	1	59, 26			1 1				1		1				6/12 5/12			Brain Lung	1 1
Serai 1985[29]	1	1		42			1				1					3yr				Pleura	1
Rockley & Liu 1986[46]	10	8	2		18–71	1	8		1		5	3	1	1	(2) 9 yr 14 yr		(8) 4/12 4 yr			(2) Peritoneal Pleura Lymph node	7
Hyams et al 1988[3b]	70				majority 6–7th decades																
Lukinmaa et al 1988[30]	1		1	31			1				1					28/12				Liver	
Oppenheimer & Friedman 1988[31]	1		1	29			1						1				9/12				
Smith & Soames 1989[32]	1	1		24					1		1				5 yr						
Harrison & Lund	7	4	3	48	23–67	1	5		1		5	2			20 yr 5 yr		4/12 6 yr		3		

S, surgery; S/DXT, surgery and radiotherapy; S/DXT/C, surgery radiotherapy and chemotherapy; A&W, alive and well; AWR, alive with recurrence; DOD, dead of disease; DICD, dead of intercurrent disease; METS, metastases; No FU, no follow-up; N, nose; M, maxilla; E, ethmoid; F, frontal sinus

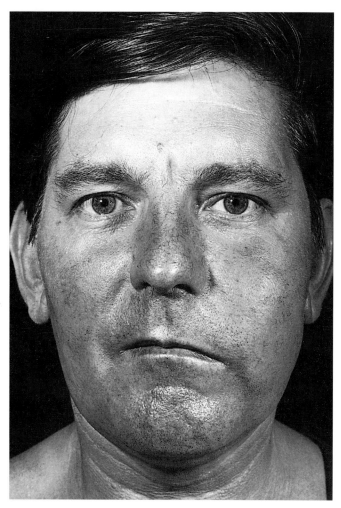

Fig. 8.2   Facial views of patient with extensive fibrosarcoma of maxilla.

Macroscopic and microscopic appearance

The lesion may be polypoid or sessile and presents an homogeneous firm white mass of tissue which is essentially non-encapsulated but may have a pseudocapsule of compressed tissues.

Microscopic appearance

Microscopically the tumour is composed of fusiform cells which are rather uniform and separated by collagen, which is prominently displayed by acid aniline dyes such as Masson's trichrome stain.[4b] A number of histologic grading systems have been devised[35,36] but the lesions can be broadly divided into well-differentiated and poorly differentiated, particularly when considering prognosis. A 'herringbone' pattern of interlacing fascicles of fibroblasts can be seen in the well-differentiated lesions whereas the pattern is less organized, with less collagen and more mitoses in the poorly differentiated tumours. In the upper jaw, lesions tend to be well-differentiated. Sometimes the most well-differentiated tumours are termed 'fibromatosis' but caution should be exercised in the use of this term as it may mask the malignant potential of these lesions.[37]

Natural history

Well-differentiated fibrosarcomas tend to be locally infiltrative with frequent recurrence but rarely metastasize. The poorly differentiated lesions as expected are characterized by local aggression and secondaries. Consequently in the upper jaw, death results from local intracranial spread. The incidence of local recurrence in the literature is shown in Table 8.2. Metastases when they occur, are haematogenous rather than lymphatic,[12,38] and mainly to the lung,[12,15] though liver, brain, other bones and skin metastases have been described.[14,38] Between 18–20% of patients may develop these during the course of their disease.[14,38]

Although in the upper jaw a genuinely intraosseous origin is less likely, intraosseous lesions in the rest of the body behave more aggressively in local and distant spread than those of soft-tissue origin.

In comparison with other malignant soft tissue tumours in this region, fibrosarcomas appear to grow more slowly, infiltrate less extensively, metastasize less frequently and are consequently associated with a better prognosis.[1b]

Differential diagnosis

This diagnosis has been erroneously applied many times in the past to a wide range of pathologies so some earlier reports should be reconsidered. When Stout[13] reviewed the histology in 84 cases originally described as fibrosarcoma, he was able to confirm the diagnosis in only 85%. It is important to examine many sections and to consider the following lesions, all of which have been confused with fibrosarcoma in the past:

Benign fibromatosis, characterized by the regular appearance of the fibrocytes and abundant collagen

Table 8.2   Soft tissue fibrosarcoma in all sites: incidence of local recurrence in literature

Author	No.	Local recurrence (%)
Stout 1948[13]	144	60
Pack & Ariel 1952[39]	144	56
Mackenzie 1964[40]	205	49
Bizer 1971[41]	61	74 (Local surgery) 30 (Radical surgery)
Scott et al 1989[42]	114	42

Osteosarcoma, particularly when there is only a small amount of malignant osteoid tissue

Fibrous dysplasia, ossifying fibroma, cementifying fibroma

Leiomyosarcoma

Malignant fibrous histiocytoma[43]

Neurilemmoma (benign and malignant), neurofibroma.

Treatment

Despite the paucity of numbers, all authors are agreed that wide radical excision is the treatment of choice. Any form of more limited resection will inevitably lead to recurrence due to the infiltrative nature of the lesion, the possibility of a pseudocapsule and of finger-like extensions from the main mass and the occasional existence of satellite lesions.

Radiotherapy alone is of little benefit though there have been a few recent reports supporting the use of adjuvant radiotherapy and chemotherapy.[1b,4b,44–48] However such remissions are probably short-lived and Scott et al[42] in a recent review of 132 patients regarded the case as unproven. There may be a place for such treatment in palliation.[49]

Prognosis (Table 8.1)

Considerable attempts have been made to establish prognostic criteria for fibrosarcoma in general; notably patient age,[50] size of lesion,[28] site,[12] grade of histological differen-

tiation,[13,43,51] and the presence of tumour-free resection margin.[14,15] The last two factors unsurprisingly seem the most important though the very young patients do appear to fare better. Table 8.3 shows the overall survival in some of the larger series but comparisons must be made with care as the histologic differentiation may vary from series to series, the importance of which can be seen in Table 8.4. It should also be remembered that 5-year survival does not represent cure as recurrence can occur up to 22 years later[42] so long-term follow-up is mandatory.

As already stated, fibrosarcomas of soft tissue origin have a better prognosis than true intraosseous lesions and those in the head and neck are generally less aggressive than other mesenchymal tumours such as osteogenic sarcomas and rhabdomyosarcomas in the same situation.

LIPOMA AND LIPOSARCOMA

Definition and aetiology

A lipoma is a benign encapsulated tumour of fat though it may often be difficult to distinguish between benign neoplasia, a hamartomatous malformation and hyperplasia. The malignant form, liposarcoma, was first described by Virchow,[54,55] in 1857 and 1865 and may arise from lipoblasts or totipotential mesenchymal cells. There are 120 lipomas for every liposarcoma[56] in the body and it is thought that liposarcomas arise de novo rather than from existing lipomas.[1a]

Table 8.3 Fibrosarcoma of upper jaw: overall survival in literature

Author	Total No.	No. in head and neck	Type	Survival (%) at		
				5 yr	10 yr	20 yr
Conley et al 1967[38]	–	84	Fibroscarcoma of head & neck	33		
Van Blarcom et al 1971[50]	–	13	Fibrosarcoma of mandible	40		
Pritchard et al 1974[52]	199		Soft tissue fibrosarcoma	41	29	
Huvos & Higinbotham 1975[12]	130	19	Primary fibrosarcoma of bone	34	28	25
Russell et al 1977[36]	231	37	Soft tissuc sarcomas	48		
Scott et al 1989[42]	114	–	Soft tissue fibrosarcomas	39	33	23

Table 8.4 Fibrosarcoma of upper jaw: survival by histological differentiation in literature

Author	Histology (% survival)		
	Well-differentiated (%)	Undifferentiated (%)	Follow-up (yr)
Batsakis 1980[1b]	80	33	–
Enterline 1981[53]	80	0	10
Friedmann & Osborn 1982[37]	55	11	6

Incidence

Both the benign and malignant fat tumours are amongst the commonest neoplasms of soft tissues[57] but are rare in the head and neck and exceptional in the upper jaw despite the presence of abundant fat. No lipomas have been encountered in 27 years at the Institute of Laryngology and Otology and only a handful of cases appear in the literature (Table 8.5). Between 1958 and 1965 only four cases of liposarcoma in the head and neck were reported in the south of England.[58] In several series of liposarcomas which include head and neck lesions, none affected the upper jaw.[3c,59–61]

Age and sex variation

Lipomas can occur at any age but liposarcomas are rare under 30 years with a peak incidence in the 6th decade.[1c]

Site

Lipomas may be found in the upper gastro-intestinal tract and most commonly affect the cheek and occasionally the soft palate and pharynx. Liposarcomas usually occur in the retroperitoneal, gluteal and thigh regions but have been reported in the cheek and maxilla.

Clinical features

The non-specific clinical features of any mass may occur but in those few documented cases a polypoid or pedunculated mass may be found incidentally.[65]

Macroscopic and microscopic appearance

Lipomas may show areas of calcification if present for a long time. Liposarcomas vary from a 'jelly-like' to 'brain-like' consistency.[1c] The benign lipoma is composed of a mixture of fat cells and fibroblasts. If spindle-shaped cells are encountered the lesion may be erroneously interpreted as malignant but it should be remembered that a spindle-cell lipoma can occur.

Liposarcomas generally present with increased cellularity and nuclear polymorphism. An apparent capsule may be found, tempting the surgeon to 'shell-out' the lesion with inevitable recurrence. Four different histological subgroups have been described and attempts made to correlate these with prognosis:[68,69]

1. Myxoid
2. Round cell
3. Well-differentiated
4. Pleomorphic.

In the head and neck most liposarcomas are myxoid.

Natural history and prognosis

Those few lipomas in the literature have proved relatively easy to eradicate surgically. The malignant form will recur locally in more than half the cases irrespective of the histological subtype.[59] Duration and size of the mass do not appear to correlate with prognosis but rapid enlargement and a size greater than 12 cm increases the likelihood of metastases. Spittle et al[57] found an overall 5-year survival of 64% in 60 cases of liposarcoma throughout the

Table 8.5   Lipoma and liposarcoma of the upper jaw: in literature

Author	Sex	Age (yr)	Site	Treatment	Outcome
Lipoma					
Goldstein 1915[62]	M	42	Maxilla	Caldwell–Luc	No recurrence after 6 yr
Silbernagel 1938[63]	M	50	Maxilla	Caldwell–Luc	No FU
Hatziotis 1971[64]	F (3) M (3) unknown (3)	33–72	Hard palate	Local excision	Unknown
Fu & Perzin 1977[65]	F	34	Maxilla	Caldwell–Luc	No recurrence after 21 yr
Preece et al 1988[66]	–	1/12	Nasal septum (synchronous with lipoma of corpus callosum)	Surgical excision	No FU
Liposarcoma					
Giardino & Manfredi 1967[67]	–	–	Cheek invading maxilla	–	Unknown
Fu & Perzin 1977[65]	F	67	Maxilla – ethmoid, sphenoid & middle cranial fossa	DXT	Died 1 mth after treatment
Harrison & Lund	M	13	Orbit	Orbital exenteration, DXT, lateral craniotomy	A&W 3 yr

A&W, alive and well; DXT, radiotherapy; No FU, no follow-up

body. However, studies suggest that histological subtype can be correlated with survival and frequency of secondaries. Myxoid and well-differentiated tumours have a better prognosis of 70–80% (5-year survival) compared to less than 20% for pleomorphic and round cell types. Recurrence and incidence of secondaries also increase in these two histological subgroups. Recurrence rates rise to 73–85% and one–third show distant spread.[68]

Differential diagnosis

A lipoma should be considered in any list of congenital masses in the nasal cavity.[70]

Treatment

Surgical excision is the principle method of treatment for all fatty tumours. Some regression has been reported when radiotherapy has been given as a palliative measure in liposarcoma.[61]

MYXOMAS

Definition

Stout[71] defined the myxoma as a tumour composed of sometimes spindle-shaped cells set in a myxoid stroma containing mucopolysaccharide, through which course very delicate reticulin fibres in various directions.

Synonyms

Fibromyxoma, myxofibroma

Historical aspects

In 1871 Virchow[72] described a group of tumours which histologically resembled the mucinous substance of the umbilical cord. The earliest report in the nose appeared in 1910.[73] In 1949 Harbert et al[74] described a myxoma of the maxilla and five other reported cases.

Incidence

Myxomas are the 3rd commonest soft tissue malignancy after fibro- and liposarcoma but are uncommon in the head and neck.[71] In a series of 256 non-epithelial tumours of the nose and sinuses, there were six myxomas.[75] In Stout's series of 143 extracardiac myxomas, 22 occurred in the head and neck and of these three involved the maxilla.[71] Zimmerman & Dahlin reported 26 myxomas of the jaw, 15 of which affected the maxilla.[76]

Age, sex and ethnic variation (Table 8.6)

Myxomas can occur at any age but tend to affect younger people. Four of the six cases reported by Fu & Perzin[75] were under 25 years and Zimmerman & Dahlin's cases were between the 2nd and 4th decades.[76] No particular sexual preponderance has been found.

Site

Myxomas classically arise in cardiac muscle but can affect subcutaneous tissue or bone. In the head and neck, the tumour may occur in the soft tissues or be intraosseous affecting the facial skeleton.[77,78] Of these the mandible is the commonest site but in the upper jaw the maxilla is most frequently affected. However, it may be the cavity, external walls and alveolar bone which are involved. The nasal septum, ethmoid and body of sphenoid have also been sites of tumour. In a review of soft tissue myxomas in the head and neck,[79] ten cases affecting the palate are included.

Aetiology

No specific aetiological factors have been found though most tumours are presumed to arise in adjacent bone. An association with viral infection or trauma[80] has been largely dismissed and the suggested odontogenic origin[81] is probably co-incidental. Stout[71] believed that myxomas arose from primitive mesenchyme.

Clinical features

Most myxomas produce a swelling of the cheek, nose or mouth which may or may not be painful. If neglected, the lesion can achieve a massive size.[82]

A 14-month-old West Indian girl was noted to have a mass distorting the right side of the nose which was increasing in size (Fig. 8.3). This was biopsied via a sublabial incision and found to be a myxoma. 3 months later a lateral rhinotomy was performed though the lesion was known not to have been completely excised. The child was referred for further excision and underwent a revision lateral rhinotomy 9 months later. The lesion was found to involve the maxilla, with erosion of the anterior and superior walls. There was no evidence of recurrence for the next 7 years.

Radiology

As the tumour most frequently affects the maxilla, opacification of the sinus may be seen with varying degrees of bone resorption or erosion. Occasionally the classical 'soap-bubble' or 'honeycomb' appearances may be seen.[83]

Macroscopic and microscopic appearance

Grossly a greyish mass of variable consistency is found. Depending on the fibrous content the tumour can be gelatinous or firm. No true capsule is formed.

Table 8.6 Myxomas of the upper jaw: in literature

Author	No.	Sex	Age (yr)	Site	Treatment	Outcome
Babbitt & Pfeiffer 1937[86]	1	F	14	Hard palate – oropharynx	Wide local excision	A&W 1/12
Harbert et al 1949[74]	1	M	17	Maxilla	Excision, maxillectomy	Recurrence after 4 yr A&W 1 yr
Greenfield & Friedmann 1951[87]	1	M	2	Maxillary sinus	Enucleation	A&W 10 yr
Bruce & Royer 1952[88]	1	M	14	Maxilla (3×2 cm)	Excision	–
Attar 1956[89]	1	M	11	Maxilla (6×6×7 cm)	Radical excision	A&W 4 yr
Zimmerman & Dahlin 1958[76]	10	–	13–64, mean 29	Maxilla (2×2×3 cm–8×9×6 cm)	Enucleation & curettage	25% recurrence within 5 yr
Dutz & Stout 1961[90]	2	F	6	Maxilla (7 cm)	Excision/partial maxillectomy	A&W 3 yr
		M	9	Maxilla (1.5 cm)	Excision	A&W 9 yr
Buchner & Ramon 1965[91]	1	F	52	Maxilla	Enucleation	A&W 1 yr
Bochetto et al 1967[92]	1	F	40	Maxilla	Radical maxillectomy	A&W 5 yr
Barros et al 1969[93]	7	M	49	Maxilla (0.8 – 4 cm dia)	Local excision	–
		M	6			–
		F	45			–
		F	43			–
		M	25			–
		F	22			3/12
		F	19			15/12
Ghosh et al 1973[94]	4	F	26	Maxilla	Maxillectomy	A&W 26 yr
		F	1			A&W 22 yr
		F	30			A&W 12 yr
		M	47			A&W 9 yr
Pradhan et al 1972[95]	1	F	32	Hard palate	Wide local excision	A&W 1 yr
Faccini & Williams 1973[96]	1	M	45	Cheek & nose	Wide local excision	A&W 9/12
Canalis et al 1976[77]	4	M	32	Maxilla	Caldwell–Luc maxillectomy	A&W 1 yr
		M	47	Nose	Excision	A&W 1 yr
		M	23	Maxilla	Excision	A&W 1.5 yr
		M	2	Maxilla	Excision	A&W 3 yr
Fu & Perzin 1977[75]	6	F	15/12	Maxilla	Partial maxillectomy	A&W 9 yr
		M	9	Maxilla	Maxillectomy	A&W 4 yr
		F	23	Maxilla	6 local excisions – maxillectomy	A&W 7 yr
		M	24	Antro ethmoid, – Ant. cranial fossa	Craniofacial × 2 & extended maxillectomy, orbital clearance	A&W 5 yr
		M	45	Nose	Wide excision	AWR 2 yr
		F	52	Maxilla	Maxillectomy	A&W 7 yr
Prasad & Sharan 1983[97]	1	M	14	Maxilla		
Slootweg & Wittkampf 1986[98]	4	F	25	Maxilla (canine/premolar)	Excision	A&W 30 yr
		M	30	Maxilla (molar)	Excision	A&W 24 yr
		F	40	Maxilla (premolar)	Excision	A&W 15 yr
		F	19	Maxilla (premolar/molar)	Excision	A&W 9 yr
James & Lucas 1987[100]	1	F	11/12	Maxilla	Chemotherapy, surgical excision	A&W 13/12
Harrison & Lund	1	F	14/12	Nose	Excision – lateral rhinotomy × 2	A&W 8.5 yr

A&W, alive and well; AWR, alive with recurrent disease

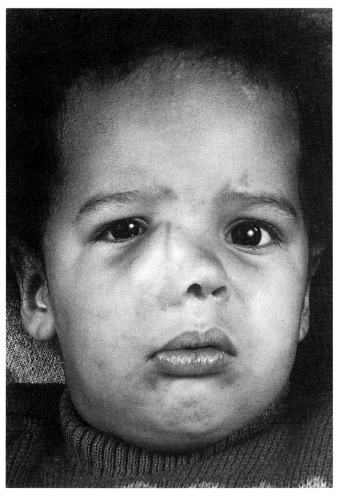 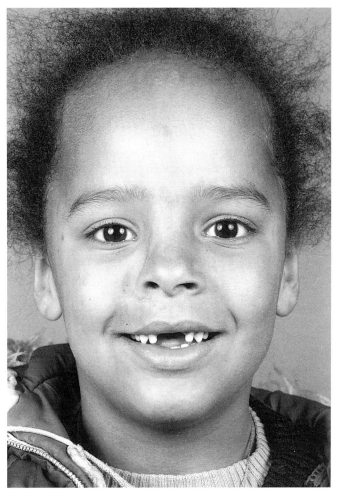

Fig. 8.3   2-year-old girl with recurrent myxoma of right maxilla (**A**).   The same child 4 years following further surgical excision (**B**).

Microscopic appearance

Microscopically the tumour is composed of characteristic stellate and spindle cells randomly distributed in a ground substance of loose mucoid stroma which also contains a delicate network of reticulin fibres. Identifying any other recognizable cellular elements excludes the diagnosis of myxoma. If collagen is abundant, the term 'fibromyxoma' is sometimes used. The tumour stains positively for mucopolysaccharides and electron microscopy shows the myxoma cells to possess the features of fibroblasts.

Natural history

Myxomas should be regarded as benign, but locally aggressive, tumours. They do not metastasize and the existence of a genuine myxosarcoma is generally doubted.[1d] However, the ability to insidiously infiltrate surrounding tissue including bone means that local excisions and 'enucleations' inevitably lead to recurrence.[84] Extensive

local spread from the upper jaw may occasionally result in death.[71]

Differential diagnosis

Many other tumours have myxoid areas so it is important to obtain a sufficiently large biopsy. The presence of any other recognizable cellular elements should suggest the following tumours; embryonal rhabdomyosarcoma, fibrosarcoma, liposarcoma, fibro–osseous lesions, neurilemmomas and pleomorphic adenomas.[1d,4c] In some retrospective reviews, several cases were reassigned on re-examination of the histology. Immunoperoxidase studies and electron microscopy may be helpful.

Treatment

Wide en bloc surgical excision is needed if recurrence is to be avoided. This usually means that some form of maxillectomy is performed. There is no evidence of radiosensitivity.[76,85]

Prognosis (Table 8.6)

With adequate surgical excision, long-term survival without recurrence can be anticipated. However, it should be remembered that recurrence can occur many years later.

MALIGNANT FIBROUS HISTIOCYTOMA

Definition

Malignant fibrous histiocytoma is one of a rare group of mesenchymal soft tissue tumours. The term 'fibrous histiocytoma' was coined by Stout & Lattes[99] in the belief that these lesions originated from the tissue histiocyte. Based on histological pattern, mitotic activity and cellular activity three main forms are now recognized:[101]

1. Benign fibrous histiocytoma
2. Fibrous histiocytoma of intermediate malignancy
3. Malignant fibrous histiocytoma.

All those occurring in the upper jaw should be regarded as potentially malignant.

Synonyms

There are a number of synonyms used,[102] which may be grouped with regard to potential malignancy.

1. Benign
   Xanthoma
   Giant cell tumour of tendon sheath
   Villonodular synovitis
   Juvenile xanthogranuloma
   Dermatofibroma
   Sclerosing haemangioma
   Fibrous xanthoma

2. Intermediate
   Dermatofibroma protuberans
   A typical fibrous xanthoma

3. Malignant
   Malignant fibrous histiocytoma
   Malignant fibrous xanthoma
   Malignant histiocytoma
   Fibroxanthosarcoma.

Historical aspects

As can be seen from the list of synonyms, a wide range of terms have been applied to this tumour. In 1973 the first two cases of 'malignant fibrous histiocytoma' in the nose and sinuses were described by Townsend et al[103] and this has been followed by a regular flow of case reports in the English literature.

Incidence

Whilst malignant fibrous histiocytoma is regarded as one of the most common soft tissue sarcomas of later life[101] where it usually affects skeletal muscle of the limbs, it is relatively rare in the upper jaw. In one of the largest series of 200 cases, only six affected the head and neck and none occurred in the upper jaw itself. However overall, 3–10% of all malignant fibrous histiocytomas occur in the head and neck region, of which one–third affect the sinonasal tract.[104]

Age, sex and ethnic variations (Table 8.7)

A broad age range may be affected by this tumour with a neonate to a 92-year-old reported in the literature. The average age is 44 years and the majority occur in the 6th decade (Fig. 8.4). Although a slight male preponderance has been suggested in the head and neck,[104] in the case reports available for the upper jaw the male to female incidence was equal.

Site (Table 8.7)

In the upper jaw the maxilla was the commonest site, accounting for over half the cases (64%), followed by ethmoid, nasal cavity and frontal. A somewhat arbitrary distinction has been made in certain case reports between those tumours arising in the maxillary sinus and those believed to originate from the bone.

Other common sites in the head and neck include the craniofacial bones (15–25%), larynx (10–15%), soft tissues of the neck (10–15%), major salivary glands (5–15%) and oral cavity (5–15%).[104–106]

Aetiology

This aspect of the tumour has been widely discussed because of the possibility of radiation induction.[107,108] Cases have been reported 19 and 36 years following treatment of retinoblastoma and chondrosarcoma respectively.[109,110]

A number of diseases such as Paget's disease of bone,[111–114] fibrous dysplasia,[111] bone infarcts[114,115] and sickle cell disease[116] have been reported to predispose to malignant fibrous histiocytoma. One case in the upper jaw occurred synchronously with an olfactory neuroblastoma.[117]

Industrial exposure to phenoxyacids has also been suggested[118] but the numbers were too low to establish a causal relationship. The majority arise de novo.[111]

Table 8.7 Malignant fibrous histiocytoma of the upper jaw: cases reported in literature

Author	Age (yr)	Sex	Site	Treatment	Outcome	Local recurrence	Lymph node metastases	Systemic metastases
Shearer et al 1973[130]	Neonate	M	Nose	S(LR)	No FU			
Townsend et al 1973[103]	3	M	Maxilla	S(LR) DXT	A&W 3/12			
	61	F	Maxilla	S(TM/O)	No FU			
Rice et al 1974[131]	13	F	Ethmoid	S	A&W 24/12			
	23	F	Maxilla	S C	AWR 6/12		+	
	82	M	Ethmoid	S	A&W 12/12			
Spector et al 1974[132]	46	M	Maxilla	S(TM/O) DXT	A&W 12/12			
Lesica et al 1975[128]	38	M	Ethmoid	S		+9 yr		
Leite et al 1977[122]	38	F	Nose	S C		+	+	
Slootweg & Muller 1977[133]	59	M	Maxilla	S(TM/RND)DXT	DICD 7/12		+	
Taxy & Hidvegi 1977[117]	16	F	Maxilla	S DXT C		+	+	
Crissman & Henson 1978[102]	65	M	Maxilla	S(PM/RND) DXT	DOD 6/12		+	Pleural
DeMoura & Yook 1978[134]	51	F	Maxilla	S DXT C	A&W 24/12	+		
Jee et al 1978[135]	53	F	Maxilla	S (×2)	A&W 27/12	+		
McDonald & Weiland 1978[136]	57	M	Frontal	S (OPF)	A&W 24/12			
Sidhu et al 1978[137]	14	F	Maxilla	S DXT C	DOD 10/12	+		
Wilmes & Meister 1978[138]	36	F	Nose	S	A&W 18/12			
	53	F	Maxilla	DXT	A&W 12/12			
Tovi & Sidi 1979[139]	60	M	Maxilla	S DXT	No FU			
Del-Rey & De-La-Torre 1980[140]	17	F	Antro-ethmoid	S(TM)	A&W 18/12			
Merrick et al 1980[141]	32	F	Maxilla	S(PM) DXT C	DOD 2/12			Bone, liver
Ogura et al 1980[129]	10	F	Antro-ethmoid	S(PM) DXT	A&W 12/12			
	46	M	Maxilla	DXT S(TM/O)	DOD 54/12			Brain
Perzin & Fu 1980[142]	28	F	Nose	S	Lost			Bone
	32	F	Maxilla	S(CL) C				
	44	F	Nose	S	A&W 24/12			
	52	M	Antro-ethmoid	S(PM, TM/O) DXT(×2)	AWR 48/12	+		
	53	F	Maxilla	S(TM) DXT	Lost			
	54	F	Maxilla	Refused	Lost			
	65	F	Maxilla	S(PM)	AWR 6/12			
	65	M	Fronto-ethmoid	S(OPF) DXT	A&W 12/12			
	67	F	Maxilla	S(CL,TM/O)	A&W 6/12			
Schaefer et al 1980[143]	33	M	Frontal sinus	S DXT C	DOD 10/12			Widespread
Sonobe et al 1980[144]	39	M	Maxilla	DXT C	DOD			Lung, stomach, kidney, bone
Ushigome & Hirota 1980[145]	24	M	Maxilla	S C	DOD 6/12			Lung
Blitzer et al 1981[104]	92	F	Fronto-ethmoid	S	A&W 6/12			
Tewfik et al 1981[146]	36	M	Ethmoid	S DXT C	DOD 12/12		+	
Brookes & Rose 1983[147]	51	M	Ethmoid	C S(×2) (CL/PM)	A&W 18/12	+		
Sasaki et al 1983[148]	30	M	Maxilla	DXT S(TM/O)	A&W 24/12			
Mugliston & Shaw 1984[124]	26	F	Maxilla	C DXT S(PM)	A&W 24/12			
	49	F	Antro-ethmoid	C DXT S	A&W 24/12			
Abdul-Karim et al 1985[149]	19	F	Maxilla	S(PM/O) DXT C	DOD 16/12	+		Lung +
	29	M	Maxilla	S(TM) DXT	A&W 27/12			Liver
	31	M	Maxilla	DXT S(PM)C	AWR 14/12	+		Brain +
	61	M	Maxilla	S(TM) DXT C	AWR 18/12	+		Bone +
	75	F	Maxilla	S(TM)	DICD 4/12			
Hayter et al 1985[150]	44	M	Maxilla	DXT	DOD 10/12	+		? Lung
Nishizawa et al 1985[110]	20	M	Maxilla	S(× 2) PM	DOD 55/12			? Brain
Barnes & Kanbour 1988[127]	54	M	Maxilla	S(TM) DXT	DOD 19/12	+		Skin, lung
	67	F	Ethmoid	S(CF)	DOD 4/12	+		
	74	M	Maxilla	S(PM)	DOD 24/12	+		
Ireland et al 1988[109]	56	M	Maxilla	S(PM/O)	DOD 6/12			? Bones
Harrison & Lund	49	M	Maxilla	S(TM/O,CF) DXT	DOD 48/12	+		Brain
	54	M	Antro-ethmoid	S(TM/O,CF)		+		
	81	F	Maxilla	S(PM)	DOD 3/12	+		

S, Surgery; DXT, radiotherapy; C, chemotherapy; O, orbital clearance; CF, craniofacial; CL, Caldwell–Luc; LR, lateral rhinotomy; PM, partial or hemimaxillectomy; TM, total maxillectomy; RND, radical neck dissection; OPF, osteoplastic flap; A&W, alive and well; AWR, alive with recurrence; DOD, dead of disease; DICD, dead of intercurrent disease; No FU, no follow-up

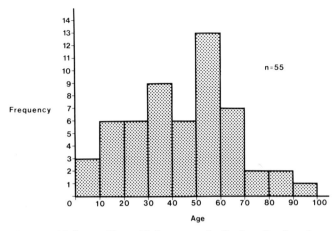

Fig. 8.4 Malignant fibrous histiocytoma: distribution of patients by age.

Clinical features

The clinical features are the non-specific ones of any malignant tumour, including nasal obstruction, epistaxis, rhinorrhoea and epiphora and proptosis when the orbit is involved. However, it is notable that several patients have initially presented to their dentists with facial pain and loosening of teeth.

A 49-year-old General Certificate Examination (GCE) examiner developed nasal obstruction and proptosis. Following biopsy, he underwent a lateral rhinotomy at another hospital. He was referred with recurrent disease a year later for craniofacial resection and orbital clearance at which the cribriform plate was found to be breached by tumour but the dura was intact. The postero-medial orbital wall was also invaded. A further recurrence was evident 5 months later, having spread through the greater wing of the sphenoid into the middle cranial fossa, for which he had a course of radiotherapy. He developed a space occupying intracerebral lesion 18 months later which would be consistent with either a cerebral secondary or abscess but no further investigation or treatment were offered in view of his general deterioration and he succumbed in a hospice after 2 months.

Radiology

The radiological appearances are non-specific and similar to fibrosarcoma with bone expansion and destruction.

Macroscopic or microscopic appearance

A fibrous soft tissue mass is found.
Microscopic appearance.
The original hypothesis that the histiocyte is a facultative fibroblast is now largely discounted.[4d,99,119] It is more likely that it derives from undifferentiated mesenchymal stem cells which then form fibroblastic and histiocytic elements in variable proportions.

The tumour is composed of histiocytic cells, foam cells and multinucleate giant cells. Five patterns have been described:[101]

storiform-pleomorphic (so-called as it resembles a rush-mat)
inflammatory
myxoid
giant cell
angiomatoid.

The histiocytes contain lipid and haemosiderin. Histological criteria for malignancy have been proposed but a good correlation between these and behaviour is lacking.[120,121]

Natural history (Table 8.8)

Malignant fibrous histiocytoma in the head and neck are said to behave more aggressively than their counterparts in the skin and of these the intraosseous tumours of the jaws and those of oral soft tissues appear potentially more aggressive. The natural history is characterized at best by frequent local recurrence and at worst by metastatic dissemination. The frequency of local recurrence was 39% in the 55 reported cases in the upper jaw compared with rates of between 40 and 73% for all those occurring in the head and neck.

Lymph node metastases were found in 12% of the case reports compared with 10–41% in the head and neck series. Systemic metastases are said to occur more commonly with malignant fibrous histiocytoma than other malignant soft tissue tumours with rates of 10–42% quoted for the head and neck. 31% of the upper jaw cases manifested these, affecting the lung and bones most commonly.

Differential diagnosis

The diagnosis is often one of exclusion as the lesion may be confused with any sarcoma (fibro-, osteo-, leiomyo- or rhabdo-) or spindle cell carcinoma, depending on which cell type predominates.[43] Immunocytochemistry may be valuable as tumour cells often contain lysosomal enzymes, such as α-1-antitrypsin and α-1-antichymotrypsin.[2]

Treatment (Table 8.7)

The majority of authors agree that radical local excision within the given anatomical constraints of the upper jaw is the most useful approach in view of the tumour's natural history (surgery alone in 38%, surgery combined with other modalities in 51%). This has included partial and total maxillectomy, craniofacial resection and orbital clearance. Radical neck dissections have been performed for clinically positive necks but not for prophylaxis. Additional radiotherapy has been given both pre- and

Table 8.8 Prognosis of malignant fibrous histiocytomas: current series vs those in literature

Author	No. of cases	Site	Local recurrences(%)	Regional lymph node metastases (%)	Systemic metastases (%)	Mortality (%)
Weiss & Enzinger 1978[108]	200	Soft tissue from all areas of body	44	12	42	40 at 2 yr
Enjoji et al 1980[151]	130	Soft tissue from all areas of body	48	2	20	39 at 2 yr
Kearney et al 1980[152]	167	Soft tissue of trunk extremities, and retroperitoneum	51	7	45	69 at 5 yr
Blitzer et al 1981[104]	87	Soft tissue and bones of head and neck	20	15	32	27 (no time interval given)
Barnes 1985[105]	63	Soft tissue and bones of head and neck	27	10	35	32 (70% of these died within 2 yr)
Bertoni et al 1985[153]	78	Soft tissue of extremities	38	4	42	64 at 5 yr
Huvos et al 1985[111]	130	Bones from all areas	—	4	44	29 at 2 yr
Barnes & Kanbour 1988[127]	12	Soft tissue and bones of head and neck	42	0	25	42 at 2 yr
Current series of case reports (1991)	55	Upper jaw	40	12	31	36 at 2 yr

postoperatively in 51% of upper jaw cases but neither in these cases nor in the head and neck as a whole does it appear to improve prognosis.

Chemotherapy has also been used in a proportion of the upper jaw lesions (24%) but never as a single modality and usually in the inoperable. The South West Oncology Group in the USA has the largest series of patients with this neoplasm receiving chemotherapy.[122] Their data reveals a 30% response of patients to adriamycin, cyclophosphamide, vincristine with or without actinomycin D or dimethyltriazenoimidazole carboxamide (DTIC) but as reported by other workers, complete response is exceptional.[104,122–126]

Prognosis

The numbers affecting the upper jaw are too few with minimal follow-up to accurately estimate prognosis. A careful analysis of cases in the head and neck by Barnes & Kanbour[127] determined a number of factors (Table 8.9) though some, such as depth of invasion, are not applicable to the upper jaw. It is evidently a truism that the presence of positive surgical margins is the most important factor in local recurrence but other histological criteria are of minimal value.[120,121]

In the upper jaw patients, 36% died of disease, the majority (82%) within 2 years. A crude survival rate of 60% is found in these patients but the follow-up is also 2 years or less in most (range 3–27 months, mean 12.9 months). Seven of the cases are known to have residual disease and both local recurrence and secondary disease can occur anything up to 9 years later.[128,129]

In Blitzer et al's review[104] of 87 head and neck lesions a mortality rate of 27% was found. Weiss & Enzinger[108] considered 200 cases throughout the body and found that 32% died of disease within the first 2 years and a further 14% during subsequent follow-up of between 3 and 12 years. Of the 76 (38%) surviving patients, 15 had evidence of recurrence.

In the upper jaw, the average survival in those patients alive with no evidence of disease is 17 months. Although the numbers are small in each group, there is no statistical difference between the different treatment groups when those treated by surgery alone are compared with the group as a whole and with those treated with additional radiotherapy and/or chemotherapy.

Table 8.9 Prognostic factors in malignant fibrous histiocytomas (MFHs) of head and neck

Factor	Effect
Age	Prognosis worsens with age: mortality ranges from 13% for patients <20 yr old to 72% for those >72 yr[104]
Pain	Tumours tend to behave more aggressively in male patients[104]
Tumour size	Usually an ominous sign associated with aggressive tumours[104]
Location of tumour	Intraosseous tumours of jaws and those of oral soft tissues are potentially more aggressive than those in other sites of head and neck[127]
Depth of tumour	Tumours that arise within subcutaneous tissue have better prognosis than those arising in bone or deep soft tissue[108]
Histologic subtype	Angiomatoid and myxoid MFHs have best prognosis and giant cell worst: inflammatory and storiform-pleomorphic variants fall between these two extremes[101]
DNA flow cytometry	Aneuploid MFHs are associated with higher incidence of local recurrence and mortality than diploid tumours[154]
Margins of resection	Positive surgical margins are most important single factor relating to local recurrence[155]
Local recurrence	80% of patients with local recurrences subsequently die of their disease[127]
Primary vs secondary	Secondary MFHs are more aggressive than those that arise de novo[111]

EWING'S SARCOMA

Definition

Ewing's sarcoma is an aggressive poorly differentiated tumour found primarily in long bones of children between the ages of 10 and 15 years.[156–160] Extraskeletal sarcoma, indistinguishable both clinically and pathologically from bony Ewing's sarcoma has been described[161–163] but is exceptionally rare in the head and neck, where it may affect the soft tissues of the face or sinonasal tract.

Historical aspects

In 1921 James Ewing[164] described a 'diffuse endothelioma' of bone occurring in the ulna of a 14-year-old girl. This lesion initially responded to radiotherapy, thus distinguishing it from osteogenic sarcoma but the patient unfortunately succumbed the following year with metastatic disease.

Incidence

Ewing's sarcoma comprises 4–6% of all primary bony tumours[165] but is rare in the head and neck region. The pelvic girdle and long bones of the lower limbs are the favoured sites of origin and the neoplasm ranks second to osteosarcoma as the most common osseous malignancy in the 2nd decade of life.[166] In the facial bones and the calvarium, the incidence of Ewing's sarcoma has been estimated at 2.5% and 0.7% respectively.[165,167] By 1983, 86 cases of Ewing's affecting the jaws had been reported[168] and in a review of 139 extraskeletal cases, Stuart-Harris et al[169] found the head and neck ranked with the chest wall in frequency (11%) behind extremities and paravertebral locations.

Age, sex and ethnic variation (Table 8.10)

Males are affected more often than females though there is no significant difference between sex and survival. Whilst the condition as a whole is one affecting the young, any age may be affected and those with maxillary disease seem to be somewhat older.

Site

In the head and neck the majority occur in the skull[165] or mandible, usually the horizontal portion.[170–174] 20 cases affecting the maxilla have been reported in the literature and only a handful describe tumour in the nasal cavity or ethmoids (Table 8.10). Cases originating in the temporal bone and orbit have also occasionally been described.[175,176] There are no known aetiological factors.

Clinical features

Patients usually present with a mass or swelling at the involved site accompanied by nasal obstruction or pain. Other symptoms and signs may result from CNS or orbital spread.

A 14-year-old Caucasian boy presented with a 2 month history of swelling and tenderness over the nasal bridge and right medial canthus accompanied by partial nasal obstruction. Examination revealed a firm mass affecting the nasal bridge, right medial canthus associated with periorbital oedema, and expansion of the superior nasal septum.

Radiology (plain X-rays, tomography and CT scanning) showed a large mass involving the ethmoid bilaterally, nasal septum and nasal cavity with erosion of the right medial orbital wall and cribriform plate (Fig. 8.5). A definite diagnosis could not be made following examination under anaesthesia and biopsy when a list of suggested possibilities included neuroblastoma, lymphoma and undifferentiated carcinoma. Subsequent electron microscopy revealed ultrastructural details consistent with Ewing's sarcoma.

In the absence of obvious metastatic spread, triple modality therapy was undertaken, comprising craniofacial resection, followed by radiotherapy and chemotherapy. The tumour was found to involve both ethmoid labyrinths, breaching the cribriform plate, and infiltrating anterior cranial fossa dura. There was a large extramedullary component subcutaneously beneath both medial canthal areas and in the right nasal fossa. En bloc resection of the main lesion was performed including the dura which was repaired with fascia lata and a split skin graft. Iliac crest bone was used to replace resected nasal and frontal bones.

4 weeks postoperatively chemotherapy was commenced, using a 3-weekly regime of vincristine and cyclophosphamide with dactinomycin and adriamycin added alternately. Sequential radiotherapy of 50 Gy was given over 5 weeks and subsequently the patient has remained well with no sign of recurrence or metastatic disease for 10 years.

Radiology

The classical appearance in the long bones of a poorly-defined infiltrating lesion with a laminated periosteal reaction, a so-called 'onion ring', is not usually apparent in the upper jaw though some lytic changes or honeycombing may be seen.[177–179]

Macroscopic and microscopic appearance

There are no specific gross appearances to the lesion and light microscopy is generally inconclusive. Consequently more reliance is placed on immunocytochemistry and ultrastructural features though even these may not be definitive. Typically the cytoplasm contains clusters of glycogen rosettes which must be distinguished from the glycogen of rhabdomyosarcoma and the pseudorosettes of olfactory neuroblastoma. There is a paucity of organelles and neither myofilaments nor specialized junctional attachments are seen.[3d,180,181] Immunocytochemistry suggests an uncommitted primary mesenchymal cell but a neuroectodermal origin is not altogether excluded.

Owing to the tumour's rarity, it continues to present difficulties in diagnosis and the histopathological spectrum of Ewing's is further broadened by the existence of an atypical or large-cell variant.[158,166]

Natural history

The tumour is locally aggressive and capable of rapid haematogenous spread, which can be asymptomatic. It is estimated that between 15 and 30% of patients have covert pulmonary or skeletal metastases at or within 6 months of diagnosis[182] and these are a common cause of death in the rare cases of extraskeletal lesions. The high

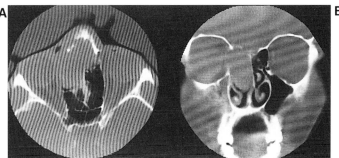

Fig. 8.5 Ewing's sarcoma arising in ethmoidal region.[181] **A**, axial and **B**, coronal scans.

Table 8.10 Ewing's sarcoma of the upper jaw: reports in literature

Author	Age (yr)	Sex	Site: Nose	Maxilla	Ethmoid	Treatment: DXT/C	DXT/C Surg	DXT/Surg	Surg/C	A&W	AWR	Outcome: DICD	DOD	Mets	Total no. of cases	No. in upper jaw
Soraluce 1958[195]			1													1
Hunsuck 1968[194]	33	M		1				1		18/12						
Roca et al 1968[194]	3	M					1			11 yr					63	2
	7	M		2				1		5 yr						
Brownson & Cook 1969[197]	6	F		1			1			No FU						
Dehner 1973[198]	6	M		1		1				2 yr						1
Fernandez et al 1974[199]				2				2							59	2
Awatagochi et al 1976[200]			1													2
				1									+			
Ferlito 1978[178]	29	M	1			1						10/12		+ (pul/bone)		
	44	M		1			1			8/12						
	43	M		1		1							8/12	+		
	44	M		1			1			8/12						
Strong et al 1979[201]				3				1		No FU					24	3
Pontius & Sebek 1981[162]	44	M	1					1		No FU						
Hossfeld et al 1982[189]				1										14	1	
Howard & Lund 1985[181]	14	M			1	1										
Siegel et al 1987[165]	14	M		1		1				10 yr						
	9	F			1	1				9 yr						
	9	M		1		1				8 yr						
	8	F		1		1				7 yr						
	15	F		1		1				11/12						
Lane & Ironside 1990[202]	7	M		1					1	No FU						

DXT, radiotherapy; C, chemotherapy; Surg, Surgery; A&W, alive and well; AWR, alive with recurrence; DICD, dead of intercurrent disease; DOD, dead of disease; Mets, Metastases; No FU, no follow-up.

degree of lethality relates to the tumour's rapid growth, often with a doubling time of under 25 days, and a considerable propensity for early dissemination.[183] This results in micrometastases long before the primary tumour has reached a diagnosable size.

Differential diagnosis

Ewing's sarcoma must be distinguished from other small cell tumours: olfactory and primitive neuroblastoma, rhabdomyosarcoma, lymphoma, retinoblastoma and anaplastic carcinoma.

Treatment

The Intergroup Ewing's Sarcoma Study (IESS) was established in the USA to compare a variety of treatment protocols and has considered over 800 cases since 1972.[165] Seven protocols have been used, all of which consist of three or four drug chemotherapy (vincristine, cyclophosphamide, dactinomycin plus adriamycin) with or without radiotherapy. Surgical resection has been performed in some of these cases. When the cases reported in the upper jaw are considered a considerable variety of treatment modalities have been employed, though the vast majority have included radiotherapy.

Prognosis

Histologically a filigree pattern with a high mitotic rate is thought to be associated with a poor prognosis[167] though this form is not usually found in the head and neck region. In 1975 pre-treatment serum lactate dehydrogenase was considered as a predictor of metastatic spread[184] though there have been no subsequent follow-up reports.

Until the 1970s results for the treatment of Ewing's were uniformly poor, with 5-year survival figures of 8% and 16% respectively in two large series published in 1967 and 1975.[185,186] Of more than 1000 cases with Ewing's sarcoma in the world literature up to 1975, approximately 100 had survived for 5 years or longer. Fortunately, the use of combined treatment has considerably improved prognosis. Formerly 75% of patients died of metastatic spread to the lung or bone, often within 1 year of diagnosis. This has been transformed into a disease-free survival of 64–80% for 3–7 years following triple therapy.[187–193]

Evaluation of prognostic indicators and therapeutic techniques have been enhanced through the collaborative efforts of the IESS and have shown that the location of the primary site is the single most important predictor of clinical behaviour. The maxilla is regarded as a prognostically better site. In Siegel et al's series[165] all four maxillary patients were free of disease at 10, 8 and 7 years and 11

months respectively. In a series of six patients[194] the four cases affecting the mandible died, whereas the two maxillary cases survived long-term.

ALVEOLAR SOFT PART SARCOMA

Definition

This rare tumour which is sometimes called organoid granular-cell tumour (misleadingly in the opinion of Batsakis et al[59]) was first described in 1952 by Christopherson et al.[203] It constitutes 0.04–1% of all soft tissue sarcomas where it usually occurs in skeletal muscle of the extremities.[101b] Only 18 cases have been reported in the head and neck, the majority of which affected the tongue.[204–208] Two cases have been reported in the nasal cavity[204,207] and two cases (one male, one female, aged 7 and 9 years respectively) have been seen at the Institute of Laryngology and Otology, London, both presenting with a mass in the orbit (Fig. 8.6).

Incidence

The lesion tends to occur in children and young adults with an average age of 25 years. Women appear to be twice as commonly affected as men and there is a curious predeliction for the right side of the body.[209]

Aetiology

The tissue of origin is unknown. Michaels[4e] considered it with muscular lesions due to the suggested relationship with rhabdomyosarcomas[210] and its occurrence in skeletal muscle. Several authors[211–213] have supported a paraganglionic origin but if this were the case, the paucity of lesions in the head and neck is surprising. Two cases have presented during pregnancy suggesting a hormonal association.[208]

Clinical features

In the two case reports of nasal lesions[204,207] the patients were women aged 15 and 21, both of whom presented with nasal obstruction and in one case facial swelling, proptosis and bilateral lymphadenopathy. The first case had a localized lesion of the middle turbinate which was removed surgically and no recurrence or secondaries occurred in the 26 months follow-up. The second more extensive case received radiotherapy and was not followed-up.

Macroscopic and microscopic appearance

The tumour appears well circumscribed with incomplete encapsulation. The cells are arranged in compact groups

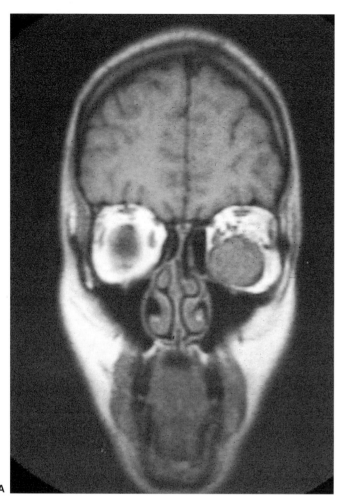

A

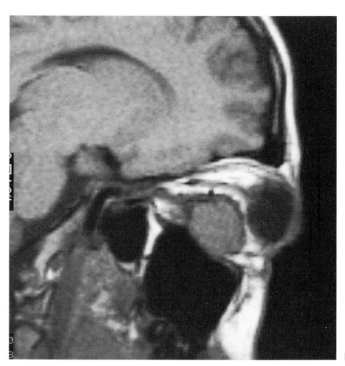

B

Fig. 8.6 A, Coronal and **B,** sagittal MR scans, T1 weighted sequence, showing orbital alveolar soft-part sarcoma lying adjacent to roof of maxilla.

of 5–50 cells which are eosinophilic with a finely granular cytoplasm and eccentric nuclei.[4e,59] Shipkey et al[214] described large crystals in the cytoplasm in 9 of 13 cases which were thought to derive from Z bands by Fisher & Reidbord,[210] hence a muscular origin.

Natural history

The lesion is slow-growing and painless and is always fatal. Distant haematogenous rather than lymphatic metastases are common, to lungs, liver and bone

Lieberman et al[209] found distant secondaries in 28 out of 46 cases. In a study of 53 cases at the Memorial Sloan-Kettering Cancer Center,[215] 82% were alive at 2 years, 59% at 5 years and 47% at 10 years but there were no survivors at 20 years.

Differential diagnosis

The differential diagnosis includes renal clear cell carcinoma, paraganglioma, granular cell tumour, and alveolar rhabdomyosarcoma.

Treatment

In the head and neck 11 of the 18 cases have been treated by surgery alone.[204–208] Of the remaining seven patients, two received radiotherapy, three chemotherapy and three a combination of modalities. It has been suggested that radiotherapy and chemotherapy should be reserved for recurrence.[216] However, with such small numbers and short follow-up, it is impossible to draw any conclusion about optimal management.

REFERENCES

1. Batsakis J G 1980 Tumors of the Head and Neck. Williams and Wilkins, Baltimore, a: pp 252–279; b: pp 145–168; c: 360–364; d: 359–360
2. Hellquist H B 1990 Pathology of the nose and paranasal sinuses. Butterworths, London, pp 134–136
3. Hyams V J, Batsakis J G, Michaels L 1988 Tumors of the upper respiratory tract and ear. Armed Forces Institute of Pathology, Washington, a: pp 112–128; b: pp 115–116; c: 117–119; d: 127–128
4. Michaels L 1987 Ear, nose and throat histopathology. Springer-Verlag, Berlin, a: pp 211; b: 212–216; c: 215–216; d: 214–215; e: 446–448
5. Fu Y-S, Perzin K H (1976) Nonepithelial tumors of the nasal cavity, paranasal sinuses and nasopharynx. A clinico-pathologic study. VI Fibrous tissues tumors (fibroma, fibromatosis, fibrosarcoma). Cancer 37: 2912–2928
6. Mackenzie D H 1972 The fibromatoses: a clinicopathologic concept. British Medical Journal 4: 277–281
7. Lloyd G A S 1988 Diagnostic imaging of the nose and paranasal sinuses. Springer-Verlag, London, pp 159

8. Enzinger F M, Weiss S H (eds) 1988 Soft tissue tumors, 2nd edn. C V Mosby, St. Louis
9. Billroth T 1872 Spindelzellensarkom in der Nase. Chirurgische Klinik (Wien 1869–1870) A Hirschwald, Berlin Band 3, p 73
10. Johnston R H 1904 Sarcomata of the nasal septum. Laryngoscope 14: 454–473
11. Portela J 1927 Fibrosarcome envahissant des fosses nasales, des deux sinus maxillaires, de l'ethmoide et des deux sinus sphenoidaux. Revue de Laryngologie 48: 530–531
12. Huvos A G, Higinbotham N L 1975 Primary fibrosarcoma of bone. A clinicopathologic study of 130 patients. Cancer 35: 837–847
13. Stout A P 1948 Fibrosarcoma. The malignant tumor of fibroblasts. Cancer 1: 30–63
14. Swain R E, Sessions D G, Ogura J H 1974 Fibrosarcoma of the head and neck: a clinical analysis of forty cases. Annals of Otology, Rhinology and Laryngology 83: 439–444
15. Jeffree G M, Price C H G 1976 Metastatic spread of fibrosarcoma of bone. A report on forty-nine cases, and a comparison with osteosarcoma. The Journal of Bone and Joint Surgery 58: 418–425
16. McKenna R J, Schwinn C P, Soong K Y, Higinbotham N L 1966 Sarcomata of the osteogenic series (osteosarcoma, fibrosarcoma, chondrosarcoma, parosteal osteogenic sarcoma and sarcomata arising in abnormal bone). An analysis of 552 cases. The Journal of Bone and Joint Surgery 48: 1–26
17. Stratton H J M 1953 A case of fibrosarcoma of the ethmoid. Journal of Laryngology and Otology 67: 631–634
18. Hoggins G S, Brady C L 1962 Fibrosarcoma of the maxilla. Oral Surgery, Oral Medicine, Oral Pathology 15: 34–38
19. Karlan M S, Kunin J 1963 Fibrosarcoma in the antrum of a child. California Medicine 99: 197–200
20. Prasad U, Kanjilal J K 1969 Fibrosarcoma of the ethmoid. Journal of Laryngology and Otology 83: 627–631
21. Richardson D, Maguda T A 1970 Fibrosarcoma of the nose and paranasal sinuses. Journal of Tennessee Medical Association 63: 829–831
22. Cronin J 1973 Fibrosarcoma of the paranasal sinuses. Journal of Laryngology and Otology 87: 667–674
23. Goepfert H, Lindberg R D, Sinkovics J G, Ayala A G 1977 Soft-tissue sarcoma of the head and neck after puberty. Treatment by surgery and postoperative radiation therapy. Archives of Otolaryngology 103: 365–368
24. Shah J P 1977 Fibrosarcoma of nasal cavity. New York State Journal of Medicine 77: 983–984
25. Agarwal M K, Gupta S, Gupta O P, Samant H C 1980 Fibrosarcoma of nose and paranasal sinuses. Journal of Surgical Oncology 15: 53–57
26. Broniatowski M, Haria C 1981 Fibrosarcoma of the nose and paranasal sinuses. Ear, Nose and Throat Journal 60: 302–306
27. Kadri Z, Pratt L 1981 Fibrosarcoma of the maxillary sinuses. Otolaryngology, Head and Neck Surgery 89: 257–289
28. Slootweg P J, Muller H 1984 Fibrosarcoma of the jaws. Journal of Maxillofacial Surgery 12: 157–162
29. Seraj A A 1985 Ethmoid sinus fibrosarcoma arising as a frontal mucocele. Ear, Nose and Throat Journal 64: 47–50
30. Lukinmaa P-L, Hietanen J, Swan H, Ylipaavalniemi P, Perkki K 1988 Maxillary fibrosarcoma with extracellular immuno-characterization. British Journal of Oral and Maxillofacial Surgery 26: 36–44
31. Oppenheimer R W, Friedman M 1988 Fibrosarcoma of the maxillary sinus. Ear, Nose and Throat Journal 67: 193–198
32. Smith M C F, Soames J V 1989 Fibrosarcoma of the ethmoid. Journal of Laryngology and Otology 103: 686–689
33. Hernandez F J, Fernandez B B 1976 Multiple diffuse fibrosarcoma of bone. Cancer 37: 939–945
34. Pettit V D, Chamness J T, Ackerman L V 1954 Fibromatosis and fibrosarcoma following irradiation therapy. Cancer 7: 149–158
35. Broders A C, Hargrave R, Meyerding H W 1939 Pathologic features of soft tissue sarcoma. Surgery, Gynecology and Obstetrics 69: 267–280
36. Russell W O, Cohen J, Enzinger F, Hajdu S I, Heise H, Martin R G, Meissner W, Miller W T, Schmitz R L, Suit H D 1977 A clinical and pathological staging system for soft tissue sarcomas. Cancer 40: 1562–1570
37. Friedmann I, Osborn D 1982 Mesenchymal soft tissue tumours of the nose and sinuses. In: Pathology of granulomas and neoplasms of the nose and paranasal sinuses. Churchill Livingstone, Edinburgh, pp 231–234
38. Conley J, Stout A P, Healey W V 1967 Clinicopathologic analysis of eighty-four patients with an original diagnosis of fibrosarcoma of the head and neck. American Journal of Surgery 114: 564–569
39. Pack G I, Ariel I M 1952 Fibrosarcoma of the soft somatic tissue. Surgery 31: 443–478
40. Mackenzie D H 1964 Fibroma: a dangerous diagnosis. British Journal of Surgery 51: 607–612
41. Bizer L S 1971 Fibrosarcoma. American Journal of Surgery 121: 586–587
42. Scott S M, Reiman H M, Pritchard D J, Ilstrup D A 1989 Soft tissue fibrosarcoma. A clinicopathologic study of 132 cases. Cancer 64: 925–931
43. Dahlin D C, Unni K, Matsuno T 1977 Malignant (fibrous) histiocytoma of bone – fact or fancy? Cancer 39: 1508–1516
44. Eilber F R, Morton D L, Eckhardt J, Grant T, Weisenburger T 1984 Limb salvage for skeletal and soft tissue sarcomas: Multidisciplinary preoperative therapy. Cancer 53: 2579–2584
45. Lindberg R D, Martin R G, Romsdahl M M 1975 Surgery and postoperative radiotherapy in the treatment of soft tissue sarcomas in adults. American Journal of Roentgenology, Radium Therapy and Nuclear Medicine 123: 123–128
46. Rockley T J, Liu K C 1986 Fibrosarcoma of the nose and paranasal sinuses. Journal of Laryngology and Otology 100: 1417–1420
47. Rosenberg SA, Glatstein E J 1981 Perspectives on the role of surgery and radiation therapy in the treatment of soft tissue sarcomas of the extremities. Seminars on Oncology 8: 190–200
48. Windeyer B, Dische S, Mansfield C M 1966 The place of radiotherapy in the management of fibrosarcoma of the soft tissues. Clinical Radiology 17: 32–40
49. Ackerman L V, Del Regato J A 1970 Cancer, 4th edn. Mosby, St. Louis
50. Van Blarcom C W, Masson J K, Dahlin DC 1971 Fibrosarcoma of the mandible. Oral Surgery, Oral Medicine, Oral Pathology 32: 428–439
51. Cunningham M P, Arlen M 1968 Medullary fibrosarcoma of bone. Cancer 21: 31–37
52. Pritchard D J, Soule E H, Taylor W F, Ivins J C 1974 Fibrosarcoma – a clinicopathologic and statistical study of 199 tumors of the soft tissues of the extremities and trunk. Cancer 33: 888–897
53. Enterline H T 1981 Histopathology of sarcomas. Seminars in Oncology 8: 133–155
54. Virchow R 1857 Ein Fall von bosartigen zum Teile in der Form des Neurons auftretenden Fettgeschwulsten. Archiv fur Pathologische Anatomie 11: 281–288
55. Virchow R 1865 Myxoma lipomatodes malignum. Archiv fur Pathologische Anatomie 32: 545–546
56. Pack G T, Pierson J C 1954 Liposarcoma: a study of 105 cases. Surgery 36: 687–712
57. Spittle M F, Newton K A, Mackenzie D H 1970 Liposarcoma. British Journal of Cancer 24: 696–704
58. Stoller F M, Davis D G 1968 Liposarcoma of the neck. Archives of Otolaryngology 88: 419–422
59. Batsakis J G, Regezi J A, Rice D H 1980 The pathology of head and neck tumors: fibroadipose tissue and skeletal muscle, Part 8. Head and Neck Surgery 3: 145–168
60. Enterline H T, Culberson J D, Rochlin D B, Brady L W 1960 Liposarcoma. Cancer 13: 932–950
61. Saunders J R, Jaques D A, Casterline P F, Percarpio B, Goodloe S 1979 Liposarcomas of the head and neck. Cancer 43: 162–168
62. Goldstein M A 1915 Lipoma of the maxillary antrum. Laryngoscope 25: 142-144
63. Silbernagel C E 1938 Lipoma of the maxillary antrum. Laryngoscope 48: 427–428
64. Hatziotis J C 1971 Lipoma of the oral cavity. Oral Surgery 31: 511–524
65. Fu Y-S, Perzin K H 1977 Non-epithelial tumours of the nasal cavity, paranasal sinuses and nasopharynx; VIII Adipose tissue tumours. Cancer 40: 1314–1317

66. Preece J M, Kearns D B, Wickersham J K, Grace A R, Bailey C M 1988 Nasal lipoma. Journal of Laryngology and Otology 102: 1044–1046

67. Giardino C, Manfredi C 1967 Liposarcoma della guancia con invasione secondaria del seno mascellare. Giornale Italiano Chirurgia 23: 743–758

68. Enzinger F M, Winslow D J 1962 Liposarcoma. Archiv fur Pathologische Anatomie 335: 367–388

69. Stout A P 1944 Liposarcoma – the malignant tumour of lipoblasts. Annals of Surgery 119: 86–107

70. Bradley P J, Singh S D 1982 Congenital nasal masses: diagnosis and management. Clinical Otolaryngology 7: 87–97

71. Stout A P 1948 Myxoma, the tumour of primitive mesenchyme. Annals of Surgery 127: 706–719

72. Virchow R 1871 Cellularpathologie in ihrer Begrundung auf physiologische und pathologische Gewebelehre. Verlag von August Hirschwald, Berlin, p 563

73. Hajek M, Polyak L 1910 Myxoma lymphangiectaticum des Nasengerustes. Archiv fur Laryngologie und Rhinologie 23: 43–56

74. Harbert F, Gerry R G, Dimmette R M 1949 Myxoma of the maxilla. Oral Surgery, Oral Medicine, Oral Pathology 2: 1414–1421

75. Fu Y-S, Perzin K H 1977 Non-epithelial tumours of the nasal cavity, paranasal sinuses and nasopharynx: a clinico-pathologic study. VII Myxomas. Cancer 39: 195–203

76. Zimmerman D C, Dahlin D C 1958 Myxomatous tumours of the jaws. Oral Surgery, Oral Medicine, Oral Pathology 11: 1069–1080

77. Canalis R F, Smith G A, Konrad H R 1976 Myxomas of the head and neck. Archives of Otolaryngology 102: 300–305

78. Kangur T T, Dahlin D C, Turlington E G 1975 Myxomatous tumors of the jaws. Journal of Oral Surgery 33: 523–528

79. Tse J J, Vander S 1985 The soft tissue myxoma of the head and neck region – report of a case and literature review. Head and Neck Surgery 8: 479–483

80. Glazunov M F, Puvkov J 1963 Uber die Sogenannten Muskelmyoxmeoun Myxosarkome des Menschen mit Zelleins. Chalussenz Krebsforsch 65: 439

81. Thoma K H, Goldman H M 1947 Central myxoma of the jaw. American Journal of Orthodontics (Oral Surgery Section) 33: 532–540

82. Adekeye E O, Avery B S, Edwards M B, Williams H K 1984 Advanced central myxoma of the jaws in Nigeria. Clinical features, treatment and pathogenesis. International Journal of Oral Surgery 13: 177–180

83. Kurt T H, Goldman H M 1960 Central myxoma of the jaw. In: Oral Pathology, (5th edn) Kimpton, London

84. Batsakis J G 1987 Pathology consultation. Myxomas of soft tissues and the facial skeleton. Annals of Otology, Rhinology and Laryngology 96: 618–619

85. Sinha S N, Yadav Y C 1970 Myxoma of the pharynx . Archives of Otolaryngology 91: 82–83

86. Babbitt J A, Pfeiffer D B 1937 Myxoma of the palate and pharynx. Archives of Otolaryngology 26: 453–458

87. Greenfield S D, Friedman O 1951 Myxoma of maxillary sinus. New York State Journal of Medicine 51: 1319–1320

88. Bruce K W, Royer R Q 1952 Central fibromyxoma of maxilla. Oral Surgery 5: 1277–1281

89. Attar S 1956 Myxoma: clinicopathologic study. American Journal of Surgery 91: 755–760

90. Dutz W, Stout A P 1961 The myxoma in childhood. Cancer 14: 629–635

91. Buchner A, Ramon Y 1965 Fibromyxoma of the maxilla. Journal of Oral Surgery 23: 145–147

92. Bochetto J, Minkowitz F, Minkowitz S, Shulman A 1967 Antral fibromyxoma presenting as a giant nasal polyp. Oral Surgery, Oral Medicine and Oral Pathology 23: 201–206

93. Barros R E, Dominguez F V, Cabrini R L 1969 Myxoma of the jaws. Oral Surgery, Oral Medicine and Oral Pathology 27: 225–236

94. Ghosh B C, Huvos A G, Gerold F P, Miller T R 1973 Myxoma of the jaw bones. Cancer 31: 237–240

95. Pradhan A C, Varma R K, Pradhan S 1972 Myxoma of the hard palate. International Surgery 57: 341

96. Faccini J M, Williams J L 1973 Myxoma involving the soft tissues of the face. Journal of Laryngology and Otology 87: 817–821

97. Prasad I B, Sharan R 1983 Fibro-myxoma of the maxilla. Journal of Laryngology and Otology 97: 549–551

98. Slootweg P J, Wittkampf A R M 1986 Myxoma of the jaws. An analysis of 15 cases. Journal of Cranio-Maxillo-Facial Surgery 14: 46–52

99. Stout A P, Lattes R 1967 Tumors of the Soft Tissues. Fascicle 1, Second Series. Atlas of Tumor Pathology, Washington: Armed Forces Institute of Pathology

100. James D R, Lucas V S 1987 Maxillary myxoma in a child of 11 months. Journal of Cranio-Maxillo-Facial Surgery 15: 42–44

101. Enzinger F M, Weiss S W 1983 Malignant fibrohistiocytic tumors. In: Enzinger F M, Weiss S W (eds) Soft tissue tumors. C V Mosby, St Louis, a: pp 166–198; b: Ch. 31

102. Crissman J D, Henson S L 1978 Malignant fibrous histiocytoma of the maxillary sinus. Archives of Otolaryngology 104: 228–230

103. Townsend G L, Neel H B, Weiland L H, Devine K D, McBean J B 1973 Fibrous histiocytoma of the paranasal sinuses. Report of a case. Archives of Otolaryngology 98: 51–52

104. Blitzer A, Lawson W, Zak F G, Biller H F, Som M L 1981 Clinical pathological determinants in prognosis of fibrous histiocytomas of head and neck. Laryngoscope 91: 2053–2070

105. Barnes L 1985 Tumors and tumorlike lesions of the soft tissue. In: Barnes L (ed) Surgical pathology of the head and neck. Marcel Dekker, New York, pp. 725–880

106. Daou R A, Attia E L, Viloria J B 1983 Malignant fibrous histiocytoma of the head and neck. Journal of Otolaryngology 12: 383–388

107. Angervall L, Johansson S, Kindblom L-G, Save-Soderbergh J 1979 Primary malignant fibrous histiocytoma of bone after irradiation. Acta Pathologica Microbiologica Scandinavia 87: 437–446

108. Weiss S W, Enzinger F M 1978 Malignant fibrous histiocytoma. An analysis of 200 cases. Cancer 41: 2250–2266

109. Ireland A J, Eveson J W, Leopard P J 1988 Malignant fibrous histiocytoma: a report of two cases arising in sites of previous irradiation. British Journal of Oral and Maxillofacial Surgery 26: 221–227

110. Nishizawa S, Hayashida T, Horiguchi S, Inouye K, Imamura T 1985 Malignant fibrous histiocytoma of maxilla following radiotherapy for bilateral retinoblastoma. Journal of Laryngology and Otology 99: 501–504

111. Huvos A G, Heilweil M, Bretsky S S 1985 The pathology of malignant fibrous histiocytoma of bone. A study of 130 patients. American Journal of Surgical Pathology 9: 853–871

112. Schajawicz F, Aranjo E S, Berenstein M 1983 Sarcoma complicating Paget's disease of bone: a clinicopathologic study of 62 cases. Journal of Bone and Joint Surgery 65: 299–307

113. Spanier S S, Enneking W F, Enriquez P 1975 Primary malignant fibrous histiocytoma of bone. Cancer 36: 2084–2098

114. Dorfmann H D, Norman A, Wolff H 1966 Fibrosarcoma complicating bone infarction in a caisson worker. Journal of Bone and Joint Surgery 48: 528–532

115. Mirra J M, Bullough P G, Marcove R C, Jacobs B, Huvos A G 1974 Malignant fibrous histiocytoma and osteosarcoma in association with bone infarcts. Journal of Bone and Joint Surgery 56: 932

116. Mirra J M, Gold R H, Marafiote R 1977 Malignant (fibrous) histiocytoma arising in association with a bone infarct in sickle-cell disease: coincidence or cause and effect. Cancer 39: 186–194

117. Taxy J B, Hidvegi D F 1977 Olfactory neuroblastoma. Cancer 39: 131–138

118. Eriksson M, Hardell L, Berg N O, Moller T, Axelson O 1981 Soft-tissue sarcomas and exposure to chemical substances: a case referent study. British Journal of Industrial Medicine 38: 27–33

119. Kauffman S L, Stout A P 1961 Histiocytic tumors (Fibrous xanthoma and histiocytoma) in children. Cancer 14: 469–482

120. Kempson R L, Kyriakos M 1972 Fibroxanthosarcoma of the soft tissues - a type of malignant histiocytoma. Cancer 29: 961–976

121. Soule E M, Enriquez P 1972 A typical fibrous histiocytoma, malignant fibrous histiocytoma, malignant histiocytoma and epitheloioid sarcoma. Cancer 29: 961–976

122. Leite C, Goodwin J W, Sinkovics J G, Baker L H, Benjamin H 1977 Chemotherapy of malignant fibrous histiocytoma. Cancer 40: 2010–2014

123. Bassett W B, Weiss R B 1978 Prolonged complete remission in malignant fibrous histiocytoma treated with chemotherapy. Cancer Treatment Reports 62: 1405–1406

124. Mugliston T A H, Shaw H J 1984 Malignant fibrous histiocytoma of the maxillary sinus. Journal of Laryngology and Otology 98: 153–157

125. Smith D K, Poon M C, Flint A 1979 Inflammatory fibrous histiocytoma: response to non-surgical therapy. A case report. Medical Paediatrics and Oncology 7: 263–267

126. Urban C, Rosen G, Huvos A G, Caparros B, Cacavio A, Nirenberg A 1983 Chemotherapy of malignant fibrous histiocytoma of bone. A report of five cases. Cancer 51: 795–802

127. Barnes L, Kanbour A 1988 Malignant fibrous histiocytoma of head and neck. A report of 12 cases. Archives of Otolaryngology, Head and Neck Surgery 114: 1149–1156

128. Lesica A, Harwood T R, Yokoo H 1975 Atypical fibroxanthoma of the ethmoid sinus. Archives of Otolaryngology 101: 506–508

129. Ogura J H, Toomey J M, Setzen M, Sobol S 1980 Malignant fibrous histiocytoma of the head and neck. Laryngoscope 90: 1429–1439

130. Shearer W T, Schreiner R L, Ward S P, Marshall R E, Stromingen D B, McAlister W H, Kissane J, Ogura J H 1973 Benign nasal tumor appearing as neonatal respiratory distress. First reported case of nasopharyngeal fibrous histiocytoma. American Journal of Diseases of Children 126: 238–241

131. Rice D H, Batsakis J G, Headlington J T, Boles R 1974 Fibrous histiocytoma of the nose and paranasal sinuses. Archives of Otolaryngology 100: 398–401

132. Spector G J, Ogura J H 1974 Malignant fibrous histiocytoma of the maxilla. Archives of Otolaryngology 99: 385–387

133. Slootweg P J, Muller H 1977 Malignant fibrous histiocytoma of the maxilla. Oral Surgery 44: 560–566

134. DeMoura L F P, Yook T S 1978 Malignant fibrous histiocytoma of the maxillary sinus. Otolaryngology, Head and Neck Surgery 86: 685–688

135. Jee A, Domboski M, Milobsky S A 1978 Malignant fibrohistiocytoma of the maxilla presenting with endodontically involved teeth. Oral Surgery 45: 464–469

136. McDonald T J, Weiland L H 1978 Fibrous xanthoma of the frontal sinus. Otology, Rhinology and Laryngology 86: 721–724

137. Sidhu S S, Bansal B P, Parkash H 1978 Primary malignant fibrous histiocytoma of the maxilla. Journal of Dentistry: 6: 261–264

138. Wilmes E, Meister P 1978 Fibrose Histiozytome der Nase und Nasennebenhohlen. Laryngologie, Rhinologie und Otologie (Stuttgart) 57: 69–72

139. Tovi F, Sidi J 1979 Malignant fibrous histiocytoma of the maxillary sinus. Journal of Oral Surgery 37: 500–503

140. Del-Rey E, De-La-Torre F E 1980 Fibrous histiocytoma of the nasal cavity. Laryngoscope 90: 1686–1693

141. Merrick R E, Rhone D P, Chilis T J 1980 Malignant fibrous histiocytoma of the maxillary sinus. Archives of Otolaryngology 106: 365–367

142. Perzin K H, Fu Y-S 1980 Non-epithelial tumors of the nasal cavity, paranasal sinuses and nasopharynx. A clinico-pathologic study XI. Fibrous histiocytomas. Cancer 45: 2616–2626

143. Schaefer S D, Denton R A, Blend B L, Carder H M 1980 Malignant fibrous histiocytoma of the frontal sinus. Laryngoscope 90: 2021–2026

144. Sonobe H, Tagushi K, Motoi M, Ogawa K, Matsumura M, Ohsaki K 1980 Malignant fibrous histiocytoma of the maxillary sinus. Acta Pathological Japonica 30: 79–89

145. Ushigome S, Hirota T 1980 Malignant fibrous histiocytoma. Acta Pathologica Japonica 30: 799–813

146. Tewfik H H, Tewfik F A, McCabe B F 1981 Malignant fibrous histiocytoma of the nose and nasopharynx. Archives of Otolaryngology 107: 191

147. Brookes G B, Rose P E 1983 Malignant fibrous histiocytoma of the ethmoid sinus. Journal of Laryngology and Otology 97: 279–289

148. Sasaki R, Sasaki S-I, Murata M, Itoh M, Honda M, Aozasa K 1983 Malignant fibrous histiocytoma in the maxillary sinus. Xanthoma-like change of the tumor after radiotherapy. Laryngoscope 93: 202–204

149. Abdul-Karim F W, Ayala A G, Chawla S P, Bao-Shing J, Goepfert H 1985 Malignant fibrous histiocytoma of jaws. A clinicopathologic study of 11 cases. Cancer 56: 1590–1596

150. Hayter J P, Williams D M, Cannell H, Hope-Stone H 1985 Malignant fibrous histiocytoma of the maxilla. Journal of Maxillo-Facial Surgery 13: 167–171

151. Enjoji M, Hashimoto H, Tsuneyoshi M et al 1980 Malignant fibrous histiocytoma: a clinicopathologic study of 130 cases. Acta Pathologica Japan 30: 727–741

152. Kearney M M, Soule E, Ivins J C 1980 Malignant fibrous histiocytoma. A retrospective study of 167 cases. Cancer 45: 167–178

153. Bertoni F, Capanna R, Biagini R, Bacchini P, Guerra A, Ruggieri P, Present D, Campanacci M 1985 Malignant fibrous histiocytoma of soft tissue. An analysis of 78 cases located and deeply seated in the extremities. Cancer 56: 356–367

154. Radio S J, Woolridge T N, Linder J 1988 Flow cytometric DNA analysis of malignant fibrous histiocytomas and related fibrohistiocytic tumors. Human Pathology 19: 74–77

155. Weber R S, Benjamin R S, Peters L J et al 1986 Soft tissue sarcomas of the head and neck in adolescents and adults. American Journal of Surgery 152: 386–392

156. Dahlin D C, Coventry M B, Scanlon P W 1961 Ewing's sarcoma: a critical analysis of 165 cases. Journal of Bone and Joint Surgery 43: 185–192

157. Dahlin D C 1978 Bone tumours: general aspects and data on 6221 cases, 3rd edn. Charles C Thomas, Springfield, Illinois, pp 274–287

158. Lombart-Bosch A, Blache R, Peydro-Olaya A 1978 Ultrastructural study of 28 cases of Ewing's sarcoma: typical and atypical forms. Cancer 41: 1362–1373

159. Mahoney J P, Alexander R W 1978 Ewing's sarcoma: a light and electron-microscopic study of 21 cases. American Journal of Surgical Pathology 2: 283–298

160. Navas-Palacios J J, Aparicio-Duque R, Valdes M D 1984 On the histogenesis of Ewing's sarcoma: an ultrastructural, immunocytochemical and cytochemical study. Cancer 53: 1882–1901

161. Angervall L, Enzinger F M 1975 Extraskeletal neoplasm resembling Ewing's sarcoma. Cancer 36: 240–251

162. Pontius K I, Sebek B A 1981 Extraskeletal Ewing's sarcoma arising in the nasal fossa. American Journal of Clinical Pathology 85: 410–415

163. Szakacs J E, Carla M, Szakacs M R 1974 Ewing's sarcoma, extraskeletal and of bone. Case report with ultrastructural analysis. Annals of Clinical Laboratory Science 4: 306–322

164. Ewing J 1921 Diffuse endothelioma of the bone. New York Pathology Society 21: 17–24

165. Siegel G P, Oliver W R, Reinus W R, Gilula L A, Foulkes M A, Kissane J M, Askin F B 1987 Primary Ewing's sarcoma involving the bones of the head and neck. Cancer 60: 2829–2840

166. Sneige N, Batsakis J G 1989 Ewing's sarcoma of bone and soft tissues. Annals of Otology, Rhinology and Laryngology 98: 400–402

167. Kissane J M, Askin F B, Foulkes M, Stratton L B, Shirley S F 1983 Ewing's sarcoma of bone: clinicopathologic aspects of 303 cases from the Intergroup Ewing's Sarcoma Study. Human Pathology 14: 773–779

168. Arafat A, Ellis G L, Adrian J C 1983 Ewing's sarcoma of the jaws. Oral Surgery, Oral Medicine, Oral Pathology 55: 589–596

169. Stuart-Harris R, Wills E J, Philips J, Lunglands A O, Fox R M, Tattersall M H N 1986 Extraskeletal Ewing's sarcoma. A clinical, morphological and ultrastructural analysis of five cases with a review of the literature. European Journal of Cancer and Clinical Oncology 22: 393–400

170. Bernstein P E, Bone R C, Feldman P S 1979 Ewing's sarcoma of the mandible. Annals of Otology, Rhinology and Laryngology 88: 105–108

171. Borghelli R F, Barros R E, Zampieri J. 1978 Ewing's sarcoma of the mandible. Journal of Oral Surgery 36: 473–475

172. Mariano A, Gastelo Acunal L, Lodd J P, Champy M 1977 The warning signals in sarcoma of the mandible. Journal of Medicine (Strasbourg) 8: 127–130
173. Mikaelian D O, Scherr S A, Delucca L E 1980 Primary Ewing's sarcoma of the mandibular ramus. Otolaryngology Head and Neck Surgery 88: 211–214
174. Rapoport A, De Andrade Sobrinho J, De Carvalho M B 1977 Ewing's sarcoma of the mandible. Oral Surgery, Oral Medicine, Oral Pathology 44: 89–94
175. Beraud R, Fortin P. 1967 Ewing's sarcoma of the temporal localisation. Canadian Medical Association Journal 97: 338–341
176. Fitzer P M, Steffey W R 1976 Brain and bone scans in primary Ewing's sarcoma of the petrous bone. Journal of Neurosurgery 44: 608–612
177. DeSantos L A, Jing B-S 1978 Radiographic findings of Ewing's sarcoma of the jaws. British Journal of Radiology 51: 682–687
178. Ferlito A 1978 Primary Ewing's sarcoma of the maxilla: a clinicopathological study of four cases. Journal of Laryngology and Otology 92: 1007–1024
179. Weir J C, Amonett M R, Krolls S O 1979 Tumorous conditions of the fibula, supraorbital area and mandible. Journal of Oral Pathology 8: 313–318
180. Friedman B, Gold H 1968 Ultrastructure of Ewing's sarcoma of bone. Cancer 22: 307–322
181. Howard D J, Lund V J 1985 Primary Ewing's sarcoma of the ethmoid bone. Journal of Laryngology and Otology 99: 1019–1023
182. Johnson R E, Pomeroy T C 1975 Evaluation of therapeutic results in Ewing's sarcoma. American Journal of Roentgenology 123: 583–587
183. Pearlman A W 1975 Ewing's sarcoma – growth rate and tumour lethal dose. Frontiers of Radiation Therapy and Oncology 10: 48–62
184. Brereton H D, Simon R, Pomeroy T C 1975 Pretreatment serum lactate dehydrogenase predicting metastatic spread in Ewing's sarcoma. Annals of Internal Medicine 83: 352–354
185. Falk S, Alpert M 1967 Five year survival of patients with Ewing's sarcoma. Surgery, Gynecology and Obstetrics 124: 319–324
186. Pritchard D J, Dahlin D C, Danphire R T, Taylor W F, Beabart J W 1975 Ewing's sarcoma. Journal of Bone and Joint Surgery 57: 10–16
187. Gasparini M, Lombardi F 1980 Adjuvant chemotherapy in Ewing's sarcoma patients. Recent Results in Cancer Research 80: 120–123
188. Goldman A 1982 Ewing's sarcoma: treatment with high dose radiation and adjuvant chemotherapy. Recent Results in Cancer Research 86: 115–119
189. Hossfeld D K, Seeber S, Siemers E, Schmidt C G, Scherer E 1982 Early results of combined modality therapy of patients with Ewing's sarcoma. Recent Results in Cancer Research 80: 124–127
190. Kinsella T J, Triche T J, Dickman P S, Costa J, Tepper J E, Glaubiger D 1983 Extraskeletal Ewing's sarcoma. results of combined modality treatment. Journal of Clinical Oncology 1: 489–495
191. Le Mevel B P 1980 Ewing's sarcoma: 5 year survival under adjuvant chemotherapy. Recent Results in Cancer Research 80: 128–133
192. Rosen G, Wollner N, Tan C 1974 Disease-free survival in children with Ewing's sarcoma treated with radiation therapy and adjuvant four-drug sequential chemotherapy. Cancer 33: 384–393
193. Rosen G, Caparros B, Mosende C, McCormick B, Huvos A G, Marcove R C 1978 Curability of Ewing's sarcoma and considerations for future therapeutic trials. Cancer 41: 88–89
194. Roca A N, Smith J L, MacComb W S, Jing B-S 1968 Ewing's sarcoma of the maxilla and mandible. Oral Surgery, Oral Medicine, Oral Pathology 25: 194–203
195. Soraluce J 1958 Ewing's sarcoma of the inferior nasal turbinate. Acta Oto-rino-laringologica Ibero-Americana 9: 50–53
196. Hunsuck E E 1968 Ewing's sarcoma of the maxilla. Oral Surgery, Oral Medicine, Oral Pathology 25: 923–928
197. Brownson R J, Cook R P 1969 Ewing's sarcoma of the maxilla. Annals of Otology, Rhinology and Laryngology 78: 1299–1304
198. Dehner L P 1973 Tumours of the mandible and maxilla in children. Cancer 32: 112–120
199. Fernandez C H, Lindberg R D, Sutow W W, Samuels M L 1974 Localized Ewing's sarcoma: treatment and results. Cancer 34: 143–148
200. Awatagochi S, Suzuki F, Hiraoka M. 1976 Ewing's sarcoma of the nasal cavity and maxilla. Journal of Otolaryngology (Japan) 79: 549–551
201. Strong L C, Herson J, Osborne B M, Sutow W W 1979 Risk of radiation-related subsequent malignant tumors in survivors of Ewing's sarcoma. Journal of the National Cancer Institute 62: 1401–1406
202. Lane S, Ironside J W 1990 Extraskeletal Ewing's sarcoma of the nasal fossa. Journal of Laryngology and Otology 104: 570–573
203. Christopherson W M, Foote F W, Stewart W 1952 Alveolar soft part sarcoma. Structurally characteristic tumors of uncertain histogenesis. Cancer 5: 100
204. Chatterji P, Purohit G N, Ramdev I N, Soni N K 1977 Alveolar soft part sarcoma of the nasal cavity and paranasal sinuses. Journal of Laryngology and Otology 91: 1003–1008
205. Evans H L 19485 Alveolar soft part sarcoma – a study of 13 typical examples and one with a histologically atypical component. Cancer 55: 912–917
206. King J B, Fee W E 1983 Alveolar soft part sarcoma of the tongue. American Journal of Otolaryngology 4: 363–366
207. Rubinstein M I, Drake A F, McClatchey K D 1988 Alveolar soft part sarcoma of the nasal cavity: report of a case and a review of the literature. Laryngoscope 98: 1246–1250
208. Spector R A, Travis L W, Smith J 1979 Alveolar soft part sarcoma of the head and neck. Laryngoscope 89: 1301–1306
209. Lieberman P H, Foote F W, Stewart F W, Berg J W 1966 Alveolar soft part sarcoma. Journal of the American Medical Association 198: 1047–1051
210. Fisher E R, Reidbord H 1971 Electron microscopic evidence suggesting the myogenous derivation of the so-called alveolar soft part sarcoma. Cancer 27: 150–159
211. Delaney W E 1975 Non-myogenic tumors involving skeletal muscle. A survey with special reference to alveolar soft part sarcoma. Annals of Clinical Laboratory Science 5: 236–241
212. Unni K K, Soule E H 1975 Alveolar soft part sarcoma. An electron microscopic study. Mayo Clinic Proceedings 50: 591–598
213. Welsh R A, Bray D M, Shipkey F H, Mayer A T 1972 Histogenesis of alveolar soft part sarcoma. Cancer 29: 191–204
214. Shipkey F H, Lieberman P H, Foote F W, Stewart F W 1964 Ultrastructure of alveolar soft part sarcoma. Cancer 17: 821–830
215. Miser J S, Pizzo P A 1985 Soft tissue sarcomas in childhood. Pediatric Clinics of North America 32: 779–800
216. Olson R A J, Perkins K D 1976 Alveolar soft part sarcoma in oral cavity: report of case. Journal of Oral Surgery 34: 73–76

9. Vasoform tumours

These cover a wide range of benign and malignant conditions not all of which can be clearly differentiated as true 'tumours'. The choice of lesions to be discussed within this chapter has been primarily influenced by their clinical behaviour within the upper jaw and follows the classification proposed by Batsakis & Rice in their 1981 survey of the pathology of head and neck tumours.

1. Benign
   (i) Localized
      a. Haemangiomata (capillary, cavernous or mixed)
      b. Angiofibroma
      c. Aneurysmal bone cyst
      d. Angiomyolipoma
   (ii) Inflammatory
      a. Granuloma pyogenicum
      b. Granuloma graviderum
   (iii) Angiomatous syndromes
      a. Familial haemorrhagic telangiectasia

2. Malignant
      a. Angiosarcoma
      b. Kaposi's sarcoma
      c. Haemangiopericytoma

3. Pericyte-like
      a. Paraganglioma
      b. Glomus.

Even though a predominant cell of origin can be identified for most of these conditions, many are associated with other vascular components. There is still much to learn regarding the histopathology and biological behaviour of these comparatively rare, but interesting conditions.

HAEMANGIOMA

Definition

Over half of all haemangiomata occur within the head and neck region comprising in children the commonest tumour within this area. Most of the lesions involute spontaneously by the age of 7 years and it is likely that most are hamartomas rather than true neoplasms.[1]

In adults the incidence is less, but in all age groups haemangiomatous lesions may develop in the skin or anywhere in the mucosal lining of the upper aero-digestive tract. The congenital lesions are usually treated conservatively and Illingworth, reviewing a large series of children, considered that no more than 2% of these required active therapy. Most enlarged early in life then ceased to grow and subsequent cosmetic surgery could then be left until puberty.[2] However, within the larynx, obstruction may necessitate early intervention.

Mucosal haemangiomas within the upper airway behave in a manner more characteristic of a benign neoplasm, occurring after puberty particularly in the 4th to 5th decades of life. Histological classification is based upon the size of the proliferating vascular spaces; *capillary, cavernous* and a *mixed group*.[3]

Incidence

Fu & Perzin's analysis of 156 benign non-epithelial tumours involving the nasal cavity, paranasal sinuses and nasopharynx, found that 20% were capillary haemangiomata exceeded in number only by juvenile angiofibroma.[4] Within the maxilla, haemangioma behave differently however, and will be considered separately.

Capillary haemangioma

The literature suggests that few cases occur below the age of 16 years giving an average age at diagnosis of 40 years and no clear sexual preponderance. Presenting symptoms are nasal obstruction and epistaxis in over 80% of patients as the primary site of origin is the mucosa covering the anterior end of the nasal septum. This is a region of considerable vascularity and the characteristic reddish-purple appearance with a lobulated smooth polypoidal mass has given this lesion the term 'bleeding polyp of the septum'.

Less frequent are haemangiomas growing from the inferior turbinates but at no site are these tumours usually larger than 2 cm, possibly because, with such a prominent mass, diagnosis is early.

Macroscopic and microscopic appearance

Although the morphological picture is one of a lobulated mass with capillary channels mixed with occasional larger vessels, inflammatory infiltration may lead to a diagnosis of granuloma pyogenica. The latter are usually reactions to local trauma being characterized by exuberant granulation tissue. Despite the similarity to capillary haemangiomata both the natural history and aetiology is different and the alarming growth of granulation tissue is due to an increased rate of cellular division, as in intubation granulomata.

Batsakis & Rice consider that in many patients, histological differentiation is possible although Michaels disagrees considering that 'treatment is the same for both'.[3,5] Treatment is by local excision but with angiomata it is essential to remove an area surrounding the base of the tumour with underlying cartilage to avoid rapid recurrence. Although relatively easy on the septum, partial resection is needed with lesions on the turbinates.

Cavernous haemangioma

There are far less common within the nasal cavity and tend to occur in patients over the age of 40 years most often on the nasal turbinates.

Dilated, thin-walled blood channels may invade underlying bone with endothelially-lined spaces actually within the marrow. The turbinate will be enlarged rather than carrying a pedunculated tumour and biopsy will cause profuse bleeding. Where feasible, local resection gives a good long-term result but extensive involvement may cause confusion with primary haemangioma of the maxilla or an angiosarcoma.

Venous haemangioma

These are usually broad-based, rarely exceeding 3 cm in diameter and grow from the nasal vestibule. Microscopically, they are composed of thick-walled venous channels and larger feeding vessels lined with flat endothelial cells. Extension into surrounding muscle or cartilage may present problems in excision.

There is no longer justification for treating any of these lesions with radiotherapy, injection of sclerosing agents or systemic steroids. Local cryosurgery may be useful as can be the argon laser but wide excision remains the procedure of choice in most instances.

NASAL GRANULOMA GRAVIDARUM (Fig. 9.1)

Vascular haemangiomatous lesions associated with pregnancy are histologically indistinguishable from pyogenic granulomata although they are usually less ulcerated. Most common within the mouth, where they may be termed 'epulis of pregnancy', in the nose they produce epistaxis. As the lesion grows, the epistaxis increases as does nasal obstruction and eventually a bleeding mass may present at the anterior nares.

McShane & Walsh[6] in reporting three patients found that diagnosis was usually made during the 3rd trimester and most patients were multiparous. Examination shows a reddish-brown mass of variable size, usually ulcerated, growing from the mucosa of the anterior end of the septum or inferior turbinate. The histological picture is identical with that found in granuloma pyogenicum[7] or epulis of pregnancy,[8] although its relationship with pregnancy and spontaneous resolution after delivery, suggests a hormonal dependence.

In 1959 Harrison discussed the effect of exogenous oestrogen on the nasal mucosa of the guinea-pig and human[9] and his findings were later developed by Taylor who demonstrated increased thickness and vascularity of the nasal mucosa with dilated subepithelial blood spaces.[10]

Helmi & El-Ghazzawi in 1975 also working with guinea-pigs given oral oestrogen, found this increased vascularity.[11] Combination between an 'oestrogen primed' mucosa together with local trauma may be the explanation for this exaggerated granulomatous response. Local removal is preferable to reduce symptoms and should present little problem under local anaesthesia. Extensive lesions are better left to await spontaneous resolution, if persisting after parturition then formal removal may be needed.

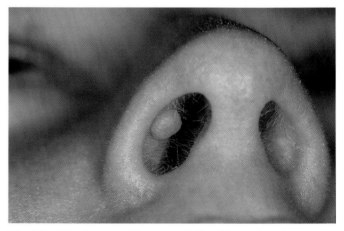

Fig. 9.1 Granuloma graviderum atypically arising on lateral vestibular wall.

Haemangioma of the maxilla

Approximately half of all bone haemangiomata occur within the vertebra where they are considered to be hamartomas. At other sites however, they are thought to be true neoplasms characterized radiologically by new bone formation. Involvement of the jaws is rare although in the 60 cases reported by Batsakis & Rice,[3] 20 were sited within the maxilla. Females apparently are affected more than males and all age groups are susceptible.

Bucy & Capps in 1930[12] first described primary haemangioma of bone but found that only 10% of all lesions within the skull were haemangiomata and these tumours are undoubtedly uncommon.

Besides a slowly progressive, painless swelling, haemangiomas may cause loosening of the teeth, bleeding or even nerve damage when situated within the maxilla (Fig. 9.2). The case reported by Ghosh et al had expansion of the maxilla with proptosis, palatal bulging and fullness in the alveolar-buccal sulcus.[13] Radiologically, there was opacity of the maxillary sinus and gross expansion of the maxilla but no 'honeycomb or soap-bubble' appearances. Biopsy via a Caldwell–Luc was reviewed by several pathologists with diagnoses ranging from fibrous dysplasia to haemangioma. Eventually, the tumour was removed by total maxillectomy with subsequent confirmation of the haemangioma. Bleeding was said to be minimal confirming suggestions that these lesions do not connect directly with main blood vessels.[14]

Nishimura et al in 1990[15] described a patient presenting with a maxillary haemangioma which also involved the zygoma. This 69-year-old male gave a 5-year history of facial swelling. CT showed an expansive soft-tissue mass within the left maxillary sinus and an irregularly mineralized matrix expanding the orbit and zygoma. MRI showed the lesion to be a low-signal intensity mass with high-signal intensity in T1 and T2 weighted images. Enhancement with gadolinium diethylenetriamine pent-

acetic acid (Gd-DTPA) showed the tumour to be similar to haemangiomata seen elsewhere in the body. Arteriography confirmed that the internal maxillary artery was a prime feeder (as it is to the normal maxilla) and this was embolized prior to biopsy via a Caldwell–Luc. Haemangioma was confirmed and this was removed by partial maxillectomy with reconstruction of the malar with a vascularized outer-table calvarial bone flap.[15]

Most maxillary haemangioma are said to be basically cavernous although a capillary component may be present. Although standard radiology may not help in definitive diagnosis both CT and MRI are clearly useful in defining vascularity as well as bone destruction.

Differential diagnosis lies between odontogenic tumours such as ameloblastoma, giant cell granuloma and myxoma.

FAMILIAL HAEMORRHAGIC TELANGIECTASES

Definition

This condition is typically characterized by the triad of multiple telangiectases, haemorrhage and a familial occurrence.

Although the most common synonym is perhaps the 'Osler-Rendu-Weber disease', Harrison[16] has suggested that there is good evidence that Benjamin Guy Babington, should have priority. In most North American publications familial is replaced by hereditary.

Historical aspects

It is generally accepted that Sutton in 1864 reported some 'curious cases of recurrent epistaxis associated with internal haemorrhages and telangiectases of the skin'.[17] The following year Babington, who also constructed the first glottiscope, published in the Lancet the clinical history of a family suffering from an inherited tendency to epistaxis.

Mrs L, a native of Lincolnshire in England, was during the whole of her early years and up to the day of her marriage, the subject of frequent and violent epistaxis. She had four children, two of whom (a male and female) likewise had habitual and severe epistaxis during all of their lives. One of them, who is my informant, had six children two of whom (both females) had frequent nose bleeds. The elder now has a son aged 19 years who has severe epistaxis, the other-unmarried continues to have frequent epistaxis.

Although habitual epistaxis was therefore noted in five generations, no mention was made of telangiectases.[18]

In 1896, Rendu reported the case of a 52-year-old man who had repeated epistaxis and small superficial angiomata on the skin of face, neck and thorax as well as the oral mucous membrane. The patient's mother and brother were similarly affected and he called this condition 'pseudohaemophilia'.[19]

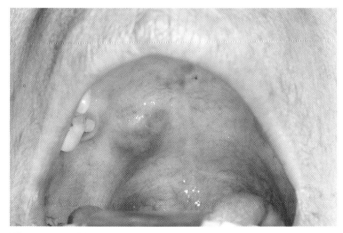

Fig. 9.2 Maxillary haemangioma.

Osler's paper in 1901 entitled 'On a family form of recurring epistaxis associated with multiple telangiectases of skin and mucous membrane', clearly describes the clinical condition that we recognize today.[20]

Weber in 1907[21] and Hanes 2 years later[22] made additional individual contributions in clarifying the clinical and pathological characteristics of this disease and it was Hanes who suggested the descriptive terminology of familial haemorrhagic telangiectasia instead of the clearly inaccurate Osler–Rendu–Weber disease.

Incidence

The hereditary nature of the vascular defect responsible for the telangiectases has been established as single, autosomal dominant, non sex-linked. Since the condition can therefore be transmitted by either sex, it is a dominant inheritance which does not permit atavism. A striking example of this was described by Wintrobe in the Mormon community. One male had 22 children by four wives, 10 of the children were affected by haemorrhagic telangiectases and transmitted the disease through four generations. Eventually, 82 affected descendants from the original progenitor were traced.[23]

Such intermarriage is of course highly dangerous for, if the genetic defect occurs in the heterozygous form in the parents, it could be transmitted by both to siblings producing the invariably fatal homozygous form.

Despite these genetic assumptions 'skipped generations' do occur but telangiectases may not appear until late in life, so long-term follow up is needed before concluding that any susceptible individual is free.

Age, sex and ethnic variation

The clinically established condition has been recognized in all European races and probably has a world-wide incidence although the skin lesions may be difficult to recognize in pigmented individuals.

Epistaxis is common in children and when occurring in families who already suffer from familial haemorrhagic telangiectases, leads to urgent consultation.

Harrison's experience of 118 patients within 38 families, all with well established disease, has demonstrated the difficulty of diagnosing this condition before the age of 20 years, although anecdotal reports of younger patients are available.[24] Suspicious mucosal lesions can be seen, particularly on the nasal mucosa, but previous cauterization makes evaluation difficult. Women appear to be more frequently affected with epistaxis and the number of telangiectases increases after the menopause.

The large personal series of patients reported by Harrison[16] found that 80% of his patients had serious bleeding by the age of 30 years and there was a female preponderance of 5:1.

Site

Diagnosis is made on the association of recurrent epistaxis, present in at least 90% of afflicted patients, cutaneous and/or mucosal telangiectases and usually a family history of the disease. Determination of the last demands time and patience but 'senior' members of the family frequently possess much 'forgotten' information regarding the illnesses of distant relatives. Although severe unexpected bleeding is usually recalled, the presence of obvious telangiectases is less so and inherent inaccuracies is inevitable in retrieval of this material.

Although any cutaneous or mucosal surface can be the site of telangiectases, it is those most susceptible to trauma that tend to bleed most often. Tongue, skin and beneath the nails show visible lesions but tend to be 'protected', whilst the nasal passages, lips or gastrointestinal tract are vulnerable to trauma. The dangers from gastro-intestinal telangiectases has been described by Baker (1953) in a family of 32 individuals, 12 of whom had familial haemorrhagic telangiectases. Five of these, all adults, had gastro-intestinal bleeding producing melaena or haematemesis. None had died at the time of the report with the eldest patient then being 52 years.[25]

Associated with this genetic-induced disability are isolated or multiple arteriovenous fistulae. Within the liver these can be fatal and in the lung produce central cyanosis.

A 41-year-old male was seen in June 1956 complaining of severe epistaxis since late childhood.[26] Many attempts had been made to control the bleeding by cauterization and nasal packing. Several close relatives, including his mother and two sisters, also suffered from epistaxis and like himself, had widespread cutaneous and mucosal telangiectases. Despite an invitation to attend for treatment his next visit was in July 1957, when in addition to increasing epistaxis he complained of increasing dyspnoea, walking being limited to 20 metres. He was a non-smoker and had no cough or haemoptysis.

Examination showed multiple telangiectases on lips, palate, dorsum of nose, finger tips, pinnae and on the nasal and oral mucosa. A localized systolic murmur was heard to the right of the midline in the 6th interspace 1 inch (2.5 cm) from the sternum. Radiology of the chest showed a sharply defined mass about 3 inches (7.5 cm) in diameter in the medial segment of the right middle lobe and a possible leash of vessels extending from the mass to the right hilum. In addition there was emphysema of the right lung. Tomography confirmed the abnormal vascular communication between hilum and mass and a selective angiocardiogram confirmed that despite the large arteriovenous fistula, arterial saturation was only slightly reduced. The dyspnoea was therefore thought to be largely the result of the emphysema, although the possibility of inadequate ventilation of the right lung was not discounted.

It was decided to delay surgical removal of the fistula and the patient was started on high-dose oestrogen therapy. His epistaxis was controlled but within 1 year the dyspnoea had increased and a lobectomy with removal of the fistula was carried out in August 1958. There has been a marked improvement in both breathing and nasal bleeding with no further arteriovenous fistulae diagnosed.

Clinical features (Figs 9.3–9.5)

The typical cutaneous lesion is purplish-red in colour, often elevated but sharply demarcated from surrounding skin. Lesions blanch on pressure, and bleed, the colour returning once the pressure is removed. The appearances are not dissimilar from acquired arterial spider naevi although usually more widespread. Although occasionally seen in the young, most telangiectases appear after puberty, becoming more numerous with increasing age, particularly after the male climacteric or menopause.[27]

Careful inspection, which can be difficult with pigmented skin, reveals numerous lesions throughout the body but generally most visible within the oral cavity and

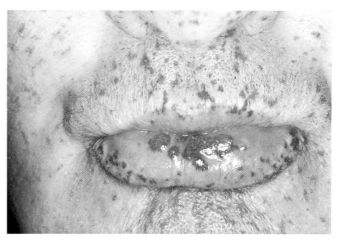

Fig. 9.4 Clinical photograph showing lips and tongue in the patient in Figure 9.3.

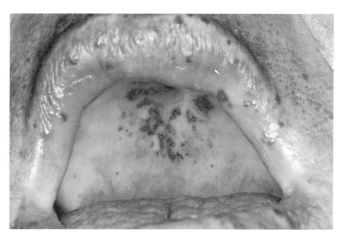

Fig. 9.5 Palatal lesions in same patient as in Figures 9.3 and 9.4.

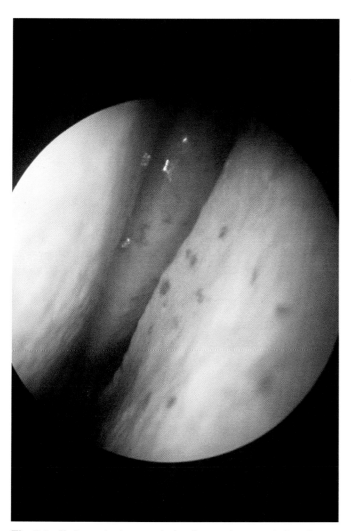

Fig. 9.3 Endoscopic photograph showing nasal mucosa in hereditary haemorrhagic telangiectasia.

particularly in the nasal passages. The anterior end of the inferior and middle turbinates and the nasal septum are common sites and these are both easily seen and traumatized.

Epistaxis occurs in more than 90% of patients although less than 70% have a well-defined family history. Bleeding is sudden and often unexpected although sneezing or nose blowing can produce severe, uncontrolled haemorrhage.[28] Intracranial, gastro-intestinal, vaginal bleeding or bleeding from other less accessible sites will be of serious consequence although within the stomach the lesions can be treated gastroscopically with laser or cryoprobe. Within the cranial cavity fatal strokes have been reported.[25]

The association between pulmonary hypertension and familial haemorrhagic telangiectasia was recorded by Sapru et al in 1969 when they reviewed patients with pulmonary arteriovenous fistulae.[29] Possibly 10% of patients with clinically established haemorrhagic telangiectases will ultimately develop an A–V fistula in liver or lung, but this may not be diagnosed for many years (Fig. 9.6).

Macroscopic and microscopic appearance (Fig. 9.7)

Hanes' original description was of superficial vessels lined by a single layer of endothelium but deficient in muscular or elastic tissue.[22] More recently, electron microscopy has developed this account showing that these large vascular channels, dilated venules of capillary or postcapillary type, are lined with a single layer of endothelial cells of varying thickness on a continuous basement membrane. Although the smooth muscle cells are elongated they do not form a continuous coat around the vessels and no elastic tissue is present in relation to the vascular spaces. It is concluded that the altered vessels are part of a systemic vascular disorder being primarily weak rather than thinned due solely to vascular dilatation. This inherited defect involves not only terminal but large vessels as is suggested by the associated finding of arteriovenous fistulae.[30,31]

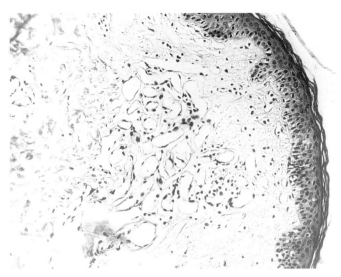

Fig. 9.7   Histology section through inferior turbinate showing large vascular spaces in patient with hereditary haemorrhagic telangiectasia.

It is of some interest that the studies of Menefee et al included some patients previously treated with exogenous oestrogen. They found that post therapy biopsies in these individuals showed reconstruction of vascular integrity without any endothelial gaps or degenerative changes.[31]

Natural history

Even in the presence of a well established family history, diagnosis is dependent upon the observation of telangiectases, for epistaxis alone is indicative of many conditions. In childhood it is primarily related to mild trauma and is rarely severe. Our personal study of the members of 38 families covering at least four generations, confirms that 'missed members' did occur even after prolonged follow-up. In addition, individuals' natural history in relation to the progression of the disease and the problems caused, varies from individual to individual, being unrelated to age at diagnosis. However, there do appear to be 'bad families' where the afflicted members suffer from progressive disease. Our understanding of this awaits more detailed genetic studies.

Koch et al in 1952 was the first to observe that in affected women, bleeding from nasal telangiectases was often worse at the end of the menstrual cycle, after ovariectomy or at the menopause – all times of low circulating oestrogen.[32] It is interesting that some woman taking the 'contraceptive pill' notice a reduction in the severity of their epistaxis.

Despite 'family guidelines' there is no sure way of anticipating whether telangiectases will appear or in what number, nor the likelihood of severe symptoms in an apparently unaffected member of an afflicted family. Every member must be followed up or at least encouraged to seek help if any symptoms appear. Harrison

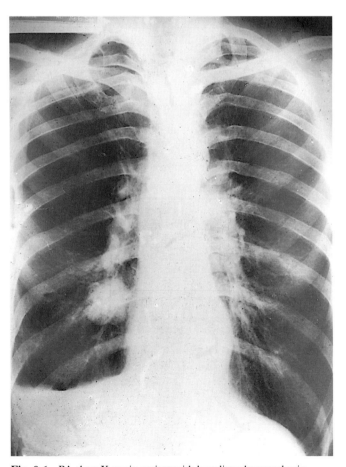

Fig. 9.6   PA chest X-ray in patient with hereditary haemorrhagic telangiectasia showing pulmonary vascular anomalies.

found that approximately 80% of his 118 patients had significant symptoms or signs by the age of 30 years, irrespective of their sex. However, Koch et al reported that the most severe symptoms were found in 68% of the women after the age of 45 years.[32] This varies with the findings of McCaffrey et al but the difference is possibly related to the patterns of referral and the longer follow-up in Harrison's personal series.[28]

Differential diagnosis

There is usually little difficulty in identifying untreated telangiectases in well established cases, although isolated lesions may be confused with spider naevi particularly in the absence of a clear family history.[27] However, epistaxis is common in many blood diseases and haematological evaluation is essential in every patient particularly since most patients with continual blood loss are anaemic. It is in fact this persistent, unexpected, uncontrolled bleeding which is the primary purpose of seeking treatment although the cutaneous telangiectases can be displeasing!

Treatment

A wide variety of therapeutic measures have been applied to the nasal, lingual and buccal lesions since they cause most of the bleeding problems, and are relatively accessible. Even the correction of the associated anaemia may present difficulties, for some patients will have had over 200 transfusions and the development of antibodies can limit suitable supplies of blood.

Applications of caustic agents, submucosal injections of sclerosing fluids, local coagulation with snake venom, even the use of irradiation have all found favour. Unfortunately, the thin-walled vascular spaces are easily traumatized by these procedures and prove difficult to seal with any degree of permanence. In addition, the inherited vascular abnormality ensures that all blood vessels are susceptible to the production of telangiectases and re-vascularization, even after radiotherapy, can see the development of new lesions.

Pressure within the nasal cavity, using a balloon rather than packing which further damages the telangiectases, offers immediate control but it is the unpredictable nature of the bleeding which affects most patients' lives.

When there are only a few lesions readily accessible within the nasal cavity, local coagulation, particularly with the potassium-titanyl phosphate laser (KTP/532) or Argon laser which offer good tissue discrimination and preferential absorption of reddish pigments, can provide reasonable short-term palliation.[33]

More troublesome cases can be offered intranasal dermoplasty as described by Saunders in 1960.[34] In essence this surgical technique consists of removing the mucosa from the anterior part of the nasal septum, nasal floor and as much of the lateral wall as proves feasible. The denuded area is then covered with a split-thickness skin graft held in place by packing. An external alar incision is often needed to provide access to more posterior septal lesions and the graft is better stuck to the bed with tissue glue thus avoiding the trauma of nasal packing. Severe operative bleeding can make this a difficult procedure although it can be assisted by the initial submucosal injection of vasoconstrictor agents prior to elevation of the nasal mucosa. This is always difficult to remove from the turbinates particularly after previous enthusiastic cauterization or laser coagulation.

Graft contraction unveiling residual lesions has been blamed on poor technique and the grafting should certainly be as large as possible to produce the best effect (Fig. 9.8). Revascularization is inevitable and carries some risk of new telangiectases although this may take 5 years or more.[24,35]

More recently midfacial degloving has provided an excellent approach to both sides of the nose at one operation enabling the affected mucosa to be removed as far posteriorly as required.

Laurian et al in 1979 recommended the use of amniotic membrane to graft the denuded area rather than skin, claiming superiority because of good adherence-haemostasis and subsequent vascular penetration.[36] They reported six patients with trouble-free follow-up for 9 to 30 months. However, this material is not easily available in the fresh state and good revascularization may prove to be a disadvantage!

With the development of effective techniques for the management of massive traumatic epistaxis using selective arteriography with embolization, it was inevitable that this procedure would find a place in the prophy-

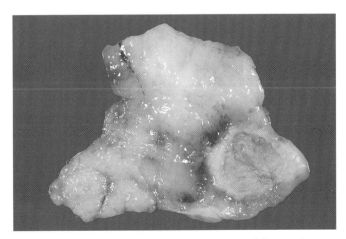

Fig. 9.8 Operative specimen: septal mucosa removed from patient with hereditary haemorrhagic telangiectasia who had undergone previous septodermoplasty. The skin graft is considerably contracted and surrounded by telangiectasia.

lactic treatment of familial haemorrhagic telangiectases. Merland et al treated 17 patients with only one failure[37] and Strother & Newton also reported the use of embolization of both internal maxillary arteries in a 40-year-old man with a 14 year history of frequent hospitalization for severe nasal bleeding from 'Osler-Rendu-Weber' disease. Follow-up was only 6 months but gave good palliation.[38] However, since any of the blood supply to the nasal cavity can be the origin of telangiectases it is not feasible to destroy all the vessels thus jeopardizing normal tissues. Although reasonable palliation can be obtained by selective embolization, and the technique is repeatable, revascularization brings new vessels and of course the chance of new lesions. The procedure is time consuming, requires considerable expertise and carries a small but significant morbidity.

Following observations that there appears to be a hormonal influence on the frequency of bleeding in women with familial haemorrhagic telangiectasia, Koch et al treated a few patients with systemic oestrogen.[32] In 1955, following animal experimentation on the effects of stilboestrol implants on the nasal mucosa of guinea–pigs, Harrison treated 20 patients suffering from familial haemorrhagic telangiectasia with systemic ethinyloestradiol. Biopsies confirmed that although the lesions appeared to remain untouched, the overlying mucosa changed to the more protective squamous state.[24]

Ethinyloestradiol was chosen because of its availability in 1 mg grooved tablets allowing multiples of 0.25 mg to be prescribed as a single dose. Prior to beginning treatment the rationale is explained to each patient, particularly the inevitable side effects. In the male loss of libido, testicular atrophy and gynaecomastica. In the female 'break through' bleeding for those with a uterus but of course freedom from post-menopausal symptoms. Contraindications include previous neoplasia of the sex organs, history of venous thrombosis or liver disease and of course poor motivation! All potential patients are first evaluated by a thorough physical, haematological and biochemical examination to eliminate systemic disease that might be adversely affected by oestrogen given in large doses. Even so, selection of patients for therapy followed a rigid criteria for in 1955 the long-term effects of exogenous oestrogen were unknown. However, selected patients had all demanded relief from their frequent severe unpredictable epistaxis previously having failed to get this from other therapies.

In 1982 Harrison reported his long-term experience with 67 patients (52 female, 10 male) treated with oestrogen over a total period of 25 years. No cases of uterine, cervical or breast cancer had occurred although eight women had cervical polyps and two had hysterectomies for oestrogen-induced metropathia. Three of the men ceased treatment because of unacceptable side effects. The women's age of commencement of treatment varied between 38 and 53 years with the longest period of continuous therapy being 10 years. This patient had taken a total of 130 g of ethinyloestradiol.[24]

Improvement in the frequency and severity of epistaxis was obtained in every patient who continued with medication, although nasal crusting proved to be a persistent problem. Removal of these crusts, part of the protective mechanism, provoked bleeding and nasal packing was a disaster as it effectively removed the squamous covering.[27]

There seems no doubt that systemic oestrogen and other preparations could prove to be as effective and possibly with less side effects, and can dramatically improve nasal bleeding in many of these patients. However, the administration of large doses of oestrogen to women of any age must be viewed with caution although there is no evidence that potential dangers are dose-related.

Familial haemorrhagic telangiectases is a demoralizing, frightening, messy disease which is difficult to control in many patients. Perhaps treatment can best be summarized as 'dermoplasty for the young or accessible telangiectases – carefully controlled oestrogen for the failures or those with very extensive nasal lesions not amenable to other modalities'.

JUVENILE ANGIOFIBROMA

Definition

Although morphologically benign, this tumour can exhibit aggressive local growth extending along planes of least resistance or preformed pathways and, when large, can invade directly by bone erosion.

Prior to the development of sophisticated radiological techniques the site of origin was confidentially placed within the nasopharynx, the region where growth is most easily detected. The term nasopharyngeal angiofibroma, usually coupled with juvenile because of the young age at which diagnosis is made, is now firmly established within medical folklore, despite being proven to be inaccurate!

Historical aspects (p. 173)

Although it has been suggested, with little in the way of documentary evidence, that Hippocrates had recognized and removed this tumour presenting as a nasal polyp, Chelius[39] in 1847 described a 'fibrous nasal polyp which commonly occurs in persons around the time of puberty'! No mention was made of a male dominance or a propensity to bleed and this lesion may well have been an antrochoanal polyp. Several years later Legouest commented that these tumours occurred primarily in males[40] and Chaveau in 1906 introduced the name 'Juvenile nasopharyngeal angioma'.[41] However, not until 1940 did Friedberg add the 'Angiofibroma' following his histological studies on operative specimens.[42]

Incidence

Whilst recognizing that these are rare lesions occurring primarily in adolescent males and representing less than 0.05% of all head and neck tumours, the true incidence is speculative. Spector gives a figure of 1.6 per 16 000 ENT patients,[43] Chandler et al quote 1 per 50 000 patients[44] whilst Tandon et al give 1 per 9380 new out-patients.[45] The literature abounds with small personal series as well as collective experiences of more than 100 patients from major referral centres.

There is however, no substantive evidence of a definite ethnic susceptibility and it is likely that the large series reported from India and Egypt merely reflect local referral patterns to the few centres of expertise. Consequently, these cases tend to be more advanced failures from inadequate primary therapy or late diagnosis, thus giving an erroneous impression of variations in natural history in different ethnic groups.

There appears to be general agreement that this is a male dominated condition, although the age at diagnosis ranges widely between 5 and 50 years, the latter figure reported by Tandon et al from Delhi, India.[45] The median age is around 13 years and age association may be of importance when considering possible metamorphosis to malignancy. Makek et al found that half of the reported cases of malignant transformation, usually after previous radiotherapy or multiple surgical removals, occurred in those patients whose angiofibroma was diagnosed after the age of 25 years.[46]

It is perhaps surprising that despite differences in ethnic maturity, there is close agreement worldwide in the median age of diagnosis for it is the hormonal changes at puberty that are thought to be the primary influence on the growth of this tumour. Angiofibroma has occasionally been reported in woman. Fitzpatrick et al had two females aged 14 and 36 years in their series of 48 patients[47] and Cummings et al reported two more aged 14 and 19 years in their Canadian group of 43 patients.[48] One of the earliest and best documented cases of a female with a postnasal angiofibroma was described by Osbourne & Sokoloski in 1965.[49] The latter was an experienced head and neck pathologist and the sex and histological diagnosis were not in doubt, which is in contradistinction to some other case reports of this unusual occurrence.

Site and aetiology

It is possible that relatively unsophisticated radiological assessment together with the limited information provided by the transpalatal approach, has been responsible for the erroneous assumption that angiofibroma arise within the nasopharynx. The place of origin is clearly the area related to the superior margin of the sphenopalatine foramen which forms the junction of the sphenoidal process of the palatine bone and the pterygoid process of the sphenoid.[50] Erosion of the base of the medial pterygoid plate with enlargement of the sphenopalatine foramen is a constant radiological feature[51] and from this origin tumour can spread laterally through the pterygopalatine fissure into the fossa and infratemporal space. Extension into orbit, paranasal sinuses, nasal cavity or posteriorly to fill the empty nasopharynx is common with eventually intracranial extension along planes of least resistance or preferred pathways without necessarily producing bone erosion.

The base of the tumour may be narrow and pedunculated or broad extending over the whole entrance to the pterygopalatine fossa, making total removal impractical. Additional secondary attachments from pressure ulceration of epithelium covering bone or cartilage is common in the nasopharynx or nasal cavity causing suspicion of additional sites of origin. Such vascular adhesions are not usually seen within the pterygopalatine fossa or sphenoidal sinus.

Having established the site of origin, most of the earlier proposals regarding aetiology are now viewed as being only of historical interest. The ventral periosteum, craniopharyngeal duct and fascia basalis all attracted some attention in their time. However, in 1942 Brunner examining sections of the heads of two full-term human embryos found endothelially-lined vascular spaces within the fascia basilis in the region of the sphenoid.[52] Harrison (1987) also examined serially sectioned foetal heads (24-weeks-old) cut in the coronal and axial planes, finding large endothelially-lined spaces in the region of the sphenopalatine foramen and base of the pterygoid plates, in both male and female specimens.[53] The known male preponderance, together with the relatively restricted age at diagnosis has promoted the proposition that the aetiology of angiofibroma is a haematomatous ectopic nidus of vascular tissue, perhaps misplaced sequestrated genital tissue, awaiting the stimulus at puberty by male hormones.[54] Antonelli et al[55] analysed cytosol from the tumours of five male patients, obtaining negative values for both oestrogen and progesterone receptors but a highly positive figure for dehydrotestosterone receptors. They concluded that juvenile angiofibromata were androgen-dependent and this confirmed earlier proposals of Martin et al in 1948[40] that these tumours were hormonally influenced. Schiff[56] put forward his hypothesis in 1959 that the tumour was due to an alteration in the androgen–oestrogen axis stimulating ectopic sex-sensitive vascular tissue. Certainly, a nidus of vascular tissue appears to be sited at the known site of origin but there is no evidence of a specific endocrine abnormality in males with this tumour. Fitzpatrick et al carried out detailed endocrine assessment of 11 young males with angiofibromata without detecting any abnormality.[47] However, our understanding of the complex series of hormonal changes underlying the events of puberty remains fragmentary. Only recently have reliable techniques been developed for measuring the small changes that take place in the blood and urine during puberty. Adolescence is initiated by the brain not pituitary gland, being controlled by hormones each of which acts on a set of targets or receptors that exist in a variety of organs or tissues. Detailed evaluation of these levels in patients of all ages, and particularly in the rare female with angiofibromas, may eventually offer some explanation for variations in the aetiology and natural history of this unusual tumour.

Clinical features (Figs 9.9 and 9.10)

Early symptoms of nasal obstruction and intermittent epistaxis are found in combination or singly in over 80% of patients. As the tumour extends from its site of origin there may be additional symptoms of facial swelling, proptosis, bulging palate, deafness, sinusitis or cranial nerve paresis. Apart from nasal obstruction the frequency with which other symptoms present at diagnosis reflect variations in rate of growth, patterns of extension and the stage reached by the tumour. Epistaxis has not been a constant feature in the series of 46 males seen at the Professorial Unit, Royal National Throat, Nose and Ear Hospital, London. It was concluded that in the absence of local trauma, such as biopsy, bleeding is a reflection of the angiomatous content of the lesion which can vary from a near angioma to a non-vascular fibroma. Intracranial extension can be present however without

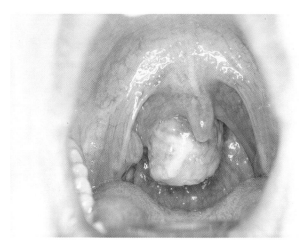

Fig. 9.10   Angiofibroma presenting in postnasal space.

any additional clinical symptoms and the real frequency of this problem cannot be determined solely on clinical grounds.[57]

Physical examination, including rhinoscopy and nasopharyngoscopy preferably using fibre optic instrumentation, invariably confirms the presence of a mass obstructing the posterior nares. The appearance depends upon the vascularity but is usually described as reddish-grey, lobulated with a smooth surface on which blood vessels may be seen. Since the degree of vascularity cannot be determined clinically, although palpation does differentiate between the 'rock hard' fibroangioma and the soft compressible angiofibroma, the dangers of excessive bleeding should preclude biopsy. Diagnosis can now be made with near certainty radiologically, which also allows accurate assessment of tumour extent and vascularity.

Radiology (Figs 9.11–9.15)

Erosion of the base of the medial pterygoid plate, associated with enlargement of the sphenopalatine foramen was demonstrated in all 46 patients reported by Lund et al[51] when examined by conventional or computerized tomography (CT). Indentation of the posterior wall of the maxillary antrum, the antral sign, shown on lateral plain X-rays, confirms a mass within the pterygopalatine fossa and has been reported as being present in over 80% of patients with angiofibromata.[51,58]

However, this can be found in any slow growing lesion in this area and is not pathognomonic of angiofibroma. Computerized tomography with contrast enhancement has added a new degree of accuracy to both diagnosis and analysis of tumour extent and must now be viewed as an essential investigation in every patient.

Involvement of sphenoid sinus, infratemporal fossa, orbit or middle cranial fossa is well demonstrated since

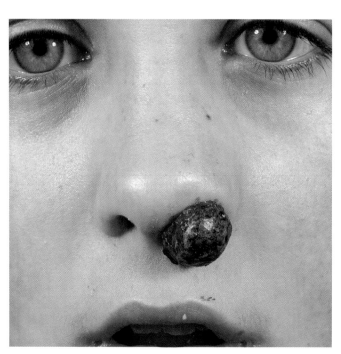

Fig. 9.9   Young boy with angiofibroma protuding from nasal cavity.

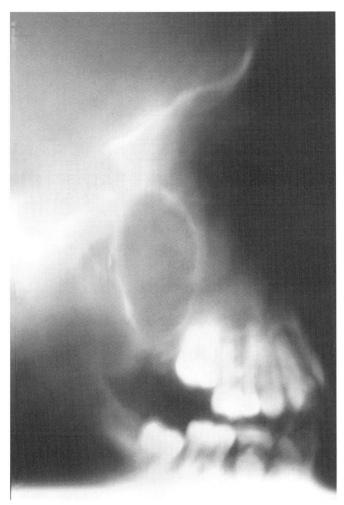

Fig. 9.11 Juvenile angiofibroma: lateral hypocycloidal tomogram showing 'antral' sign with anterior bowing of posterior maxillary wall.

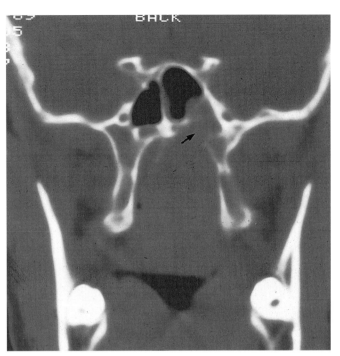

Fig. 9.12 Coronal CT scan showing erosion of medial pterygoid plate by juvenile angiofibroma (arrowed).

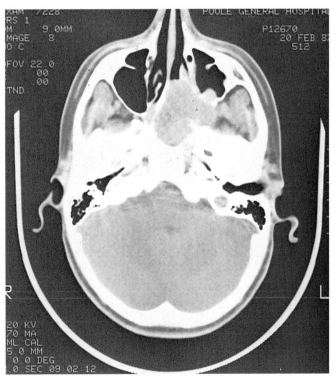

Fig. 9.13 Axial CT scan showing widening of the sphenopalatine foramen with extension of the angiofibroma into the infratemporal fossa.

surrounding tissues have smaller attenuation coefficients. Some estimate of the longest linear dimension of the tumour is possible with figures ranging from 2 to 7 cm.[59] A more accurate estimate of size relative to adjacent structures can be defined by magnetic resonance imaging (MRI) using 3-plane imaging and T2 weighted spin echo sequences. The distinction between the mass and fluid in an obstructed sinus can be made and the vascularity of the lesion   clearly indicated by signal voids from the vessels within the angiofibroma. Optimum demonstration of extent of tumour is now by gadolinium-enhanced MRI.

Routine CT forms the basis of existing classification systems and this has to some extent reduced the necessity for routine diagnostic angiography, except for preoperative embolization, the need for which remains in some doubt although favoured by Roberson et al.[60] However, if surgical removal is planned for the larger intracranial lesions, bilateral carotid angiography is essential to delineate tumour blood supply. Identification of a supply from the internal carotid artery or invasion of this vessel is important since the artery can safely be managed providing knowledge of involvement has been established preoperatively.[43] Although most angiofibroma derive their main

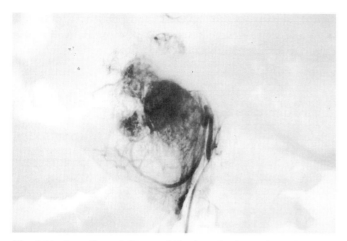

Fig. 9.14 Juvenile angiofibroma following selective angiography.

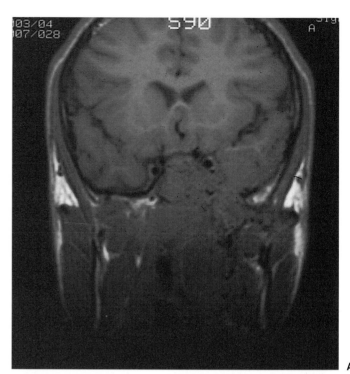

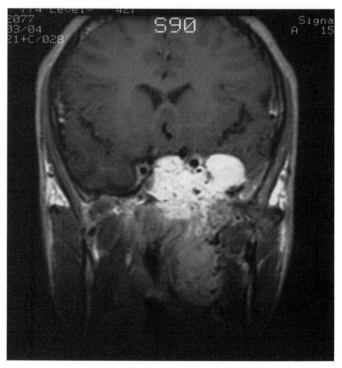

Fig. 9.15 Large juvenile angiofibroma extending into middle cranial fossa. **A**, coronal MR scan, T1 weighted sequence. **B**, same scan, post-gadolinium showing significant enhancement of tumour mass with signal voids in areas of large vessels producing classical 'salt and pepper' appearance.

blood supply from the internal maxillary artery, which is to be expected in view of their site of origin, arteriography shows that additional supplies may come from the sphenoidal and ophthalmic branches of the internal carotid as well as from the ascending pharyngeal and palatal branches of the external carotid artery. The distinction between real and false supply from the internal carotid is important.[61] Intrasphenoidal extension frequently recruits a vascular supply from the capsular vessels. Posterior ethmoidal arteries provide a supply from the ophthalmic artery and numerous anastomoses exist between the cavernous part of the internal carotid and distal maxillary artery branches giving a false impression of tumour extent as well as significant blood supply.[50] Routine angiography however, has confirmed that in large tumours a substantial blood supply comes from the arteries on the contralateral side from the tumour, thus limiting the potential value of embolization or balloon catheterization, except during surgery.

Biller[62] limits embolization to large tumours which are shown to be fed by both the internal and external carotid systems or in only partially resectable lesions. Routine angiography, bearing in mind the potential morbidity, is not necessary if CT or MRI is available, unless there is suspected intracranial extension.

Staging systems

Although not strictly comparable with classifications for malignant neoplasms most authors have recognized the value of a classification system in planning and assessing treatment regimes for angiofibroma. Session's system described in 1981 was based upon anatomical location, being similar to that used for nasopharyngeal carcinoma.[63] However, this proved to be imprecise, particularly with more extensive lesions and failed to consider patterns of growth. Chandler et al in 1984 modified this system but again failed to consider the complexities of intracranial

extension, possibly because of limited experience of modern radiological techniques.[44] These defects became more apparent as surgical techniques themselves improved and Andrews et al in 1988[64] proposed a staging system that attempted to follow the growth and spread of these tumours as revealed by the experience of Ugo Fisch.[65]

Class 1 lesions. These are confined to their site of origin at the sphenopalatine foramen and may extend into the nasopharynx or nasal cavity.

Class 2 lesions. The next sequence of extension involves the pterygopalatine fossa or paranasal sinuses.

Class 3 lesions. These involve the infratemporal fossa or orbit with the subdivision 3a for those remaining extracranial and 3b for lesions with involvement of the parasellar region.

Class 4 lesions. These are again divided with 4a being extradural and 4b being reserved for the most extensive aggressive angiofibromata. These will have grown into the cavernous sinus, pituitary fossa or optic chiasma.

This has proven to be the most logical and practical system to date with close correlation to the difficulty of tumour extirpation and is now in general use.

Macroscopic and microscopic appearance

When viewed in situ angiofibroma are red, but on palpation are of variable consistency depending upon the ratio between angiomatous and fibrous elements within the tumour. Following excision, they are seen as lobulated masses with a base of varying width, and a grey or pinkish-grey appearance (Fig. 9.16). Dilated vessels may be seen on the surface and bleeding from these may be responsible for the continued blood loss during surgical exposure.[66]

Microscopically, angiofibroma have a characteristic structure of blood vessels set in a stroma of fibroblasts and collagen. Michaels has described the histology as showing the deeper vessels as thickened but superficially

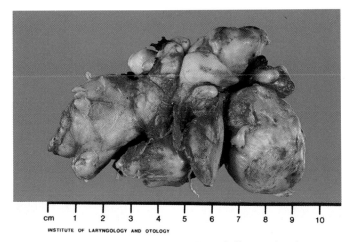

Fig. 9.16 Operative specimen of juvenile angiofibroma showing lobulations which extend into the sphenoid, nasopharynx and infratemporal fossa.

the vessel walls may be thin with little or no muscle fibres. Endothelial cells in the vessel walls have been called 'angioblasts' with the suggestion that stromal fibroblasts are derived from them, although immunological stains dispute this hypothesis.[5]

Organized thrombi of varying ages are commonly seen within the lumen of vessels and there is some evidence that the volume of collagen is related to the age of the patient. Serial sections through the tumour show varying amounts of angiomatous tissue and stroma, making objective assessment of the relative quantity of each impossible to make with accuracy. However, some lesions are predominantly fibrous and may be considered as the end stage of involution.

Spontaneous malignant change has not been verified although sarcomas do occur following repeated surgical removals as well as high dose irradiation. Makek et al[46] described the development of a fibrosarcoma after four operations and two courses of irradiation, 17 years after a transpalatal removal of a proven angiofibroma. The first recurrence was treated with 4500 cGy of Cobalt-60; 5 years later another 4050 cGy was given and 2 years later a fibrosarcoma was diagnosed. This was removed surgically with a 10-year tumour-free follow-up. They reviewed five other case reports of malignant change all of whom had multiple operations as well as radiotherapy, the dosage varying from 3000 cGy to a massive 12 000 cGy. The interval between the irradiation and diagnosis of malignancy varied from 11 months to 21 years. The neoplasm was in most cases a fibrosarcoma but in one patient it was called a malignant fibrous histiocytoma.[67–70] Makek et al commented in their paper that it appeared likely that the fibrous component of the angiofibroma was the source of the neoplastic change.[46] These stellate fibrocytes or myofibroblasts within the connective tissue matrix are often multinucleated and can show some hyperchromatism. Hubbard[71] noted that there is often an apparent increase in fibrous tissue within the angiofibroma of older patients and this may play some part in any subsequent malignant change following radiotherapy.

It is of particular interest that amongst the 55 patients treated by Cummings et al with radiotherapy for angiofibroma,[48] two later developed malignant tumours within the head and neck. One thyroid carcinoma occurred 14 years after receiving 3500 cGy and the other, a basal cell carcinoma followed two doses of 3500 cGy separated by an interval of 8 years. The latter was diagnosed 13 years after the initial irradiation.

Natural history

Despite the considerable interest shown in this unusual tumour there is little factual evidence to support a common belief that with increasing age angiofibroma will show spontaneous involution. Patients are diagnosed when presenting with symptoms which require treatment and only an untreated control series, followed up with regular radiological assessment would confirm that eventually involution does occur. Meanwhile of course extension into inaccessible sites would produce increasing symptoms – an unethical situation. However, reports by Jacobsson et al[72] and Stansbie & Phelps[73] have confirmed by radiological follow-up that even intracranial extensions can cease to grow after cessation of unsuccessful surgical excision. The absence of a true capsule together with a broad base of attachment to the base of the pterygoid plates inevitably leads to some remnants of tumour left in situ, even after an apparently radical removal. Since many angiofibromas are in fact fibro-angiomas, reduction in the blood supply to a largely fibrous tumour will result in minimal symptomless regrowth. Changes in the 'stimulating androgen' levels, if this be the prime initiating factor, may also play some part in involution. None of this can however be anticipated and there is no proven relationship between age and 'tumour aggressiveness'. Consequently, all untreated cases must be viewed as possessing potential for continued growth. There is some largely anecdotal evidence that with increasing age there is a reduced tendency for angiofibromas to bleed, possibly from reduction in the angiomatous content. However, we have experienced continued growth of an extremely vascular lesion in a man aged 29 years and there are many variations in natural history.

The routine use of CT shows that even in symptomless patients following apparently successful excision, small recurrences are common although frequently slow to grow. In the absence of any reliable evidence to the contrary it must be assumed that all untreated angiofibromas possess potential for aggressive growth.

Evaluation of residual tumour will therefore take into account the histopathology of operative specimens, site of recurrence and rate of growth as shown by radiological assessment.

Differential diagnosis

Symptoms of nasal obstruction and epistaxis in male adolescents when associated with a nasal or postnasal mass and radiological evidence of bone destruction in the region of the sphenopalatine foramen is pathognomonic of angiofibroma. Nasal obstruction alone within this age group can indicate adenoids or an antrochoanal polyp, neither of which produce these changes on radiology. Any slow growing tumour within the pterygopalatine fossa can produce bowing of the posterior antral wall. Neurilemmoma, haemangiopericytoma or rhabdomyosarcoma can all mimic the vascular changes seen on MRI or even arteriography, and biopsy may be needed to differentiate between angiofibroma and these neoplasms.

However, thorough radiological evaluation has now replaced routine biopsy of suspected angiofibromata, which frequently, in a predominately fibrous lesion, proved both dangerous and unhelpful.

Treatment

For purposes of treatment planning, it is essential to evaluate not only the site of origin of this tumour but the pathways of potential extension. Failure to appreciate these factors has resulted in a high incidence of incomplete removal together with significant morbidity, even mortality, for patients who die do so as the result of treatment, not from their tumour![74]

The proportion of vascular 'angiomatous' tissue to surrounding avascular stroma varies within individual tumours as well as between patients, although possibly less so with increasing age. Since the tumour is uncapsulated, total removal is not only related to accessibility but also to the ease with which the base can be detached from underlying bone or surrounding structures. With the advent of superior diagnostic imaging modalities, surgical techniques have moved away from the earlier 'routine transpalatal' approach to a state where the operation is chosen to fit each individual tumour and all its ramifications. With lesions involving the skull base, excision demands special expertise for, as with most malignant tumours, the greatest chance of success lies with the first operation.

Despite the many papers detailing treatment strategies uniformity has not been reached as to the most practical classification system or the most appropriate surgical technique for individual stages of tumour extension. 'Success rate or cure' are inappropriate terms when evaluating treatment modalities in this instance since the presence of asymptomatic disease cannot necessarily be considered failure of treatment. However, persistent or recurrent symptomatic tumour does require further intervention and may be the most realistic measure of therapeutic effectiveness.[75] Consequently, the frequency with which specific operations are advocated or practised will reflect not only an individual's surgical experience but the type of case requiring treatment. Secondary referrals are frequently more extensive requiring more complex surgery. Wide exposure is the key to safe and complete removal yet the transpalatal approach, historically the first and possibly still the most commonly used, only exposes the anterior and caudal surfaces of the angiofibroma.[76]

Neither the base nor posterior surfaces can be seen and the use of 'forceps avulsion' is followed by considerable blood loss. Lateral extension into the pterygopalatine fossa, too small for radiological detection, will be left in situ. In many patients this operation is combined with an additional transantral or fronto-ethmoid approach.[77] Success in managing early lesions by this means has been reported by Sardana,[76] Neel et al,[78] Gill et al,[79] and Economou et al[75] but failure to visualize the tumour base and difficulties in controlling haemorrhage are serious disadvantages.

A more logical approach to the pterygoid plates, pterygopalatine fossa or maxillary sinus utilizes a lateral rhinotomy incision. The value of this operation had been underestimated until Harrison in 1977 discussed its use for a wide range of pathologies within the nasal cavity and paranasal sinuses.[50] Medial maxillectomy, a term which evolved shortly after publication of this paper, has little meaning since lateral rhinotomy is an incision not an operation! For removal of angiofibromata it is necessary not only to remove the medial wall of the maxillary antrum but also much of the medial wall of the orbit. Neel et al gives a detailed description of the technicalities of this approach and it was the primary method of treatment used in the Mayo Clinic for 85 patients[78] and for 31 patients operated upon by the Professorial unit at the Royal National Throat, Nose and Ear Hospital, London. A Weber–Fergusson extension may be needed to give adequate exposure of the infratemporal fossa.

Although this approach gives direct visualization of the tumour base and its extracranial extensions, some facial scarring and occasional epiphora is unavoidable. Complications of the transpalatal approach are minimal with a small number of palatal dehiscences and short-lived rhinolalia.

The midfacial degloving operation, first published by Casson et al in 1974[80] gives excellent access to the whole of the nasosinal area without the need for a facial incision. Although the concept was developed in the mid 1960s, acceptance of the intrinsic value of this operation in removing angiofibroma has been tardy. The pterygoid musculature and plate, posterior wall of sphenoidal sinus and the clivus are the posterior limits of excision. Superiorly, removal is limited by the cribriform plate, whilst laterally dissection reaches as far as the coronoid process of the mandible. Inferiorly lies the palate. Control of the internal maxillary artery is easy and, apart from infraorbital numbness, complications are limited to postoperative crusting and occasional vestibular stenosis. Extension into the cheek is readily managed and exposure of maxillary, ethmoidal and sphenoid sinuses is far superior to a transpalatal approach whilst avoiding the facial scarring of a lateral rhinotomy. This operation has been used in the last 14 patients treated at the Throat, Nose and Ear Hospital and is now the procedure of first choice.

The real incidence of late stage angiofibroma with intracranial invasion is impossible to quantify since it is dependent on adequate radiological assessment and tends to be localized to institutions experienced in skull base surgery. Andrews et al reported a 75% incidence of intracranial invasion in their series of 51 angiofibromas, 37% of whom had compression or infiltration of the cavernous sinus.[64] Close et al also had a 35% incidence of cavernous sinus involvement in 17 patients.[57] In our group of 46 patients there were no primary cases of late stage involvement, whereas Economou et al[75] had a 21% incidence of late stage tumours, 17 in a total of 44.

In the past, failure to establish effective surgical management for these large tumours led to the routine use of radiotherapy or a policy of 'watchful optimism'. Development of a magnified approach to the anterior cranial fossa and skull base has resulted in a reappraisal of the surgical possibilities in many of these extensive angiofibromata.[57,64] Following delineation with high-resolution CT and MRI, angiography is needed to determine not only tumour blood supply but particularly the role played by the internal carotid artery. Preoperative embolization and when required balloon catheter occlusion of the artery, provides essential information prior to surgical excision, particularly with reference to morbidity rates associated with sacrifice of the internal carotid. Combinations of a lateral infratemporal approach with midfacial degloving or fronto-ethmoid removal gives excellent visualization of the extradural aspects of the margins of the cavernous sinus.[57] Most of these tumours are extradural and can be dissected free from dural attachments. Bleeding from the venous cavernous plexus and temporary damage to the abducens (cranial nerve VI) is possible but this technique is both safe and effective.

Embolization

When contemplating the surgical excision of any vascular lesion it is desirable to reduce the blood supply if possible to facilitate removal and thus minimize operative morbidity. Embolizing the vascular bed may be preferable to ligating feeding vessels, many of which may be inaccessible. If intravascular thrombosis is to be obtained careful choice of embolic material, accurate angiographic assessment as well as the timing of subsequent surgery, is essential. Prior to the availability of CT and MRI, angiography was used primarily to verify diagnosis or, less often, as a means of embolization of tumour blood supply. Its success has been quantified as producing 'reduction in operative blood loss' rather than the more informative 'percentage of total blood volume lost'. Anecdotal accounts of reduction in the expected amount of bleeding may simply be related to a more accessible, largely fibrous lesion, whereas quantity of blood replaced will be related to individual blood volume. There is some disparity regarding the role of embolization in the management of angiofibromas, except when there is evidence of intracranial extension.[61]

Robertson et al were the first to recommend its use either as an adjunct to surgery or a definitive treatment.[60] Although external carotid ligation is of little value, due to the extensive collateral circulation, the internal maxillary artery is accessible for ligation via both the lateral rhinotomy or midface degloving approach. Since much of the support for embolization is anecdotal there is as yet no clearly defined policy for its routine use except when radiology confirms intracranial extension. However, McCombe et al[81] have commented on a potential disadvantage of preoperative embolization. Shrinkage of the tumour may result in incomplete removal by allowing small areas of tumour to remain undetected although potentially active. In six patients embolized before apparently successful surgery all developed local regrowth, all within 10 months. Both the incidence and speed of regrowth were independent of original tumour size.

At the age of 13 years, Stephen had an adenoidectomy with bilateral myringotomies for severe nasal obstruction, occasional nose bleeds and a suspected bearing loss.

1 year later his symptoms had worsened; examination revealed unilateral secretory otitis media and a swelling filling the nasopharynx. Fluid was aspirated from the ear and the postnasal mass was biopsied. This produced moderate haemorrhage and an inconclusive report!

He was referred in March 1985 following a CT scan which confirmed the mass filling the nasopharynx which extended into the nasal cavity deviating the nasal septum. The posterior wall of the maxillary antrum was pushed anteriorly and there was some suspicion of erosion of the greater wing of the sphenoid. The absorption measure of the mass prior to contrast was 20.8 EMI which rose to an average of 45 units after contrast.

Prior to surgical excision May 1985, a carotid angiogram with embolization of the ascending pharyngeal and branches of the maxillary artery was performed. 2 days later, following recovery from this exhausting experience, the angiofibroma was removed completely via a lateral rhinotomy approach. The base was attached to the pterygoid plates, bleeding minimal with a measured loss of only 200 ml. Within 6 months fluid had collected again within the right middle ear and regrowth of angiofibroma was visible in the region of the right sphenopalatine fissure. CT scanning showed this to be extending into the infratemporal fossa pushing the buccal fat pad forward beneath the right cheek.

In December 1985 this regrowth was approached via a Weber–Fergusson incision. Bony defects were found in the floor of the orbit as well as the posterior and posterolateral walls of the maxillary sinus. The internal maxillary artery was tied and the mass removed by avulsion with a blood loss of 1800 ml.

In July 1986 he was re-examined because of recurrent epistaxis, biopsy confirmed a small regrowth on the right lateral wall of the postnasal space. Arteriography showed that both the ascending pharyngeal and internal maxillary arteries were greatly enlarged and both were once again embolized. Ligation of the right external carotid and accessible branches was carried out prior to further excision of the tumour via a lateral rhinotomy.

Despite continuing minor epistaxis, fibreoptic nasendoscopy showed no regrowth but considerable crusting. His complaint of blurred vision was attributed to myopia but by December 1988 there was evidence of right proptosis together with swelling of the cheek. CT scan showed a large regrowth filling the infratemporal fossa and extending through the floor of the middle cranial fossa with compression of the brain stem (Fig. 9.17).

It was considered that removal was not possible without risk to both vision and life. Radiotherapy using the 5 Mev linear accelerator giving a tumour dose of 3960 cGy in 22 fractions over 30 days was given in April 1989. This was followed by an improvement in colour vision and visual acuity in the right eye. Proptosis was reduced to 2.5 mm with full extraocular movement.

CT scan in January 1990 showed a considerable reduction in size of the tumour and by the following October there was almost complete resolution of the middle cranial lesion. When last examined January 1991 the only remaining symptom was crusting in the large operative defect and minimal nose bleeds.

Pathological examination of all the operative specimens has shown little variation over the whole period with areas of fibrotic stroma intermixed with marked vascular spaces.

The problems experienced in the management of this boy's angiofibroma obviously cannot be blamed on the use of embolization and there is clearly a place for this procedure although it is difficult to determine an exact criteria. It requires both time and expertise as well as close co-operation between radiologist and surgeon. In addition there is a definite, although small, associated morbidity attached to this procedure which must be considered in each individual patient.

Hormonal therapy

The rationale for prescribing preoperative hormone therapy appears to stem from the paper by Schiff in 1959.[56] His article contained a number of unsubstantiated concepts and hypotheses based upon random biopsies from two patients with angiofibromata receiving 15 mg of diethylstilboestrol per day for 1 month. In view of the well recognized random distribution of collagen and vascular spaces within individual tumours, this uncontrolled study was of little value.

Similar criticism might be applied to the report of Walike & MacKay[82] who also based their impressions of 'worthwhile improvements' on one uncontrolled report of

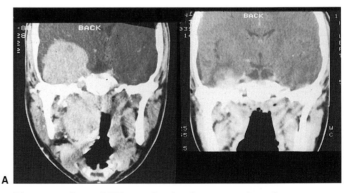

Fig. 9.17 Coronal CT scan showing **A**, recurrent juvenile angiofibroma in middle cranial fossa and **B**, taken 1 year later showing resolution following radiotherapy.

a boy receiving 5 mg of diethylstilboestrol per day for a month.

Although there is evidence supporting testosterone dependence,[54] and 25 mg of testosterone a day increases rate of growth of angiofibroma, there is no objective evidence that giving oestrogen materially effects the vasculature of this lesion.[83] The dosage previously recommended was 15 mg per day for 1 month. 3 mg per day will reduce plasma testosterone to female levels within 2 weeks, and puberty is the time of maturation of testicular function. Testicular atrophy occurs within a month for males taking 1 mg ethinyloestradiol, which is roughly equivalent to 2 mg of diethylstilboestrol.[50] Fortunately, enthusiasm for preoperative therapy has diminished in recent years as surgical expertise has increased.

Historical note[84]

In 1841 a case report appeared in the Lancet of 8 October concerning an operation carried out by Mr Liston of University College, London, on a 21-year-old male from Gibraltar. For over 3 years this man had suffered from intermittent nasal bleeding associated with a large mass projecting from his left nostril. Not only was this increasing in size but it had grown into the cheek and mouth by, it was suspected, absorbing bone. Several attempts had been made by ligation to destroy the tumour but each sloughing was accompanied by haemorrhage and regrowth. On 6 September 1841 at 2 pm, without the benefit of general anaesthesia, the mass was removed along with the whole maxilla but preserving the eye. The dissection of all soft tissue attachments was completed by 6 pm and the estimated blood loss was 8 to 10 ounces.

24 days postoperatively, the Lancet reported that 'progress of the recovery has been most satisfactory and uninterrupted; he is now eating a mutton-chop daily'. Despite this satisfactory situation he died three and a half months postoperatively from erysipelas of the scalp!

In May 1987 the operative specimen was retrieved from the pathology museum of University College School of Medicine (Fig. 9.18) and sectioned by Myhre & Michaels.[84] Microscopically it showed large, thin-walled, anastomosing vascular channels embedded within a collagenous stroma containing stellate stromal cells with nuclei showing single central nucleoli. No mitotic activity and the picture was of a typical angiofibroma, removed 5 years before the availability of ether anaesthesia!

Role of radiotherapy

Anxiety over the technical and haemorrhagic problems associated with large angiofibromata has led to the use of radiotherapy as primary or secondary therapy for many years. Both the dosage and regimes have varied from implantation of radon seeds, 270 or 400 Kv to modern day megavoltage external beam irradiation. Cummings et

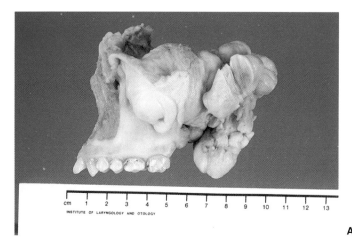

A

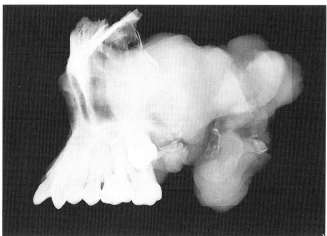

B

Fig. 9.18 **A**, Surgical specimen of maxilla and **B**, X-ray of specimen removed by Liston in 1841.

al (1984) in Toronto, Canada have been the most enthusiastic proponents of primary radiotherapy reporting a series of 55 patients given either 3000 cGy or 3500 cGy in 14 to 16 fractions over 3 weeks by external beam megavoltage.[48] Permanent control of symptoms was obtained in 80% of these patients with failure blamed upon inadequate treatment volumes. Regression following irradiation, which was the same for both the 3000 and 3500 cGy regimes, was slow with half the patients showing macroscopical tumour within 6 months of treatment. Although some patients took 3 years or longer for complete involution, a visible mass persisting for longer than 2 years carried a probability of 50% eventual symptomatic regrowth. They concluded that with accurately determined irradiation fields, a dosage of 3000 cGy is both safe and effective – eventually! This is not supported by Economou et al (1988). 13 of their patients received primary external beam megavoltage irradiation at doses greater than 3000 cGy with three failures. However, all of these 13 patients had advanced tumours and the value of this primary irradiation must be viewed against the hazards of attempted surgical excision.[75]

Although Cummings has succinctly discussed the relative risk factors in irradiating angiofibromas[85] confirming that no disorders of the facial skeleton, pituitary gland or orbit should occur, anxiety over the risk of late malignant change persists, particularly since most of these patients are young. Two of his 55 patients developed neoplasms, one papillary thyroid carcinoma 14 years later and a basal cell 8 years post-irradiation. Makek et al reported a patient developing a nasopharyngeal fibrosarcoma 22 years after treatment of an angiofibroma with several surgical excisions as well as a total of 8550 cGy of Cobalt-60. They included in their paper details of five other cases from the literature, four of whom developed fibrosarcoma and one a malignant fibrous histiocytoma. Dosage of radiotherapy had varied from a single course of 3000 cGy to a mammoth 12 000 cGy given in three courses over a 20 year period.[46]

Irradiation as a cause of cancer is well recognized with a possibility that least 7% of all who are exposed to irradiation develop thyroid cancer within a latent period of between 3 and 35 years. There is also a small, but definite risk of an irradiation-induced bone sarcoma within the site of a treated angiofibroma, although for this the latent period may be as short as a year.[86] If irradiation is to be used either as primary therapy or for recurrence then life-long follow-up is essential. The risk may be reduced by limiting a dosage to 3000 cGy and avoiding repeated surgical removals by using more effective surgical approaches. However, some cases continue to defeat even the most enthusiastic skull base surgeons and radiotherapy will continue to play an important part in treatment strategy.

Chemotherapy

Whilst accepting the problems in treating the recurrent or advanced angiofibromata Goepfert et al in 1985 offered no explanation for their rationale in giving five patients a variety of chemotherapeutic agents. Doxorubin, dacartrazine, vincristine, dactinomycin, cyclophosphamide and cysplatin were combined into two regimes and objective regression was obtained in all patients.[87] They wisely advocated controlled trials to elucidate the logic and possible long-term benefits of these regimes, which appear to be a unique contribution to the management of angiofibromata!

Prognosis

Despite a natural history which bears some resemblance to a malignant tumour, assessment of treatment success in any patient with an angiofibroma is realistically measured by freedom from troublesome symptoms. Regular post-treatment examination, particularly with MRI assessment, reveals an uncomfortably high rate of local regrowth. This must be expected when dealing with an uncapsulated tumour, arising in the region of bone or muscle and possessing a capability for aggressive growth.[59,75,86,88] Figures range from 0% to over 30% which themselves reflect frequency of detailed follow-up, secondary referral and presentation of results. All are regrowths of residual tumour and the most accurate figure will be affected by a combination of pathological, therapeutic and regional factors.

The procedure which allows the greatest and safest access to effect thorough surgical excision must be considered as offering individual patients their best chance of avoiding frequent and rapid regrowth. As yet no standard regime has proved to be universally successful.

ANEURYSMAL BONE CYST

Because of its occasional occurrence within the maxilla and the problems of differentiation from cavernous haemangioma, osteoclastoma or fibrous dysplasia, mention must be made of this cystic vascular osseous tumour, which both destroys and expands bone.

Called at one time or other, *expansive haemangioma, ossifying haematoma, haemangiomatous bone cyst, aneurysmal giant cell tumour* and much else, it was first described in the jaws in 1958.[89] Most occur within the long bones with no more than 1% in the facial skeleton where the mandible is the favoured site. Gruskin & Dahlin described 13 cases, four of which were in the maxilla, with an age incidence within the first 30 years of life and no sex predilection.[90] Giddings et al in reporting one patient with a mandibular lesion reviewed the historical aspects of the terminology and also found that the average age at diagnosis was 17 years with a range between 6 and 59 years.[91]

The initial symptoms were a facial or mandibular mass with some pain in about 25% of cases. Delay in diagnosis was in most patients less than 1 month, although the 13-year-old girl reported by Hady et al in 1990 had a 1 year history of a slowly growing painless swelling in the region of the cheek.[92] It appears that the growth rate of these tumours is variable and there may be a sudden increase in activity, causing attention.

Radiology can show some bone destruction but the appearances are not specific, a circumscribed mass can be seen on CT (Fig. 9.19). Elsewhere in the body, MRI shows the lesions to have a high signal intensity within the tumour although arteriography shows the cysts to be hypovascular. On gross examination the tumour is firm with a smooth surface. The normal architecture is however destroyed, being replaced by large cavernous spaces filled with unclotted blood. Histologically, there are frequent multinucleated giant cells throughout a fibrous stroma, the fibroblasts being the commonest cell within aneurysmal bone cysts.

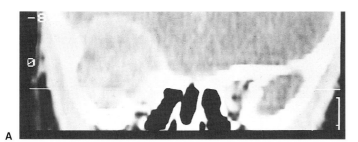

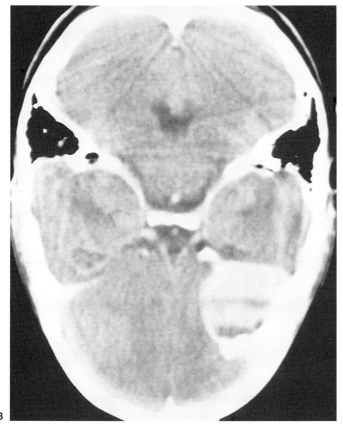

Fig. 9.19 Extensive aneurysmal bone cyst with fluid levels, arising in lateral orbital roof. **A**, coronal CT scan; **B**, axial CT scan of same (Courtesy of D.J. Howard).

Aetiology is unknown although trauma, vascular anomaly or the residuum of a primary bone lesion destroyed by haemorrhage have all been suggested.[91] However, these tumours have been found in association with other pathology such as fibrous dysplasia, giant cell granuloma and cementifying fibroma and care is needed to avoid misdiagnosis.[93] Yarrington et al described a case of aneurysmal bone cyst of the maxilla in association with a central giant cell reparative granuloma.[94]

Curettage has been advocated within the mandible with a reported 20% recurrence rate. This compares with a 10% figure for radical resection. Within the maxilla enucleation has proved successful for the small number of reported cases and it is doubtful if radical surgery is justified at this site.[91,92]

NASAL ANGIOMYOLIPOMA

Definition

Although recognized as a rare but definitive entity within the kidney, where it may be associated with tuberculosis,[95] this tumour has only been reported as occurring within the nasal cavity once. Vascular hamartomata can be expected anywhere within the body and angiolipoma do occur occasionally within the upper jaw. However, the rarity of angiolipoma may in part be related to histological differentiation since they contain a mixture of proliferating blood vessels, some thick walled smooth muscle as well as fat cells.

A 52-year-old Yemeni male complained of a 1 year history of right-sided nasal obstruction with epistaxis.[96] A fleshy mass was visible at the anterior nares which had pushed the nasal septum to one side and had also distorted the medial wall of the maxillary sinus. There was no evidence of bone destruction but biopsy produced severe bleeding.

A carotid angiogram substantiated that this was a vascular tumour, the blood supply coming primarily from the facial artery at the level of the naso-labial fold. The CT scan, with enhancement added little extra information and after ligation of the facial artery the tumour was removed intranasally – with brisk bleeding!

Follow up 1 year later showed no recurrence.

The tumour was firm and lobulated with a smooth surface and a thick pedicle by which it had been attached to the lateral nasal wall. Histologically, this was a benign vascular tumour showing a mixture of vascular, smooth muscle and adipose elements justifying a diagnosis of angiomyolipoma. This was not dissimilar in many clinical and pathological features from the angioleiomyomas considered under muscle tumours of the upper jaw.

ANGIOSARCOMA

Definition

Malignant tumours arising from blood vessels are rare and consequently reliable epidemiological data is unavailable. Given the rarity of these tumours, confusion regarding terminology is not surprising although division into low- and high-grade is now generally accepted as being a realistic classification. Well-differentiated malignant vascular tumours have however been called haemangioendotheliomata with angiosarcoma reserved for the poorly-differentiated high-grade malignancies.[97] Other pathologists refer to all of these tumours as haemangioendotheliomas, but then divide them into various grades of malignancy.[98] Malignant angioendothelioma has also been used to describe all variants but Batsakis & Rice in 1980 finalized discussion by dividing angiosarcoma into low and high grades and this relates reasonably well to ultimate prognosis.[99]

Incidence

Although Wold et al in 1982 described 112 patients with angiosarcoma of bone, only three had disease in the mandible or maxilla.[98] The commonest site is in fact the scalp and facial soft tissues, with over half of all angiosarcoma found at these sites.[100] Panje et al in 1986 reported 11 cases with head and neck lesions but only one arose within the nose and ethmoids.[101] Whilst of the 100 non-epithelial malignant tumours sited within the nasal cavity, paranasal sinuses and nasopharynx reported by Fu & Perzin, only two were angiosarcoma.[102] Within the upper airway, primary angiosarcoma are uncommon and Bankaci et al in 1979 could find only 14 published cases situated within the nasal cavity.[103] In the same year five patients with primary maxillary antrum or maxillary bone angiosarcoma were described by Sharma & Mawalicha.[104]

Angiosarcoma also arises within bone with an incidence of about 0.5%.[105] Within the head and neck the skull and mandible are the commonest sites. Zachariades et al in 1980 found 46 cases of oral angiosarcoma, in six of these patients the maxilla or maxillary sinus was thought to be the site of origin.[106] Isolated cases with upper jaw angiosarcoma have been published more recently but the numbers remain too small for meaningful confirmation of treatment policies.[107–111]

Age, sex variation

Any age group, sex or nationality can be affected although the greatest incidence occurs within the 5th decade of life. However, two maxillary cases were reported by Henry in babies under 6 months and apparently the diagnosis was confirmed by several histopathologists.[108]

Within the skin however, there is a marked predominance of males over females by a ratio of 4:1 and all cases occur in the elderly.

Site and aetiology

Aetiological theories are abundant and in 1950 McCarthy & Pack enthusiastically suggested that angiosarcomas developed from granulation tissue capillaries in traumatized tissues.[112] The same authors also reported three patients whose previously benign angioma had become malignant following radiotherapy. In 1975 Duck found that in 30 individuals with angiosarcoma of the liver, vinyl chloride was a possible aetiological agent.[113] Heath calculated that the increased risk of hepatic angiosarcoma in plant workers exposed to polyvinyl chloride (PVC) is 400-fold over the general population.[114] A similar risk may also occur with those who work with PVC products for manufactured PVC contains 200–400 ppm of vinyl chloride monomer (VCM) and in animals exposure to 50 ppm of VCM for 4 hours daily for 5 days a week produced hepatic angiosarcoma.[115]

Most of the recorded cases of upper jaw angiosarcoma however, do not give an occupational link with PVC. Williamson & Ramsden in 1988 described a 48-year-old man who had handled or been exposed to vinyl chloride for 6 years prior to developing a low grade angiosarcoma of the upper jaw from which he died 27 months from initial diagnosis. Permission for necropsy was unfortunately refused but there was no clinical evidence of hepatic involvement and death was attributed to intracranial invasion from uncontrolled local disease. Although it proved impossible to quantify the degree of exposure of this patient to VCM dust, his working conditions were poorly ventilated and with such a rare disease, this occupational hazard cannot be ignored.[110]

Clinical features

Most patients present with a short history of a few months spontaneous nasal bleeding, obstruction, facial pain and, with extension to orbit or maxilla, proptosis and facial swelling. Such symptoms are common to most upper jaw neoplasms and even the observance of a friable, vascular mass is not pathognomonic of angiosarcoma.

Local bone invasion, cervical lymphadenopathy or metastasis can all occur early in the disease and because of multicentricity, the limits of this tumour are often indeterminable. The lesion is poorly circumscribed and within the scalp may spread beneath the dermis for considerable distances. With bone invasion no clear line of demarcation is possible.

Tumours apparently confined to the inferior turbinate and middle meatus, presenting as a polypoidal mass, have been described by Kurien et al[109] but this does not necessarily indicate a limited origin as the patient reported by Williamson & Ramsden with a nasoantral wall mass proved to have considerable underlying bone destruction and responded poorly to radical treatment.[110]

Macroscopic and microscopic appearance

Angiosarcoma are malignant tumours of the vascular endothelial cells with low-grade lesions showing diffuse proliferation of inter-anastomosing atypical capillaries lined by large endothelial cells, with papillary fronds into the lumen and hyperchromatic nuclei. High-grade tumours are diffusely cellular with areas of undifferentiated cells with pleomorphism and multiple mitoses. Many of these atypical cells are spindle-shaped and no longer form vascular channels. These tumours may be difficult to distinguish from undifferentiated carcinomata or malignant melanoma.[99]

Associated with both grades of angiosarcoma may be changes in vessels at a distance from the main lobules of the neoplasm. In well differentiated lesions, the neoplastic cells may in fact be identical to normal endothelium but can give a positive reaction in their cytoplasm for factor VIII antigen by the immunoperoxidase method. The formation of primitive lumina as an index of angio-genesis is an important ultrastructural finding but most tumours, however will show wide variation in histological appearances and careful search, together with a high index of suspicion, is needed to identify areas or foci typical of angiosarcoma.

These diagnostic difficulties are greater with primary bone angiosarcoma where differentiation from well-vascularized metastatic carcinoma (kidney, liver or thyroid) ameloblastoma or osteogenic sarcoma can be exacting.

Natural history

It is impossible to lay down precise guide lines for treatment, or analyse with confidence, factors which relate to long-term prognosis. The commonest problem with angiosarcoma within the upper jaw is local control, although better control might well lead to an increase in later metastasis! It does appear however, from the small number of well-documented cases in the literature and where follow-up has been reasonably long, that upper jaw tumours do have a better prognosis than those within the scalp. If this be so, then it may be due to early presentation with epistaxis or more likely, a greater preponderance of well-differentiated tumours. Radical excision is no more feasible within this region than in the soft tissues of face or head.

Over one half of all patients with scalp angiosarcoma will die within 5 years of diagnosis, most with metastases.[103] With primary bone lesions the prognosis is little better possibly because of the multicentric nature of these tumours.[116]

Treatment and prognosis

Irrespective of the histological grading of the tumour, present consensus of opinion agrees that a combination of surgery and radiotherapy offers the best hope of local control with long-term survival always a possibility. Where feasible, surgery should be radical although with a multicentric lesion and the near impossibility of obtaining clear margins within the upper jaw, excision must be tempered with judgement. Postoperative irradiation should be given at cancercidal dosage with chemotherapy remaining experimental in the absence of prospective controlled trials.

There are few reported 5-year survival figures for primary angiosarcoma of the upper jaw, although the two babies remained alive and free from tumour for over 2 years following wide excision of their maxillae.[108] It must be considered therefore as having an extremely poor long-term prognosis.

KAPOSI'S SARCOMA

Definition

Despite considerable controversy over the histogenesis of Kaposi's sarcoma, Batsakis & Rice conclude that this neoplasm arises from vasoformative cells.[99] Warner & O'Loughlin in 1975 theorized that the tumour developed from a chronic immunological interaction between normal and antigenically altered or transformed lymphocytes, resulting in the formation of an angionetic factor which in turn evoked a proliferation of mesenchymal and endo-thelial cells. These eventually produced the sarcoma.[117] Certainly, lymphoma-like changes as well as definable lymphoma in patients with this tumour lend support to a host-vs-graft response theory.

Historical aspects

Kaposi's sarcoma was first described by him in 1872 as 'multiple idiopathic pigmented sarcoma of skin'.[118] For the next 70 years it was viewed as yet another dermato-logical curiosity but with an unusual ethnic and geographical distribution. In Europe it favoured Ashkenazi Jews and Italians from the Po Valley, and was normally an indolent disease. Within the USA, it was the immigrants from Eastern Europe who were initially affected although it soon spread to involve the black population.

Following the establishment of cancer registries in southern Africa, it became clear that Kaposi's sarcoma was endemic in Zaire and Uganda accounting for 11% of all adult malignancies.[119] However, despite this concentration in specific ethnic groups there is no apparent regular form of inheritance.

Incidence

Long before the present epidemic of AIDS (Acquired Immunodeficiency Syndrome) Kaposi's sarcoma was seen in patients who were immunosuppressed. Renal-transplanted patients on immunosuppressive therapy have a high incidence of cytomegalovirus (CMV) excretion as well as Kaposi's sarcoma as do many patients with lymphoid tumours.[119]

All AIDS patients now show a remarkable tendency to develop this sarcoma, indeed AIDS has been defined by the American Centre for Disease Control as 'the appearance of Kaposi's sarcoma in individuals younger than 60 years, and/or life-threatening opportunistic infections with no known predisposing cause for these infections'.[120]

At least 35% of these tumours present within the mouth and/or pharynx, but all mucosal disease is usually advanced and generalized. Abramson & Simons consider that the head and neck dermis, including the nasal skin to be the most frequent site for non-mucosal lesions.[121]

Clinical features

Although the oropharynx and larynx are areas of predilection for lesions of the mucous membrane, within the oral cavity the palate is the commonest site involving the upper jaw. The lesions here may be solitary or multiple, red–purple macules, plaques or nodules although many palatal tumours appear angiomatous. Lymphadenopathy in all AIDS patients is universal, particularly in the cervical region, and this is accompanied by a low-grade persistent fever. Other symptoms include headache, malaise, weakness, myalgia and arthralgia, all of which will attract attention in patients with isolated palatal lesions. Low white cell count, anaemia and a moderately raised erythrocyte sedimentation rate are significant in reaching a diagnosis. 20% of AIDS patients show anergy to skin testing for mumps, candida or tuberculosis; evidence of immune deficiency.[122]

Macroscopic and microscopic appearance

Light microscopy shows a proliferation of atypical spindle cells and vascular channels. The dominant tumour cell is spindle-shaped with a tendency to form vascular slits, some containing red blood cells. Lymphocytes and plasma cells may infiltrate the tumour.

A histological classification based upon well established lesions, for early tumours are notoriously difficult to diagnose, is useful in predicting response to treatment in patients with locally aggressive tumours.[123] Mixed-cell neoplasms, characterized by small capillary slits with intervening spindle cells interspersed with well formed vascular spaces, usually respond to therapy. Anaplastic tumours do not! The vascular spaces appear to be more sensitive to chemotherapy than the spindle cells and the general prognosis for Kaposi's sarcoma alone can be good. Clinical classification into nodular, locally aggressive and generalized is also of some prognostic value. Local nodal involvement with a locally aggressive tumour carries a poor prognosis, as does bone involvement.

Treatment

Even though the treatment of AIDS consists primarily of medical care for opportunistic infections, a more direct attack upon locally troublesome Kaposi's sarcoma requires oncological support. Patients may be suitable for chemotherapy and vinblastine used as a single agent has been reported as producing partial or total remission in 37% of patients. However, this is accompanied by a high incidence of concurrent infection and alpha interferon probably produces a more durable and trouble-free response.[124]

Regression of palatal lesions with radiotherapy, 2500–4000 rad has been reported and there is a place for local tumour destruction with the CO_2 laser. However, whereas the isolated Kaposi's sarcoma responds to treatment most of these tumours are now diagnosed in patients with AIDS and this new variant tends to affect the viscera carrying with it a universally poor long-term prognosis. Management then of the rare single palatal lesion requires careful evaluation of the long-term prognosis and the potential benefit likely to be gained by instituting a regime of immunosuppressive chemotherapy or radiotherapy.

HAEMANGIOPERICYTOMA

Definition

Whilst studying the histology of the cat's eye, Rouget in 1873 was the first to describe the pericyte, and for many years they were referred to as 'Rouget cells'.[125] This special type of amoeboid cell present in the pericapillary space of many vertebrates were at one time called 'cellules adventices', but in 1923 Zimmermann described the same cell wrapped around the capillaries and named them pericytes.[126] Acceptance that these pericytes, widely distributed throughout the vascular system could be the source of an unusual tumour did not take place until 1942. Stout & Murray reviewed the literature on vascular tumours and then described nine patients with what they called a 'haemangiopericytoma'.[127] After prolonged tissue culture studies, they recognized this as a true pathological entity and in fact one of their patients had a pedunculated mass arising from the infra-auricular area. Stout's second publication in 1949 contained two head and neck cases amongst the 25 patients, on the base of the tongue and in the nasal cavity.[128] It was this paper which eventually led to the general acceptance of haemangiopericytoma as a definitive diagnosis and a clinical entity. Stout & Murray's original tissue cultures had suggested that the tumours were closely related to glomus tumours, although their literature search had suggested the existence of a unclassified vascular tumour whose natural history differed significantly from glomus and other lesions. Discussion related to the nature of haemangiopericytomas has continued ever since!

Incidence

As with other rare conditions, no accurate figures are available for the incidence of haemangiopericytomata within the head and neck. Possibly representing only 1% of all vasoform tumours and with less than 25% of haemangiopericytomas occurring within the head and neck, the largest series reported is by Compagno & Hyams from the Armed Forces Institute of Pathology, USA and this was a collective series.[129] Even so, they qualified their histological diagnosis to 'haemangiopericytoma-like'. However, many small personal series of patients have described the clinical behaviour of these tumours when they arise within the nasal cavity or maxillary sinus, as well as the large series relating to the commoner sites in the extremities, retroperitoneum and pelvis.[130]

Age and sex variation

Within the head and neck region most patients are adults between the 6th and 7th decades of life and without an obvious sexual weighting. Cases have been reported in patients as young as 40 years of age. Of particular interest are the infantile or congenital haemangiopericytomas which occur exclusively during infancy. They present primarily within the subcutis with a predilection for the head and neck, and are said to be particularly benign.[131] However, Kauffman & Stout reported a 35% poor prognosis for this age group in 1960 but this may reflect variations in histological interpretation.[132] Multiple congenital haemangiopericytomas occurring in a newborn were removed by Seibert et al in 1978 from the scalp and nasopharynx. They reported an excellent long-term success.[133]

Aetiology and clinical features

Trauma, steroid therapy and hormonal imbalance have all been implicated as causative agents. The spontaneous disappearance of one tumour following pregnancy was attributed to such changes but with such an unusual tumour a clearly recognizable aetiology is unlikely.[134]

It is doubtful if haemangiopericytoma can ever be diagnosed clinically for their commonest presenting symptoms of nasal obstruction, epistaxis, proptosis or epiphora are found in most nasal and sinus malignancies. As with most neoplasms the mode of presentation is related to the site of origin (Table 9.1, Figs 9.20 and 9.21). The mass is usually painless, being well circumscribed whilst the surface is described as lobulated or even nodular with a soft, spongy, firm or friable feel, the consistency depending, as with angiofibroma, on the degree of vascularity. Biopsy can therefore produce severe bleeding, uncontrollable in some inaccessible sites. Within the upper jaw, tumours have been found within the nasal cavity where they may arise from the septum, lateral nasal wall or nasal roof. They also grow from the maxillary antrum although these may be extensions from ethmoidal primaries. The small number of well documented cases make it impossible to extract reliable data regarding behaviour patterns of the natural history or even the expected response to treatment.[99,134–140]

It is rare for patients to present with cervical lymph nodes or metastases and the duration of significant symptoms may be long-standing, ranging from months to over 10 years.[140] Since there is little that can be considered as specific either in clinical or radiological assessment, diagnosis depends upon histological evaluation of a biopsy.

Macroscopic and microscopic appearance

A distinction between malignant and benign haemangiopericytoma is not always possible with absolute certainty but there are features which characterize those tumours which are likely to pursue an aggressive behaviour. Large tumours (over 6 cm diameter) occurring outside the head and neck with mitosis, cellular anaplasia, necrosis and haemorrhage, do badly.[139] The basic pattern of vascular channels and pericytes show considerable variation. McMaster et al suggested that some prophylactic predictability can be achieved however, by dividing tumours into histologically benign (low-grade), borderline (intermediate) and malignant (high-grade).[130] Low-

Table 9.1 Locations of haemangiopericytoma of nasal cavity and sinuses: cases in the literature

Author	No. of cases			
	Spheno-ethmoid	Nasal cavity	Nasopharynx	Maxillary region
Walike & Bailey 1971[141]	2	5	1	–
Compagno & Hyams 1976[129]	10	13	–	–
Gorenstein et al 1978[140]	1	8	1	3
Chawla & Oswal 1987[134]	14	7	6	1
Harrison & Lund	2	1	–	2
Total No.	29	34	8	6

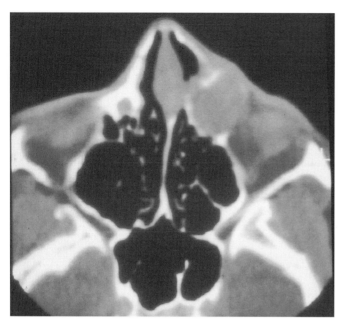

Fig. 9.20 Axial CT scan showing haemangiopericytoma arising in nasolacrimal region.

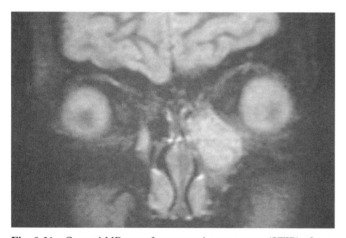

Fig. 9.21 Coronal MR scan, fat suppression sequences (STIR) of case in Figure 9.20.

grade have a prominent vascular pattern with scant areas of compressed vascular spaces. The pericytes are spindled in shape and there are minimal mitotic figures. Intermediate-grade tumours are more cellular with a less prominent vascular pattern. Here the pericytes are plump, less spindly but there are more mitosis. High-grade lesions are characterized by increased anaplasia, more mitosis and considerable compression of the vascular spaces.[125] Survival of patients is also said to be worse if the biopsy shows a lack of lymphocytic infiltration, fibrosis or desmoplasia.

Both McMaster et al[130] and Enzinger & Smith[131] found good correlation between this histological grading and long-term survival, although 5-year follow-up does not adequately reflect overall survival rates for both local

recurrence and metastases can occur within 20 years of treatment.

A less aggressive biological behaviour for these tumours when arising within the head and neck is reported by Compagno & Hyams.[129] This may be related to a higher frequency of low-grade tumours or to what these pathologists call 'haemangiopericytoma-like neoplasms'. They report that this particular lesion shows little in the way of nuclear or cytoplasmic pleomorphism, minimal or no mitosis, no necrosis or haemorrhage. In fact a benign haemangiopericytoma! However, local recurrence is well documented even in these cases, with figures of 25 to 40% and systemic metastases in between 5 and 10%. With really long-term follow-up the final mortality may be as high as 50%.[135,141]

Natural history

There is now clear evidence that histological grading of these tumours bears a reasonably close relationship to eventual survival providing that the primary lesion is adequately removed. Long-term follow-up is imperative since recurrence or metastases can occur after more than 5 years 'disease free interval'. As with adenoid cystic and malignant melanomata, follow-up is for life!

Barwinkle & Diddam reported that recurrence rate increased with increasingly long follow-up. In the orbit, mouth and nasopharynx there was a 4.7% recurrence rate in the first year, 19% from 1 to 2 years and 33% at 5 years.[142] Chawla & Oswal reviewed 23 patients with nasal tumours, not graded, and had 11 recurrences within 2 years.[134] Only a lengthy comprehensive follow-up can adequately evaluate the real natural history and treatment effectiveness of this unusual tumour but some guidance is available from histological grading.

Differential diagnosis

There are a wide variety of 'haemangiopericytomata-like' intranasal tumours which must be excluded by the histopathologist. Glomus, haemangioendothelioma, undifferentiated or metastatic carcinoma, Kaposi's or Ewing's sarcoma, most nasopharyngeal tumours, olfactory neuroblastoma and juvenile angiofibroma. Ultrastructural studies by Batsakis et al have described the criteria for identifying neoplastic pericytes, although it is admitted that they can be variable in appearance.[143] They concluded that haemangiopericytoma originates from cells of a perivascular nature and that some typical features can be found in most cases to confirm the diagnosis.

Treatment

As with most other sinonasal tumours, wide local excision is advocated with radiotherapy reserved for inoperable or surgically incomplete lesions. Lateral rhinotomy is useful when the tumour is confined to the lateral nasal wall but may need to be extended to a full craniofacial resection for less accessible tumours as is illustrated in the following case.

A 69-year-old female presented in January 1989 with a history of unilateral nasal obstruction for 3 years and recent mild epistaxis. A polypoidal mass was removed from the left nasal passage and initially diagnosed as an olfactory neuroblastoma. This was changed to low-grade haemangiopericytoma after consultation, with less than 2 mitoses per 10 high power fields and no necrosis.

CT scans showed the lesion to be localized to the upper nasal cavity with involvement of the posterior ethmoids and sphenoid sinus. A left craniofacial resection confirmed that the lesion was confined to the nasal cavity but that the sphenoid was filled with mucus not tumour. The cribriform plate was removed with the specimen and the dural defect closed primarily.

There has been no evidence of local or systemic disease 2 years postoperatively.

A wide margin of excision is rarely possible within the upper jaw, although radical maxillectomy was used by Caldarelli & Sperling for a primary antral haemangiopericytoma in a 66-year-old woman.[138] She was reported as being alive without disease at 2 years. Small local recurrences can be treated with radiotherapy or even cryosurgery. High dose irradiation, giving between 7500 cGy and 9000 cGy in 30 to 60 days has been described but in view of the imprecise natural history, the effectiveness of these regimes remains unconfirmed.[136,144] Chemotherapy, in the form of a cocktail using adriamycin, vincristine, cyclophosphamide and actinomycin D has been used speculatively for both local recurrence and metastases, but without objective relief.[145]

Prognosis

Apart from the rare 'congenital haemangiopericytoma', long-term prognosis must be guarded even in patients where wide field excision within the upper jaw is feasible. However, with proven low-grade tumours, which appear to be more common within the head and neck, together with adjuvant radiotherapy for doubtful margins, good local control can be expected for at least 5 years. After this time both recurrences and metastases may occur without warning.

NASAL PARAGANGLIOMA

Definition

Unfortunately, there are a variety of names in common use describing those tumours that arise from the paraganglionic chemoreceptor cells. 'Glomus tumour' is clearly incorrect since there is no relationship with the glomus bodies found throughout the body. 'Non-chromaffin' paraganglioma was based upon the intense 'chromaffin' reaction used to test these tumours for catecholamine. However, it is now appreciated that when using more sophisticated tests for catecholamines, extra-adrenal paraganglionic tumours do contain catecholamines but only in small concentrations.

Only the term 'paraganglioma' adequately describes all of these lesions and prefacing by site of origin, e.g. carotid body paraganglioma, should avoid confusion. Within the head and neck, all paragangliomata are uncommon. In the 60 000 patients reviewed within the Sloan-Kettering Cancer Centre 1937–1975 only 69 tumours were diagnosed as paragangliomata. Within the same period in 13 400 autopsies only one unexpected carotid body tumour was found.[146]

However, increasing interest in skull base surgery together with developments in radiology has led to reports of 1000 or more cases of temporal bone paraganglioma.[147] Despite this, few patients have been recorded with paragangliomas arising within the upper jaw. Talbot in 1990 when reviewing the literature found 12 possible cases involving the nasal cavity with three more originating within the maxillary sinus. He added one more patient to the latter group (Table 9.2).[148]

Age, sex and ethnic variation

Within the small number of published cases there appears to be a distinct female preponderance although the age at diagnosis ranged from 17 to 89 years. Although it is often said that paragangliomata may be characterized by a tendency towards multicentricity and familial inheritance, there has been no evidence of this occurring in upper jaw tumours. However, prolonged follow-up is needed to ensure that patients with controlled local lesions do not ultimately develop further tumours for delay in diagnosis may be over 2 years.[146]

Symptoms are similar to those found in most upper jaw malignancies; epistaxis, nasal obstruction, facial swelling or epiphora. The presence of a vascularized tumour growing within the nasal passages, particularly when associated with radiological evidence of sinus opacity or bone destruction, indicates a need for open biopsy.

Macroscopic and microscopic appearance

Macroscopically, many of these tumours present as polyps, being well-encapsulated and of a grey or purple appearance.[149]

Histologically, they are characterized by 'Zellballen', i.e. aggregates of tumour cells having epithelioid features. The cytoplasm is finely granular and the tumour nests surrounded by blood vessels. Nuclear pleomorphism and cellular hyperchromatism are common though not mitosis.[148]

Table 9.2   Nasal paraganglioma: cases in the literature

Author	Sex	Age	Site	Treatment	Outcome (yr A&W)
Apple & Kreines 1962[154]	F	50	Ethmoid	DXT	6
Moran 1962[155]	F	89	Anterior nares	Excision ($\times$ 3)	2
Lack et al 1977[156]	F	50	Polyp	Excision ($\times$ 3)	11
	F	50	Middle turbinate	Excision	–
	M	8	Middle turbinate	Excision	8
Himelfarb et al 1983[146]	M	41	Middle turbinate	Excision	2
Ueda et al 1985[157]	F	31	Ethmoid	Excision ($\times$ 2)	2
Watson 1988[158]	F	56	Polyp	Excision, DXT	3
Talbot 1990[148]	F	17	Middle turbinate	Excision	1
Harrison & Lund	F	42	Polyp	Excision, DXT	9

A&W, alive and well; DXT, radiotherapy

No consistent focus of paraganglionic tissue is found within the upper jaw and paraganglionic cell distribution is more extensive in the foetus and newborn.[150] It is possible that nasal paragangliomas arise therefore in vestigial cell nests. Girgis & Fahmy found paraganglionic tissue in close proximity to the terminal branches of the internal maxillary artery giving some credence to this hypothesis.[151]

There is some similarity between paragangliomata and neuroendocrine carcinoma which also show 'Zellballen'. Both tumours express general neuroendocrine markers although only the large cell neuroendocrine carcinomata mark for both cytokeratin and calcitonin. Milroy et al investigating these tumours arising within the larynx, identified sustenacular cells in the paraganglioma cases and they marked for both S-100 protein and glial fibrillary acidic protein.[152] Differentiation using immunohistochemistry is essential, since large cell neuroendocrine carcinomas are highly malignant.

Kameya et al have reported two patients with upper jaw paraganglioma which behaved in a malignant manner, both demonstrated neurosecreting functions and death occurred 6 and 8 years after radical excision.[153]

Treatment

As with the majority of other upper jaw neoplasms, complete excision offers the best prospect of long-term control. Radiotherapy alone has been said to produce a good initial response but is associated with a high probability of late regrowth.

Surgical excision of even apparently localized lesions, such as a polyp, may be followed by recurrence and clear margins are essential. However, these tumours are highly vascular and preoperative embolization is recommended to assist in radical excision. Where clear margins are not obtained postoperative radiotherapy is advocated. In all patients, long-term follow-up is necessary and the

published cases suggest that even when repeated surgical excision are needed, eventual control is possible.

GLOMUS TUMOUR

Definition

Glomus bodies are found in the dermis throughout the body, being most numerous in the digits, pinnae and nasal cavity. Most probably a hamartoma, the glomus is a specialized anastomosis between an arteriole and a primary venule being lined by endothelium. It is surrounded by smooth muscle cells interspersed with several layers of glomus cells. With its related vessels and nerves, the whole body, sometimes called a glomangioma, is enclosed within a connective tissue capsule.[4] Originally, this tumour was thought to be of pericytic origin but it has now been established as originating from smooth muscle.[159]

Glomus tumours are believed to result from a proliferation of the various elements of the glomus body with either a cellular or vascular component dominating. It is also thought that the cellular forms are most symptomatic, producing pain. However, these lesions must not be confused with chemodectomas, which erroneously are often called 'glomus tumours'.

Although the size may vary from 0.2 to 4 cm, most are less than 1 cm in diameter and are commonly found beneath the finger nails. All are uncommon and in 500 consecutive soft-tissue tumours of the extremities reported by Soule et al,[160] only 1.6% were glomus tumours. Within the head and neck cavity, reported cases are rare and Table 9.3 records the available data confirming a female preponderance and the nasal septum as the commonest site.

A 48-year-old male complained of intermittent moderate left-sided epistaxis for several months. Examination showed a 0.5 cm raised lesion on the anterior part of the nasal septum

Table 9.3 Intranasal glomus tumours: cases in the literature

Author	Sex	Age	Site	Symptoms
Pantazopoulos 1965[161]	F	45	Inferior turbinate	Obstruction, epistaxis
De Bord 1972[162]	F	33	Posterior choana	Obstruction
Fu & Perzin 1973[4]	F	71	Septum	Asymptomatic
Fleury & Basset 1979[163]	M	24	Septum	Obstruction
Potter et al 1984[164]	F	81	Septum	Asymptomatic
Harrison & Lund	F	61	Septum	Obstruction, epistaxis
	M	48	Septum	

which was dark red and friable. The lesion bled on touching was dark red and friable. The lesion bled on touching and was excised under local anaethesia with underlying cartilage. Histology confirmed a glomus tumour without mitotic activity or cytological atypia. There has been no recurrence.

Despite the frequency with which subungual glomus tumours are associated with pain on pressure, none of the patients reporting to date with nasal lesions complained of pain. However, removal should be complete where technically possible and this presents no problems when they arise from the septum.

REFERENCES

1. Weimert T A, Gilmore B B 1978 Multiple head and neck haemangiomas in the adult. Journal of Laryngology and Otology 92: 937–942
2. Illingworth R S 1976 Thoughts on the treatment of strawberry naevi. Archives of Disease of Children 51: 138–140
3. Batsakis J G, Rice D H 1980 The pathology of head and neck tumours. Vasoformative tumors. Head and Neck Surgery 3: 231–239
4. Fu Y S & Perzin K H 1974 Non-epithelial tumors of the nasal cavity, paranasal sinuses and nasopharynx. Cancer 33: 1275–1288
5. Michaels L 1987 Ear, nose and throat histopathology. Springer-Verlag, London, ch. 19
6. McShane D P, Walsh M A 1988 Nasal granuloma gravidarum. Journal of Laryngology and Otology 102: 828–830
7. Ash J E, Old J W 1950 Haemangioma of the nasal septum. Transactions of the American Academy of Ophthalmology and Otolaryngology 54: 350–356
8. Bicknell P G 1971 Granulomata arising in the nasal mucosa during pregnancy. Journal of Laryngology and Otology 85: 515–520
9. Harrison D F N 1959 The effect of systemic oestrogen upon the nasal mucous membrane and its application to the treatment of familial haemorrhagic telangiectasia. MS Thesis University of London, England
10. Taylor M 1961 Experimental study of the influence of the endocrine system on the nasal respiratory mucosa. Journal of Laryngology and Otology 85: 972–977
11. Helmi A M, El-Ghazzawi I F 1975 Effect of oestrogen on the nasal respiratory mucosa. Journal of Laryngology and Otology 89: 1229–1241
12. Bucy P, Capps C S 1930 Primary haemangioma of bone with special reference to X-ray diagnosis. American Journal of Roentgenology 23: 1–6
13. Ghosh L M, Samanta A, Nandy T 1988 Haemangioma of the maxilla. Journal of Laryngology and Otology 102: 725–726
14. Watson W L, McCarthy W D 1940 Blood and lymph vessel tumors. Report of 1056 cases. Surgery, Gynaecology and Obstetrics 71: 569–574
15. Nishimura T, Takimoto T, Umeda R 1990 Osseous hemangioma arising within the facial bone. Otology, Rhinology and Laryngology 52: 385–390
16. Harrison D F N 1956 Babington's disease, hereditary haemorrhagic telangiectasia. Guy's Hospital Reports 104: 246–266
17. Sutton H G 1864 Epistaxis as an indicator of impaired nutrition and degeneration of the vascular system. Medical Mirror 1: 769–771
18. Babington B G 1865 Hereditary Epistaxis. Letter to the Editor of the Lancet. Lancet 2: 362–363
19. Rendu M 1896 Epistaxis repetees chez un sujet posteur de petits angiones cutanes et murqueux. Bulletin Medical Society of the Medical Hospital Paris 13: 731–733
20. Osler W 1901 On a family form of recurring epistaxis associated with multiple telangiectases of skin and mucous membrane. Johns Hopkins Medical Bulletin 12: 333–337
21. Weber F M 1907 Multiple hereditary developmental angiomata of the skin and mucous membranes with recurrent haemorrhage. Lancet 2: 160–162
22. Hanes F M 1909 Multiple haemorrhagic telangiectasia causing epistaxis. Johns Hopkins Medical Bulletin 20: 63–67
23. Wintrobe M M 1951 Clinical haemotology, 3rd edn. London, England, p. 794
24. Harrison D F N 1982 Use of estrogen in the treatment of familial hemorrhagic telangiectasia. Laryngoscope 92: 314–320
25. Baker G P 1953 Hereditary haemorrhagic telangiectasia with gastrointestinal haemorrhage. Guy's Hospital Reports 102: 246–252
26. Harrison D F N 1958 A case of familial haemorrhagic telangiectases associated with pulmonary arteriovenous fistula. Journal of Laryngology and Otology 72: 153–159
27. Harrison D F N 1963 Familial haemorrhagic telangiectases. 20 cases treated with systemic oestrogen. Quarterly Journal of Medicine 33: 25–38
28. McCaffrey T V, Kern E B, Lake C F 1977 Management of epistaxis in hereditary hemorrhagic telangiectasia. Archives of Otolaryngology 103: 627–630
29. Sapru R P, Hutchinson D C S, Hall J I 1969 Pulmonary hypertension in patients with pulmonary arteriovenous fistulae. British Heart Journal 31: 559–569
30. Jahnke V 1970 Ultrastructure of hereditary telangiectasia. Archives of Otolaryngology 92: 262–265
31. Menefee M G, Flessa H C, Glueck H I 1957 Hereditary hemorrhagic telangiectasia. An electron microscopic study of the vascular lesions before and after therapy with hormones. Archives of Otolaryngology 101: 246–251
32. Koch H J, Escher G C, Lewis J S 1952 Hormonal management of hereditary hemorrhagic telangiectasia. Journal of the American Medical Association 149: 1376–1380

33. Levine H L 1989 Endoscopy and the KTP/532 Laser for nasal sinus disease. Annals of Otology, Rhinology and Laryngology 98: 46–51

34. Saunders W H 1960 Septal dermoplasty for control of nose bleeds in hereditary hemorrhagic telangiectasia. Transactions of the American Academy of Ophthalmology and Otolaryngology 64: 500–506

35. McCabe W P, Kelly A P 1972 Management of epistaxis in Osler-Rendu-Weber disease. Recurrence of telangiectases within a nasal skin graft. Plastic and Reconstructive Surgery 50: 114–118

36. Laurian N, Kalmanovitch M, Shimberg R 1979 Amniotic graft in the management of severe epistaxis due to hereditary haemorrhagic telangiectases. Journal of Laryngology and Otology 93: 589–595

37. Merland J J, Melki J P, Chiras J 1980 Place of embolization in the treatment of severe epistaxis. Laryngoscope 90: 1694–1704

38. Strother C M, Newton T H 1976 Percutaneous embolization to control epistaxis in Rendu-Osler-Weber disease. Archives of Otolaryngology 102: 58–60

39. Chelius M S 1847 A system of surgery, Vol. 2. Renshaw, London

40. Martin H, Ehrlich H E, Abels J C 1948 Juvenile nasopharyngeal angiofibroma. Annals of Surgery 127: 513–536

41. Chaveau C 1906 Histoire des Maladies du Pharynx. Balliere, Paris

42. Friedberg S A 1940 Vascular fibromas of the nasopharynx. Archives of Otolaryngology 31: 313–326

43. Spector J G 1988 Management of juvenile angiofibroma. Laryngoscope 98: 1016–1026

44. Chandler J R, Goulding R, Moskowitz L 1984 Nasopharyngeal angiofibromas: Staging and management. Annals of Otology, Rhinology, Laryngology 93:322–329

45. Tandon D A, Bahadur S, Kacker S K 1988 Nasopharyngeal angiofibroma. Journal of Laryngology and Otology 102: 805–809

46. Makek M S, Andrews J C, Fisch U 1989 Malignant transformation of a nasopharyngeal angiofibroma. Laryngoscope 99: 1088–1092

47. Fitzpatrick P S, Briant D R, Berman J M 1980 The nasopharyngeal angiofibroma. Archives of Otolaryngology 106: 234–236

48. Cummings B J, Blend R, Keane T 1984 Primary radiation therapy for juvenile nasopharyngeal angiofibroma. Laryngoscope 94: 1599–1605

49. Osbourne D A, Sokoloski A 1965 Juvenile nasopharyngeal angiofibroma in a female. Review of a case. Archives of Otolaryngology 82: 629–632

50. Harrison D F N 1977 Lateral rhinotomy - a neglected operation. Annals of Otology, Rhinology, Laryngology 86: 756–764

51. Lund V J, Lloyd G A S, Howard D J 1989 Juvenile angiofibroma–imaging techniques in diagnosis. Rhinology 27: 179–185

52. Brunner H 1942 Nasopharyngeal fibroma. Annals of Otology, Rhinology, Laryngology 51: 29-63

53. Harrison D F N 1987 The natural history, pathogenesis and treatment of juvenile angiofibroma. Archives of Otolaryngology 113: 936–942

54. Farag M M, Ghanimah S E, Ragaie A 1987 Hormonal receptors in juvenile nasopharyngeal angiofibroma. Laryngoscope 97: 208–211

55. Antonelli A R, Cappiello J, Orlandi A 1987 Diagnosis, staging and treatment of juvenile nasopharyngeal angiofibroma. Laryngoscope 97: 1319–1325

56. Schiff M 1959 Juvenile nasopharyngeal angiofibroma. Laryngoscope 69: 981–1016

57. Close L G, Schaefer S D, Mickey B E 1989 Surgical management of nasopharyngeal angiofibroma involving the cavernous sinus. Archives of Otolaryngology 115: 1091–1095

58. Holman C B, Miller W E 1965 Juvenile nasopharyngeal fibroma. American Journal of Roentgenology 94: 292–298

59. Witt R T, Shah J P, Sternberg S S 1983 Juvenile nasopharyngeal angiofibroma. American Journal of Surgery 146: 521–525

60. Roberson G W, Biller H, Sessions D G 1972 Presurgical internal maxillary artery embolisation in juvenile angiofibroma. Laryngoscope 82: 1524–1532

61. Lasjaunias P 1980 Nasopharyngeal angiofibromas: hazards of embolisation. Radiology 136: 119–123

62. Biller H F 1978 Juvenile nasopharyngeal angiofibroma. Annals of Otology, Rhinology, Laryngology 87: 630–632

63. Sessions R B, Bryan R N, Naclerio R M 1981 Radiographic staging of juvenile angiofibroma. Head and Neck Surgery 3: 279–283

64. Andrews J C, Fisch U, Valavanis A 1988 Surgical management of extensive nasopharyngeal angiofibroma with the infratemporal approach. Laryngoscope 98: 429–437

65. Fisch U 1983 The infratemporal approach to nasopharyngeal tumours. Laryngoscope 93: 36–44

66. Girgis I H, Fammy S A 1973 Nasopharyngeal fibroma: its histopathological nature. Journal of Laryngology and Otology 87: 1107–1123

67. Batsakis J G, Klopp C T, Newman W 1956 Fibrosarcoma arising in a juvenile nasopharyngeal angiofibroma following extensive radiation therapy. American Journal of Surgery 21: 786–793

68. Chen K T, Bauer F W 1982 Sarcomatous transformation of nasopharyngeal angiofibroma. Cancer 49: 369–371

69. Donald P S 1979 Sarcomatous degeneration in nasopharyngeal angiofibroma. Otolaryngology, Head and Neck Surgery 87: 42–46

70. Gisselsson L, Lindgren M, Stenram V 1958 Sarcomatous transformation of a juvenile nasopharyngeal angiofibroma. Acta Pathologica 42: 305–312

71. Hubbard E M 1958 Nasopharyngeal angiofibroma. Archives of Pathology 65: 192–204

72. Jacobsson M, Petruson B, Ruth M 1989 Involution of residual juvenile nasopharyngeal angiofibroma. Archives of Otolaryngology 115: 238–239

73. Stansbie J M, Phelps P D 1986 Involution of residual juvenile angiofibroma. Journal of Laryngology and Otology 100: 599–603

74. Sellars S L 1980 Juvenile nasopharyngeal angiofibroma. South African Medical Journal 58: 961–964

75. Economou T S, Abemayor E, Ward P H 1988 Juvenile nasopharyngeal angiofibroma. An update of the UCLA experience 1960–1968. Laryngoscope 98: 170–175

76. Sardana D S 1965 Nasopharyngeal fibroma: extension into the cheek. Archives of Otolaryngology 81: 584–588

77. Panje W R 1987 Surgical therapy for tumours of the nasopharynx. In: Thawley J E, Panje W R, Batsakis J G, Lindberg (eds) Comprehensive management of head and neck tumours Vol. 1. Saunders, Philadelphia

78. Neel H B, Whicker J H, Devine K D 1973 Juvenile angiofibroma. American Journal of Surgery 126: 547–556

79. Gill G, Rice D H, Rittr F N, Kindt G 1976 Intracranial and extracranial nasopharyngeal angiofibroma. Archives of Otolaryngology 102: 371–373

80. Casson P R, Bonnano P C, Converse J M 1974 The midface degloving procedure. Plastic and Reconstructive Journal 53: 102–113

81. McCombe A, Lund V J, Howard D 1990 Recurrence in juvenile angiofibroma. Rhinology 28: 1–6

82. Walike J W, Mackay B 1970 Nasopharyngeal angiofibroma. Light and electron microscopic changes after stilboestrol therapy. Laryngoscope 80: 1109–1121

83. Johnsen S, Kloster S H, Schiff M 1966 Action of hormones on juvenile nasopharyngeal angiofibroma. Acta Otorhinolaryngologica 61: 143–189

84. Myhre M, Michaels L 1987 Nasopharyngeal angiofibroma treated in 1981 by maxillectomy. Journal of Otolaryngology 16: 390–392

85. Cummings B J 1980 Relative risk factors in the treatment of juvenile nasopharyngeal angiofibroma. Head and Neck Surgery 3: 21–40

86. Waldman S R, Levine H L, Astor F 1981 Surgical experience with nasopharyngeal angiofibroma. Archives of Otolaryngology 107: 677–682

87. Goepfert H, Cangir C, Ya-Yen-Lee 1985 Chemotherapy for aggressive juvenile nasopharyngeal angiofibroma. Archives of Otolaryngology 111: 285–289

88. Bremer J W, Neel B H, DeSanto L W 1986 Angiofibroma: treatment trends in 150 patients, during 40 years. Laryngoscope 96: 1321–1329

89. Bernier J L, Bhaskar S N 1958 Aneurysmal bone cyst in the mandible. Oral Surgery 17: 30–41

90. Gruskin S E, Dahlin D C 1968 Aneurysmal bone cyst of the jaws. Journal of Oral Surgery 26: 523–528

91. Giddings N A, Kennedy T L, Knipe K L 1989 Aneurysmal cyst of the mandible. Archives of Otolaryngology 115: 865–870
92. Hady M R, Ghanaam B, Hady M Z 1990 Aneurysmal bone cyst of the maxillary sinus. Journal of Laryngology and Otology 104: 501–503
93. Prein J, Remangen W, Spiessel B 1985 Atlas of tumors of the facial skeleton. Springer-Verlag, Berlin.
94. Yarrington C T, Abbott J, Raines D 1964 Aneurysmal bone cyst of the maxilla. Archives of Otolaryngology 80: 313–317
95. McCullough D, Scott R, Seybold H 1971 Renal angiomyolipoma: Review of the literature and report of seven cases. Journal of Urology 105: 32–44
96. Dawlatly E E, Anim J T, El-Hassan A Y 1988 Angiomyolipoma of the nasal cavity. Journal of Laryngology and Otology 102: 1156–1158
97. Dorfman H D, Steiner G C, Jaffe H L 1971 Vascular tumours of bone. Human Pathology 2: 349–376
98. Wold L E, Ivins J C, Unni K V 1982 Haemangioendothelios-arcoma of bone. American Journal of Surgical Pathology 6: 59–70
99. Batsakis J G, Rice D H 1980 Pathology of head and neck tumours. Vasoform tumours. part 9B. Head and Neck Surgery 3: 326-339
100. Girard C, Johnson W C, Graham J H 1970 Cutaneous angiosarcoma. Cancer 26: 868–883
101. Panje W R, Moran W S, Bostwick D G 1986 Angiosarcoma of the head and neck. Laryngoscope 96: 1381–1384
102. Fu Y, Perzin K H 1974 Non-epithelial tumours of the nasal cavity, paranasal sinuses and nasopharynx. A clinico-pathologic study. Cancer 33: 1381–1384
103. Bankaci M, Myers E N, Barnes L 1979 Angiosarcoma of the maxillary sinus: literature review and case report. Head and Neck Surgery 1: 274–280
104. Sharma B G, Mawalicha P L 1979 Angiosarcoma of the maxillary antrum: report of a case. Journal of Laryngology and Otology 93: 181–186
105. Dahlin D C 1967 Vascular tumours. In: Bone tumours, 2nd edn. Charles C Thomas, Springfield USA, p 100
106. Zachariades N, Papdakou A, Koundouris C 1980 Primary haemangioendotheliosarcoma of the mandible. Review of the literature and case report. Journal of Oral Surgery 38: 288–291
107. Brook I M, Martin B A 1980 Angiosarcoma metastasis to the maxilla and mandible. British Journal of Oral Surgery 18: 266–271
108. Henry F A 1949 Angiosarcoma of the maxilla in a 3-month-old infant. Journal of Oral Surgery 7: 250–253
109. Kurien M, Nair S, Thomas S 1989 Angiosarcoma of the nasal cavity and maxillary antrum. Journal of Laryngology and Otology 103: 874–876
110. Williamson I G, Ramsden R T 1988 A case of angiosarcoma following exposure to vinyl chloride. Journal of Laryngology and Otology 102: 464–467
111. Zakrzewska J M 1986 Angiosarcoma of the maxilla – case report and review of the literature including angiosarcoma of the maxillary antrum. British Journal of Oral and Maxillofacial surgery 24: 286–292
112. McCarthy W D, Pack G T 1950 Malignant blood vessel tumours. A report of 56 cases of angiosarcoma and Kaposi's sarcoma. Surgery, Gynecology and Obstetrics 91: 465–470
113. Duck B W 1975 Proceedings: Vinyl chloride carcinogenesis. British Journal of Cancer 32: 260–263
114. Heath C W 1975 Characteristics of cases of angiosarcoma of the liver amongst vinyl chloride workers in the United States. Annals of the New York Academy of Science 246: 231–236
115. BMJ Leader 1974 More facts on vinyl chloride and cancer. British Medical Journal, November 30: 486–487
116. Garcia-Moral C A 1972 Malignant haemangioendothelioma of bone. Review of the world literature and report of a case. Clinical Orthopaedics 82: 70–79
117. Warner T F, O'Loughlin S 1975 Kaposi's sarcoma: a byproduct of tumour rejection. Lancet ii: 687–689
118. Kaposi M 1872 Idiopathic multiple pigmentsortum der Haut. Archives of Dermatology and Syphilology 4: 265–273
119. Marcusen D C, Sooy C D 1985 Otolaryngologic and head and neck manifestations of AIDS. Laryngoscope 95: 401–405
120. Update: Acquired Immunodeficiency Syndrome – United States 1982 Mortality, Morbidity Weekly Report 31(37): 507–508
121. Abramson A L, Simons R L 1970 Kaposi's sarcoma of the head and neck. Archives of Otolaryngology 92: 505–507
122. Rosenberg R A, Schneider K L, Cohen N L 1984 Head and neck presentation of acquired immunodeficiency syndrome. Laryngoscope 94: 642–646
123. O'Connell K M 1977 Kaposi's sarcoma: histopathological study of 159 cases in Malawi. Journal of Clinical Pathology 30: 687–695
124. Ammann A J, Dritz S K, Volberding P 1984 AIDS: The multidisciplinary enigma. Western Journal of Medicine 140: 66–81
125. Berdsis C 1957 Transplantable and metastasizing haemangiopericytoma in the rat. Oncologica 10: 336–337
126. Zimmermann K W 1923 Der feineire bau der Blutcapillaren. Zoologica Anatoma Entwicklungsqesch 68: 29–109
127. Stout A P, Murray M R 1942 Haemangiopericytoma – vascular tumour featuring Zimmermann's pericytes. Annals of Surgery 116: 26–33
128. Stout A P 1949 Haemangioperiocytoma: a study of 25 new cases. Cancer 2: 1027–1054
129. Compagno J, Hyams V J 1976 Haemangiopericytoma-like intranasal tumours. A clinicopathological study of 23 cases. American Journal of Clinical Pathology 66: 672–683
130. McMaster M J, Soule E H, Wins J C 1975 Haemangiopericytoma – A clinicopathologic study and longterm follow up of 60 patients. Cancer 36: 2232–2244
131. Enzinger F M, Smith B H 1976 Haemangiopericytoma – analysis of 106 cases. Human Pathology 7: 61–82
132. Kauffman J L, Stout A P 1960 Haemangiopericytoma in children. Cancer 13: 695–710
133. Seibert S S, Seibert R W, Weisenburger D S 1978 Multiple congenital haemangiopericytomas of the head and neck. Laryngoscope 88: 1006–1012
134. Chawla D P, Oswal V H 1987 Haemangiopericytoma of the nose and paranasal sinuses. Journal of Laryngology and Otology 101: 729–737
135. Al-Khalifa S, Paulose K O, Sharma R K 1988 Haemangiopericytoma of the nasal septum. Journal of Laryngology and Otology 102: 1161–1163
136. Benveniste R S, Harris H H 1973 Nasal haemangiopericytoma. Archives of Otolaryngology 98: 358–359
137. Brown J A 1977 Nasal haemangiopericytoma. Southern Medical Journal 70: 359–360
138. Caldarelli D D, Sperling R L 1976 Haemangiopericytoma of the maxilla. Archives of Otolaryngology 102: 47–50
139. Compagno J 1978 Haemangiopericytoma-like tumours of the nasal cavity – a comparison with haemangiopericytoma of soft tissue. Laryngoscope 88: 460–469
140. Gorenstein A, Jacer G W, Weiland L H 1978 Haemangiopericytoma of the nasal cavity. Otorhinolaryngology 86: 405–415
141. Walike J W, Bailey B 1971 Head and neck haemangiopericytoma. Archives of Otolaryngology 93: 345–353
142. Barwinkle K D, Diddon J A 1970 Haemangiopericytoma – report of a case and a comprehensive review of the literature. Cancer 25: 896–907
143. Batsakis J G, Jacobs J B, Templeton A C 1983 Haemangiopericytoma of the nasal cavity. Journal of Laryngology and Otology 97: 361–368
144. Bermond G, Garein M, Bonnaud G 1975 Les haemangiopericytes de la sphere ORL. Journal Francais d'Otologie, Rhinologie et Laryngologie 24: 381–386
145. Ortega J A, Finklestein J Z, Hittle R 1971 Chemotherapy of malignant haemangiopericytoma of children. Cancer 27: 730–735
146. Himelfarb M Z, Ostrzega N L, Samuel J 1983 Paraganglioma of the nasal cavity. Laryngoscope 93: 350–351
147. Zak F G and Lawson W 1982 The paraganglioma chemoreceptor system – physiology, pathology and clinical medicine. Springer-Verlag, New York
148. Talbot A R 1990 Paraganglioma of the maxillary sinus. Journal of Laryngology and Otology 104: 248–251
149. Sykes J M & Ossoff R H 1986 Paragangliomas of the head and neck. Otolaryngologic Clinics of North America 19: 755–767

150. Glenner C G, Grimley P M 1974 Tumors of the extra-adrenal paraganglioma system (including chemoreceptors). In: Atlas of Tumor Pathology. Second series. Fascicle 9. Armed Forces Institute of Pathology, Washington.

151. Girgis I H, Fahmy S A 1973 Nasopharyngeal fibroma: its histopathological nature. Journal of Laryngology and Otology 87: 1107–1123

152. Milroy C M, Rode J, Moss E 1991 Laryngeal paragangliomas and neuroendocrine carcinomas. Histopathology 18: 201–209

153. Kameya T, Shinesato Y, Adachi I 1980 Neuroendocrine carcinoma of the paranasal sinuses: a morphological and endocrine study. Cancer 45: 330–339

154. Apple D & Kreines S 1962 Non-chromaffin paraganglioma of the nasal cavity. Laryngoscope 72: 201–216

155. Moran T E 1962 Non-chromaffin paraganglioma of the nasal cavity. Laryngoscope 72: 201–216

156. Lack E E, Cublla A L, Woodruff J M 1977 Paraganglioma of the head and neck region. Cancer 39: 397–409

157. Ueda N, Yoshida A, Fukunshi R 1985 Non-chromaffin paraganglioma of the nose and paranasal sinuses. Acta Pathologica Japonica 35: 489–495

158. Watson D S 1988 Nasal paraganglioma. Journal of Laryngology and Otology 102: 526–529

159. Stout A P 1956 Tumors featuring pericytes: glomus tumors or hemangiopericytoma. Laboratory Investigation 5: 217–223

160. Soule E H, Ghormley R K, Bulbulian A H 1955 Primary tumours of the soft tissues of the extremities exclusive of epithelial tumours: An analysis of 500 cases. Archives of Surgery 70: 462–474

161. Pantazopoulos P E 1965 Glomus tumour of the nasal cavity. Archives of Otolaryngology 81: 83–86

162. De Bord B A 1972 Glomus tumors - unusual presentation in otolaryngology. Surgical Clinics of North America 52: 473–483

163. Fleury I, Basset J M 1979 Tumeurs rares de la cloison – Huit cas rapportes. Annals Otolaryngology Surgery Cervicofacial 96: 767–779

164. Potter A J, Khatib G, Peppard S B 1984 Intranasal glomus tumours. Archives of Otolaryngology 110: 755–756

10. Tumours of muscle origin

Tumours of smooth and skeletal muscle are exceptionally rare in the upper jaw, though the head and neck in general is a frequent site for these lesions and orbital rhabdomyosarcoma is one of the commonest malignant tumours in children. The previously dismal prognosis of this condition has been markedly improved by a better understanding of its natural history, improved clinical staging and effective combined oncology regimes but these efforts are still confounded by failure on the part of clinicians to suspect the diagnosis. Tumours covered in this group are:

1. Leiomyoma, leiomyoblastoma and leiomyosarcoma
2. Rhabdomyoma
3. Rhabdomyosarcoma.

LEIOMYOMA, LEIOMYOBLASTOMA AND LEIOMYOSARCOMA

Definition

These are all neoplasms of smooth muscle cells showing varying degrees of differentiation.

Historical aspects

In 1958 Dobben[1] published a case of leiomyosarcoma in the nasal cavity of a 69-year-old woman and this has been followed by a sporadic number of case reports.

Incidence

Whilst the head and neck are not uncommon sites for superficial smooth muscle tumours, these are exceptionally rare in the upper jaw itself.[2] The total number in the literature is just under 50 (Tables 10.1 and 10.2). In 76 cases of smooth muscle tumours in children[3] none occurred in this area and Mindell et al[4] found two in the sinonasal tract out of 31 leiomyosarcomas affecting the head and neck. The malignant tumours are slightly more common than the benign leiomyomas but there is only one case report (of our own patient) with a leiomyoblastoma in the nose.

Age, sex and ethnic variation

The cases of leiomyoma range from 5–76 years (average 48 years), with a slight female preponderance (7:4) (Table 10.1). The leiomyosarcomas cover a similar age range (18–75 years; average 52 years) with an equal male to female ratio (Table 10.2). It may be of significance that a number of case reports have emanated from Japan.

Site

Smooth muscle tumours are usually found in the uterus, gastro-intestinal tract and subcutaneous tissues, though they can occur wherever smooth muscle occurs. The paucity of smooth muscle within the sinonasal tract may account for their rarity here, where they mainly arise in the nasal cavity.

Aetiology

The likeliest source of smooth muscle is found in the vasculature of the region though it has also been suggested that the tumours arise from multipotential mesenchymal cells.

One case of leiomyosarcoma reported by Fu & Perzin[5] had received radiotherapy 22 years previously for chronic sinusitis. Lalwani & Kaplan[6] also published a case which occurred 6 years after radiation and cyclophosphamide. Whilst there is no evidence that leiomyomas become malignant, Fu & Perzin[5] also found one case of leiomyosarcoma containing an area with the pattern of leiomyoma, suggesting this possibility.

Clinical features and radiology

Some leiomyomas are found incidentally when 'polyps' are removed. Two of eight cases[7] presented in this way,

Table 10.1 Leiomyomas of upper jaw: in the literature

Author	Sex	Age (yr)	Site	Treatment	Outcome
Maesaka et al 1966[21]	F	49	Vestibule	Local excision	A&W 1 yr
Cherrick et al 1973[22]	M	53	Palate	Local excision	
	M	56	Palate	Local excision	
	M	47	Palate	Local excision	No FU
	F	28	Palate	Local excision	
Schwartzman & Schwartzman 1973[23]	M	57	Maxilla, ethmoid, sphenoid	Trans-antral ethmoidectomy	No FU
Wolfowitz & Schmaman 1973[24]	F	42	Inferior turbinate	Local excision	–
Fu & Perzin 1975[5]	M	46	Nasal cavity	Polypectomy	Lost
	F	60	Nasal cavity	Polypectomy	A&W 7 yr
Rhatigan & Kinus 1976[25]	F	71	Alveolus	Local excision	–
McCaffrey et al 1978[26]	F	76	Inferior turbinate	Local excision	No FU
Mechlin et al 1980[27]	F	21	Alveolus	Caldwell–Luc, partial maxillectomy	No FU
Lijovetsky et al 1985[28]	M	73	Vestibule	Local excision	No FU
Hanna et al 1988[29]	F	64	Inferior turbinate	Local excision	A&W 1 yr
Tang & Tse 1988[7]	M	56	Inferior turbinate	Transpalatal excision	A&W 1 yr
Zijlker & Visser 1989[30]	M	33	Ethmoid	Lateral rhinotomy	A&W 2 yr
Barr et al 1990[31]	F	44	Nasal septum	Local excision	No FU
Harrison & Lund	F	5	Middle turbinate	Polypectomy, lateral rhinotomy (×3), craniofacial resection	12 yr since diagnosis, 18/12 since last operation A&W
	F	55	Middle meatus, nasolacrimal duct	External ethmoidectomy	No FU

A&W, alive and well; No FU, no follow-up

half presented with epistaxis, and two had facial pain. Those with leiomyosarcoma also frequently had epistaxis, nasal obstruction and facial pain and in addition facial swelling and proptosis may occur.

Radiologically there are no specific features other than those common to benign and malignant lesions in this area (Fig. 10.1).

A 5-year-old girl was first seen in June 1979 for recurrent epistaxis. On examination a polypoid mass was found and removed from the left nasal cavity, which histology showed to be a leiomyoblastoma. She was well until February 1980 when epistaxis and nasal obstruction recurred and a further pedunculated mass was seen arising from the middle turbinate. Tomograms suggested an origin from the ethmoid region and she underwent a lateral rhinotomy. A friable vascular tumour 1.5 × 1 × 1 cm was removed from the anterior ethmoidal region and histology again confirmed a leiomyoblastoma. Further recurrences have occurred in September 1981 and August 1985, each being excised via a lateral rhinotomy approach.

In July 1989 when she developed further symptoms at the age of 15, a craniofacial resection was performed to radically clear the ethmoid and cribriform plate region. The tumour was firmly adherent to the undersurface of the nasal bones, with a separate deposit on the septum. She has been well with no sign of recurrence for the last 2 years.

A 41-year-old man presented with a 6 month history of facial pain which had been empirically treated as sinusitis by his general practitioner with antibiotics. 3 months later he developed epistaxis, numbness in the left upper teeth and nasal obstruction. 1 month later a nasal mass became apparent and he was found on examination and imaging to have an antro-ethmoidal lesion which had breached the orbit. Biopsy of a friable polyp showed a leiomyosarcoma and he was referred for radical excision, by total maxillectomy and orbital clearance. He has had no sign of recurrence after 5 years, follow-up.

Macroscopic and microscopic appearance

In all cases the lesions are well-circumscribed and greyish-white or reddish-white in colour.

Microscopically, leiomyomas have baton-shaped nuclei and contain myofibrils which can be shown with routine staining[8a,9,10] such as phosphotungstic acid haematoxylin. The lesions have a variable degree of vascularity and have been divided into vascular and non-vascular lesions by Stout & Lattes.[11] It has been suggested that the vascular lesions may be malformations rather than tumours or represent the end-point in a progression from haeman-

Table 10.2 Leiomyosarcomas of upper jaw: in the literature

Author	No.	Sex	Age (yr)	Site	Treatment	Outcome
Dobben 1958[1]	1	F	69	Nasal cavity, nasopharynx	Local excision	A&W 1 yr
Lukes & Rauchenberg 1959[35]	–	–		Nasal cavity, paranasal sinus	–	–
Ogiba 1962[32]	1	M	29	Nasal cavities, R&L	DXT, neck dissection & maxillectomy	DOD 17/12 Lung 2°s
Canciullo & Nucci 1963[33]	1	F	61	Nasal cavity	Surgery	No FU
Pimpinella & Marquit 1965[20]	1	M	56	Nasal cavity, maxilla, nasopharynx	Local excision, recurrences, 9 yr later lateral rhinotomy, 5 yr later lateral rhinotomy	14 yr from diagnosis 4/12 since last op. A&W
Maesaka et al 1966[21]	1	F	53	Nasal cavity, nasopharynx	–	A&W 1 yr
Kawabe et al 1968[19]	2	M	60	Maxilla	Local excision, recurrence & cervical lymphadenopathy treated DXT/C	DOD 7/12
		M	52	Nasal cavity, maxilla	Maxillectomy, DXT/C for recurrence with cervical lymphadenopathy	DOD 1 yr
Fu & Perzin 1975[5]	6	F	18	Nasal cavity	Polypectomy; Caldwell–Luc maxillectomy/orbit; further excision, DXT	A&W 1 yr from last op.
		F	37	Nasal cavity	Lateral rhinotomy; maxillectomy at 14/12; surgical excisions ×3 for further recurrences during next 28/12; C	DOD 3.5 yr Lung 2°s
		M	36	Nasal cavity, maxilla	Surgery; DXT	DICD 18/12
		M	56	Nasal cavity; all sinuses, nasopharynx, orbit	Polypectomy 14 yr before Surgery; recurrence 18/12, DXT	DOD 3 yr
		F	40	Antro-ethmoid, nasal cavity	Caldwell–Luc; surgery for recurrence 3/12; DXT	DOD 1 yr
		M	45	Nasal cavity, maxilla	Polypectomy 16 yr before; maxillectomy/orbital clearance, DXT	DICD 6/12
Mindell et al 1975[4]	1	M	70	Maxilla	Caldwell–Luc	A&W 2 yr
Dropkin et al 1976[16]	1	M	75	Nasal cavity, maxilla	Polypectomy; recurrence, lateral rhinotomy; recurrence, maxillectomy	A&W 26/12 from last op
Jakobiec et al 1978[17]	1	M	39	Maxilla, orbit, nasopharynx, pterygo-palatine fossa	C, DXT, radical surgery 1 yr later	AWR 3 yr
Kurvilla et al 1990[34]	9	M	22	Nasal septum	Radical excision	A&W 15/12
		F	68	Lateral nasal wall	Medial maxillectomy	A&W 9 yr
		M	86	Inferior turbinate	Excision	A&W 9 yr
		F	72	Inferior turbinate	Medial maxillectomy	A&W 20/12
		M	66	Antro-nasal	Radical excision, DXT/C	DOD 6 yr
		F	51	Antro-nasal	Partial excision	AWR 3/12
		F	28	Ethmoid & nasal cavity	Excision	A&W 9/12
		F	43	Ethmoid & nasal cavity	Medial maxillectomy & ethmoidectomy	A&W 19/12
		F	60	Ethmoid & nasal cavity	Craniofacial resection	A&W 19/12
Lalwani & Kaplan 1990[6]	1	M	66	Antro-nasal	Partial excision, DXT/C	AWR 9/12
Harrison & Lund	2	M	47	Antro-ethmoid	Maxillectomy & orbital clearance	A&W 5 yr
		F	54	Antro-ethmoid		

A&W, alive and well; AWR, alive with recurrence, DOD, dead of disease; No FU, no follow-up; 2°s, secondaries; DICD, dead of intercurrent disease; DXT, radiotherapy; C, chemotherapy

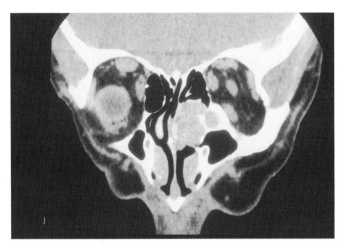

Fig. 10.1   Coronal CT scan showing leiomyoma arising in the nasolacrimal region.

Leiomyosarcoma are distinguished by increased cellularity, mitoses and cellular and nuclear irregularity.[13] In the rest of the body, e.g. uterus, even without cytological atypia the number of mitoses/high power field (HPF) is indicative of potential behaviour.[14] Less than 5/10 HPF suggests a benign lesion, 5–10/10 HPF intermediate activity and >10/10 HPF malignancy. In the presence of atypia, the incidence of mitoses is less important,[7,15] particularly in other areas of the body.

Natural history

Leiomyomas can achieve a large size but are cured by complete excision. Leiomyosarcoma are characterized by local invasion in 75% of cases.[9,16,17] The majority, though arising in the nasal cavity, usually involved an adjacent sinus and local recurrence is mainly responsible for death, in half the cases between 1 and 3.5 years later. Less than 10% develop lymph node metastases[4,18] but haematogenous secondaries are commoner (20%),[4] most often to the lungs (5/6)[19] and lead to an earlier demise within 18 months.

Differential diagnosis

Smooth muscle tumours must be distinguished from other spindle cell tumours such as haemangiopericytoma, malignant schwannoma and fibrosarcoma. Electron microscopy generally demonstrates the myofibrils in characteristic focal condensations and immunoperoxidase staining for desmin is positive indicating muscular differentiation.

Treatment

The benign lesions are cured by local excision but will recur if this is inadequate as evidenced by our own case.

Surgery is also the treatment of choice for leiomyosarcomas, though because of their infiltrating nature often prove more difficult to eradicate and may recur several times, even over long periods of time.[20] Radiotherapy and chemotherapy have been used, particularly for recurrence but are largely ineffective.[16]

Prognosis

Cure can be achieved with leiomyoma though there are few cases with long term follow-up. By contrast, there are few cases of leiomyosarcoma surviving beyond 5 years and even with adequate surgery, local recurrence and distant metastases occur. In Mindell's series of 31 cases in the head and neck 19 survived without evidence of disease for 4 months to 12 years (average 4 years) but eight died of disease, six with secondaries. In the literature (Table 10.2) 15 patients were alive and well 12–26 months from diagnosis, three having had additional treatment for recurrences. One further case had two recurrences after 9 and 5 years. Seven patients had died of disease between 7 months and 6 years from diagnosis (four with obvious metastases) and two had died of intercurrent disease.

RHABDOMYOMA

This benign tumour of skeletal muscle has a predilection for the head and neck but is virtually unknown in the upper jaw. It is most commonly encountered in cardiac muscle where it is thought that the majority are developmental harmatomatous malformations. Some are associated with glycogen storage diseases such as tuberosclerosis and two forms have been described: adult and fetal.[8b,18] The latter must be distinguished from rhabdomyosarcoma.

26 cases have been reported in the head and neck of adults, affecting the tongue, oral cavity and larynx. Fu and Perzin[36] included one case in the nasopharynx which impinged on the posterior nasal cavity. They can occur at any age and may be slightly commoner in men. They present a well-defined mass which is cured by complete excision.

RHABDOMYOSARCOMA

Definition

Rhabdomyosarcoma is a neoplastic analogue of embryogenesis of skeletal muscle.[8b] The rhabdomyoblast, the primitive muscle cell, recapitulates the normal development from a primitive round cell to spindle cell to multinucleated muscle fibres, but in a highly disorganized manner.

Historical aspects

Weber[37] recognized a malignant tumour of skeletal muscle in 1854 and Bard[38] discussed it further in 1885. The first large series of rhabdomyosarcomas was reported by Rakov[39] in 1937 and in 1946 Stout[40] described the pleomorphic variety. The embryonal type had been reported in 1894[41] and was more fully discussed by Stobbe & Dargeon in 1950.[42] Riopelle & Theriault[43] described the alveolar type in 1956 and the botryoid form was initially mentioned in 1854.[44]

Incidence

In adults, rhabdomyosarcoma is most frequently found affecting the extremities and torso. By contrast in children it is commonest in the urogenital region and head and neck where it is the most common malignant soft tissue neoplasm in this age group.[45] King & Clatworthy[46] found it to constitute 51.4% of all soft tissue sarcomas in children and Farr[47] reported 198 head and neck sarcomas, of which 96 (48.5%) were rhabdomyosarcomas. Between 34% and 43% of rhabdomyosarcomas occur in the head and neck[48,49] but the majority of these affect the orbit. The nose and paranasal sinuses are uncommonly affected (Table 10.3).

Age, sex and ethnic variation

The lesion can occur at any age, from birth to 80, but in the head and neck it is the first decade which is predominantly affected. This is in contrast to the 5th to 6th decades when the tumour occurs in other parts of the body. In a series of 166 cases in the head and neck, 77% were 12 years or less at the time of diagnosis, of which half were younger than 6 years.[8b] The average age in Fu & Perzin's patients was 7 years.[36]

There is said to be a slight male preponderance[50,51] of 1.37–1.5:1 and whilst ethnic information is not always available, the lesion is much less common in Negroes.

Site

In the head and neck, the orbit is most frequently the site, followed by the soft tissues of the neck. The upper jaw is rarely primarily affected (Table 10.3) but may be secondarily involved by spread from the nasopharynx or orbit. Of 777 rhabdomyosarcomas, 8.2% occurred in the nose and sinuses[52] where the nasal cavity and maxilla are most commonly affected.

Aetiology

Despite considerable research, there does not appear to be a familial risk, with the concordance rate in siblings being lower than for a number of other childhood malignancies. The rarity in Negroes has, however, led to speculation about possible genetic factors.[53] Friedmann[9,54] reported that the tumour could be induced experimentally in animals by the injection of nickel sulphide but this seems an unlikely aetiological factor given the age group affected. More recently viral induction has been suggested by some studies.[50,55]

The absence of skeletal muscle in the mucous membrane of the nose and sinuses implies that the lesion arises from immature muscle tissue or undifferentiated mesenchyme.

Clinical features

Moderately rapid growth leads to presentation with a mass, epistaxis, nasal obstruction, facial swelling or pain. Orbital involvement produces proptosis and decreased visual acuity. Spread to the skull base can result in cranial nerve palsies (III–VII).[36]

A 32-year-old female accounts clerk had presented to the ophthamologist with a medial canthal mass. This was accompanied by nasal obstruction, blood-stained rhinorrhoea, infraorbital pain and blurred vision and she was referred to us via Moorfields Eye Hospital. A biopsy showed an embryonal rhabdomyosarcoma and imaging with CT and MRI confirmed an extensive left antro-ethmoid lesion.

At craniofacial resection, disease was found in the frontal, ethmoid, sphenoid and antrum with invasion of the orbit and cribriform plate. Orbital clearance was therefore performed. Fine needle aspiration of a cervical lymph node was also positive and she then commenced a course of radiotherapy and chemotherapy. 8 months later she developed a recurrence in the frontal lobes and received further chemotherapy and radiotherapy but sadly she succumbed to widespread metastases, notably in the spine after 4 months.

Radiology (Figs 10.2 and 10.3)

Bone destruction is observed relatively early.[56] In nine of our cases whose plain sinus X-rays and CT scans were reviewed by Lloyd,[57] all had affected the nasal cavity and maxilla, and the majority had spread into the orbit and ethmoids at presentation. Five of the nine had also infiltrated the sphenoid and frontal sinuses, though there was no evidence of calcification or new bone formation. The lesion presents a high-intensity signal on T2 weighted spin echo sequences of MRI and the use of the three-plane multislice technique can show unsuspected involvement of the parapharyngeal space.

Macroscopic and microscopic appearance

The tumour may appear as a grape-like polypoid mass or 'botryoid' though the term 'sarcoma botryoides' is not endorsed by some pathologists.[58] The lesion may also

Table 10.3   Rhabdomyosarcoma of the upper jaw: in the literature

Author	No.	Sex	Age (yr)	Site	Histology	Treatment	Outcome
Cooper 1934[74]	1	M	67	Maxilla	Pleomorphic	DXT/lateral rhinotomy	No FU
Pastore et al 1950[75]	1	M	46	Maxilla	Pleomorphic	Surgery, DXT	A&W 7 yr
Riopelle & Theriault 1956[43]	1	M	22	Maxilla	Alveolar	DXT	DOD 5/12
Koop & Tewarson 1964[76]	1	–	–	Nasal cavity	Alveolar	Maxillectomy	A&W 7 yr
Masson & Soule 1965[77]	14	–	–	Nasal cavity		–	–
	7	–	–	Maxilla	Embryonal	–	–
Dabezies & Naugle 1968[78]	1	M	26	Ethmoid	Alveolar	DXT/C	No FU
Henny & Downs 1968[79]	1	M	4	Maxilla	Embryonal	Triple therapy	A&W 31/12
	1	F	12	Maxilla	Embryonal	Triple therapy	AW R 20/12
Donaldson et al 1973[56]	5		12			DXT/C	DOD, lung 2°s
			3	All maxilla	All embryonal	DXT/C	AWR
			5			Triple therapy	A&W
			10	Both nasal cavity		DXT/C	A&W
			9			DXT/C	AWR, cervical 2°s
Ghavimi et al 1975[63]	1	M	6	Maxilla	Embryonal	Triple therapy	A&W 28/12
Makishima et al 1975[80]	1	M	25	Ethmoid	Alveolar	Triple therapy	DOD 6/12
Fu & Perzin 1976[36]	16	10M 6F	10/12–28 yr (mean 7 yr)	Nasal cavity (12) Maxilla (2) Ethmoid (2) Nasopharynx (6) Sphenoid (1) Multiple sites affected	Embryonal (10) Botryoid (5) Alveolar (1)	5 (inoperable) DXT 4 small – triple therapy (with localized surgery) 4 moderate – triple therapy (with inadequate but more radical surgery) 3 – triple therapy (extensive radical surgery)	All 5 DOD, 4–15/12 1 No FU 3 DOD 9/12 10/12, 7 yr 1 No FU 3 DOD 14–18/12 1 DOD 8/12 1 A&W 8 yr 1 A&W 7 yr
Murakami 1978[81]	1	M	2	Nasal cavity	Embryonal	Triple therapy	A&W 9/12
Healy et al 1979[69]	1	–	–	Maxilla	–	Triple therapy	A&W 1 yr
Pandhi et al 1980[82]	4	F	2	Maxilla	Embryonal	C/DXT	A&W 15/12
		M	3.5	Antro-ethmoid & CLN	Embryonal	DXT/C	No FU
		M	12	Antro-ethmoid & CLN	Embryonal	DXT/C	DOD 5/12
		F	45	Antro-ethmoid	Pleomorphic	DXT/maxillectomy	A&W 18/12
Kanegaonkar et al 1981[83]	1	F	27	Maxilla & CLN	Mixed embryonal & alveolar	DXT/C	Distant 2°s 10/12 Further C/DXT No FU
Feldman 1982[55]	2	M	27	Maxilla	Embryonal	Triple therapy	A&W 6 yr
		F	28	Maxilla	Alveolar	DXT/C	No FU
Proops & Mann 1984[84]	1	–	child	Maxilla	–	Triple therapy	–
Suzuki et al 1984[85]	1	F	22	Maxilla, ethmoid, sphenoid	Pleomorphic	C/Surgery	A&W 8/12
Kraus et al 1990[86]	2	1	child	Both paranasal sinus	–	Triple therapy	Both DOD, 2°s
		1	adult				
Harrison & Lund	14	M	4	Nasal cavity	Embryonal	Triple therapy; Surgery (lateral rhinotomy)	No FU
		F	9	Nasal	Embryonal	DXT/C	DOD
		M	10	Nasal cavity	Embryonal	DXT/C	DOD
		M	20	Antro-ethmoid	Embryonal	Triple therapy	No FU
		F	32	Antro-ethmoid	Embryonal	Maxillectomy/orbital clearance Craniofacial/C	DOD 22/12
		M	44	Ethmoid	Pleomorphic	Triple therapy Craniofacial	DICD 10/12
		F	41	Ethmoid	Pleomorphic	DXT/lateral rhinotomy	DOD
		M	70	Maxilla	Pleomorphic	Maxillectomy/orbital clearance	A&W 5/12
		F	4	Orbit	Embryonal	Triple therapy	No FU
		F	6	Orbit	Embryonal	Orbital clearance	No FU
		M	8	Orbit	Embryonal	Orbital clearance/C	A&W 13 yr
		F	16	Orbit (& CLN)	Embryonal	DXT/C	A&W 6/12
		M	53	Orbit	Embryonal	DXT/C	A&W 11 yr
		F	20	Orbit (submandibular node)	Embryonal	Biopsy DXT/C	No FU

Triple therapy: chemotherapy, radiotherapy, radical surgery: A&W, alive and well; AWR, alive with recurrence; No FU, no follow-up; DXT, radiotherapy; C, chemotherapy; CLN, cervical lymphadenopathy; 2°s, secondaries; DOD, dead of disease; DICD, dead of intercurrent disease

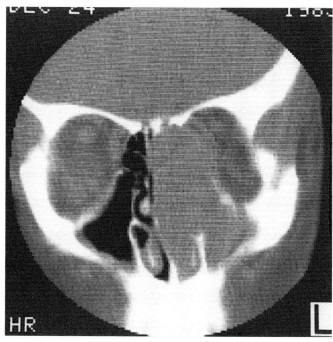

Fig. 10.2 Coronal CT scan showing extensive rhabdomyosarcoma of the left maxilla.

appear as a red-gray mass, for example when seen in the vestibule, though an apparent pseudo-encapsulation belies the lesion's infiltrating nature.[10b,59]

The tumour attempts to recapitulate the embryonic process but in a disorganized fashion. Four histological varieties have been described: *pleomorphic*; *embryonal*; *alveolar*; *botryoid*. The last is discounted by some as a separate group and a mixture of patterns can be observed. In the head and neck the embryonal type is commonest and has the appearances of muscle in a 7–10 week fetus. The pleomorphic lesions are the most differentiated with the most obvious cross-striations and is found mainly in older individuals.

The presence of cross-striations however, is not essential to the diagnosis. In their absence, electron microscopy can be helpful and may show distinct regularly spaced Z bands with an hexagonal arrangement of thick (myosin, 120–150 A) and thin (actin, 60–80 A) filaments.[48] In difficult cases desmin has proven the most useful antibody[60] due to its early expression but vimentin, myoglobulin, antimyosin and antiactin antibodies have also been used for characterization.[58,68]

Natural history

Rhabdomyosarcoma is locally aggressive if untreated and is associated with early haematogenous spread to lungs, bone, brain, skin, pleura and abdominal viscera. Okamura et al[61] reported a 20% incidence of distant metastases at the time of presentation and Fu & Perzin[36]

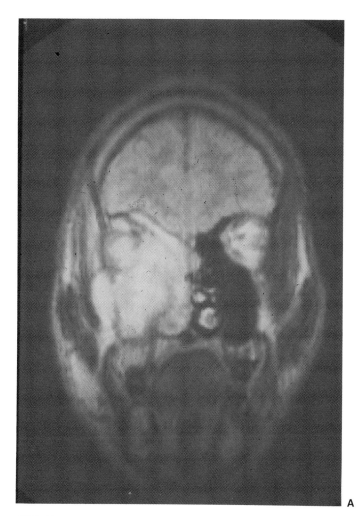

A

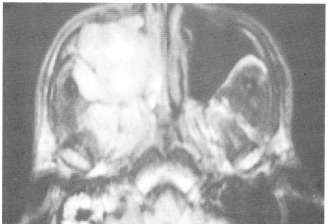

B

Fig. 10.3 Rhabdomyosarcoma of maxillary sinus extending into the pterygoid region. **A**, coronal and **B**, axial MR scans.

found them in two-thirds of patients during the course of the disease. Involvement of lymph nodes is also moderately common compared with other sarcomas, though less so with the head and neck lesions than those in the extremities. Half the upper jaw cases in Fu & Perzin's series had cervical lymphadenopathy.[36]

Differential diagnosis

The list of lesions with which rhabdomyosarcoma can be confused both clinically and histologically is lengthy. Polyps and angiofibromas are possible clinical alternatives whereas neuroblastomas (olfactory and metastatic), retinoblastomas, melanoma, fibrosarcoma, adenocarcinoma, lymphoma and Ewing's sarcoma are some of the pathologies which must be eliminated. 'No other tumour of childhood is so often misdiagnosed.'[62]

Treatment

The previously uniformly poor outlook for this condition has been transformed by the use of triple modality therapy,[56,63,64] combining surgery, radiotherapy and multiple agent chemotherapy, first reported by Pinkel & Pickren in 1961.[65] Even when en bloc excision is not possible there is evidence that the efficacy of the radiotherapy and chemotherapy is enhanced by reducing the tumour burden so some form of debulking is recommended.[64] There is however, no indication that prophylactic neck dissection is of value.[66]

A large number of treatment regimes are employed, usually based upon tumour staging though it should be emphasized how difficult this can be due to the infiltrating nature of the lesion. A number of chemotherapy agents are used of which vincristine, actinomycin D and cyclophosphamide (VAC) are most popular but many others including adriamycin and dimethyltriazenoimidazole carboxamide (DTIC) are reported.[67,68]

Prognosis

There is no doubt that the triple therapy approach has dramatically improved prognosis but overall results are still difficult to assess due to the different staging systems, the accuracy of staging and the different therapeutic combinations. There is some disagreement as to the effects of age, sex and histological type on prognosis with some concluding that they are not determinants in the response to treatment or survival[8b,18] whilst Sutow et al[64] found that cases of the alveolar subtype and the older children did worse. Hawkins & Camacho-Velasquez[48] have stressed the correlation between cellular anaplasia and poor outcome.

The extent of disease and therefore, clinical staging seems the most important factor if it can be accurately assessed.[36,56,64,66] As a consequence, lesions of the orbit generally did better than in the sinuses with a 91% 3-year relapse-free survival compared with 75% for the rest of the head and neck lesions.[70] The survival curves for children receiving surgical therapy plus chemotherapy and/or radiotherapy were practically identical. However the survival of children who did not have any surgical treatment at all was distinctly inferior to the others. All of these had tumours in the head and it is noteworthy that in both the series of Donaldson et al[56] and Fu & Perzin[36] only 3/19 and 3/16 tumours respectively could be successfully excised.

Previously only 12% (6/49) were alive at 5 years of whom four ultimately died of disease, three with widespread metastases.[8b,71] Between 1960 and 1970 a 3-year survival of 23% was found in head and neck rhabdomyosarcomas.[63] Between 1970 and 1974, all those receiving triple therapy survived, increasing 3-year survival to 67%, with failures only occurring in the group who did not receive surgery. It should be remembered, however that the tumour can recur even after 12 years.[72] Furthermore, if initial treatment fails, the outcome is still poor, and with distant metastases survival is usually less than 12 months. There is also a price to be paid even with successful treatment which can result in serious local effects on the orbit, pituitary, dentition and bone and may induce second primaries.

ORBITAL RHABDOMYOSARCOMA (Figs 10.4 and 10.5)

This constitutes one of the commonest malignant tumours in children, over 90% of which occur under 15 years of age. Although they present with rapid proptosis, usually with a mass in the upper inner quadrant they are almost always treated as an infection and are rarely diagnosed at the initial ophthalmological consultation. Fortunately dissemination occurs late, reflecting the lymphatic drainage of the area and 5-year survival (75%) is considerably better than for the rest of the head and neck. The majority (40/55 cases)[8b] are embryonal in type.

Treatment has tended to rely on a combination of radiotherapy and chemotherapy but there is a definite place for orbital clearance if residual disease is suspected

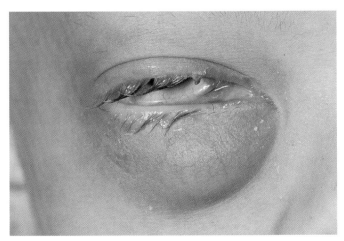

Fig. 10.4 Child with orbital rhabdomyosarcoma.

and especially when the globe is rendered blind and painful. Five cases have been managed on the Unit, three with orbital clearance (Table 10.3). Patients may present to the otolaryngologist with an interest in head and neck problems to exclude the possibility of sinus pathology particularly as cervical lymphadenopathy may be found.[73] Local spread into adjacent ethmoids may also provide a route for biopsy.

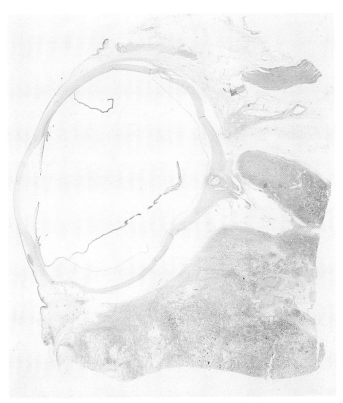

Fig. 10.5 Surgical specimen of orbital clearance showing rhabdomyosarcoma infiltrating around globe.

REFERENCES

1. Dobben G D 1958 Leiomyosarcoma of the nasopharynx. Archives of Otolaryngology 68: 211–213
2. Stout A P, Hill W T 1958 Leiomyosarcoma of the superficial soft tissues. Cancer 11: 844–854
3. Yannopoulos K, Stout A P 1962 Smooth muscle tumors in children. Cancer 15: 958–971
4. Mindell R S, Calcaterra T C, Ward P H 1975 Leiomyosarcoma of the head and neck: a review of the literature and report of two cases. Laryngoscope 85: 904–911
5. Fu Y-S, Perzin K H 1975 Nonepithelial tumors of the nasal cavity, paranasal sinuses and nasopharynx: a clinicopathologic study. IV Smooth muscle tumors (leiomyoma, leiomyosarcoma). Cancer 35: 1300–1308
6. Lalwani A K, Kaplan M J 1990 Paranasal sinus leiomyosarcoma after cyclophosphamide and irradiation. Otolaryngology, Head and Neck Surgery 103: 1039–1042
7. Tang S O, Tse C H 1988 Leiomyoma of the nasal cavity. Journal of Laryngology and Otology 102: 831–833
8. Batsakis J G 1980 Tumors of the head and neck. Williams and Wilkins, Baltimore, a: pp 354–356; b: pp 280–290
9. Friedmann I, Osborn D A 1982 Pathology of granulomas and neoplasms of the nose and paranasal sinuses. Churchill Livingstone, Edinburgh, pp 289–299
10. Michaels L 1987 Ear, nose and throat histopathology. Springer-Verlag, Berlin, a: pp 207–209; b: pp 257–259
11. Stout A P, Lattes R 1967 Tumors of the soft tissues. Armed Forces Institute of Pathology, Washington DC, pp 58–63
12. Papavasiliou A, Michaels L 1981 Unusual leiomyoma of the nose (leiomyoblastoma). Journal of Laryngology and Otology 95: 1281–1286
13. Ranchod M, Kempson R L 1977 Smooth muscle tumors of the gastrointestinal tract and peritoneum. Cancer 39: 255–262
14. Hendrickson M R, Kempson R L 1980 Surgical pathology of the uterine corpus. W B Saunders, Philadelphia, pp 468–529
15. Fields J P, Helwig E B 1981 Leiomyosarcoma of skin and subcutaneous tissue. Cancer 47: 156–169
16. Dropkin L R, Tang C K, Williams J R 1976 Leiomyosarcoma of the nasal cavity and paranasal sinuses. Annals of Otology, Rhinology and Laryngology 85: 399–403
17. Jakobiec F A, Mitchell J P, Chauan P M, Iwamoto T 1978 Mesectodermal leiomyosarcoma of the antrum and orbit. American Journal of Ophthalmology 85: 51–57
18. Hyams V J, Batsakis J G, Michaels L 1988 Tumors of the upper respiratory tract and ear. Armed Forces Institute of Pathology, Washington, pp 150–162
19. Kawabe Y, Kondo T, Hosoda N 1968 Two cases of leiomyosarcoma of the maxillary sinuses. Archives of Otolaryngology 90: 492–495
20. Pimpinella R J, Marquit B 1965 Leiomyosarcoma of nose, nasopharynx and paranasal sinuses. Annals of Otology, Rhinology and Laryngology 74: 623-630
21. Maesaka A, Keyaki Y, Nakahashi T 1966 Nasal angioleiomyoma and leiomyosarcoma: report of two cases. Otologia (Fukuoka) 12: 42–47
22. Cherrick H M, Dunlap C L, King O H 1973 Leiomyomas of the oral cavity. Oral Surgery 35: 54–66
23. Schwartzman J, Schwartzman J 1973 Leiomyoma of the paranasal sinuses (Case Report). Laryngoscope 83: 1856–1858
24. Wolfowitz B L, Schmaman A 1973 Smooth muscle tumours of the upper respiratory tract. South African Medical Journal 47: 1189–1191
25. Rhatigan R M, Kinus Z E 1976 Leiomyoma arising adjacent to maxillary tooth socket: an intraosseous leiomyoma presenting as an odontogenic lesion. South Medical Journal 69: 493–494
26. McCaffrey T V, McDonald T J, Unni K 1978 Leiomyoma of the nasal cavity: report of a case. Journal of Laryngology and Otology 92: 817–819

27. Mechlin D C, Hamasaki C K, Moore J R, Davis W E, Templer J 1980 Leiomyoma of the maxilla - report of a case. Laryngoscope 90: 1230–1233

28. Lijovetsky G, Zaaura S, Gay I 1985 Leiomyoma of the nasal cavity: report of a case. Journal of Laryngology and Otology 99: 197–200

29. Hanna G S, Akosa A B, Ali M H 1988 Vascular leiomyoma of the inferior turbinate – report of a case and review of the literature. Journal of Laryngology and Otology 102: 1159–1160

30. Zijlker T D, Visser R 1989 A vascular leiomyoma of the ethmoid. Rhinology 27: 129–135

31. Barr G D, More I A R, McCallum H M 1990 Leiomyoma of the nasal septum. Journal of Laryngology and Otology 104: 891–893

32. Ogiba Y 1962 Leiomyosarcoma of nasal cavity (one case report). Otologia (Fukuoka) 12: 42–47

33. Canciullo D, Nucci C 1963 One case of leiomyosarcoma of the nasal fossae. Archivio Italiano delle Malattie dell'Apparato Digerente 30: 605–619

34. Kurvilla A, Wenig B M, Humphrey D M, Heffner D K 1990 Leiomyosarcoma of the sinonasal tract. A clinicopathologic study of nine cases. Archives of Otolaryngology, Head and Neck Surgery 116: 1278–1286

35. Lukes A, Rauchenberg M 1959 Leiomyosarkom nosu a vedlejsich dutin nosnich (leiomyosarcoma of the nose and paranasal sinuses). Ceskoslovenska Otolaryngologie 8: 1–7

36. Fu Y-S, Perzin K H 1976 Nonepithelial tumors of the nasal cavity, paranasal sinuses and nasopharynx. A clinicopathologic study. V. Skeletal muscle tumors (rhabdomyoma and rhabdomyosarcoma). Cancer 37: 364–376

37. Weber C O 1854 Anatomische Untersuchung Einer Hypertrophischen Zunge nebst Bemekungen uber die Neubildung querquestreifter Muskelfusern. Virchow Archivs fur Pathologie und Anatomie 7: 115

38. Bard L 1885 Anatomie pathologique generale des tumeurs. Archives de Physiologie normale et Pathologique 5: 247–265

39. Rakov A I 1937 Malignant rhabdomyoblastomas of skeletal musculature. American Journal of Cancer 30: 455–476

40. Stout A P 1946 Rhabdomyosarcoma of skeletal muscles. Annals of Surgery 123: 447–472

41. Berard M 1894 Tumeur embryonnaire du muscle strie. Lyon Medecine 77: 52

42. Stobbe G D, Dargeon H W 1950 Embryonal rhabdomyosarcoma of the head and neck in children and adolescents. Cancer 3: 826–836

43. Riopelle J C, Theriault J P 1956 Le rhabdomyosarcome alveolaire. Annales d'Anatomie pathologique 1: 88–111

44. Guersant M P 1854 Polypes du vagin chez une petite fille de treize mois. Moniteur Hopitaux 2: 187

45. Soule E H, Mahour G H, Mills S D, Lynn H B 1968 Soft tissue sarcomas of infants and children: a clinico-pathologic study of 135 cases. Mayo Clinic Proceedings 43: 313–326

46. King D R, Clatworthy W 1981 The pediatric patient with sarcoma. Seminars in Oncology 8: 215–221

47. Farr H W 1981 Soft part sarcomas of the head and neck. Seminars in Oncology 8: 185–189

48. Hawkins H K, Camacho-Velasquez J V 1987 Rhabdomyosarcoma in children. Correlation of form and prognosis in one institution's experience. American Journal of Surgical Pathology 11: 531–542

49. Russell W O, Cohen J, Enzinger F, Hajdu S I, Heise H, Martin R G, Meissner W, Miller W T, Schmitz R L, Suit H D 1977 A clinical and pathologic staging system for soft tissue sarcomas. Cancer 40: 1562–1570

50. Green D M, Jaffe N 1978 Progress and controversy in the treatment of childhood rhabdomyosarcoma. Cancer Treatment Reviews 5: 7–27

51. Young J L, Miller R W 1975 Incidence of malignant tumors in US children. Journal of Pediatrics 86: 254–258

52. Barnes L 1985 Tumors and tumorlike lesions of the soft tissues. In: Barnes L (ed) Surgical pathology of the head and neck. Marcel Dekker, New York, pp 724–780

53. Miller R W, Dalager N A 1974 Fatal rhabdomyosarcoma among children in the United States 1960–1969. Cancer 34: 1897–1900

54. Friedmann I, Bird E S 1969 Electron microscope investigation of experimental rhabdomyosarcoma. Journal of Pathology 97: 375–382

55. Feldman B A 1982 Rhabdomyosarcoma of the head and neck. Laryngoscope 92: 424–440

56. Donaldson S S, Castro J R, Wilbur J R, Jesse R H 1973 Rhabdomyosarcoma of head and neck in children. Cancer 31: 26–35

57. Lloyd G A S 1988 Diagnostic imaging of the nose and paranasal sinuses. Springer-Verlag, London, pp 143–147

58. Batsakis J G, Rice D H, Howard D R 1982 The pathology of head and neck tumors: spindle cell lesions (sarcomatoid carcinomas, nodular fasciitis and fibrosarcoma) of the aerodigestive tracts, Part 14. Head and Neck Surgery 4: 499–513

59. Hellquist H B 1990 Pathology of the nose and paranasal sinuses. Butterworths, London, pp 131–133

60. Seidal T 1988 Rhabdomyosarcomas – definition and diagnosis. Medical Dissertation, Gothenburg University, Sweden

61. Okamura J, Sutow W W, Moon T E 1977 Prognosis in children with metastatic rhabdomyosarcoma. Medical and Pediatric Oncology 3: 243–251

62. Pinkel D, Pratt C 1973 Embryonal rhabdomyosarcoma. In: Holland J F, Frei E (eds) Cancer medicine. Lea and Febiger, Philadelphia, pp 1900–1907

63. Ghavimi F, Exelby P R, D'Angio G J, Cham W, Lieberman P H, Tan C, Mike V, Murphy M L 1975 Multidisciplinary treatment of embryonal rhabdomyosarcoma in children. Cancer 35:677–686

64. Sutow W W, Sullivan M P, Ried H L, Taylor H G, Griffith K M 1970 Prognosis in childhood rhabdomyosarcoma. Cancer 25: 1384–1390

65. Pinkel D, Pickren J 1961 Rhabdomyosarcoma in children. Journal of the American Medical Association 175: 295–298

66. Maurer M, Moon T, Donaldson M, Fernandez C, Gehan E, Denman H, Hay S D, Lawrence W, Newton W, Ragab A, Soule E H, Sutow W W, Tefft M 1977 The Intergroup Rhabdomyosarcoma Study: a preliminary report. Cancer 40: 2015–2026

67. Cangir A, Morgan S K, Land V J et al 1976 Combination chemotherapy with adriamycin (NSC-123127) and dimethyl-triazeno imidazole carboxamide (DTIC)(NSC-45388) in children with metastatic solid tumors. Medical and Pediatric Oncology 2: 183–190

68. Roholl P J M, de Jong A S H, Ramaekers F C S 1985 Application of markers in the diagnosis of soft tissue tumours. Histopathology 9: 1019–1035

69. Healy G B, Jaffe N, Cassady J R 1979 Rhabdomyosarcoma of the head and neck: diagnosis and management. Head and Neck Surgery 1: 334–339

70. Sutow W W, Lindberg R D, Gehan E A, Abdelsalam H R, Raney R B, Ruymann F, Soule E H 1982 Three-year relapse-free survival rates in childhood rhabdomyosarcoma of the head and neck. Cancer 49: 2217–2221

71. Dito W R, Batsakis J G 1963 Intraoral, pharyngeal and nasopharyngeal rhabdomyosarcoma. Archives of Otolaryngology 77: 123–128

72. Wei W I 1985 Rhabdomyosarcoma of the soft palate: a case of late relapse. Journal of Laryngology and Otology 99: 1029–1033

73. Harrison D F N 1980 The ENT surgeon looks at the orbit. Journal of Laryngology and Otology Suppl. 3: 1–43

74. Cooper K G 1934 Plasmacytoma and rhabdomyoma of the paranasal sinuses. Archives of Otolaryngology 20: 329–339

75. Pastore P N, Sahyoun P F, Mandeville F B 1950 Rhabdomyosarcoma of the maxillary antrum. Archives of Otolaryngology 52: 942–947

76. Koop C E, Tewarson I P 1964 Rhabdomyosarcoma of the head and neck in children. Annals of Surgery 160: 95–103

77. Masson J K, Soule E H 1965 Embryonal rhabdomyosarcoma of the head and neck. American Journal of Surgery 110: 585–591

78. Dabezies O H, Naugle T C 1968 Alveolar rhabdomyosarcoma of paranasal sinuses and orbit. Archives of Ophthalmology 79: 574–577

79. Henny F A, Downs J R 1968 Treatment of embryonal rhabdomyosarcoma of the maxilla with combined therapy. Journal of Oral Surgery 26: 316–320

80. Makishima K, Iwasaki H, Horia A 1975 Alveolar rhabdomyosarcoma of the ethmoid sinus. Laryngoscope 85: 400–410
81. Murakami Y 1978 Rhabdomyosarcoma in children, a report of two cases. Otolaryngology (Tokyo) 50: 685–692
82. Pandhi S C, Mehra Y N, Malik A K 1980 Rhabdomyosarcoma of the head and neck. Journal of Laryngology and Otology 94: 337–345
83. Kanegaonkar G, McDougall J, Grant H R 1981 Rhabdomyosarcoma of the maxillary antrum in an adult. A case report with ultrastructural observations. Journal of Laryngology and Otology 99: 863–872
84. Proops D W, Mann J R 1984 The presentation of rhabdomyosarcomas of the head and neck in children. Journal of Laryngology and Otology 98: 381–390
85. Suzuki M, Kobayashi Y, Harada Y, Kyo T, Dohy H, Kuramoto A, Etoh R 1984 Rhabdomyosarcoma of the maxillary sinus. A case report. Journal of Laryngology and Otology 98: 405–415
86. Kraus D H, Roberts J K, Medendorp S V, Levine H L, Wood B G, Tucker H M, Lavertu P 1990 Nonsquamous cell malignancies of the paranasal sinuses. Annals of Otology, Rhinology and Laryngology 99: 5–11

11. Cartilaginous tumours

Although a variety of cartilaginous tumours are recognized in this region, all such lesions should be regarded as having malignant potential. Histologically well-differentiated lesions and a slow indolent growth pattern can create a false sense of security. Even those that do not manifest metastatic spread, pose significant problems of management by infiltrating the skull base. A tumour capable of causing bilateral blindness and death could not be regarded as 'benign' and requires radical treatment from the outset. They include:

1. Chondroma
2. Benign chondroblastoma
3. Chondrosarcoma
4. Mesenchymal chondrosarcoma.

CHONDROMA

Definition

The diagnosis of a benign cartilaginous tumour in this area should be regarded with circumspection as all cartilaginous tumours behave in a malignant or locally aggressive manner.[1] Chondroma is also known as *ecchondroma*.

Historical aspects

The first chondroma occurring within a cavity was described in 1836 by Muller.[2] Trerneuil published a case affecting an 11-year-old boy in 1868[3] and Howarth reported a case in the nasal septum in 1930.[4] Ringertz reviewed 50 cases in the literature affecting the nose and sinuses and concluded that it was frequently misdiagnosed.[5] 2 years later, Hickey published a case occurring in the ethmoid associated with florid sinusitis.[6]

Incidence

Given the large amounts of hyaline cartilage in the anterior nasal septum, chondromas in this region are surprisingly rare. In Ringertz's review of 391 tumours of the nose and sinuses,[5] he found two chondromas and in 1974 Fu & Perzin found 7 out of 256 non-epithelial tumours in this area.[7] A review of the literature in 1987 demonstrated 140.[8]

Age, sex and ethnic variation (Table 11.1)

The age range in Fu & Perzin's series was 10 to 46 years (mean 26 years), a younger group than those affected

Table 11.1 Chondromas of the upper jaw: in the literature

Author	No.	Sex		Age (yr)	Site	Treatment	Outcome
		M	F				
Howarth 1930[4]	1	1		35	Nasal septum	Lateral rhinotomy	No FU
Hickey 1940[6]	1		1	56	Ethmoid	Excision via Lynch–Howarth approach	A&W 2 yr
Fu & Perzin 1974 (own cases)[7]	7	1	6	10–46 (26 av.)	3 – septum 4 – nasopharynx	Local excision	No recurrence
Kilby & Ambegaokar 1977[9]	2		1	58	Nasal septum	Lateral rhinotomy × 4	DICD 10 yr 3 recurrences
			1	10	Ethmoid	Lateral rhinotomy	No FU

A&W, alive and well; DICD, dead of intercurrent disease; No FU, no follow-up

199

by its malignant counterpart.[7] Males and females are equally affected.[9]

Site

In 128 cases, the most common site was the ethmoid (50%) followed by maxilla (18%) and nasal septum (17%), then hard palate (6%) and nasopharynx (6%), with a small number affecting the alar cartilages.[9]

Aetiology

The more common occurrence of chondromas in non-cartilaginous tissue suggests that they may arise from focal hypertrophy of heterotropic islands of cartilage within the mucosa.

Clinical features and radiology

The majority are asymptomatic incidental findings.[10] They are not usually radio-opaque.

Macroscopic and microscopic appearance

A polypoid smooth-surfaced lesion of between 0.5–2.0 cm in diameter is found which may be translucent. Few grow larger than 3 cm and the overlying mucosa is usually intact. The tumour has a 'ripe-pear' consistency and is notoriously difficult to distinguish from a low-grade well-differentiated chondrosarcoma and even from normal cartilage, being composed of mature hyaline cartilage without atypia or mitoses.[9,11,12]

Treatment and prognosis

Adequate surgical excision results in cure often via a lateral rhinotomy. It has been suggested that radiotherapy may provoke malignant transformation[9,13] though given the histological difficulties this may simply represent a case of initial misdiagnosis.

BENIGN CHONDROBLASTOMA

This benign and distinct variant of chondroma is extremely rare in the sinonasal region. Apart from an occasional case report,[14] in the 200 cases in the literature, of which 12 occurred in the cranial bones, none affected the upper jaw.[15] The lesion originates in cartilage 'germ cells' or epiphyseal cartilage cells[16] which may represent rests (congenital remnants) of fetal cartilage.[17] It affects the young (5–25 years) and is slightly commoner in men.[15] Cure is generally achieved by local excision and/or currettage, though the lesion can sometimes act more aggressively. Radiotherapy is again not recommended because of the potential risk of provoking malignant transformation.

The first case report in the maxilla concerned a 13-year-old Iraqi girl with an alveolar swelling which was managed by curettage and who remained well for 18 months postoperatively.[14]

CHONDROSARCOMA

Definition

The term chondrosarcoma is generally applied to malignant tumours arising from hyaline cartilage. A rare variant, *mesenchymal chondrosarcoma* has been described which is discussed at the end of this section.

Historical aspects

A cartilaginous tumour of the nostril of a 15-year-old boy was described by Morgan in 1836.[18] It recurred several times following excision and the patient died 15 years later. Another case affecting a metacarpal was published by Volkmann in 1855,[19] from which the patient died with secondaries in the lung. In 1870 Paget reported a malignant cartilaginous tumour arising in the innominate bone which reached the enormous proportion of 20 kg.[20]

In 1887 Heath[21] described four cartilaginous tumours occurring in the sinonasal region of which three behaved in a malignant fashion and in 1916 a case with tumour in the antro-ethmoid region which invaded the orbit of a 19-year-old girl, who succumbed postoperatively, was reported by Mollison.[22]

Chondrosarcoma as a separate entity was established by Phemister in 1930[23] and 9 years later Ewing confirmed the separation of chondrosarcoma from other osteogenic tumours.[24]

Incidence

The lesion is generally uncommon in the upper jaw although it constitutes 10% of all primary bone tumours in the body. Chondrosarcoma of the jaw has been estimated to comprise 1.25% of all chondrosarcomas[1] and it is less common than osteosarcoma[11] in the sinonasal tract. In 1974 Fu & Perzin found 15 reported cases to which they added 10 cases.[7] Kragh et al[25] found 10 cases at the Mayo over a 50-year period and Sato reviewed 35 cases in the Japanese literature occurring over a similar period.[26]

A review of the world literature reveals some 125 cases (Table 11.2) to which we have added 15 further cases, 3% of our sinonasal tumours.

Age, sex and ethnic variation

Overall chondrosarcoma affects patients in their 6th decade, but in the head and neck the patient population

Table 11.2 Chondrosarcoma of the upper jaw: in the literature

Author	No.	Male	Female	Age (yr)	Site	Treatment	Outcome
Miles 1950[39]	2	1	1	47 51	Maxilla Maxilla	Wide local excision DXT	DOD 1 yr DOD 4.5 yr
Pantazoupoulos 1950[40]	1	1		16	Hard palate	Wide local excision, DXT	DICD 4.5 yr
Link 1954[41]	1	1		28	Maxilla	Local excision	A&W 9/12
Sandler 1957[42]	1	1		45	Maxilla	Partial maxillectomy Total maxillectomy	Recurrence 9/12 A&W 5 yr
Jibiki 1958[43]	1		1	43	Nasal septum	Excision, DXT	No FU
Chaudhry et al 1961[44]	1	1		55	Maxilla	Excision	No FU
Norikane & Ogata 1961[45]	1	–	–		Nasal septum	Excision	No FU
Takeuchi et al 1966[46]	1	1		46	Nasal septum	Excision, DXT	A&W 2 yr
Aretsky et al 1970[47]	1	1		57	Septum, bilateral maxillae & hard palate	Maxillectomy & orbital clearance	A&W 10/12
Arlen et al 1970[48]	1				Maxilla		
Gallagher & Strome 1972[49]	3	1 1	1	28 16/12 42	Maxilla Orbit and ethmoid Septum, ethmoid & orbit	Partial maxillectomy Maxillectomy & orbital clearance, C Lateral rhinotomy, bilateral ethmoidectomy, C	A&W 5 yr DOD 13/12 DOD 4.5 yr
Grewal et al 1972[50]	1		1	45	Maxilla	DXT, maxillectomy	A&W 1 yr
Lott & Bordley 1972[51]	1		1	49	Sphenoid, ethmoid	Excision DXT	Recurrence 6 yr AWR 10.5 yr
Jones 1973[52]	2		1 1	67 79	Nasal septum Sphenoid	Local excision Local excision	DOD 9/12 DOD 15/12
Wolfowitz 1973[53]	2	1	1	45 20	Maxilla Palate	Maxillectomy & orbital clearance Maxillectomy	A&W 3.5 yr
Fu & Perzin 1974[7]	10	6	4	36.5 mean (20/12–69 yr range)	Antro-ethmoid, sphenoid Nasal septum, maxilla Nasal septum, middle turbinate Maxilla Middle turbinate Nasal cavity, maxilla Nasal vestibule Maxilla, sphenoid, postnasal space Base of skull Sphenoid, postnasal space	Maxillectomy Radical excision Lateral rhinotomy, partial maxillectomy Maxillectomy Local excision Local excision Local excision Maxillectomy, orbital clearance, DXT (2 courses) Biopsy, DXT Radical excision	A&W 11 yr, no recurrence A&W 3 yr 9/12, no recurrence A&W 3 yr, no recurrence A&W 2 yr 4/12, no recurrence A&W 13 yr, no recurrence DOD 18 yr, 9 recurrences A&W 6.5 yr, no recurrence DOD 4 yr 3/12, 3 recurrences DOD 13/12 DOD 6/12
Fu & Perzin 1974[7] review of literature[22,25,27–38]	15	6	9	47 (mean) (15–76 yr range)	Upper jaw 5 Maxilla 6 Nasal cavity 3 Ethmoid 1	Local excision – alone 3 & DXT 1 Radical excision – alone 2 & DXT 4 DXT alone 2 Unknown 3	DOD 11 AWR 4 A&W 8 DICD 2

Table 11.2   Chondrosarcoma of the upper jaw: in the literature *(contd)*

Author	No.	Male	Female	Age (yr)	Site	Treatment	Outcome
Coates et al 1977[54]	13	1		44	Nasal septum	Excision	A&W 19 yr
		1		44	Nasal septum	Excision, DXT for recurrence	DICD 20 yr
			1	33	Nasal septum	Excision, lateral rhinotomy	Recurrence 19/12 A&W 2 yr
			1	60	Antro-ethmoid	Lateral rhinotomy, craniotomy after 7 yr DXT after 8 yr	5 recurrences in 3–10 yr, DOD 10 yr
			1	63	Maxilla	Caldwell–Luc, DXT (2 courses)	Recurrence (×2) DOD 6 yr
		1		63	Nasal cavity, ethmoid, frontal, orbit	Lateral rhinotomy	DICD 1/12
		1		76	Nasal cavity	Caldwell–Luc	DOD 4 yr
		1		38	Nasal cavity	Excision, DXT	Recurrence DOD 4 yr
		1		70	Maxilla	Maxillectomy	A&W 23 yr
			1	50	Base of skull Ethmoids	Lateral rhinotomy Craniotomy (after 8 yr), DXT	Recurrence 8 yr A&W 15 yr
			1	69	Nasal cavity Sphenoid	Lateral rhinotomy Lateral rhinotomy (after 11 yr)	Recurrence 11 yr A&W 16 yr
			1	61	Maxilla	Maxillectomy	A&W 19 yr
			1	18	Maxilla	Maxillectomy, DXT	DOD 2 yr with 2°s pelvis
Sato et al 1977[26]	21	9	12	41.3 (mean)	Maxilla (12) Nose (5) Ethmoid (2) Palate (2)	Radical surgical excision (17) & DXT (5)	10/17 DOD <1yr
Buchner et al 1979[55]	1		1	33	Maxilla	Partial maxillectomy	No FU
Chattopadhyay et al 1979[56]	1		1	55	Nasal septum	Excision	A&W 2 yr
Endo et al 1979[57]	1	1		71	Nasal septum	Excision	A&W 10/12
Myers & Thawley 1979[58]	2	1		45	Nasal septum	Maxillectomy & septectomy	A&W 2 yr
		1		59	Maxilla	Maxillectomy	A&W 3 yr
Peppard & Matz 1979[59]	1	1		33	Nasal septum & antrum	Ethmoidectomy & medial maxillectomy, fast neutrons	A&W 14/12
Zusho et al 1979[60]	1	1		58	Nasal septum	Excision, DXT	A&W 12/12
McCoy & McConnel 1981[61]	1		1	59	Nasal septum	Craniofacial	A&W 5 yr
Waga et al 1981[62]	1		1	27	Ethmoid	Craniofacial	No FU
El Ghazali 1983[63]	1		1	60	Ethmoid	Lateral rhinotomy	A&W 4 yr
Hornibrook & Sleeman 1983[64]	1		1	65	Hard palate, nasal septum	Bilateral radical maxillectomy	A&W 3 yr
Beneck et al 1984[65]	1	1		89	Nasal septum	En bloc excision	A&W 6/12
Finn et al 1984[66]	11		1	48	Maxilla hard palate	Partial maxillectomy	A&W 29 yr
			1	47	Nasal cavity	Maxillectomy	A&W 19 yr
			1	44	Hard palate	Radical excision	A&W 6 yr
			1	16	Spheno-ethmoid	Craniofacial	DOD 1 yr
			1	71	Maxilla	Partial maxillectomy	A&W 11 yr
			1	17	Maxilla, ethmoid, sphenoid	Local excision (×6)	AWR 10 yr
			1	40	Nasal septum	Maxillectomy & septectomy	A&W 3 yr
			1	50	Upper alveolus	Partial maxillectomy	A&W 6/12
			1	15	Nasal cavity, sphenoid, ethmoid	C	AWR?

Table 11.2 Chondrosarcoma of the upper jaw: in the literature *(contd)*

Author	No.	Male	Female	Age (yr)	Site	Treatment	Outcome
Finn et al (contd)			1	23	Maxilla, ethmoid, nasal cavity	DXT, total maxillectomy & orbital clearance	A&W 2 yr
			1	20	Frontal, orbit, anterior cranial fossa	C, craniofacial, DXT	No FU
Nishizawa et al 1984[67]	1	1		61	Nasal septum	DXT (pre and post op.), local excision, C	A&W 8 yr
Randall & Gray 1984[68]	1	1		56	Ethmoids & orbit	Bilateral ethmoidectomy & orbital clearance	DOD 7 yr
Vener et al 1984[69]	3			av. 36	Maxilla	Excision	? All DOD
Barton 1985[70]	1	1		88	Inferior turbinate	Lateral rhinotomy	Malignant melanoma 1 yr later
Ishida et al 1986[71]			1	54	Ethmosphenoid	Local excision (×2)	DOD 2 yr 7/12
Ishikawa et al 1986[72]			1	80	Nasal septum	DXT	No FU
El-Silimy et al 1987[73]	1	1		42	Nasal septum	Surgical excision	DOD 8 yr Local recurrence Bony 2°s
Massarelli et al 1988[74]	1			35	Maxilla	Subtotal maxillectomy	A&W 2 yr
	1			32	Maxilla	Local excision (×2), subtotal maxillectomy 3 yr later	Lost to FU after 12 yr
Harrison & Lund	14	1		12	Fronto-ethmoid	Osteoplastic flap, craniofacial 3/12 later, DXT	A&W 1 yr
		1		25	Ethmosphenoid	Craniofacial, orbit, maxillectomy, 2 yr 3/12 later. 3 further local excisions	AWR 4 yr
		1		39	Nasal septum, base of skull	Lateral rhinotomy, craniofacial 2/12 later. MCF exploration 3 yr later. 3 further craniofacial resections	DOD 12 yr
			1	43	Ethmoid	Craniofacial, DXT	A&W 8 yr
			1	48	Nasal cavity, orbit	Lateral rhinotomy, craniofacial 3 yr 2/12 later	A&W 8 yr 2/12
			1	53	Nasal septum, ethmoid	Craniofacial	No FU
			1	57	Nasal cavity, maxilla, postnasal space	Craniofacial	AWR 5 yr 4/12
			1	62	Ethmoid	Craniofacial, orbital clearance	A&W 2 yr 2/12
			1	63	Ethmoid	Craniofacial, DXT	A&W 1 yr 2/12
			1	71	Nasal septum	Craniofacial, revision 6 yr later	A&W 7 yr
			1	68	Nasal septum	Midfacial degloving	AWR 3 yr
		1		41	Maxilla	DXT, maxillectomy and orbital clearance	A&W 12 yr
		1		30	Maxilla	DXT, maxillectomy and orbital clearance	DOD 8/12
			1	20	Ethmosphenoid, base of skull nasopharynx	Craniofacial Diagnosed Ollier's disease 4 yr later	A&W 5 yr 8/12

A&W, alive and well; AWR, alive with recurrences; DOD, dead of disease; DICD, dead of intercurrent disease; 2°s, secondaries; DXT, radiotherapy; C, chemotherapy; MCF, middle cranial fossa; No FU, no follow-up tends to be younger (range 16 months to 89 years; 46 years mean)(Fig. 11.1). The literature gives variable male to female ratios. It would appear to be 1:1.2 in the cases reported (Table 11.2).

Site

In the jaws, the maxilla is more commonly affected than the mandible. The anterior maxilla is an area of predilection, with the palate and alveolus in the vicinity of the lateral incisors and canines being common sites.[10] It is again notable, given the distribution of hyaline cartilage, that the nasal septum alone is less frequently affected and if so, it is more usually the posterior septum which is involved.[67]

However, the extent of the lesion at presentation may preclude the identification of accurate origins as the tumour has often spread from antrum to both ethmoids, nasal septum, sphenoid and nasopharynx when first seen. It is this potential involvement of the skull base which so frequently compromises surgical excision.

Aetiology

Myers & Thawley[58] have classified chondrosarcomas into three types:

1. Primary chondrosarcomas arising from undifferentiated perichondrial cells
2. Secondary chondrosarcomas arising from previously benign cartilaginous lesions
3. Mesenchymal chondrosarcoma arising from primitive mesenchymal cells.

The origin of chondrosarcoma from specific areas of the upper airway has led to considerable speculation over the tissue of origin.[10] Vestigial cartilaginous rests are the favoured theory[58] related to the cartilaginous phase in the development of the nasal capsule, ethmoid and sphenoid.

Previous irradiation has been implicated in a number of cases[75,76] but none have occurred in the upper jaw. Malignant transformation provoked by incomplete excision of chondroma has also been reported[34] and although it has been claimed that 10% of benign lesions may dedifferentiate,[77,78] it is probable that malignant potential existed ab initio.

Although in the literature there have been no cases in the upper jaw with hereditary multiple exostoses and ecchondromatosis (Ollier's disease) which in other sites predisposes to chondrosarcoma[7] there is one case in our series. An Italian girl of 20 presented with extensive involvement of the ethmo-sphenoid and skull base for which she underwent craniofacial resection and developed multiple systemic lesions 4 years later, when the diagnosis of Ollier's was made.

Clinical features

Presenting symptoms vary, the percentage incidence in our personal series is given in parentheses. One of the commonest presenting symptom is that of swelling of the facial bones, possibly with displacement of the orbit (45%) and a visible mass in the nose or palate. This may be accompanied by premature eruption of the teeth, and loosening or displacement of dentition. Trismus, pain and cranial nerve palsies, with sensory loss are sometimes experienced (18%). Nasal symptoms such as obstruction and epistaxis frequently occur (64%) and visual disturbance can accompany displacement (36%). The spread of the tumour across the skull base can sadly result in bilateral blindness in a number of cases as the orbital apices and chiasma are ultimately involved in sphenoidal disease.[37]

Occasionally however the patients may be asymptomatic and the tumour can occur in association with ostensibly benign polyps emphasizing the need once again of submitting all such tissue for histology.

A 39-year-old Caucasian maintenance foreman in good general health presented with nasal obstruction;
he had apparently sustained a fractured nose 2 years previously and since that time had become aware of intermittent nasal blockage which had become constant and bilateral in the last 9 months.
Examination revealed complete obstruction of both nasal airways, with a gross septal deviation to the left and a pale mass occupying the postnasal space. There was no cervical lymphadenopathy. Sinus X-ray revealed almost complete

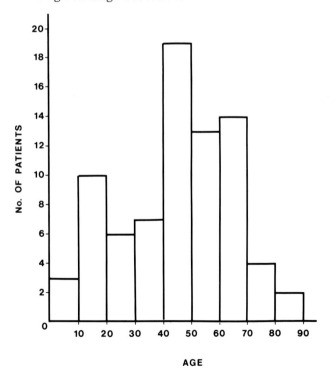

Fig. 11.1 Chondrosarcoma: distribution of cases in literature by age.

opacification of the right maxillary antrum consistent with an antrochoanal polyp. At examination under anaesthesia, a nasopharyngeal mass was found arising from the posterior end of the nasal septum with erosion of the vomer. Histology demonstrated chondrosarcoma and CT scanning showed a large mass occupying the nasal cavities and nasopharynx, invading the maxillary antrum, orbit, ethmoid and sphenoid, eroding the floor of the middle cranial fossa.

At this point the patient was referred to London for craniofacial resection. The tumour was removed en bloc with the cribriform plate and ethmoid labyrinths. The sphenoid sinuses were cleared of disease and although the postero-superior bony walls were intact, there was extensive involvement of the basisphenoid. The patient subsequently returned to work and was well for 6 months when he began to suffer from headaches. A middle cranial fossa exploration was performed at the National Hospital for Nervous Diseases 2 years later. The patient continued to be reasonably well and remained at work for a further 3 years when he underwent a revision craniofacial resection at which both orbital apices were decompressed.

Massive recurrence necessitated a further revision a year later at which the right orbit was cleared and the left optic nerve again decompressed (Fig. 11.2). Three more revisions to debulk the maxilla, infratemporal fossa, pterygopalatine fossa and orbit were performed at which obvious disease was found infiltrating the middle and posterior cranial fossa. The temporal bone was widely involved and indeed disease was lasered in the middle ear cavity. Despite these multiple procedures during the 12 years of his illness, the patient was able to continue working up until a few months ago which included regular scaffolding work and required only minimal analgesia during the major part of his illness. The patient died at Christmas 1991 with a massive haemorrhage from the craniofacial cavity.

Radiology (Figs 11.3 and 11.4)

Lloyd[79] reviewed all of our cases at the Royal National Throat, Nose and Ear Hospital, the vast majority of whom had had CT scanning and three of whom had had MRI. 73% demonstrated mottled calcification within the soft tissue mass on both plain X-ray and CT scanning. This ranged from one or two punctate areas, to multiple confluent calcification, forming characteristic dense irregular plaques.

93% involved the naso-ethmoidal region, with half the lesions being centrally located. There was spread into the orbit in 60% and two-thirds showed intracranial extension.

The MR characteristics combined with the typical calcification seen on CT are diagnostic of chondrosarcoma. High signal occurs on T2 weighted sequences with differential enhancement after gadolinium-DTPA. The enhancement is at the vascular periphery of the tumour and the avascular central oedematous core does not enhance.

Macroscopic and microscopic appearance

The tumour presents as a firm lobulated mass which can achieve large proportions. The surface is often glistening and the texture of the tumour varies from calcified and firm to soft and gelatinous in areas. Lichtenstein & Jaffe[80]

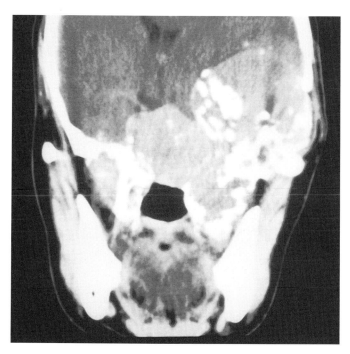

Fig. 11.2 Coronal CT scan showing extensive recurrent chondrosarcoma invading middle cranial fossa. Tumour shows typical multiple areas of confluent calcification (courtesy of D. J. Howard).

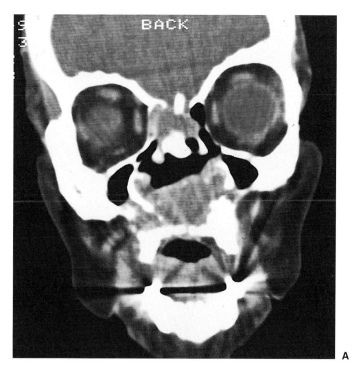

Fig. 11.3 Coronal CT scan showing recurrent chondrosarcoma affecting both superior and inferior portions of the nasal septum.

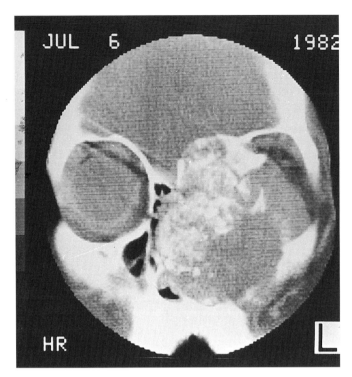

Fig. 11.4   Coronal CT scan showing massive chondrosarcoma of the upper jaw.

formulated certain criteria for the diagnosis of chondrosarcoma which essentially are too many cells, which are too irregular and too darkly staining. The cells are often multi-nucleated or binucleate and may show some atypia but Batsakis[28] has emphasized that the absence of mitoses does not preclude the diagnosis of malignancy. Fu & Perzin[7] divided the lesions into three grades based on the resemblance to normal cartilage and Evans et al[78] devised a similar classification based on mitotic rate, cellularity and nuclear size. The majority in the upper jaw are well-differentiated which renders any diagnosis of a benign chondroma open to debate. The lesion may be markedly calcified or even ossified, especially at the edge where it may represent reactive change in adjacent tissue.

Natural history

Chondrosarcoma tends to act less aggressively than other sarcomas but nevertheless pursues a slow and intractably progressive course which ultimately kills the patient in many cases. The history is therefore long, punctuated by many local recurrences as evidenced by our case report. Uncontrolled local spread throughout the skull base is responsible for the patient's demise and this is unfortunately accompanied by blindness in a proportion of cases. Distant metastases are relatively rare occurring in only 8%[7,78,81,82] principally to the lungs, compared with 54% from extrafacial sites.[82]

Differential diagnosis

The well-differentiated lesion must be distinguished from benign chondroma and can also be confused with pleomorphic adenomas which have a prominent pseudo-cartilaginous pattern.[10] Chordomas can also present similar features and also affect similar sites within the skull base.[7,83] Other sarcomas of bone and fibrous tissue can also have some common features.

It is always important to provide a sufficiently large representative biopsy material. In difficult cases immuno-cytochemistry may be helpful. Chondrosarcoma is immunoreactive to vimentin and S-100, but negative to cytokeratins and alkaline phosphatase.[11]

The literature contains one case of a synchronous tumour in the breast with chondrosarcoma of the upper jaw,[73] and one metachronous malignant melanoma.[70]

Treatment

Radical surgery offers the primary treatment modality and craniofacial resection offers the most oncologically satisfactory approach which was employed in 11/14 of our own cases. Not surprisingly the tumour will always recur if it extends to the edge of the resection.[7] Nishizawa et al[67] reported the use of pre- and postoperative radiotherapy, and chemotherapy in one case, and some regression has been noted with radiotherapy when given for recurrent disease.[31,36,51,82] One-third of our patients had received radiotherapy prior to referral.

The orbital effects of the disease can prove the most distressing, 4/14 underwent orbital clearance at initial surgery, two of whom ultimately went blind in the remaining eye despite decompression of the optic canal. However, this manoeuvre was successful in prolonging useful vision for a considerable period, can be repeated and has so far avoided visual loss in two other individuals.

Prognosis

The prognosis for chondrosarcoma is generally worse than with osteosarcoma[28] and the term 'cure' must be used with considerable reservation. The outcome is directly related to:

1. The cytologic differentiation with well-differentiated doing better than poorly-differentiated lesions
2. The location of the primary, with the nasopharynx, posterior nasal cavity and sphenoid doing worse than anterior lesions, principally due to
3. The adequacy of the primary surgical excision. Thus the craniofacial offers a significant advance and a localized septal lesion, albeit less common, is most likely to be cured.

When Fu & Perzin[7] examined the lesions by grade, one of six Grade 1 lesions died of disease after 18 years with multiple recurrences; two of three Grade 2 lesions died of disease and the one case of Grade 3 also died of disease. No correlation could be demonstrated between recurrence and histological grading as this is more dependent on the adequacy of the surgical excision. However, Evans et al[78] showed a definite association between metastatic spread and overall survival (Table 11.3). Fu and Perzin[7] found a 62% 5-year survival in their sinonasal lesions which should be compared with 54% for chondrosarcoma from extrafacial sites.[82] (Half the patients with moderately and well-differentiated disease got complete remission for 3–5 years in Finn et al's[66] and Harwood et al's[84] series.) However survival must be considered over a lifetime. In Fu & Perzin's series[7] of 25 cases, 44% were dead of disease, 38% alive and well, 16% alive with disease and 8% dead of intercurrent disease. Whilst six cases died within 5 years of presentation, the other five survived 5, 6, 7, 9 and 13 years later.

In our own series, 12 individuals are available for assessment excluding one lost to follow-up and the case of Ollier's disease. Only one has died of disease (at 8 months) and the remaining 11 are alive, four with evidence of recurrence (one of whom is about to undergo craniofacial resection). The follow-up ranges from 1–12 years (50% >5 years) and demonstrates how patients can live for many years with residual disease, undergoing repeated surgery as clinically appropriate. Regular imaging will indicate progress of the disease but will not necessarily dictate intervention in the absence of symptoms. The craniofacial approach offers the optimum surgical access to the skull base and orbital apices in the majority of cases and its success is evidenced by our results.

MESENCHYMAL CHONDROSARCOMA (Table 11.4)

This is a rare, very malignant tumour with a particular morphological pattern. It was first reported by Lichtenstein & Bernstein in 1959[87] and has a biphasic pattern of undifferentiated small round cells and islands of chondroid tissue. It can occur in skeletal and extraskeletal forms and has a predilection for facial bones and ribs. A third can occur in soft tissue such as the orbit and occasionally the maxilla and nasal cavity.[85,86,88–90]

The maxilla (including upper alveolus and hard palate) is more commonly affected than the nasal cavity in the 11 reported cases affecting the upper jaw. There is a slight female preponderance, and over a third occur in the 2nd and 3rd decades. Treatment is by surgical excision, to which radiotherapy and chemotherapy have sometimes

Table 11.3 Prognosis in chondrosarcoma: all sites[78]

Grade	I	II	III	All
5 yr survival (%)	90	81	43	77
10 yr survival (%)	83	64	29	67
Metastases (%)	0	10	71	
Local recurrence (%)	40	60	47	

Table 11.4 Mesenchymal chondrosarcoma of the upper jaw: in the literature

Author	Sex	Age (yr)	Site	Treatment	Outcome
Salvador et al 1971[85]	M	26	Hard palate	Excision DXT (after 6/12) Excision, DXT (after 19/12) Pneumonectomy (after 11 yr) Laminectomy (after 13 yr)	DOD 13.5 yr Widespread 2°s
	F	27	Hard palate	DXT Excision, C for recurrence (after 4 yr)	DOD 5 yr Widespread 2°s
	F	46	Maxilla	Excision Excision of retro-peritoneal 2° (after 18.5 yr) Maxillectomy (after 9 yr 3/12)	DOD 9.5 yr Widespread 2°s
Bloch et al 1979[86]	M	18	Upper alveolus	DXT, radical maxillectomy & orbital clearance	A&W 7 yr
	F	24	Middle turbinate	Lateral rhinotomy, DXT	AWR 15 yr
Harrison & Lund	F	19	Maxilla	Lateral rhinotomy, orbital clearance DXT, C	No FU

A&W, alive and well; AWR, alive with recurrence; DOD, dead of disease; No FU, no follow-up; DXT, radiotherapy; 2°s, secondaries been added. All modalities were employed in our one case of a 19-year-old girl with extensive disease but unfortunately no follow-up is available. If excision is inadequate, recurrence, haematogenous pulmonary metastases and death from disease occurs, even after many years.

The clinical course is thus rather variable, with survival ranging from 6 months to 15 years and again the patient can never be regarded as cured.

The lesion must be distinguished from angiofibroma, haemangiopericytoma and synovial sarcoma.[85]

REFERENCES

1. Batsakis J G, Solomon A R, Rice D H 1980 The pathology of head and neck tumors: neoplasms of cartilage, bone, and the notochord, Part 7. Head and Neck Surgery 3: 43–57
2. Muller M 1870 Die Chondrom. Archiven fur Klinische und Experimentelle Ohren, Nasen und Kehlkopfheilkunde (Berlin) 12: 323
3. Trerneuil, cited by Uffenorde W 1908 Die Chondrome der Nasenhohle und Mitteilung eines Falles von Enchondrom des Siebbeins mit allgemeines Besprechung der Operations methoden fur die Nasennebenhohlen. Archiv fur Laryngologie und Rhinologie 20: 255–279
4. Howarth W 1930 Chondroma of the nasal septum. Journal of Laryngology and Otology 45: 191–192
5. Ringertz N 1938 Pathology of malignant tumors arising in the nasal and paranasal cavities and maxilla. Acta Otolaryngologica Suppl. XXVII
6. Hickey H L 1940 Chondroma of the ethmoid. Archives of Otolaryngology 31: 645–652
7. Fu Y-S, Perzin K H 1974 Non-epithelial tumors of the nasal cavity, paranasal sinuses and nasopharynx: a clinicopathologic study. III. Cartilaginous tumors (chondromas, chondrosarcomas). Cancer 34: 453–463
8. Takimoto T, Miyazaki T, Yoshizaki T, Masuda K 1987 Chondroma of the nasal cavity and nasopharynx - a case of chondroma arising from the nasal septum. Auris, Nasus, Larynx (Tokyo) 14: 93–96
9. Kilby D, Ambegaokar A G 1977 The nasal chondroma: 2 case reports and a survey of the literature. Journal of Laryngology and Otology 91: 415–426
10. Hyams V J, Batsakis J G, Michaels L 1988 Tumors of the upper respiratory tract and ear. Armed Forces Institute of Pathology, Washington DC, pp 163–170
11. Hellquist H B 1990 Pathology of the nose and paranasal sinuses. Butterworths, London, p 130
12. Michaels L 1987 Ear, nose and throat histopathology. Springer-Verlag, Berlin, p 220
13. Lawson L J 1956 Intranasal chondrosarcoma, supplemental case report. Archives of Otolaryngology 64: 331–334
14. Al-Dewachi H S, Al-Naib N, Sangal E C 1980 Benign chondroblastoma of the maxilla: a case report and review of chondroblastomas in cranial bones. The British Journal of Oral Surgery 18: 150–156
15. Dahlin D C, Ivins J C 1972 Benign chondroblastoma. A study of 125 cases. Cancer 30: 401–413
16. Jaffe H L, Lichtenstein L 1942 Benign chondroblastoma of bone: a reinterpretation of the so-called calcifying or chondromatous giant cell tumor. American Journal of Pathology 18: 969–991
17. Levine G D, Bensch K G 1972 Chondroblastoma - the nature of the basic cell. Cancer 29: 1546–1562
18. Morgan 1836 Exostosis of the bones of the face. Guy's Hospital Reports 1: 403–406
19. Volkmann R 1855 Akutes schmerzhaftes Enchondrom des Metacarpus; Enchondrom der Lunge. Deutsche Klinik 7: 577–578
20. Paget J 1870 Cartilaginous tumours. Lectures on surgical pathology, 3rd edn. Longmans Green and Co, pp 498–528
21. Heath C 1887 Lectures on disease of the jaws. British Journal of Dental Science 30: 756–761
22. Mollison W M 1916 Some cases of growth of the upper jaw and ethmoidal region. Dental Records 36: 44–47
23. Phemister D B 1930 Chondrosarcoma of bone. Surgery, Gynecology and Obstetrics 50: 216–233
24. Ewing J 1939 A review of the classification of bone tumors. Surgery, Gynecology and Obstetrics 68: 971–976
25. Kragh L V, Dahlin D C, Erich J B 1960 Cartilaginous tumors of the jaw and facial regions. American Journal of Surgery 99: 852–856
26. Sato K, Nukaga H, Horikoshi T 1977 Chondrosarcoma of the jaws and facial skeleton. Journal of Oral Surgery 35: 892–897
27. Batsakis J G, Dito W R 1962 Chondrosarcoma of the maxilla. Archives of Otolaryngology 75: 55–61
28. Batsakis J G 1980 Tumors of the head and neck. Williams and Wilkins, Baltimore, pp 364–366, 383–387
29. Coyas A J 1965 Chondrosarcoma of the nose. Journal of Laryngology and Otology 79: 69–72
30. Dahlin D C, Henderson E D 1956 Chondrosarcoma, a surgical and pathological problem. Journal of Bone and Joint Surgery 38: 1025–1038
31. Harmer W D 1935 Treatment of malignant disease of the upper jaw. Lancet 228: 129–133
32. Hofman L 1926 Contribution a l'etude histologique et clinique des osteo et chondrosarcomas du maxillare superieur. Annales des Maladies de l'Oreille et Larynx (Paris) 45: 433–457
33. Lapidot A, Ramm C, Fani K 1966 Chondrosarcoma of maxilla. Journal of Laryngology and Otology 80: 743–747
34. Lawson L J 1952 Intranasal chondrosarcoma. Archives of Otolaryngology 55: 559–565
35. Menne F R, Frank W W 1937 So called primary chondroma of the ethmoid. Archives of Otolaryngology 26: 170–178
36. Paddison G M, Hanks G E 1971 Chondrosarcoma of the maxilla. Report of a case responding to supervoltage irradiation and review of the literature. Cancer 28: 616–619
37. Soboroff B J, Lederer F L 1955 Chondrosarcoma of the nasal cavity. Annals of Otology, Rhinology and Laryngology 64: 718–727
38. Wakumoto F, Ishikawa G 1953 Autopsy case of chondrosarcoma of cranial bases and upper jaw. Gann 44: 248–250
39. Miles A E W 1950 Chondrosarcoma of the maxilla. British Dental Journal 88: 257–269
40. Pantazoupoulos P E 1950 Primary chondrosarcoma of the hard palate. Journal of Laryngology and Otology 79: 650–655
41. Link J F 1954 Chondrosarcoma of the maxilla. Oral Surgery 7: 140–144
42. Sandler H C 1957 Chondrosarcoma of the maxilla. Oral Surgery 10: 97–103
43. Jibiki T 1958 Chondrosarcoma of the nasal septum. Journal of Otolaryngology (Japan) 61: 315–317
44. Chaudhry A P, Robinovitch M R, Mitchell D F 1961 Chondrogenic tumors of the jaws. American Journal of Surgery 102: 403–411
45. Norikane S, Ogata S 1961 Chondrosarcoma of the nasal septum. Journal of Otolaryngology (Japan) 64: 1471–1473
46. Takeuchi M, Shiroto N, Takehisa M 1966 A case of chondrosarcoma of the nasal septum. Practical Otology (Kyoto) 59: 179–183
47. Aretsky P J, Kantu K, Freund H R, Polisar I A 1970 Chondrosarcoma of the nasal septum. Annals of Otology, Rhinology and Laryngology 79: 382–388
48. Arlen M, Tollefsen H R, Huvos A G, Marcove R C 1970 Chondrosarcoma of the head and neck. American Journal of Surgery 120: 456–460
49. Gallagher T M, Strome M 1972 Chondrosarcomas of the facial region. Laryngoscope 82: 978–984
50. Grewal B S, Nirola A, Lumba S P 1972 Chondrosarcoma of maxilla. Journal of Laryngology and Otology 86: 741–745

51. Lott S, Bordley J E 1972 A radiosensitive chondrosarcoma of the sphenoid sinus and base of the skull. Report of a case. Laryngoscope 82: 57–60
52. Jones H M 1973 Cartilaginous tumours of the head and neck. Journal of Laryngology and Otology 87: 135–151
53. Wolfowitz B L 1973 Osteosarcoma and chondrosarcoma of the maxilla. Journal of Laryngology and Otology 87: 409–416
54. Coates H L, Pearson B W, Devine K D, Unni K 1977 Chondrosarcoma of the nasal cavity, paranasal sinuses and nasopharynx. Transactions of the American Academy of Ophthalmology and Otology 84: 919–926
55. Buchner A, Ramon Y, Begleiter A 1979 Chondrosarcoma of the maxilla. Journal of Oral Surgery 37: 822–825
56. Chattopadhyay A K, Ashok Kumar M S 1979 Chondrosarcoma of the nasal septum. Indian Journal of Cancer 16: 63–65
57. Endo T, Uchida Y, Katoh T 1979 Chondrosarcoma of the nasal septum, a report of a case. Otology, Rhinologie, Laryngology (Tokyo) 22: 273–278
58. Myers E M, Thawley S E 1979 Maxillary chondrosarcoma. Archives of Otolaryngology 105: 116–118
59. Peppard S B, Matz G J 1979 Chondrosarcoma of the nasal septum extending into the maxillary sinus. Otolaryngology, Head and Neck Surgery 87: 635–639
60. Zusho H, Tokito S, Takeuchi M 1979 Chondrosarcoma of the nasal septum. Jibinkoka Tokyo 51: 179–183
61. McCoy J M, McConnel F M S 1981 Chondrosarcoma of the nasal septum. Archives of Otolaryngology 107: 125–127
62. Waga S, Hiroshi T, Yamagiwa M, Nishioka H 1981 Chondrosarcoma of the ethmoid sinus extending to the anterior fossa. Surgical Neurology 16: 324–328
63. El Ghazali A M S 1983 Chondrosarcoma of the paranasal sinuses and nasal septum. Journal of Laryngology and Otology 97: 543–547
64. Hornibrook J, Sleeman M 1983 Chondrosarcoma arising in the nasal septum. Journal of Laryngology and Otology 97: 1163–1168
65. Beneck D, Seidman I, Jacobs J 1984 Chondrosarcoma of the nasal septum: a case report. Head and Neck Surgery 7: 162–167
66. Finn D G, Goepfert H, Batsakis J G 1984 Chondrosarcoma of the head and neck. Laryngoscope 94: 1539–1544
67. Nishizawa S, Fukaya T, Inouge K 1984 Chondrosarcoma of the nasal septum. Laryngoscope 94: 550–553
68. Randall C J, Gray R 1984 Nasal septal chondrosarcoma. Journal of Laryngology and Otology 98: 635–638
69. Vener J, Rice D H, Newman A N 1984 Osteosarcoma and chondrosarcoma of the head and neck. Laryngoscope 94: 240–242
70. Barton R P E 1985 Metachronous chondrosarcoma and malignant melanoma of the nose. Journal of Laryngology and Otology 99: 497–500
71. Ishida M, Ashida K, Matsunaga T, Wakasa K, Sakurai M 1986 Chondrosarcoma of the ethmoidal and sphenoidal sinuses. Otology, Rhinology and Laryngology 48: 174–179
72. Ishikawa K, Hanazawa S, Yamada M, Ito E, Itani O, Konno A, Togawa K 1986 Chondrosarcoma arising in the nasal septum: a case report. Auris Nasus Larynx (Tokyo) 13: 35–41
73. El-Silimy O E, Harvey L, Bradley P J 1987 Chondrogenic neoplasms of the nasal cavity. Journal of Laryngology and Otology 101: 500–505
74. Massarelli G, Gandolfo L, Tanda F, Ghisella F, Mannuta V 1988 Maxillary chondrosarcoma. (Report of two cases) Journal of Laryngology and Otology 102: 177–181
75. Hatcher C H 1945 Development of sarcoma in bone subjected to roentgen or radium irradiation. Journal of Bone and Joint Surgery 27: 179–195
76. Cohen J, d'Angio G J 1961 Unusual tumors after roentgen therapy of children. American Journal of Roentgenology 86: 502–512
77. Erlandson R A, Huvos A G 1974 Chondrosarcoma. A light and electron microscopic study. Cancer 34: 1642–1652
78. Evans H L, Ayala A G, Romsdahl M M 1977 Prognostic factors in chondrosarcoma of bone. A clinicopathologic analysis with emphasis on histologic grading. Cancer 40: 818–831
79. Lloyd G A S 1988 Diagnostic imaging of the nose and paranasal sinuses. Springer-Verlag, London, pp 162–166
80. Lichtenstein L, Jaffe N L 1943 Chondrosarcoma of bone. American Journal of Pathology 19: 553–589
81. Friedmann I, Osborn D A 1982 Pathology of granulomas and neoplasms of the nose and paranasal sinuses. Churchill Livingstone, Edinburgh, pp 245–253
82. Henderson E D, Dahlin D C 1963 Chondrosarcoma of bone: a study of 288 cases. Journal of Bone and Joint Surgery 45: 1450–1458
83. Heffelfinger M J, Dahlin D C, MacCarty C S, Beabout J W 1973 Chordomas and cartilaginous tumors at the skull base. Cancer 32: 410–420
84. Harwood A R, Drajbich J L, Fornasier V L 1980 Radiotherapy of chondrosarcoma of bone. Cancer 45: 2769–2777
85. Salvador A H, Beabout J W, Dahlin D C 1971 Mesenchymal chondrosarcoma - observations on 30 new cases. Cancer 28: 605–615
86. Bloch D M, Bragoli A J, Collins D N, Batsakis J G 1979 Mesenchymal chondrosarcomas of the head and neck. Journal of Laryngology and Otology 93: 405–412
87. Lichtenstein L, Bernstein D 1959 Unusual benign and malignant chondroid tumours of bone. Cancer 12: 1142–1157
88. Olszewski W 1969 Chondrosarcoma mesenchymale. Patologia Polska 20: 23–27
89. Wirth J E, Shimkin M B 1943 Chondrosarcoma of nasopharynx simulating juvenile angiofibroma. Archives of Pathology 36: 83–88
90. Dahlin D C, Henderson E D 1962 Mesenchymal chondrosarcoma - further observation on a new entity. Cancer 15: 410–417

12. Odontogenic tumours

Descriptions of tumours arising in relationship with the teeth were available in the 18th century[1] but the first attempt at classification, based upon stages of tooth development was not published until 1868 by Broca.[2] Despite this, most odontogenic tumours continued to be termed either adamantinomas or odontomas until as late as 1946, when Thoma & Goldman divided them by their tissue of origin; epithelial, mesenchymal and mixed odontogenic.[3] This division has been the basis of all subsequent modifications of classification. However, these tumours are variable in growth, behaviour and histology leading to difficulties in evaluation and confusion in nomenclature. Pindborg & Clausen in 1958 emphasized the value of classifying these lesions on embryological principles, that is the influence that cells of one tissue exert upon the cells of another or 'inductive changes'.[4] This led eventually to the elimination of mixed odontogenic lesions from future considerations. The present World Health Organization (WHO) classification is largely based upon that of Pindborg & Clausen, recognizing only benign and malignant tumours. Despite this there is a wide range of separate conditions that can be recognized both clinically and histologically, most of which are benign. Their differentiation from the locally-recurring ameloblastoma is important although not always easy because of pathological similarities.

Occasionally, malignant changes develop within cysts and benign neoplasms but ameloblastic fibrosarcoma and odontosarcoma occur as definitive entities.[5] All of these conditions are found within the upper jaw, although in many cases less commonly than in the mandible. Many are extremely rare with only the occasional patient discussed in the literature. Consequently, this chapter is primarily based upon personal experience and the conditions discussed are those that may be seen and treated by the head and neck surgeon.

AMELOBLASTOMA

Definition

This is a histologically benign tumour originating from epithelial components of the embryonic tooth, arrested developmentally prior to enamel formation. Clinically it is locally invasive, potentially lethal and occasionally shows malignant features with systemic metastases.

Historical aspects and synonyms

It is impossible to list all the wide variety of names which have been attached to this tumour which was first recognized clinically in the 19th century by Cusack.[6] The name 'epitheline adamantin' was coined by Malassez in 1885,[7] prior to this the tumour had been classified as an epithelial cyst or because of its frequent close relationship with the basal layer of the oral mucosa, a 'basiloma'.

Multicystic jaw tumour, epithelial odontoma, odontogenic epithelioma, epithelioma ameloblastoides, central epithelium, cystoma, embryoplastic odontoma, adamantinomas, chorioblastoma, proliferating cysts of the jaw, are just a few of the many titles used until Ivy & Churchill in 1930 coined the more acceptable 'ameloblastoma'.[8] For many years the favoured word had been adamantinoma but since this tumour does not produce enamel this name is no longer acceptable. The WHO monograph on International Histological Classification of Tumours now recognizes ameloblastoma, but divides it into benign and malignant as well as separating it from ameloblastic fibroma and myxoma, ameloblastic fibrosarcoma and calcifying epithelial odontogenic tumour.[9]

Incidence

As with most other rare neoplasms it is difficult to obtain an accurate assessment of the true incidence. Whereas Gorlin et al quote a figure of 1% of all odontogenic tumours or cysts,[10] Regezi et al found 78 cases in a total of 706 odontogenic neoplasms, an 11% incidence[11] and Bhaskar quoted 18%.[12] Such wide variations are probably dependent upon selective referral patterns but the two largest series of maxillary ameloblastomata only total 20–24 patients.[13,14] This is somewhat surprising since by 1987 1152 patients with ameloblastoma of the jaws had been reported with a quoted incidence for the upper jaw of 20%![15]

Age, sex and ethnic variation

In the group of patients with ameloblastoma of the upper jaw 62.5% occurred in patients between the age of 20–49.[15] Remaining patients covered a wide age range with Bredenkamp et al reporting 12 cases of maxillary ameloblastoma with ages ranging from 15 to 81 years.[16]

There appears to be no sex predominance in the small number of patients with disease localized to the upper jaw although Iko et al writing from Nigeria found not only a high incidence of 19% in 57 odontogenic tumours and cysts but a 2.6:1 female to male ratio.[17] Their average age was in the 4th decade but no range was published although Onuigbo also recording Nigerian patients, included a child of 7 years.[18] He concluded that native Africans tended to present with all jaw tumours at an early age and this particularly applied to Nigerians and Ugandans.[19] This propensity does not appear to apply to the black population in the USA.

Site

Maxillary ameloblastomata are most commonly found posterior to the canine tooth with 47% sited in the molar region, 15% within the antrum and nasal floor, 9% in the premolar area, 9% in the canine fossa and only 2% in the hard palate.[20] Because of the complex anatomical relationships of the posterior aspect of the maxilla, ameloblastoma arising in this region usually reach a large size before diagnosis, expanding into the antrum, cheek or palate. Many of the reported cases have extension into the infratemporal fossa, orbit or even intracranially and it is not surprising that removal is associated with a high recurrence rate.[21]

Most have originated centrally within the upper jaw and extraosseous or peripheral ameloblastoma are uncommon. Both the palate and molar-retromolar gingiva[22] have been recorded as sites for these tumours where it poses problems in clinical diagnosis because of their atypical appearance.[23]

Clinical features (Table 12.1)

Since ameloblastomata originate centrally within bone, early symptoms are minimal. Painless swelling of the cheek, gingiva or palate was the commonest presenting symptom in 19/20 patients reported by Shedev et al from the Memorial–Sloan Kettering Cancer Center, USA.[13] Although Mehlisch et al found that a third of their patients did complain of pain, these all had recurrent tumour usually with infection.[24]

Keay et al had two patients who presented with nasal polyps in association with epistaxis and intermittent swelling of the face. In both cases there was radiological evidence of destruction of the lateral nasal wall with extension into the antrum[25] and nasal obstruction invariably indicates extensive disease.

Loose teeth, ill-fitting dentures or malocclusion are usually second to bone expansion and these tumours may vary in size from 1 cm up to a massive 16 cm in diameter, the average being for the maxilla of about 5 cm.[26]

Delay in the diagnosis of upper jaw ameloblastomata is common and averages 5 years although 32% are said to have significant symptoms for less than 2 years.[24] This may not necessarily indicate variations in growth rate but rather differences in 'noticeability' for some sites are more obvious and some patients more concerned about changes in normality!

The peripheral (or extraosseous) ameloblastoma may present as an epulis-like growth being sessile or pedunculated and covered by a red granular mucosa. They tend to affect an older age group and in the upper jaw are localized to the palate or molar-retromolar gingiva.[23] Siar et al in 1990 described a 35-year-old Malay woman with a 3 month history of a firm painless palatal swelling adjacent to the molar teeth. There was no radiological evidence of underlying bone erosion and excision of this ameloblastoma, measuring 3 × 2.7 cm in size gave good control.[23]

Because of variations in consistency, with solid and cystic areas, palpation is unhelpful for diagnosis although an 'egg-shell' crackling has been recognized by Chaudhuri.[27] If exposed the tumour may ulcerate simulating a malignant neoplasm, so in all cases diagnosis is dependent upon biopsy.

Radiology (Fig. 12.1)

Despite the use of CT scanning, now an essential part of head and neck diagnosis and assessment, there are no pathognomonic changes for ameloblastoma. Resorption of tooth roots in the region of the 3rd molar was at one time viewed as specific for this tumour but is seen with odontogenic sarcoma and other neoplasms. Occasionally, there is a multiloculated or honeycomb radiolucency but this may also be unilocular, and when related to a tooth is not dissimilar to a dentigerous cyst. A monocystic cavity in the region of the maxillary tuberosity and adjacent to a molar tooth must be viewed as suspicious. Recurrent disease is said to be osteosclerotic, but with areas of osteolysis and tumour expansion from its origin within the maxilla, soft tissue changes in the cheek, nasal cavity or pterygoid space will become visible, particularly with enhancement. Opacity of the maxillary sinus, whether from infection or tumour extension, is common to most upper jaw neoplasms and cannot be considered as diagnostic.[17]

Table 12.1   Summary of well documented cases of maxillary ameloblastoma

Author	Age (yr)	Sex	Site – invasion	Treatment	Outcome
Chaudhuri 1975[27]	52	M	Oroantral fistula from extracted L8./X-ray: cystic swelling posterior aspect of jaw	DXT 5500 rad – Recurrence 8 yr later – partial maxillectomy	A&W 10 yr
	44	M	Painless smooth cystic swelling posterior alveolus, opaque antrum	Enucleation via partial maxillectomy External DXT 6000 rad in 21 days	A&W 14 yr
	74	M	6/12 history facial swelling, blood-stained nasal discharge. Firm swelling of maxilla – fleshy mass in nasal cavity. Tomography – opaque antrum, ethmoids, expansion of antral walls	External DXT 4500 rads in 20 days	A&W 1 yr
Atkinson et al 1984[28]	77	M	Upper alveolus ulcerated with radiological bone erosion	Co[60] 4000 rad in 14 days – complete resolution	Died 6 wk of cerebral infarction
	40	M	Ulceration posterior alveolus, opaque antrum erosion of alveolus	Co[60] 5000 rad in 25 days Recurrence 3 yr on antral floor – partial maxillectomy	A&W 4 yr
	43	M	Alveolus & maxillary antrum	Local excision 6/12 recurrence – maxillectomy & Co[60] 5000 rad in 4 wk	A&W 3 yr
	62	M	Alveolus & maxillary antrum	25 MEV 4400 rad in 4 wk & maxillectomy	A&W 3 yr
Keay et al 1988[25]	76	F	10 mth history of facial swelling, blood-stained nasal discharge, expansion of maxilla Malignant oroantral fistula, mass in nose CT scan – showed destruction of bony walls of maxilla	Caldwell–Luc approach with enucleation of tumour	A&W 18 mth
	63	M	Nasal polyp for 1 mth, headaches CT scan – opaque antrum, loss of medial, posterior, lateral walls	Caldwell–Luc approach. Trans-antral ethmoidectomy with ?clearance	A&W 3 yr
Bredenkamp et al 1989[16]	53	M	Nasal obstruction 4/12, epistaxis Maxilla, orbit, middle cranial fossa extension – fungating mass in nose	DXT 6400 rad	AWD 1 yr
	15	M	Swelling face X-ray – mass in antrum with expansion of walls	Caldwell–Luc with enucleation of mass Recurrence 2 yr, with invasion of orbit – maxillectomy Recurrence 2 yr – DXT 6500 rad & implantation iridium wires Recurrence 3 yr, chemotherapy	Died 15 yr after diagnosis
	37	F	Swelling face	Curetted Recurrence 1 yr – partial maxillectomy & DXT ? dose 3 yr later recurrence in nasal antral region – maxillectomy, intracranial extension	Died 8 yr after diagnosis
	43	M	Dental pain – extraction, oroantral fistula 12 yr later malignancy in unhealed fistula Bony destruction lateral-inferior walls of antrum	Maxillectomy Recurrence 3 yr nose & orbit – local resection Recurrence 1 yr in cavity, palate & nasopharynx – cryosurgery	AWD 11 yr after diagnosis
	59	F	Nasal polyp with mass in maxilla	Polypectomy. 4 mth later maxillectomy	A&W 5 yr
Harrison & Lund	60	M	Oroantral fistula 10 yr prior to facial swelling Destruction posterior & roof of antrum with thinning of anterior and medial walls	Caldwell–Luc with partial removal Recurrence 8 yr later – maxillectomy	A&W 10 yr
	80	M	Nasal blockage. Swelling region of zygoma 2 mth. Fungating mass alveolus	220 kV 5000 rad Recurrence 2 yr – partial maxillectomy Recurrence in cavity 6 mth – local removal, involvement of orbit	DOD 3 yr after diagnosis
	16	M	Posterior alveolus 3 mth	Partial maxillectomy with postop. DXT, ?220 kV	A&W 30 yr

A&W, alive and well; AWD, alive with disease; DOD, dead of disease; DXT, radiotherapy

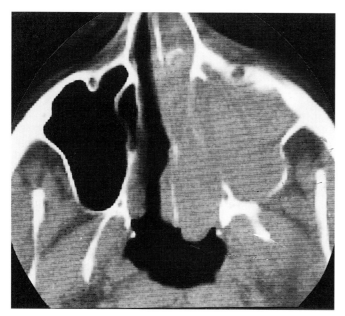

Fig. 12.1 Axial CT scan of an ameloblastoma of the maxillary antrum, extending into the nasal cavity (Lloyd 1988[29]).

Macroscopic and microscopic appearance

Macroscopically, ameloblastomata are described as varying in colour from yellow to greyish-white, predominantly firm but with areas of necrosis and cystic degeneration.

Microscopically, several types can be identified although there is no substantial evidence to suggest that individual variants are related to prognosis.

In the follicular form, islets of epithelial cells surrounded by a palisade of tall columnar cells resembling ameloblasts, are embedded in a connective tissue stroma. The internal part of the islets are composed of a loose network of stellate cells the whole resembling the enamel organ. The larger these epithelial cells, the more likely are cystic changes.

The plexiform type differs in that the epithelium is arranged in anastomosing strands which resemble the dental lamina. Cyst formation is likely in both the connective tissue stroma as well as epithelium, and this is the commonest pattern found within the upper jaw.[14]

Acanthotic changes may be seen with squamous metaplasia within the epithelial islets causing some confusion with squamous carcinoma. This has been called 'acanthomatous ameloblastoma' and irradiation of these tumours is thought to be a possible cause of malignant change.

An abundance of granular cells leads to replacement of the reticulum within the islets with large, round cells containing PAS-positive and acidophilic granules. These are thought to be products of degeneration but have no clinical significance as a prognostic sign.[5,15]

Despite the recognition of these histological variants, different morphological patterns can exist within individual tumours. The usual criteria for malignancy, mitosis and hyperchromasia, are rare in ameloblastomata and differentiation into benign and malignant poses problems for the pathologist, particularly in the absence of metastases. However, unlike the unilocular or peripheral lesions, multicystic or solid tumours are clinically invasive with a high rate of local recurrence.[16]

Other variants such as adeno-ameloblastoma, ameloblastic fibroma and ameloblastic odontoma behave benignly and do not metastasize but are extremely rare within the upper jaw and may be 'histological curiosities'.

A small number of malignant ameloblastomas have been reported although Carr & Halperin in analysing 21 of these reports found errors in diagnosis in 16 biopsies. (Confused with adenoid cystic, adeno and squamous carcinoma.) None of the definite cases showed metastases at initial presentation and the common factor was inadequate therapy with several recurrences.[30]

Singleton in 1971 reported the case of a 70-year-old woman who gave a 30 year history of facial swelling for which she had three separate operations. Ten years previously a chest X-ray had shown what was suspected to be a metastasis in the right lung. Examination showed an ulcerated palatal mass confirmed on biopsy as an ameloblastoma and she was referred for irradiation having refused surgery. 2 years later the chest picture was unchanged as was her extensive palatal lesion.[31] Whether the chest mass was really secondary to the palatal ameloblastoma is unknown but there are well documented reports of metastases to the cervical lymph nodes as well as the skeleton despite the absence of histological evidence of malignancy and this tumour must be considered as potentially lethal.[32]

Natural history and differential diagnosis

The rarity of these tumours combined with a varying histological appearance and absence of agreed classification and nomenclature, makes it impossible to rationalize behaviour patterns with any degree of certainty. Local aggressiveness, delay in diagnosis and the anatomical complexities of the upper jaw has led to a high rate of local recurrence. Even when excision appears to have been adequate, recurrence is common and this may yet prove to be related to histological variation. This propensity for regrowth after many years necessitates prolonged follow-up in every patient.

Differentiation from reparative giant-cell granuloma, odontogenic fibroma, myxoma or adenomatoid odontogenic tumour is only possible on histological grounds and this also applies to non-odontogenic tumours such as adenoid cystic carcinoma. This is of particular importance with 'mixed odontogenic tumours' for these have a younger age incidence and rarely recur, simple enucleation being curative.[26]

Treatment

There was a time when the preferred treatment for upper jaw ameloblastomata was conservative being restricted to curettage. Recurrence in all but the very small lesions was close to 100% with no more than 35% being salvaged by secondary radical excision.[13,14] Radiotherapy was said to be little better with recurrence rates around 50–70%[33] and it gradually became clear that where technically possible, and despite its benign histological appearance, maxillary ameloblastoma should be treated radically at the first opportunity.

The form this surgery should take is dictated by clinical and radiological assessment varying from partial to radical maxillectomy with extension to cover invasion of orbit or skull base. Microinvasion of cancellous bone is shown in most operative specimens and 'margins of excision' are largely irrelevant with this tumour. Excision should not be limited by false impressions, rather by anatomical confinement and this ensures that many patients are therefore ultimately incurable.[34]

A man aged 80 years was seen in August 1961 with a short history of left-sided nasal obstruction and a mildly discomforting swelling over the left zygoma. Examination revealed a proliferative mass in the alveolar-buccal sulcus and in the left nasal airway above the middle turbinate. There was a firm mass overlying the left zygoma and biopsy from the oral mass confirmed ameloblastoma. X-ray showed destruction of the posterolateral wall of the maxilla and zygoma with opacity of the antrum.

The patient refused surgery and was given 5000 rad at 220 kV to the ethmoid, orbit, maxilla and zygoma. There was considerable reduction in the size of the swelling over the zygoma and intraorally but the resulting oroantral fistula caused difficulty in eating.

By February 1962 the zygomatic swelling had returned but the fistula was clean with no obvious tumour. With antibiotics the swelling subsided and the patient remained symptom-free until June 1963 when a local recurrence within the oro-antral fistula was confirmed as ameloblastoma. 1 month later a partial maxillectomy was performed including ethmoidectomy and curettage of the region within the zygoma. By February 1964 there was further disease within the antral cavity which was curetted but proptosis developed within 3 months. No further treatment was given and he died in October 1964, just over 3 years from diagnosis.

The reappraisal of the role of radiotherapy by Atkinson et al in the management of ameloblastomata is moderately encouraging, particularly in the elderly or advanced cases. However, two of his patients had combined treatment whilst another was subsequently salvaged by surgery following recurrence of tumour. Follow-up of the 10 patients, three of whom had tumour in the maxilla, varied from 1 to 10 years. Average age at presentation was 45 years with a sex predilection of 2.5:1 favouring males.[28]

Their comments that previous reports of radiation resistance were based on outdated techniques not using megavoltage, is reasonable and the real place of irradia-

tion remains to be seen. However, since most upper jaw ameloblastomas are diagnosed only when the neoplasm has extended to surrounding structures, combination of radical excision and postoperative irradiation would appear to be the most logical approach at the present time.

CALCIFYING ODONTOGENIC CYST

Definition

Although uncommon, this is an interesting tumour since it features both as a cyst and odontogenic tumour showing calcification and keratinization.

Historical aspects and synonyms

Oral tumour of Malherbe, atypical ameloblastoma, keratinizing ameloblastoma, calcifying ghost cell odontogenic tumour and Gorlin cyst have all been used in the past. The last bears credit to its first description by Gorlin et al who in 1962 separated this lesion from other odontogenic tumours.[35] Prior to this, cases subsequently confirmed as calcifying odontogenic cysts were classified as 'atypical ameloblastoma' or even 'cholesteatoma'.

Incidence

Altini & Farman quote an incidence of less than 2% of their 411 odontogenic tumours, the maxilla being equally affected as the mandible.[36] They also found an equal sex incidence with one-third of the patients being in the 2nd decade of life. Freedman and colleagues reviewing 70 cases found an age range of 7 to 82 years (mean 38.4 years) with half of their patients being younger than 31 years of age.[37] Most of these lesions were intraosseous and localized to the region of the first molar tooth.

Clinical features and radiology (Fig. 12.2)

As with many other odontogenic lesions, presentation is with a slowly growing, painless facial swelling producing expansion of the upper jaw rather than destruction of bone.

Radiologically, this tumour invariably appears as a circumscribed unilocular area of radiolucency varying in size from 1 to 8 cm. Cortical expansion, resorption of roots or even association with an unerupted tooth have all been reported, making differentiation from ameloblastoma, keratocyst or calcifying epithelial odontogenic tumour difficult.

Macroscopic and microscopic appearance

Microscopically, differentiation from the calcifying epithelial odontogenic cyst (Pindborg tumour) is important

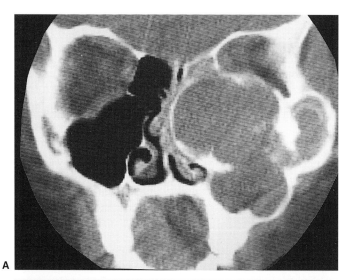

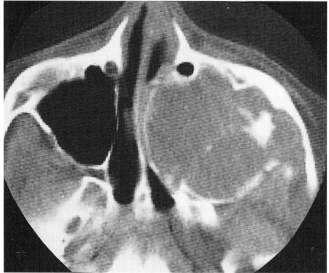

Fig. 12.2 Calcifying odontogenic cyst. **A**, coronal and **B**, axial CT scans. The cyst appears as a huge multilocular expansion of the maxillary antrum (Lloyd 1988[29]).

although both have features in common. The calcifying odontogenic cyst cavity is lined with squamous epithelium with a basal layer of stellate cells similar to those found in the enamel organ of the developing tooth. Within this layer are the characteristic 'ghost cells', which are the shadows of necrosed stellate cells. Inside these may be seen mineralization, dentinoid or even melanin pigmentation. In contrast to this, the Pindborg tumour contains amyloid-like material staining red with alkaline Congo red and showing a greenish refraction in polarized light.[38]

Most calcifying odontogenic cysts are a mixture of cysts and solid areas leading to supposition that this is a true tumour; consequently differentiation from ameloblastoma is essential from a therapeutic standpoint.

A 12-year-old boy was first seen in June 1984 with a 3 month history of headaches, right-sided nasal blockage, facial swelling and 2 weeks previously right proptosis. There was loosening of an upper molar tooth with swelling of the adjoining alveolus. The medial antral wall was pushed laterally blocking the nasal passage without evidence of proliferative tumour.

Radiology showed a mass in the right antrum which had displaced the medial wall against the septum and eroded the anterior and posterior walls. The CT scans showed that the mass was largely cystic with a fluid level. Superiorly, it was pushing up into the orbit, the floor of which was largely destroyed. Posteriorly, the soft tissue edge of the mass could be seen in the infratemporal fossa although the pterygoid plates were intact.

Following removal of the loose tooth, the antrum was explored via a Caldwell-Luc approach revealing a large cyst filled with thin fluid. Biopsy of granulation tissue within the tooth socket showed no serious pathology and the cyst was marsupialized. Extension into the pterygopalatine fossa made this difficult and loss of the orbital floor as well as the tuberosity and lateral antral wall was recorded.

Postoperatively, proptosis continued for several months before subsiding.

In December 1986 there was a recurrence of the facial swelling occurring over the previous 4 months and accompanied by proptosis and some 'bulging' in the region of the missing tuberosity. The maxillary sinus was reopened and surprisingly, much of the missing bone in the anterior maxilla had been replaced. This was removed allowing dissection of the underlying cyst wall and its removal. The orbital floor had reformed with thick bone but the cyst had encroached into the pterygoid region once more and the cyst contained clear fluid and calcified debris.

Histological report dated January 1987 stated 'The cystic lesion is lined with squamous cells, ghost cells and areas of calcification. Fine strands of this epithelium extend down into the surrounding connective tissue and may account for this recurrence'. Diagnosis was a calcifying odontogenic cyst.

An ophthalmic opinion at this time stated that vision was 6/6 right, 6/5 left; exophthalometry showed 13 mm on either side with no ocular displacement. In view of this no further treatment was advised. However, cheek swelling continued with intermittent pain. Tomography in December 1989 showed complete opacity of the right upper jaw with absence of both medial and posterolateral walls, possibly from previous surgery and/or the cyst.

In June 1990 another right upper molar became loose and facial swelling associated with a visible nasal cystic mass confirmed recurrence. A midfacial degloving procedure confirmed once again a thick-walled cyst extending into the infratemporal fossa surrounded by unusually thick new bone which was radically cleared via the improved exposure. The patient has been symptom-free since that time.

Prognosis

Despite the relative benignity of many odontogenic lesions, accessibility within the upper jaw together with a reluctance to perform major resections particularly in the young, frequently leads to a high rate of recurrence. Long-term follow-up is therefore essential to deal with these problems and also to determine realistic figures for control. Availability of cosmetically acceptable operations such as the midfacial degloving approach enables effective radical clearance to a degree not previously possible.

ODONTOGENIC KERATOCYST

Definition

Odontogenesis is a complicated process in which cells in varying stages of differentiation participate in a complex predetermined manner. After completion, remnants of epithelium may persist being derived from various sources such as tooth germ, dental lamina, enamel organ, etc.[39] Occasionally, in response to an unknown stimulus, these cell 'rests' proliferate to form odontogenic cysts or tumours. Keratocysts have distinctive histological characteristics which differentiate them from the other cysts which originate within the jaws.

Synonyms

Primordial cyst, epidermoid cyst of the jaws, cholesteatoma of the jaw.

Historical aspects

Most authorities agree that Philipsen introduced the term 'odontogenic keratocyst' in 1956 as a variant of odontogenic cysts.[40] A detailed account of the clinical and radiological features followed in 1963 by Pindborg & Hensen[41] who stressed the aggressive behaviour of this condition and its tendency to recur. Since then, there have been numerous publications usually relating to the mandible, supporting this concept but with little agreement regarding management.

Incidence and site

Although agreeing that keratocysts occur more frequently within the mandible than maxilla, the ratio being 2:1, the prevalence within all odontogenic cysts varies between a low of 5.5%[40] and 16.5%.[42] In the maxilla it is the region of the canine that appears to be the commonest site of origin and the largest series reported by Brannon showed a slight male predominance with an age at diagnosis averaging 37 years.[43] The youngest patient in this series of 312 cases was however, 7 years and the oldest 93.

Some mention must be made of the Basal Cell Naevus Syndrome, first described by Gorlin & Goltz.[44] This is characterized by:

1. Basal cell carcinoma at an early age
2. Multiple odontogenic keratocysts in the jaws
3. Bifid ribs and other skeletal anomalies
4. Frontal and parietal bossing
5. Broad base of nose
6. Calcification of the falx cerebri
7. Palmer and planter pits.

This is an autosomal dominant inheritance with marked penetration and odontogenic keratocysts are present in over 65% of these patients.[45] Multiplicity of cysts is common and the patients may be as young as 6 years old although symptoms are more usually first recognized at adolescence. Within the upper jaw the 2nd molar region is the commonest site of occurrence and recurrence occurs within 2 years of removal in more than 85% of patients.[46]

Multiple odontogenic keratocysts have also been reported in association with Marfan's and Noonan's syndromes.[47]

Clinical features

As with other odontogenic lesions, presentation within the maxilla is usually as a painless facial swelling together with nasal obstruction if the tumour is large. Shenoi et al described the clinical history of a 28-year-old Asian male with a 1 year history of nasal obstruction and swelling of the cheek from a proven odontogenic keratocyst. This had displaced the inferior turbinate medially, destroyed the anterior wall of the maxilla and extended as a soft cystic swelling up to the medial canthus.[48] This is a typical presentation and occasionally there may be loosening of teeth. If the cyst is opened then it is found to contain a malodorous cheesy material, not unlike cholesteatoma.

Radiology

Keratocysts are mostly well circumscribed, mono or multicystic and may be related to an impacted tooth or root apex. Considerable expansion of the upper jaw can suggest an odontogenic tumour, for such changes can be found in many of the lesions which co-exist with an unerupted tooth (follicular cyst) or root absorption (ameloblastoma or calcifying odontogenic cyst).

Macroscopic and microscopic appearance

The cyst lining is extremely thin, readily tearing and making effective enucleation difficult to achieve. It is between 4-10 cells in thickness, the basal lining of which resembles ameloblasts. Daughter and satellite cysts found at the periphery of the main lesion may be incompletely removed and although cellular atypia and mitosis are said to be uncommon, cyst lining left in situ will rapidly regrow.[49]

Natural history

The recurrence rate quoted varies with different authors, ranging from zero[50] to 62%[41] but this disparity probably relates to variations in site, treatment policies and length of follow-up. Recurrence may occur 20 years or more after apparently successful removal[51] and Oikarinen in 1990 reported two patients with recurrences 16 and 21 years following surgical removal.[52]

Differential diagnosis

Both the macroscopical and microscopical appearances are characteristic of this tumour so that errors in diagnosis are unlikely. However, as with calcifying odontogenic cysts, keratocysts can occur in association with other odontogenic tumours. Both unerupted teeth and root absorption are not unique to keratocysts and careful search must be made in all patients for the possibility of concurrent pathology.

Treatment

The fundamental criteria for treating this condition is complete removal of all the cyst wall. Without this, recurrence is inevitable and there is also a small, but verified risk of malignant change in inadequately treated lesions.[53] Toller found that 6 of 13 instances of carcinoma developing within cyst walls occurred with odontogenic keratocysts.[1] However, Stoelinga believes that recurrence may be due to invasion of surrounding bone by the cyst wall epithelium and this is supported by instances of invasion of bone grafts utilized to fill postoperative cavities.[54] Whatever be the aetiology, late recurrence occurs in 33 to 62% of patients with maxillary odontogenic keratocysts.[41]

Within the upper jaw, the lesion is usually multilocular and expansive at diagnosis, making complete removal problematic. Shenoi et al used a Caldwell-Luc approach followed by curettage of the bony wall.[48] Recurrence occurred within 2 months controlled by further curettage. However, at every operation effective removal becomes more difficult and long-term palliation is more feasible than cure!

A 64-year-old lady was seen in November 1983[55] with a history extending back to 1939 of a recurring dental 'abscess' which had been drained on many occasions. In 1946 the left upper last molar had been extracted and in 1972 she had a formal operation on her maxillary sinus for an odontogenic keratocyst.

Her complaint of a swelling localized to the left upper maxilla and lateral aspect of the orbit dated from 1976 and there was a discharging fistula in this region. Clinically and radiologically there was a large cyst with surrounding bone destruction involving the maxilla and orbit which included the root of the zygoma (Figs 12.3 and 12.4). Left partial maxillectomy confirmed dehiscence of the orbital floor and malar bone with the cyst wall projecting into the maxillary antrum and extraperiosteally into the left orbit. Most of the lateral orbital wall appeared to be soft and involved and was removed.

Postoperatively the fistula healed and there was no evidence of recurrence until 1987 when a swelling reappeared at the lateral aspect of the left orbit with inferior displacement of the

eye. In July 1987 a lateral orbitotomy showed recurrence of the keratocyst the wall of which was firmly attached to the orbital periosteum. The cyst was multiloculated and removed piecemeal.

The final histology report read 'The specimens from the orbit, lateral orbital wall and maxillary antrum show numerous cysts in soft tissue and bone. These cysts vary in size and contain much keratin. There are also small islets of odontogenic epithelium, some of which show early cyst formation. There is some chronic inflammatory reaction with new bone formation and this condition is a odontogenic keratocyst.'

This was our last contact with this patient who at that time possibly had a total history time of 48 years!

Prognosis

The clinicopathological problems which are inherent in comparing treatment modalities, recurrence rates and the risk of neoplastic change in aggressive cysts of the jaws have been studied by Stoelinga & Bronkhurst in some

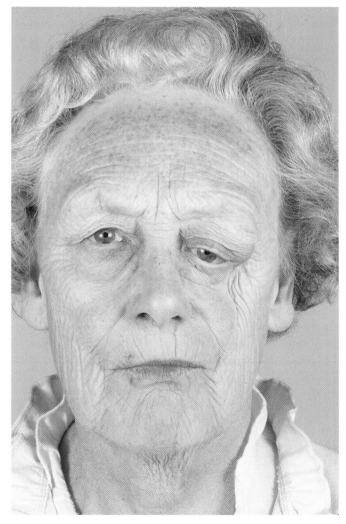

Fig. 12.3 Patient with recurrent odontogenic keratocyst of maxillary antrum, causing orbital displacement.[55]

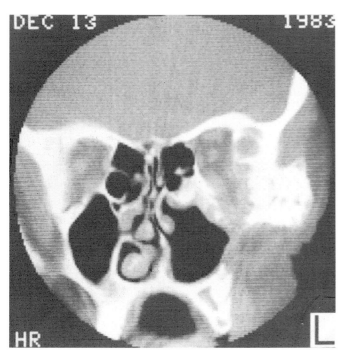

Fig. 12.4 Coronal CT scan of patient in Figure 12.3 showing involvement of floor of orbit by odontogenic keratocyst.

detail.[56] When discussing keratocysts they explain the variations in recurrence rates published by Voorsmit, 2.5 to 62.5%,[57] as relating to follow-up period, treatment modality and the methods used to calculate success rates. The lowest figure primarily based on the mandible, includes patients where excision included an area of overlying mucosa, rarely possible in the upper jaw. Indeed, most publications do relate to the more accessible mandible but in the upper jaw, resection is more difficult and follow-up must be indefinite for Oikarinen recorded recurrence after a 37-year period.[52]

CALCIFYING EPITHELIAL ODONTOGENIC TUMOUR

Synonyms

Unusual ameloblastoma, ossifying ameloblastoma, Pindborg's tumour, cystic odontoma and adenoid adamantinoma.

Historical aspects

Although already recognized as a distinct histological entity, it was Pindborg in 1958 who first accurately described this benign tumour emphasizing the rarity of recurrence and its characteristic features.[58] Early descriptions by Thoma & Goldman[59] had failed to recognize the individuality of this rare lesion but by 1976 over 100 cases had been reported in the literature.[60,61]

Incidence and site

This is clearly an unusual odontogenic tumour with a reported ratio to ameloblastoma of 1:17.[58] Franklin & Pindborg analysed 117 cases gathered from the world's literature in 1976 calculating that 1% of all odontogenic tumours were calcifying epithelial odontogenic; by 1982 this figure had risen to 1.8%.[60] Both sexes are equally affected with an average age of 40 years and a range of 8 to 92 years. The maxilla is the primary site of origin in one-third of patients, 11 but only a small number of patients with upper jaw involvement have been recorded. In these, an unerupted tooth is frequently associated with the tumour. This is said to occur in over half the cases although originally it was thought to be universal.[60]

Most of these neoplasms are intraosseous and the molar and premolar areas most commonly the primary site. When attached to an unerupted tooth, it is the enamel organ that has been suggested as the tissue of origin.

Clinical features

The usual presentation is a painless, slowly growing swelling of the maxilla accompanied by nasal obstruction from encroachment into the nasal passages.

A 51-year-old male had a 2 year history of a painless swelling of the left side of his nose without complaint of obstruction or epistaxis.[38] A firm swelling was situated at the anterior edge of the nasal bone and the nasal passage was in fact, blocked by medial displacement of the lateral nasal wall.

Radiology showed a fully developed ectopic tooth lying within a cystic cavity surrounded by calcification. There was no obvious bone destruction on tomography and via a Caldwell–Luc approach the tooth, cyst and thin bony capsule was removed from the maxillary antrum. Histology confirmed the diagnosis of a calcified epithelial odontogenic tumour and there has been no recurrence after a lengthy follow-up.

Radiology

The classical radiological appearance is a well defined area of osteolysis which may be uni- or multilocular with some calcification. However, depending on the stage of development, other tumours may present an opaque appearance, ranging from small flakes to irregular areas of calcification. With the presence of an unerupted tooth, radiology may be interpreted as a follicular cyst, calcifying odontogenic cyst, ameloblastoma or reparative giant-cell granuloma.

Macroscopic and microscopic appearance

The typical histological picture is one of sheets or islands of epithelial cells with prominent borders, intracellular bridges and occasional calcification. The nuclei are polymorphic, cytoplasm eosinophilic and mitosis rare. A characteristic feature is the homogeneous masses of amyloid like material within the epithelial cell clusters. This has been said to be derived from degenerated cells and has the staining properties of amyloid.[62] However, there is not universal agreement regarding the nature or origin of this material and Mori & Makino after histochemical studies concluded that this substance had much the same composition as enamel matrix and was not amyloid.[63]

Considerable variation in the epithelial component is found with multinucleated or pleomorphic cells which may be arranged in cribriform or adenoid patterns. However, these variations appear to be unrelated to any potential for recurrence but may cause some difficulty in diagnosis.

Treatment

The largest recorded series of patients, most being within the mandible, gave a recurrence rate after conservative management by curettage of 14%.[60] Within the upper jaw tumours tend to be larger and frequently associated with an unerupted tooth but with bony displacement rather than erosion. Total removal is advocated and best achieved by a Caldwell-Luc or midfacial degloving approach rather than potentially damaging 'blind' curettage. Although only a small number of well-documented cases have been published this philosophy appears to combine minimal structural damage with the best possibility of achieving a low rate of recurrence.

REFERENCES

1. Toller P A 1967 Origin and growth of cysts of the jaw. Annals of the Royal College of Surgeons, England 40: 306–336
2. Broca P P 1868 Recherches sur un nouveau groupe de tumeurs designees sous le nom d'odontames. Gazette Heb Medical Surgery 8: 113–115
3. Thoma K H, Goldman H M 1946 Odontogenic tumours. A classification based on observations of the epithelial, mesenchymal and mixed varieties. American Journal of Pathology 22: 433–471
4. Pindborg J J, Clausen F 1958 Classification of Odontogenic tumours. Acta Odontologica Scandinavia 16: 293–301
5. Prein J, Remagen W, Spiessl B 1986 Tumours of the facial skeleton, odontogenic and nonodontogenic tumours. Springer-Verlag, Berlin
6. Cusack J W 1827 Report of the amputation of parts of the lower and upper jaw. Dublin Hospital Records 4: 1–6
7. Malassez L 1885 Sur le role des debris epitheliaux paradententairis. Archives Physiology and Normal Pathology 5: 309–340
8. Ivy R H, Churchill H R 1930 The need of a standardized surgical and pathological classification of the tumour and anomalies of dental origin. American Association of Dental School Transactions 7: 240–245
9. International Classification of Tumours No. 5 1971 Histological typing of odontogenic tumours and cysts. World Health Organization, Geneva
10. Gorlin R J, Chaudury A P, Pindborg J J 1961 Odontogenic tumours. Cancer 14: 73–101
11. Regezi J A, Keer D A, Courtney R M 1978 Odontogenic tumors – analysis of 706 cases. Journal of Oral Surgery 36: 771–778
12. Bhaskar S N 1971 Synopsis der Mundkrankheiten Medica. Stuttgart, Wein Zurich
13. Shedev M K, Huvos A G, Strong E W 1974 Ameloblastoma of maxilla and mandible. Cancer 33: 324–333
14. Tsaknis P J, Nelson J F 1980 The maxillary ameloblastoma. An analysis of 24 cases. Journal of Oral and Maxillofacial Surgery 38: 336–342
15. McDaniel R K 1987 Odontogenic cysts and tumours. Chapter 57. In: Thawley I E Panje W R (eds) Comprehensive management of head and neck tumours. Saunders, Philidelphia
16. Bredenkamp S K, Zimmerman M C, Mickel R A 1989 Maxillary ameloblastoma. Archives of Otolaryngology 115: 99–104
17. Iko B O, Myers E M Onyekewere O 1985 Ameloblastoma of the jaws: Radiological diagnosis and follow up. British Journal of Oral and Maxillofacial Surgery 23: 333–340
18. Onuigbo W I B 1977 Jaw tumours in Nigerian Igbos. British Journal of Oral Surgery 15: 223–226
19. Dodge O G 1965 Tumours of the jaw. Odontogenic tissues and maxillary antrum (excluding Burkitt lyphoma) in Uganda Africans. Cancer 18: 205–215
20. Small I A, Waldron C A 1955 Ameloblastoma of the jaws. Oral Surgery, Oral Medicine, Oral Pathology 8: 281–297
21. Komisar A 1984 Plexiform ameloblastoma of the maxilla with extension to the skull base. Head and Neck Surgery 7: 172–175
22. Buchner A, Scuibea J J 1987 Peripheral epithelial odontogenic tumours. Oral Surgery, Oral Medicine, Oral Pathology 3: 688–697
23. Siar C H, Kok Han N G, Chon Hee Ngui 1990 Atypical peripheral ameloblastoma of the palate. Journal of Laryngology and Otology 104: 252–254
24. Mehlisch D R, Dahlin D C, Masson J K 1972 Ameloblastoma - a clinicopathologic report. Journal of Oral Surgery 30: 9–14
25. Keay D G, Kerr A G, McLaren K 1988 Ameloblastoma presenting as nasal obstruction. Case report. Journal of Laryngology and Otology 102: 530–533
26. Hansen L S, Ficarra G 1988 Mixed odontogenic tumours. Analysis of 23 new cases. Head and Neck Surgery 10: 330–343
27. Chaudhuri P 1975 Ameloblastoma of the upper jaw. Journal of Laryngology and Otology 89: 457–465
28. Atkinson C H, Harwood A R, Cummings B J 1984 Ameloblastoma of the jaw. Cancer 53: 869–873
29. Lloyd G A S 1988 Diagnostic imaging of the nose and paranasal sinuses. Springer Verlag, Berlin
30. Carr R R, Halperin V 1968 Malignant ameloblastomas from 1953-1966. Oral Surgery 26: 514–522
31. Singleton J McL 1971 Malignant ameloblastoma. British Journal of Surgery 8: 154–158
32. Takahashi K, Kiitasima T, Lee M 1985 Granular cell ameloblastoma of the mandible with metastases to the third thoracic vertebra. Clinical Orthopaedics 197: 171–180
33. Becker R, Pertl A 1967 Zur therapie des ameloblastomas. Deutsch Zeitschrift Inlund Kiferheilkd 49: 424–436
34. Gardner D G, Pecak A M J 1980 The treatment of ameloblastoma based on pathologic and anatomic principles. Cancer 53: 869–873
35. Gorlin R S, Pindborg J J, Clausen F P 1962 The calcifying odontogenic cyst - a possible analogue of the cutaneous calcifying epithelium of Mahlherbe. Oral Surgery 15: 1235–1243
36. Altini M, Farman A G 1975 The calcifying ghost cell odontogenic tumour - or calcifying odontogenic cyst. Oral Surgery 40: 751–759
37. Freedman P D, Lumerman H, Gee J K 1975 Calcifying odontogenic cyst. Oral Surgery 40: 90–94
38. Baunsgard P, Lontoft E, Sorensen M 1983 Calcifying epithelial odontogenic tumor (Pindborg tumor): an unusual case. Laryngoscope 93: 635–638
39. Shear M 1960 Primordial cysts. Journal of the Dental Association of South Africa 15: 211–217
40. Philipsen H P 1956 Om Keratoyster (kolesteatomer) Kalberne. Tandlaegebladet 60: 936–969
41. Pindborg J J, Hensen J 1963 Studies on odontogenic cyst epithelium. Acta Pathologica Microbiologica Scandinavica 58: 283–284
42. Radden B G, Reade P C 1973 Odontogenic keratocysts. Pathology 5: 325–334
43. Brannon R B 1976 The odontogenic keratocyst - a clinicopathological study of 312 cases. Oral Surgery 42: 54–72
44. Gorlin R S, Goltz R W 1960 Multiple naevoid basal cell epithelium jaw cysts. New England Journal of Medicine 269: 908–911

45. Southwick G S, Schwartz R A 1979 The basal cell naevus syndrome. Disasters amongst a series of 36 patients. Cancer 44: 2294–2302
46. Donatsky O, Hansen E, Philipsen H P 1976 Clinical, radiological and histopathological aspects of 13 cases of nevoid basal cell carcinoma syndrome. International Journal of Oral Surgery 5: 19–23
47. Connor J M, Price-Evans D A, Goose D W 1982 Multiple odontogenic keratocysts in a case of Noonan's Syndrome. British Journal of Oral Surgery 20: 213–216
48. Shenoi P, Paulose K O, Al-Khalifa S 1988 Odontogenic keratocyst involving the maxillary antrum. Journal of Laryngology and Otology 102: 1168–1171
49. Chuong R, Donoff R B, Guralnick W 1982 The odontogenic keratocyst. Journal of Oral and Maxillofacial Surgery 40: 797–802
50. Voorsmit R A, Stoelinga P 1979 Recurrence of odontogenic keratocysts in relation to clinical and histological features. A 20 year follow-up of 72 patients. International Journal of Oral Surgery 28: 47–49
51. Rudd J, Pindborg J J 1973 Odontogenic keratocysts - a follow up study of 21 cases. Journal of Oral Surgery 27: 323–330
52. Oikarinen V S 1990 Keratocyst recurrence at intervals of more than 10 years: Case reports. British Journal of Oral and Maxillofacial Surgery 28: 47–49
53. Ramsden R T, Barret A 1975 Gorian Syndrome. Journal of Laryngology and Otology 89: 615–617
54. Stoelinga P J W 1976 Studies of dental lamina related to the aetiology of cysts and tumours. Journal of Oral Pathology 5: 65–73
55. Lund V J 1985 Odontogenic keratocyst of the maxilla: a case report. British Journal of Oral and Maxillofacial Surgery 23: 210–215
56. Stoelinga P W, Bronkhurst T 1988 The incidence, multiple presentation and recurrence of aggressive cysts of the jaws. Journal of Cranio Maxillofacial Surgery 16: 184–195
57. Voorsmit R A 1985 The incredible keratocyst, a new approach to treatment. Deutsch Zahnarztl Zeitschrift 40: 641–648
58. Pindborg J J 1958 A calcifying epithelial odontogenic lesion. Cancer 11: 838–843
59. Thoma L H, Goldman H M 1946 Odontogenic tumors: classification based on observations of epithelial, mesenchymal and mixed varieties. American Journal of Pathology 22: 433–438
60. Franklin C D, Pindborg J J 1976 The calcifying epithelial odontogenic tumour. Oral Surgery 42: 753–765
61. Vap D R, Dahlin D C, Turlington E G 1970 Pindborg tumour – the so-called calcifying epithelial odontogenic tumour. Cancer 25: 629–636
62. Ranlou P, Pindborg J J 1966 The amyloid nature of the homogenous substances in the calcifying epithelial odontogenic tumour. Acta Pathologica Microbiology Scandinavia 68: 169–174
63. Mori M, Makino M 1980 The histochemical nature of homogenous amorphous materials in odontogenic epithelial tumours. Journal of Oral Surgery 38: 96–102

13. Neoplasms and other lesions related to bone

Although a variety of tumours characterized by replacement of normal bone architecture by tissue composed of varying amounts of collagen, fibroplasts, osteoid and giant cells, occur within the upper jaw, there remains considerable controversy over their diagnosis and management. Because histological similarities exist between the various lesions, classifications based somewhat arbitrarily upon relative amounts and character of their constituents has enhanced confusion whilst ignoring often marked differences in natural histories.

Some of these tumours are clearly benign, others frankly malignant, whilst a group clearly fall between these two extremes.

Terminology has on occasions been misleading and the classification adopted by the World Health Organization (WHO) in 1971 suffers from lack of consideration of the biological potential of many lesions.[1]

Makek in 1981[2] proposed a 'working' classification of fibro-osseous lesions aimed at eliminating redundant terminology whilst taking account of the biological potential of the tumours. Despite efforts to agree nomenclature, whilst at the same time avoiding the use of fibro-osseous as a collective description of a variety of differing conditions, histological diagnosis is hampered by 'unrepresentative biopsies'. Differential diagnosis in most instances must rely upon a correlation between histopathology, radiology and assessment of relevant clinical features.[3] This chapter is concerned with those tumours most commonly encountered within the upper jaw and is based upon a classification designed specifically for this purpose.

1. Fibromatosis
   Ossifying fibroma
2. Developmental disorders
   Fibrous dysplasia
3. Reactive–reparative lesions
   a. Giant-cell granuloma and tumour
   b. 'Brown tumour'
   c. Paget's disease

4. Neoplasms
   a. Osteoma
   b. Osteoid osteoma
   c. Osteoblastoma
   d. Osteogenic sarcoma.

FIBRO-OSSEOUS LESIONS

The term 'fibro-osseous lesion' has for many years been used as a general description for a group of tumours and proliferative disorders which affect the jaws. They comprise a number of specific clinical entities in which the clinical, radiological and histological features often overlap, causing confusion to both pathologists and clinicians in diagnosis and therapy.

The common denominator shared by these conditions is the replacement of normal bone architecture by tissue composed of collagen, fibroblasts and varying amounts of osteoid or bone. Lesions may vary from extensive disfiguring processes to small asymptomatic areas found accidentally on routine radiology. Despite much interest by many specialities over several decades, disagreement regarding terminology, histological interpretation and treatment persists. However, increasing personal experience rather than the collection of inadequate data from multicentric sources, has led to more distinctive classifications, particularly with regard to the two commonest conditions affecting the upper jaw – ossifying fibroma and fibrous dysplasia.[3]

A bewildering variety of names have been given to lesions within the fibro-osseous group. These include *fibrous dysplasia, osteitis fibrosa cystica, fibrous osteoma, osseous dysplasia, osteofibrosis, periapical cementoma, cementifying fibroma, juvenile ossifying fibroma, osteoblastoma* and *osteoid osteoma*. This multiplicity of names, frequently applied to the same pathological condition, has created confusion with regard to diagnostic criteria and misunderstanding of individual biological behaviour.

Makek[2] suggests that this is primarily because histological similarities between lesions comprising marrow fibrosis and bone formation have been regarded as sufficient justification for assigning biologically incompatible conditions to single groups. However, his own classification which is designed to avoid such errors by bridging the gap between morphological and descriptive diagnosis, proposes entities and pathological characteristics which are at variance with accepted nomenclature as proposed in the World Health Organization publication by Pindborg & Kramer.[1]

Evolutionary progress in our understanding of these unusual conditions is not necessarily accompanied by increased comprehension of differences in their biological behaviour and the WHO classification remains the most acceptable system, whilst not necessarily being the most accurate!

OSSIFYING FIBROMA

Definition

An encapsulated benign neoplasm consisting of fibrous tissue and containing varied amounts of metaplastic bone and mineralized masses having rounded outlines and few entrapped cells.[1]

Historical aspects

Menzel in 1872[4] has been credited with the first clinical description of an ossifying fibroma which occurred in the mandible of a 35-year-old woman and had been present for over 25 years.

The term 'ossifying fibroma' was first used by Montgomery in 1927[5] who described three patients with what may have been fibrous dysplasia, a term not introduced until 1942 by Lichtenstein & Jaffe.[6] An enduring controversy has persisted ever since as to whether these two conditions are variants of the same basic process[7] or as now appears more likely, two separate conditions difficult to distinguish histologically.[8–10] This view is supported in the authoritive WHO manual by Pindborg & Kramer[1] and by Harrison[3] based upon extensive clinical experience.

Incidence

Although there have been many publications of fibro-osseous lesions involving the mandible and maxilla, accurate data for specific incidence rates have been bedevilled by confusion in terminology and histopathological diagnosis. Schmaman et al[11] found 36 cases in a 13-year period in Baragwanath Hospital, South Africa which has 2400 beds serving a population of 700 000 patients. Five were diagnosed as having fibrous dysplasia,

11 with ossifying fibromata. Coley in 1960 estimated the incidence of fibrous dysplasia as 2.5% of all bony neoplasms and 7% of all benign bony tumours.[12] However, the term fibrous dysplasia did not appear in the Index Medica until 1967 and most authorities now consider it as an abnormal tissue development rather than a true neoplasm.

Some indication of the related incidence between fibrous dysplasia and ossifying fibroma has been given by Eversole et al in 1972.[8] They evaluated 841 patients with fibro-osseous conditions, 309 were diagnosed as having fibrous dysplasia, 225 ossifying fibroma and in 307 no definitive distinction was made! It would appear that the criteria for distinguishing between monostotic fibrous dysplasia and ossifying fibroma within the jaws is empirical and varied, despite clinical differences.

Age, sex and ethnic variation

Age distribution is best recorded at the time of diagnosis rather than the onset of symptoms and signs, since many publications fail to record the total duration of the disease. Ossifying fibromata are usually diagnosed in the 3rd to 4th decade of life being about 10 years later than monostotic fibrous dysplasia. A more aggressive variant, which has been called 'juvenile ossifying fibroma' occurs in the young. Although recognized clinically as possessing the potential for rapid, even fatal extension intracranially, no well-documented series has as yet been published and many pathologists regard this tumour either as a low-grade osteogenic sarcoma or a cementoblastoma.[13,14]

Langdon et al evaluating 39 patients with benign fibro-osseous lesions of the jaws found a high incidence in females in the 10 patients with ossifying fibromata.[15] Other publications list a male preponderance or an equal ratio. This illustrates the problems in evaluating inadequate data and it is likely that there is no major difference in the sex incidence.

Accounts of jaw tumours in black Africans from Nigeria indicate that fibro-osseous lesions are common and often gigantic in size. Centralization of expertise and facilities is usual in countries poorly provided with health care and Williams & Faccini reported only one ossifying fibroma in seven cases of fibro-osseous lesions seen in Nigeria in 1973.[16] Adekeye et al found three cases in a total series of 13 fibro-osseous lesions from Kaduna, Nigeria seen in 1980.[17] However, in every country, incidence of ossifying fibromata depends on both ethnic mix as well as diagnostic differentiation. Dehner reviewed 40 jaw tumours seen within 20 years at Washington University, USA finding that 60% were fibro-osseous and half of these, ossifying fibromas.[18] Greer & Mierau however, found only four of these tumours in 191 lesions of the jaws in children with an 8-year period at the University of Colorado, USA,[19] and Khanna & Khanna estimated that 28.5% of 122 African children with primary jaw tumours had cemento-ossifying fibromata.[20]

This appears to confirm a higher incidence of fibro-osseous lesions in black populations, although care must be taken in delineating specific lesions because of problems in terminology and clinicopathological differentiation.

Site and aetiology

Ossifying fibromata mainly affect bones which are ossified in membrane, possibly from cells within the bone-forming mesenchyme. There is a marked preference for the mandible rather than the maxilla[20] and the lesions usually develop in the premolar and molar region. Hamner et al in 1968 reviewing 249 patients with benign fibro-osseous tumours of the jaws commented that the fibrous connective tissue of the periodontium contained mesenchymal blastic cells with potential for forming cementum, alveolar bone and fibrous tissue.[21] They recognized histological variants of ossifying fibroma, e.g. cemento-ossifying fibroma, which have become grouped separately within the WHO classification of odontogenic lesions under the generic term 'Cementoma'.[1] However, although this particular condition is usually found in relation to the teeth, cases have been reported as originating within the ethmoid sinuses, possibly from ectopic periodontal membrane, primitive mesenchymal cell rests, or incomplete migration of the medial part of the nasal analage.[22]

Tumours diagnosed as ossifying fibroma have also been found within the nasal bones, orbit, sphenoid sinus and long bones.[23] This presents difficulties in accepting Waldron's belief that ossifying fibromata arise from the periodontal membrane.[14]

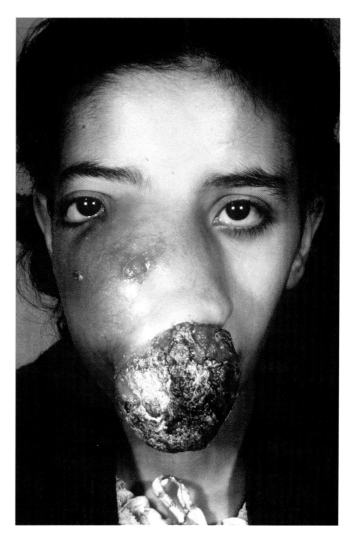

Fig. 13.1   Massive ossifying fibroma.[26]

Clinical features

Presentation and associated symptoms relate to the anatomical site of origin and the commonest complaint is of a painless swelling of the face. Expansion of bone may eventually produce hyperaesthesia or pain and nasoethmoidal tumours cause nasal obstruction or proptosis.[22]

Growth is slow and the duration from first-related symptom to diagnostic biopsy or removal varies from 6 months to 10 years, with an average of around 5 years.[14] However, these are benign tumours and they continue to grow without regard to skeletal maturity occasionally reaching considerable size (Fig. 13.1).

Juvenile ossifying fibromata, defined by Reed & Hagy as 'a localized actively growing destructive lesion occurring predominantly in children and characterized histologically by trabeculae of woven bone showing focal lamellar bone replacement in a cellular stroma'[13] grow more quickly and may mimic a malignant neoplasm.

Apart from variations in the age incidence and long-term natural history, there is no apparent difference between the clinical presentation of monostotic fibrous dysplasia and ossifying fibromata. Differentiation must be made by utilizing evidence provided by clinical, radiological and histological examination.

Radiology (Figs 13.2–13.4)

Sherman & Sternbergh describe the radiological appearances as oval or spherical with a distinct boundary and thinning of cortical bone producing an egg-shell appearance. Density is usually less than the surrounding bone and older lesions may exhibit calcification.[24] This tumour is well marginated, partly osteolytic and osteoblastic but with no periosteal reaction. In its early state the tumour appears cystic but with time there is increased mineralization producing opacity. This may be associated

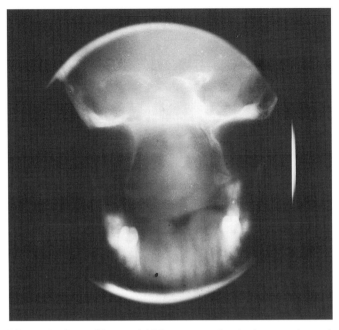

Fig. 13.2 Coronal hypocycloidal tomogram showing bony erosion and expansion caused by ossifying fibroma in Figure 13.1.

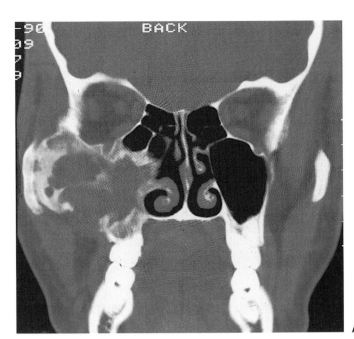

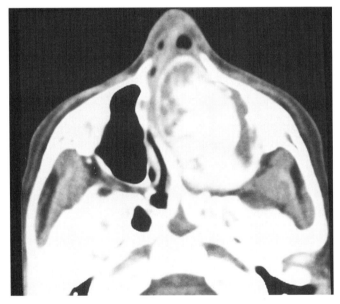

Fig. 13.3 Axial CT scan showing extensive ossifying fibroma of right maxilla.

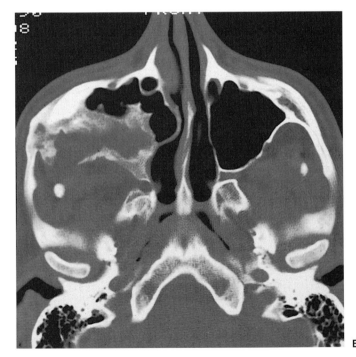

Fig. 13.4 Cementifying ossifying fibroma of right maxilla. **A,** coronal and **B,** axial CT scans.

with the 'ground glass' appearance seen in fibrous dysplasia.

Radiology shows the location of the tumour, involvement of adjacent teeth, whether it is solitary or multiple and the degree of bone expansion. In most instances the mass is surrounded by smooth, well-defined cortical bone which differentiates it from fibrous dysplasia where 'blending' into the surrounding bone is universal. 85% of the lesions identified radiologically by Waldron &

Giansenti were less than 4 cm in diameter but this may have represented early diagnosis for much larger tumours are not uncommon.[25]

Bone scintigraphy with[99m] Tc polyphosphate, although widely used in the diagnosis of skeletal disease, provides little additional information to routine CT scanning in ossifying fibromata. The lucent cortical expansion with or without central opacities of the well-developed lesions, represents the radiological feature of most of these tumours, although individual appearances will reflect variations in the amount of osteoid, bone and fibrous stroma, mimicking many other fibro-osseous lesions.[10]

Macroscopic and microscopic appearance

This tumour has a firm-to-hard consistency depending on the degree of mineralization. With increasing size, central areas of necrosis may occur although in the inactive, well-calcified masses there is usually considerable bone. Shanmugaratnam defined ossifying fibromata as 'consisting of spindle-shaped fibroblastic cells usually arranged in a whirled pattern containing islands and spicules of metaplastic woven bone and mineralized masses. It is usually encapsulated and mitosis may be present. The bony spicules show a lamellar structure peripherally rimmed by osteoblasts.'[26]

The histological picture is one of a cellular fibrous stroma containing collagen and bony trabeculae of irregular shape and disposition. These are both fibre and lamellar bone which polarizes, showing widely spaced parallel lines of bifringence. The fibrous tissue contains isomorphic spindle cells with minimal mitosis but in older lesions, bone is predominant being characterized by calcification occurring not in plates and trabeculae but in spherical globules.[15] These have been described as cementoid and similar lesions termed cemento-ossifying fibromata. This distinction however, is for practical purposes academic, playing no part in the biological behaviour of this tumour.

Natural history

Despite some variations histologically, which appear to be related to the age of the tumour, ossifying fibromata may be indistinguishable from fibrous dysplasia. However, clinically it usually develops in an older age group, is circumscribed and encapsulated and continues to grow after skeletal maturity is reached. Its behaviour is that of a benign neoplasm as illustrated in the following case report.

A 15-year-old boy was first seen in June 1981 with a 6 month history of a left-sided painless swelling of the face. Biopsy had already been performed 1 month previously which resulted in some dental pain and an equivocable report. The teeth on the side of the lesion had been displaced by a large, firm, maxillary-palatal mass which had not extended into the nasal cavity. The alkaline phosphatase was slightly elevated and tomography revealed expansion of the left maxilla with displacement of the pterygoid plates.

Biopsy via the alveolar-buccal sulcus revealed a hard mass easily cut and the report read 'mainly fibrous tissue within which are areas of calcification and ossification. The tumour is surrounded by a rim of normal lamellar bone which shows new bone formation. Diagnosis: ossifying fibroma.'

It was considered that wide resection at this time was inadvisable but by November 1985 the swelling had greatly increased in size producing an unacceptable (to the patient) cosmetic deformity. Reduction of the mass was performed via a Caldwell–Luc approach. The histological report now suggesting a more active lesion because of increased number of osteoblasts.

In March 1986 regrowth necessitated further removal using the same approach. Although the tumour was encapsulated the considerable expansion of the maxilla made complete removal unlikely and to avoid future problems a sub-total maxillectomy sparing the orbital floor was performed in June 1986. This was 5 years from initial diagnosis and there has been no further recurrence.

A Proplast implant to improve the cosmetic facial appearance was carried out in June 1988 with a good result to date.

Differential diagnosis

The most important feature distinguishing ossifying fibroma from fibrous dysplasia is the former's circumscribed nature and encapsulation. Although this is not apparent clinically or histologically, unless the growing edge is biopsied, it is frequently seen radiologically.

Many histologists have attempted to quantify specific features which might distinguish these two lesions but intrinsic variations secondary to age serve only to confuse the issue. Clinically, fibrous dysplasia can be expected to 'mature' following cessation of skeletal growth whilst the ossifying fibroma continues to grow. Since the time scale cannot be determined with any certainty, diagnosis and treatment must be related to individual patients.

Radiologically, the appearances are similar to many other upper jaw lesions such as osteoblastoma, odontogenic cyst and true neoplasms. Biopsy is therefore essential.

Treatment

Early lesions can be effectively removed by enucleation with curettage of all surrounding bone to ensure the removal of any remaining 'capsule'. This may be difficult within the upper jaw because of the size and extension of the tumour. Major resection may be required with subsequent cosmetic disability and, in the older patient, partial removal with the likelihood of further operations may be more acceptable. Much depends on the site of the tumour at diagnosis as is illustrated in the following case report.

A 15-year-old Arab boy was seen in January 1989 with a 2 year history of left-sided nasal obstruction and intermittent epistaxis. CT scan had shown a large non-homogeneous mass filling the left nose and nasopharynx and extending into the middle cranial fossa, sphenoid, ethmoid and maxillary antrum. The size was estimated radiologically as about 50 mm in diameter and biopsy confirmed a diagnosis of cementing ossifying fibroma.

Removal was carried out by a craniofacial approach which showed elevation of the planum sphenoidale between the optic canals. This huge tumour was however, encapsulated and removed in toto from the face of the clivus and first three cervical vertebra as well as the ethmoidal sinuses. Removal was judged to be complete and there has been no recurrence.

This case is similar to that reported by Fujimoto et al in 1987 in that the origin appeared to be in the region of the ethmoid-cribriform plate[22] and an even more dramatic patient was reported by Lund in 1982.[27]

A 14-year-old Iraqi girl was seen in June 1981 with a 1 year history of nasal obstruction from a progressively enlarging mass which completely distorted the nose and was now displacing the right eye and producing epiphora. Following a biopsy in her own country she had been given an unknown dosage of radiotherapy. A massive lesion occupied the right side of the nose, expanding it laterally, and protruding from the anterior nares was a large, ulcerated crusted mass (Fig. 13.1). The overlying skin was thinned, there was no intraoral extension although the mass was visible in the nasopharynx. Although displaced laterally by the lesion the right eye had normal vision and range of movements.

Plain sinus X-rays and tomography showed a huge soft-tissue growth causing expansion of the nasal cavity and maxillary antrum and there was virtually complete destruction of the right ethmoid (Fig. 13.2). The tumour had extended superiorly, thinning the planum sphenoidale and eroding the right wall of the sphenoid sinus. It was thought that there was contact between the tumour and dura of both the anterior and middle cranial fossa, the changes being consistent with pressure erosion rather than malignant invasion.

Biochemical investigations were unhelpful and the tumour, 13×7×6 cm in size was removed via a right lateral rhinotomy. It was encapsulated, a finding substantiated on radiological review, and attached primarily to the area of the cribriform plate where it was possible to dissect it free from the underlying dura (Fig. 13.5). There was considerable bony loss due to pressure erosion and the alveolae were 'free-floating' due to loss of the whole hard palate. Loss of much of the right maxilla, ethmoid and face of the sphenoid together with most of the nasal septum had also taken place and on subsequent questioning it was clear that this lesion had been present for several years. The incision was closed following removal of redundant skin and some attempt to refashion a nasal septum.

Postoperative recovery was uneventful with no leakage of cerebrospinal fluid. An oral prosthesis was introduced at the completion of the operation to support the flaccid palate thus allowing oral feeding. Stabilization occurred within 6 months and subsequently the depressed nasal bridge has been reconstructed to give an excellent cosmetic result. There has been no recurrence of the tumour. Histologically, the tumour was composed of spindle cells, some of which were fibroblasts and fibrocytes. Osteoblasts formed dense groups and throughout the tissues were calcified particles and areas of newly woven bone. In the centre of the tumour there was considerable necrosis and the periphery was surrounded by a fibrous capsule in which newly formed bone is seen. There were no mitotic figures.

Irradiation is contraindicated, as it is in all benign fibro-osseous lesions of the upper jaw,[28] and radical removal is advocated where technically feasible for continuous growth can be anticipated in this otherwise benign tumour.

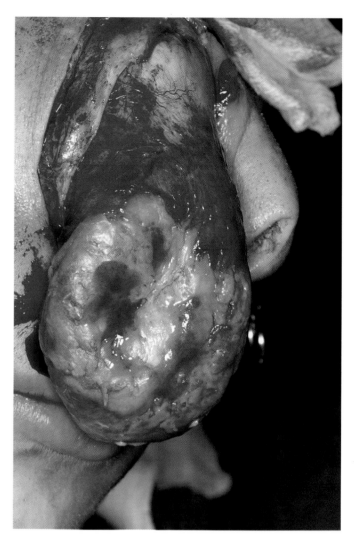

Fig. 13.5 Intraoperative photograph showing exposure of ossifying fibroma in patient shown in Figure 13.1.

FIBROUS DYSPLASIA

Definition

A benign localized bone disorder of unknown aetiology in which endocrinopathologies, abnormal pigmentation of the skin and mucous membranes may form part of the disease.[29]

Synonyms

When the term was first coined by Lichtenstein & Jaffe in 1942, there were 33 synonyms in their paper.[30] More recent names have included ossifying fibroma, focal fibrosis of bone, bone cyst, Jaffe-Lichtenstein-Uehlinger disease, osteodystrophia fibrosa, osteofibroma, fibrous osteoma, fibrous chondroficans, osteitis fibrosis localis and cystofibromatosis.[31]

Historical aspects

In 1891 von Recklinghausen reported three groups of bone diseases, one of which contained patients with what is now recognized as polyostotic fibrous dysplasia.[29] Jaffe suggested in 1926 that certain forms of the bony lesion then diagnosed as osteitis fibrosa generalisata that were not associated with altered serum calcium levels or parathyroid adenomata, represented a specific type of disease.[31] However, it was not until 1937 that Albright et al described a syndrome characterized by bony lesions, skin pigmentation and female precocious puberty.[32] He used the old name 'osteitis fibrosa generalisata' whilst McCune & Bruch in the same year chose 'osteodystrophia fibrosa' for the same condition.[33] Lichtenstein in 1938 described the pathology of eight cases of fibro-osseous bone disease without extraskeletal manifestations using the present day terminology of 'polyostotic fibrous dysplasia'.[34] In Europe, Vehlinger (1940) independently chose the term 'osteofibrosis deformans juvenilis' and he had already recognized that these lesions were not endocrine-related and that both monostotic and polyostotic forms existed.[35] The monostotic form was described as a distinct entity by Lichtenstein & Jaffe 2 years later.[6]

For many years however, fibrous dysplasia was not distinguished from primary hyperparathyroidism both being described pathologically and radiologically as osteitis fibrosa cystica. Pritchard in 1952 reviewed 31 patients with fibrous dysplasia all of whom had been fruitlessly explored for a parathyroid tumour.[36] Hunter & Turnbull in 1931 in their paper on hyperparathyroidism had already described a localized fibrous bony lesion not associated with abnormalities of calcium or phosphate metabolism. They called it 'osteitis fibrosa' adding yet another name to an already confusing situation.[37]

The separation of fibrous dysplasia from other disseminated bony diseases such as hyperparathyroidism and multiple neurofibromatosis was initiated by the studies of Albright in 1947[38] and Jaffe in 1953.[39] Nevertheless, it was believed for many years that fibrous dysplasia and ossifying fibroma of the facial skeleton were variants of the same disease. Today, the main consensus of opinion favours a clear distinction with fibrous dysplasia belonging to the category of dysplasia whilst ossifying fibroma fits more logically into the classification of benign tumours.[3,8,40–42]

Incidence

Fibrous dysplasia is essentially a disease of the young, being usually diagnosed in early childhood or even infancy. Coley estimated that 2.5% of all bony lesions are fibrous dysplastic, but no reliable data are available for population prevalence and this condition must be considered as rare.[34]

Within the upper jaw the monostotic form is most common, 84% of the 48 cases of fibrous dysplasia included in "The Atlas of Tumours of the Facial Skeleton" by Prein et al were monostotic[31] and this form is said to be 30 times more common than polyostotic fibrous dysplasia.[6] Most series however, are numerically small, showing equal sex distribution, although there appears to be a female preponderance in the polyostotic variety.[30]

Site

Polyostotic fibrous dysplasia most commonly affects the ribs, femur and tibia with craniofacial involvement in most severe polyostotic disease.[33] Although solitary lesions within the maxilla are said to be commoner than the mandible, this may reflect reference selectivity. Certainly, early recognition is likely since facial deformity is more noticeable in the young.[43] Within the head and neck region the areas most frequently involved in the monostotic form are maxilla, frontal bone, mandible, parietal, occipital and temporal bones. However, isolated cases where the lesion appears to have originated in the ethmoid sinuses have been reported, presenting problems in both diagnosis and management.[44]

As with many other bony lesions of the upper jaw there is some evidence of an increased incidence amongst black Africans but this may represent centralization of data.

Aetiology

There is no general agreement as to the aetiology of the disease which appears to have no familial, hereditary or congenital basis. Firat & Stutzman in 1968 published an account of two cases of familial hyperparathyroidism associated with fibrous dysplasia in a mother and daughter. In both instances removal of the parathyroid adenoma had little appreciable effect on the fibrous dysplasia.[45] Ehrig & Wilson (1972) described two patients with fibrous dysplasia and hyperparathyroidism and again there was no change following parathyroidectomy.[46]

Lichtenstein & Jaffe thought that fibrous dysplasia represented a 'congenital anomaly of development' with defective activity of bone-forming mesenchyme. This would certainly explain the young age at diagnosis.[6] Schlumberger noting that proliferation of connective tissue is a basic response to injury, suggested that this lesion was a reparative process[47] whilst hormonal imbalance may explain Albright's disease.[32] Changus postulated a hyperplasia of osteoblasts in response to an unidentified stimulus[48] and Edgerton et al, a mutant gene.[49] The most readily accepted theory appears to be abnormal activity of mesenchymal cells which describes the pathological changes but not why they occur!

Clinical features (Fig. 13.6)

The commonest presentation within the upper jaw is a slow-growing, asymmetrical, painless swelling which may only be detected at examination. In some instances large areas of the skull may be involved[50,51] and oral examination frequently shows a smooth fusiform expansion of the alveolar ridge and adjacent maxilla. The covering mucosa is invariably normal in appearance and non-ulcerated whilst the teeth, although within the lesion and displaced, are not loosened. The hard palate is rarely involved but the maxillary mass may extend into the nose producing obstruction, or the orbit causing proptosis. Involvement of the antro-ethmoid region may cause a frontal sinus mucocoele by duct obstruction and although the lesion is usually unilateral it may cross the midline. Compression of the optic nerve results in visual loss, and excessive vascularity within active fibrous dysplasia may produce symptomatic arteriovenous fistulae, as in Paget's disease.

Contrary to most authors' experience, Boysen et al found that in all of their 15 fibro-osseous lesions of the craniofacial bones, five of which were fibrous dysplasia, the patients complained of pain.[52] This has not been our experience with 61 fibro-osseous lesions and it is difficult to explain unless it was subsequent to secondary infection or neoplastic change.

Although elevation of the alkaline phosphatase is said to indicate an actively-growing lesion with osteoclastic bone resorption, this is a common finding in young children and apart from excluding hyperparathyroidism, biochemical estimations play little part in diagnosis. Clinically, fibrous dysplasia is little different from ossifying fibroma except perhaps occurring in a younger age group. However, there is good evidence that growth slows down after puberty but may continue intermittently up to the 4th decade of life. Smith, a histopathologist, describes three types of fibrous dysplasia according to microscopical activity, the last of which represents an inactive stage. This can however, only be surmised by

radiological evidence of cessation of growth over a long period of time.[42]

Radiology (Fig. 13.7)

The most characteristic, but not necessarily pathognomonic feature of monostotic fibrous dysplasia within the

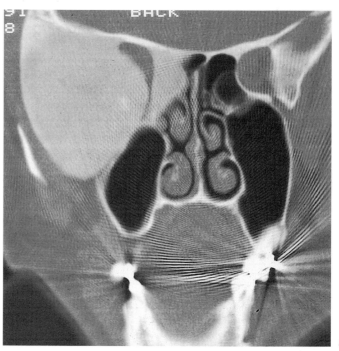

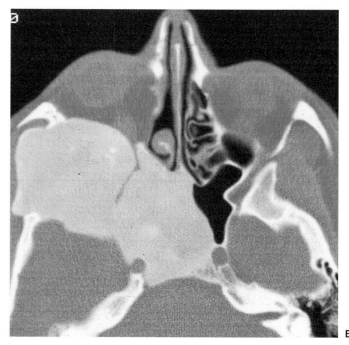

Fig. 13.7   Extensive fibrous dysplasia of sphenoid; **A**, coronal and **B**, axial CT scans.

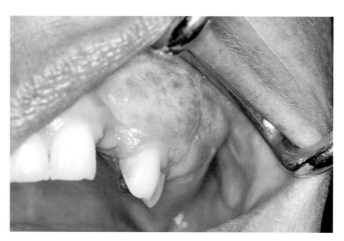

Fig. 13.6   Gingival mass of fibrous dysplasia arising in the upper jaw.

upper jaw, is the radiological appearance. Although non-specific, its features depend upon the age of the lesion and degree of metaplastic bone formation. All lesions have diffusely blending margins in marked contradistinction to the sharply demarked ossifying fibromata.

Sherman & Glauser have classified fibrous dysplasia of the jaws into three radiological groups. Type 1 is usually seen in the maxilla and shows a diffuse uniform sclerosis which follows bony contours as well as enlarging the bone. Type 2 is lytic and the most commonly seen, appearance producing cortical expansion and multiloculation. Type 3 is the rare unilocular lesion.[9]

Fries has also attempted to classify the various radiological patterns, the first being termed 'Pagetoid' with bone expansion and areas of radiodensity or radiolucency. This is said to occur in patients over the age of 30 years with long histories of disease. The second pattern is sclerotic with bone expansion and a homogeneous radiodensity whilst the third is cystic with sclerotic borders. This is said to be most common in younger patients averaging 20 years of age with short clinical histories.[53]

Depending on the age of the lesion, all zones may appear uniformly opaque (the ground-glass effect), cystic or multiloculated and the thinned overlying bone showing reactive periosteal new bone. Without clinical and histological support, attempts at diagnosing let alone classifying such a variable condition must be considered as 'unwise'. Perhaps the evidence of peripheral diffusion and the extent of the visible lesion is all that radiology can be expected to contribute although radionuclide imaging does show the high degree of vascularity in the active stage of growth which could be of value in planning treatment.

Macroscopic and microscopic appearance

The gross morphology varies but within the upper jaw the lesion is composed of grey to reddish-brown fibrous tissue that has enough osteoid to give a firm gritty consistency which cuts easily.

The basic histological component is an overgrowth of fibrous tissue within cancellous bone. This stroma may have abundant spindle cells with many capillaries and within this stroma are metaplastically formed fibre bone trabeculae. Both the trabeculae and poorly formed membranous bone is irregularly distributed within the fibrous tissue and there may be nests of multinucleated giant cells close to areas of vascularity. The lesions are not encapsulated and there is fusing and blending between normal and abnormal bone, making the margins of this lesion impossible to verify.

Reed believed that fibrous dysplasia represents a permanent maturation arrest in the woven bone stage and suggested that demonstration of lamellar bone transformation negated a diagnosis of fibrous dysplasia.[54] Schmaman et al in compiling a table of differentiating factors to distinguish fibrous dysplasia from ossifying fibroma, giant cementoma and chronic osteomyelitis, also commented on the importance of the absence of lamellar bone in fibrous dysplastic lesions.[11]

However, the question of osseous differentiation beyond the woven bone stage remains controversial. Boysen et al found both lamellar bone formation and osteoblastic rimming in lesions which met both clinical and radiological criteria for fibrous dysplasia.[52] Lamellar bone may of course represent pre-existing host bone which has become incorporated into the lesion. However, Kwee has suggested that in older 'quiescent' lesions, lamellar bone can form and in discussing this question, the age of the lesion and its activity must be considered.[55]

Woven bone is structurally inefficient and is normally found in the early stages of intramembranous ossification and in the periosteal growth of bones formed by endochondral ossification. Because of its association with the early stages of skeletal growth it has been called 'immature' although it is also found in the early stages of many reparative processes. In fibrous dysplasia the stages of cellular differentiation and cellular by-products such as collagen, osteoid and bone, are all the result of faulty development and abnormal cellular formation. However, this appears to cease after puberty with possible maturation of the lesion. Consequently, biopsies taken from non-representative areas or at different time scales of growth may well show varying histological pictures, causing diagnostic confusion.[3,52]

Natural history

Fibrous dysplasia is primarily a disease of children and adolescents with most active growth taking place in the first two decades of life. It is likely that it represents an error of development in the bone-forming mesenchyme[31] and growth can be expected to slow or stop after puberty in monostotic disease. As yet there is no reliable means of ensuring that this has taken place other than comparative radiological assessment and possibly the presence of lamellar bone in biopsies! Differentiation between this lesion and ossifying fibroma is however, important since the latter being a benign neoplasm will continue to grow.

Differential diagnosis

Variations in histological and radiological appearances in monostotic fibrous dysplasia in the upper jaw can lead to confusion with osteoma, ossifying fibroma, meningioma, osteoblastoma, giant cell granuloma, ameloblastoma and cysts. Polyostotic disease must be separated from hyperparathyroidism, Paget's disease and neurofibromatosis.

Treatment

There is no reliable evidence to suggest that anything other than surgery is effective in reducing the size of the lesion. Total excision, except in very small masses, is not feasible because of the absence of distinct margins and the blending of the lesion into surrounding bone. Radiotherapy is contraindicated because of the risk of sarcomatous change.[56] Malignant change has been recorded to occur spontaneously being said to take place more frequently in polyostotic disease. Both osteo- and fibrosarcoma were found by Williams & Thomas who gave an incidence of 0.4%.[57] This is far less than in Paget's disease but rapid increase in size or pain in a pre-existing fibrous dysplastic lesion requires urgent biopsy. Schwartz & Alpert also gave a 0.5% chance of malignant change, but after irradiation.[58]

The timing of surgical reduction is important since active lesions are highly vascular and regrowth is often rapid. An aggressive form of fibrous dysplasia exists although not differentiated histologically. Progression is rapid after biopsy or reduction and Schofield reported a case in a 7-year-old girl where three operations were performed within 18 months before controlling growth.[59]

Small lesions may be removed completely but are rarely diagnosed. However, the mere presence of an area of fibrous dysplasia does not in itself indicate a need for interference. Partial removal to improve appearance or more urgently if functions such as vision are threatened are reasonable. Jackson et al however, argues that within the cranio-orbital region, radical surgery is indicated because of the high rate of recurrence following partial removal.[60] The diffuse nature of this lesion and its variable rate of growth together with bleeding during the active phase, suggests that major surgical interference should be reserved for those few patients with a serious threat to vital functions.

As with most other fibro-osseous lesions of the upper jaw, each patient must be viewed individually with careful assessment of the extent, histology and symptoms before advising surgery of any nature.

A 9-year-old boy was first seen in October 1986 with a gradual swelling of the left face. There was expansion of the maxilla and alveolar region substantiated by tomography and a partial maxillectomy was performed. The maxillary antrum was filled with a diffuse, yellowish mass with only a small residual cavity left within the antrum. This was enlarged by removing as much of the mass as possible with careful preservation of the tooth apices. Bleeding was minimal and after fashioning a large antrostomy the Weber-Fergusson incision was closed.

The histological report reads, 'trabeculae of woven bone forming thin, elongated, twisted shapes separated by fibroblasts and vascular spaces. In a few places fibroblasts are abundant and bone fragments small and round. The bony trabeculae show some areas of osteoblastic rimming and the appearances are consistent with fibrous dysplasia.'

By February 1988 the depression over the left maxilla had been maintained suggesting that no major regrowth had occurred but by April 1990 there was both clinical and radiological evidence of considerable regrowth in the maxilla, zygoma, ethmoid and sphenoid sinuses. A full mid-face degloving approach enabled most of the firm mass to be removed by drilling and curettage. To avoid damage to the left optic nerve the posterior ethmoid cells and sphenoid sinus were untouched although the orbit was decompressed. Bleeding was minimal but the diffuse nature of the lesion and absence of a capsule confirmed the original diagnosis of fibrous dysplasia; the histology was unchanged.

Prognosis

Apart from the exceptional case where spontaneous neoplastic change takes place, the principal problem with fibrous dysplasia is the need for timing of any 'reduction surgery'. The modern mid-face degloving approach offers in selected cases the possibility of removing safely much of even extensive lesions with minimal cosmetic defect. However, with a condition which ceases to grow spontaneously the need for anything but minimal interference must be considered in all but those patients whose disease is aggressive or where serious functions are threatened.

GIANT CELL GRANULOMA AND GIANT CELL TUMOUR

Definition

At least three distinct varieties of giant cell lesions occur within the facial skeleton; giant cell reparative granuloma, the brown tumour of hyperparathyroidism and the true giant cell tumour or osteoclastoma. Although distinctly individual in their clinical manifestations, they share many common histological characteristics causing problems in both diagnosis and terminology.

Historical aspects

According to Ewing[61] Ambroise Pare deserves the credit for first describing the giant cell tumour in the 16th century. In 1934, Albright et al described a variety of giant cell tumour secondary to hyperparathyroidism which was termed 'brown tumour' because of its macroscopic appearance.[62] Prior to 1952 the term giant cell tumour had covered a variety of differing conditions. Jaffe coined the name 'giant cell reparative granuloma' to represent a type of giant cell lesion found exclusively in the jaws where areas of osteoid deposition alongside areas of destruction give an appearance of attempted repair.[39]

A third variety then became obvious, the 'true' giant cell tumour, although this is both vague and unscientific since all these lesions could be considered as tumours and contain giant cells! Osteoclastoma is possibly a better expression for this tumour the features of which have been clearly described by Jaffe in 1953[63] and Lichtenstein in 1959.[64]

Although this concept is now generally recognized there remains doubt as to whether the reparative granuloma and giant cell tumour are really separate entities, identical processes or part of a spectrum of giant cell lesions which might include cherubism and the aneurysmal bone cyst?

Incidence

Whereas giant cell tumours of any variety are uncommon, the reparative granuloma is the commonest, accounting for 3.5% of all the benign tumours found in this region.[65] The giant cell tumour or osteoclastoma, is rare with Dahlin reporting that in a series of 6221 bone tumours occurring throughout the body only 3 (4.2%) giant cell tumours were in the head and neck area, all within the sphenoid.[66] Quick et al[67] reviewing giant cell tumours of the maxilla in children found seven previous cases and added three more of their own. They commented that since these tumours were rare, individual cases were more likely to be reported, which was in contradistinction to the commoner reparative giant cell granuloma. Certainly, accurate incidence rates for both these lesions are difficult to extrapolate from the literature because of confusing terminology. There has been a tendency for 'giant cell lesion and giant cell tumour' to be used interchangeably without attempts at classification.

Burnam et al found 13 previously reported patients with a giant cell tumour originating in the ethmoid sinuses adding one new case.[68] However, much of the data and pathological characteristics referring to this tumour are extrapolated from lesions localized to the epiphysis of the long bones rather than the small number of cases occurring in the upper jaw.

Age and sex variation

It appears reasonably conclusive that the giant cell granuloma is predominantly a disease of childhood and young adults with approximately 75% of lesions being diagnosed within the first two decades of life. There is a modest female preponderance and an occasional patient aged over 80 years of age.[69] Giant cell tumours (osteoclastoma) affect an older age group when the long bones are involved; 85% of Dahlin's 266 patients were in the 2nd to 3rd decade.[66] Burnam et al say that within the maxilla this neoplasm never occurs under the age of 18 years although this is open to question (see the case report).[68] However, there are insufficient reliable data to provide conclusive guidance as to age span and nothing recorded to substantiate ethnic susceptibility.

Site and aetiology

The giant cell granuloma is a non-neoplastic reparative reaction to haemorrhage, possibly secondary to trauma or inflammation. It occurs most frequently in the mandible and Batsakis has suggested that it originates from injury to the periodontal membrane, odontogenic mesenchyme or dental sac.[70] Whatever the aetiology, most pathologists consider them reactive, which is in contradistinction to the giant cell tumour. Within the long bones the cell of origin is the osteoclast which is indistinguishable from the 'giant' cell of the upper jaw lesion. Burnam et al believe that all true giant cell tumours arise from cartilaginous bone, possibly from centres of ossification.[68] Geschickter & Copeland[71] support this contention emphasizing that this neoplasm's origin is at the site of bone which has been formed in cartilage and is related to the normal resorptive process of bone osteoclasts which takes place in the histogenesis of these bones.

The occipital, sphenoid, ethmoid and petrous part of the temporal bone are all cartilaginous in origin whilst the maxilla and most of the mandible ossify in membrane. This is in accord with our existing knowledge in that giant cell tumours when occurring in the head and neck, are found in the sphenoid, ethmoid and temporal bone, with a few cases in the maxilla or frontal bones (possibly extensions from the ethmoid).[72]

However, differences in terminology and histological interpretation may have led to some of the tumours found in unusual sites being actually giant cell reparative granulomata, or in areas secondary to unsuspected Paget's disease of hyperparathyroidism. It is doubtful if 'true giant cell tumours occur elsewhere in the head and neck although Bullock & Luck described 'giant cell-like tumours' adding additional confusion to an already complicated situation.[73]

Clinical features

Reparative giant cell granulomata produce a painless swelling which is frequently undetected until facial deformity or nasal obstruction occurs. Loosening or displacement of teeth can occur when teeth become embedded in loose granulation tissue. In edentulous patients the lesion may proliferate into the oral cavity giving the appearance of a carcinomata. The three patients recorded by Quick et al[67] all had palatal swellings with friable masses in the nasal airways causing epistaxis. The duration of symptoms varies from 2 months to a year in published cases and pain is unusual unless there is secondary infection. Burnam et al when discussing giant cell tumours[68] found that many complained of a dull ache and their origin within the spheno-ethmoid region was frequently associated with proptosis or visual disturbance. The duration of symptoms was shorter than with reparative granulomata as might be expected when considering a true neoplasm, but reliable data regarding this remains scarce.

Radiology

There are no pathognomonic radiological features to differentiate reparative giant cell granulomata from the giant cell tumour. Small spicules of bone may be seen within the former or a thin calcified rim around the periphery of this lesion. The margins of the giant cell tumour merge into surrounding bone and may be unusually vascular.[64] Both lesions can show uni- or multilocular osteolytic areas with resorption of tooth roots.

Macroscopic and microscopic appearance

Although it has been said that reparative giant cell granuloma is histologically indistinguishable from the giant cell tumour this is not supported by Batsakis,[70] Jaffe[63] or Lichtenstein.[64]

Reparative granulomata are composed of multiple haemorrhagic fragments of soft tissue showing a fibrillar stroma with many spindle-shaped connective tissue cells. Irregularly interspersed in this matrix are multinucleated giant cells and there are areas of haemorrhage with haemosiderin as well as lipid-laden histiocytes. Typically, spicules of osteoid deposition give an appearance of attempted repair. This is indistinguishable from the brown tumour of hyperparathyroidism.[68] Batsakis says that giant cell tumours do not usually show osteoid formation and are devoid of haemorrhage, haemosiderin or lipid-laden histiocytes.[70] Hiyeda et al studied the ultrastructure of these tumours and suggested that the giant cells were formed by the fusion of stroma cells, which were themselves indistinguishable from osteoclasts.[74] Steiner & Ghosh believe that the cells originate from fusion of mononuclear cells and that the bulk of the tumour comes from undifferentiated bone marrow connective tissue.[75]

The supposition that these neoplasms arise from hyperplastic osteoclasts remaining after normal histogenesis of endochondral bone appears erroneous since osteoclasts are not confined to endochondral bone. Growth of bone is a dynamic process whether it be of membranous or cartilaginous origin.[67]

Histological differentiation between the reparative giant cell granuloma and giant cell tumour is clearly often difficult. Both contain giant cells and stromal cells interspersed with varying amounts of matrix. However, differences do occur and correlation between the clinical history, laboratory investigations, radiological assessment and histological appearances should allow accurate delineation, essential for treatment planning.

Natural history

Since giant cell granulomata are considered to be essentially a reparative process and benign, local excision or curettage is the usual form of treatment with local recurrence reduced by meticulous haemostasis. However, local recurrence rates vary from 10%[76] to 69%[18] and aggressively behaved lesions do occur. Malignancy only occurs following irradiation.[77]

Ablative surgery in the form of total excision is recommended for proven giant cell tumours as failure to remove all disease is followed by a high recurrence rate. Jaffe reported a figure of 55% in his series of 60 patients although most of these had long bone tumours.[39]

Differential diagnosis

Lesions with similar appearances to reparative giant cell granulomata include hyperparathyroidism, aneurysmal bone cyst, fibrous dysplasia, Paget's disease, cherubism and the true giant cell tumour or osteoclastoma.

Histologically, brown tumour of primary or secondary hyperparathyroidism and reparative granuloma are identical but can be distinguished by serum calcium and phosphate estimations.

Cherubism is a rare autosomal dominant condition affecting the jaws of children. Although the histopathology is similar, it is not identical and differentiation is helped by variations in clinical presentation. Cherubism is a painless, bilateral swelling of the jaws first apparent about the age of 10 years. Progress may be rapid and radiologically this lesion is multilocular with bone expansion. Other lesions presenting problems in differential diagnosis have been discussed elsewhere and present varying degrees of difficulty in establishing a definitive diagnosis.

Treatment

Aggressive curettage of reparative granulomata must include surrounding bony walls with meticulous removal of all disease including that surrounding involved teeth. There is invariably considerable bleeding and good haemostasis is essential to ensure disease is not left in situ. The bony cavity can be packed with autologous cancellous bone if very large but occasionally there is widely spread disease and the cavity is then best left open to facilitate early detection of local recurrence. Giant cell tumours may also follow a relatively benign course but never subside spontaneously. Lichtenstein has said that less than one half will be permanently controlled after the first operation even when radically excised. At least 10% will behave malignantly and metastasize to the lungs.[68] Grading is not feasible because of the frequency of variations in histology and site of origin and most authors report a high local recurrence rate.

Primary or postoperative irradiation has not been shown to be of value and carries a risk of about 20% of subsequent sarcomatous change.[66] The most effective therapy is wide local excision.

A 15-year-old boy when seen early in 1982 was complaining of nasal blockage, purulent rhinorrhoea and disturbance of vision. There was radiological evidence of a mass situated in both the ethmoid and sphenoid sinuses and extending into the left orbit as well as the nasal cavity. Biopsy confirmed a diagnosis of giant cell tumour and a craniofacial resection of the cribriform plate with ethmoidal block was performed preserving the eye. Most of the disease was situated posteriorly within the spheno-ethmoidal region but had involved the anterior fossa dura.

There has been no evidence of local recurrence 7 years post-surgery.

'BROWN' TUMOUR (HYPERPARATHYROIDISM)

Definition

A benign slow growing tumour, identical histologically with giant cell granuloma but associated with hyper-parathyroidism.

Historical aspects

The diagnosis of hyperparathyroidism and its surgical treatment originated in Austria and Boston, USA in the mid 1920s.[78] Initially regarded as a severe disease of bone it gradually became clear that renal stones were the commonest complication of this condition, rather than osteitis. In recent years, automated clinical chemistry has led to an increased detection of patients with primary hyperparathyroidism, many of which are asymptomatic. Consequently, advanced skeletal disease has become rare, particularly within the facial-maxillary region.[79] However, as cases are now discovered earlier in their disease, clinical presentation becomes more subtle. Initial presentation with a brown tumour of the jaw although uncommon, presents a challenge in both detection and diagnosis.

Incidence

It is now recognized that primary hyperparathyroidism is quite common with incidence rates of between 25 and 28 cases per 100 000 population per year. This figure rises sharply beyond the age of 40 years and after the age of 60 reaches 200 cases per 100 000 population per year in women and 100 per 100 000 population per year in men.[80]

Most patients are diagnosed after the age of 30 years with a female to male ratio of 2:1. Many of these individuals however, have few or no symptoms with only a mild elevation of serum calcium. Facio-maxillary brown tumours are rare and affect the mandible more than the maxilla. Even in 1950 when Black & Ackermann reviewed 23 severe cases of parathyroid adenomata, maxillary involvement was uncommon.[81] Robinson & Woodhead reported one case in 1988 and could find only one other patient presenting with maxillary disease, and this was dated in 1984.[82] These two patients had advanced bony disease.

Today renal stones are said to occur in 30% of hyperparathyroid patients, abdominal and non-specific symptoms in about 65% and symptomatic bone disease in only 5%. In 3% of patients the cause is a parathyroid carcinoma![83] Secondary hyperparathyroidism in patients on long-standing haemodialysis may eventually result in an increase in brown tumours of the jaws although as yet this has not materialized.

Aetiology and clinical features

Increase in the production of parathyroid hormone produces 'demineralization' with pathological and radio-logical changes in the jaws which are similar to other giant cell lesions in this region. Hellquist suggests that brown tumours may in fact represent reparative scarring in an area already damaged by the effects of hyper-parathyroidism.[84]

Elsewhere in the body bone pain, pathological fractures and skeletal deformities assist in clinical diagnosis. Within the upper jaw painless swelling of the face with nasal ob-struction from bony distortion are more likely symptoms. There is no loosening of the teeth and diagnosis is by a combination of biopsy and laboratory investigations.

Radiology

Opacity of the maxillary antrum together with expansion and erosion of its bony walls may suggest a malignant neoplasm. However, these features are more typical of pressure erosion rather than neoplastic destruction and must be viewed as non-specific. The maxillary lesion has been described as osteolytic and expansive although this tumour is composed of solid connective tissue, multinu-cleated giant cells, haemorrhage and haemosiderin which partly enhances on CT scanning. Most patients with a maxillary brown tumour will already have established skeletal expansive lytic lesions and possibly nephro-calcinosis. At least 20% have spinal osteopenia and 36% cortical erosion in the radial aspect of the middle phalanges of the hands.[85]

Macroscopic and microscopic appearance

Increase in parathyroid hormone produces a fibrous and osteoclastic reaction throughout the skeleton but particularly in the jaws. This is associated with a giant cell reaction representing the focal lesion of hyperparathyroidism. In the jaws it is termed a brown tumour because of the characteristic macroscopical appearance of brown, yellow or haemorrhagic tissue. Osteoblastic activity is not however impaired, and evidence of bone regeneration may be seen on histological examination. Since these features are common to other giant cell conditions which affect the jaw, diagnosis is dependent upon biochemical studies even when there is radiological evidence of skeletal lytic lesions.

The classical laboratory findings are hypercalcinaemia. Elevation of serum calcium in the absence of malignancy, sarcoidosis, hypervitaminosis D and some other rare conditions, can be considered as primary hyperparathyroidism.

The pathogenesis of brown tumour is not clearly defined although it appears to be a complication of severe progressive hyperparathyroidism associated with large parathyroid adenomas with high parathyroid hormone levels.[86]

Natural history

Following the successful removal of the causative adenoma (or adenomata) brown tumours slowly resolve, eventually remineralizing according to Robinson & Woodhead in a 6 month follow-up of one patient with a maxillary tumour.[82] The time taken will be related to whether there is a single or multiple glandular enlargement, the degree of renal damage, preoperative parathyroid hormone levels and surgical success.

Differential diagnosis

Brown tumours are identical to reparative giant cell tumours of the jaws and may be manifestations of the same reparative process. Diagnosis is dependent on biochemical estimations confirming an underlying hyperparathyroidism which itself must be differentiated from hypercalcinaemia arising from malignancy, sarcoid or thiazide therapy. With malignancy there is usually advanced disease, severe hypercalcinaemia and a poor prognosis. Sarcoid granulomata are thought to be producers of vitamin D metabolite which is the underlying cause of the abnormal calcium metabolism. Pulmonary lesions are common and brown tumours of the jaws unreported!

Treatment

Once a diagnosis has been made, treatment relies on reducing the hyperparathyroidism by surgical extirpation of the adenoma or adenomata.

Robinson & Woodhead described a 40-year-old male patient presenting with a short history of a painless swelling of the right cheek with nasal obstruction.[82] This was associated with severe occipital headaches. Examination revealed a tumour of the right maxillary sinus which had displaced the lateral nasal wall producing obstruction. Biopsy confirmed this to be a giant cell tumour and the serum calcium was 3.79 mmol/l (normal 2.20 to 2.60 mmol/l) with a hypophosphataemia of 0.34 mmol/l (normal 0.7 to 1.5 mmol/l). The serum parathyroid level was 340 ng/l, confirming the associated hyperparathyroidism.

Radiologically, there was a partially enhancing mass expanding the maxillary sinus and obstructing the homolateral nasal passage. There was also an occipital lesion obstructing the 4th ventricle producing hydrocephalus. Skeletal survey revealed lytic lesions within the pelvis, abdomen and hands together with bilateral nephrocalcinosis.

Following the removal of a solitary large parathyroid adenoma and the introduction of a ventriculo-peritoneal shunt, this patient's headaches subsided with a gradual reduction in the size of the facial swelling.

PAGET'S DISEASE (OSTEITIS DEFORMANS)

Definition

A disease characterized by a disordered pattern of bone formation and resorption.

Incidence

Despite its recognition since 1877 when it was first described by Paget,[87] little attention has been paid to the effect of this disease on the jaws, since most symptoms are related to other sites such as skull, pelvis, vertebral column and femur. Otologists have considered Paget's disease of the temporal bone[88] but facial manifestations are described primarily in the dental literature. Fisher reported two patients with rhinological symptoms[89] and included five other patients previously published between 1923 and 1962 (Table 13.1).

Paget made no mention of maxillary involvement in his original paper but later reports of patients with 'leontiases ossea' probably included some cases of Paget's disease. Patients with polyostotic Paget's do have maxillary involvement although the real incidence is uncertain since examination of this region has not been considered an essential part of clinical evaluation, unless there are symptoms referable to this area.

Stafne & Austin examined the jaws radiologically in 138 patients with skeletal Paget's finding jaw involvement in 23 instances (17%).[90] Estimations of the incidence of Paget's disease vary with age, 1% in the 5th decade to 10% in the 10th, with one patient in every 100 individuals over the age of 45 years. 80% of these have some symptoms referable to this disorder on questioning but most do not seek help until bone pain, pathological fracture or neurological complications ensue.[89]

Subclinical Paget's is becoming more common because of an ageing population where skeletal X-rays used routinely for many common complaints detect unexpected bony changes. However, symptomatic disease

Table 13.1 Reported cases of Paget's disease affecting the upper jaw

Author	Age (yr)	Sex	Symptoms	Signs
Knaggs 1923[98]			Nasal obstruction	Bony masses
Harris 1948[99]	64	F	Nasal obstruction, facial deformity	Total obstruction from bony masses
Harrison 1949[93]	69	F	Nasal obstruction, facial deformity	Enlarged maxilla, displaced teeth
Fuller 1961[92]	64	F	Nasal obstruction	Enlarged turbinates, obliterated sinuses
Drury 1962[100]	53	M	Nasal obstruction, facial deformity	Enlarged right turbinate
Fisher 1990[90]	66	F	Facial deformity, nasal obstruction	Bilateral bony masses, obstructed nose, skull lesion
	58	F	Epistaxis, facial swelling	(Osteogenic sarcoma)
Harrison & Lund	80	M	Nasal obstruction	Bilateral fronto-ethmoidal mucocoele associated with bilateral proptosis, fistula in upper lid. Enlarged turbinates, deviated nasal septum

in the jaws remains rare and when present is always part of a more generalized condition.

A small male preponderance is suggested from the published data but no information is available regarding variations in ethnic susceptibility.

Site and aetiology

The paucity of published cases makes it difficult to verify anecdotal preponderance of the maxilla over the mandible when the jaws are involved in this disease. Slow progression, unless malignancy supervenes, ensures that it is the disabling symptom, such as ill-fitting dentures, nasal obstruction, progressive facial swelling or loosening of teeth, that ultimately leads to diagnosis of jaw involvement in established cases of Paget's disease.

The cause remains uncertain although the finding of virus-like structures within osteoclasts has prompted a suggestion that the disease may be of viral aetiology.[91]

Clinical features

The commonest presenting symptom of upper jaw involvement is facial deformity accompanied by a feeling of warmth, possibly secondary to increased blood flow through this well vascularized tumour. Deformity of the nose or nasal obstruction[89,92,93] is frequently accompanied by distortion of the alveolar ridge leading to retroclination of the incisor teeth and palatoversion of posterior teeth. Interference with the fitting of dentures is a common reason for seeking advice and palatal ulceration can result from pressure of submucosal bony masses on loosely fitting dentures.[94]

Rapid growth accompanied by pain and epistaxis in pre-existing Paget's disease must raise a suspicion of a malignant change, thought to occur in 10% of all patients.[95]

Radiology (Fig. 13.8)

Radiological changes vary according to stage reached by the disease ranging from radiolucency to sclerosis. Osteoporosis is the initial finding but gradually the blending of small radiolucent areas with areas of increased osteoblastic activity produces the typical 'cotton wool' appearance.

Skeletal survey and isotope scintigrams may provide evidence of other bony involvement, frequently in the femurs, pelvis and spine. High resolution CT scans may demonstrate involvement of the labyrinthine capsule or

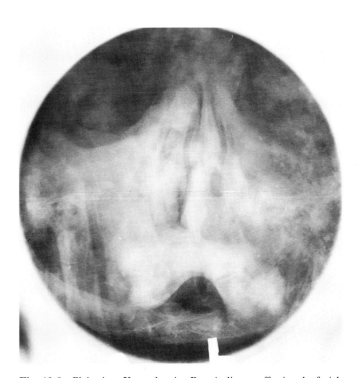

Fig. 13.8 Plain sinus X-ray showing Paget's disease affecting the facial skeleton.

cochlea offering an explanation for any associated hearing or vestibular disorders.

Profuse bleeding from a biopsy of the alveolus or after dental extraction may suggest malignancy but is secondary to the intense arteriovenous shunt which exists within the bones affected by Paget's disease. The sclerotic phase of the disease can reduce resistance to infection and can result in local areas of osteomyelitis following dentral extraction.[95]

Macroscopic and microscopic appearance

The main pathological change is one of active bone formation proceeding alongside active bone destruction. During the initial stage or osteoporotic phase, large amounts of new bone are seen in a loose vascular connective tissue stroma. In the fully developed disease there is simultaneous osteoblastic and osteoclastic activity and it is this that gives the bone its characteristic mosaic pattern. This is the result of the formation of curved cement lines and depressions on the surface of the bone. As the disease becomes less active the marrow becomes fibrotic and less vascular with both osteoblasts and osteoclasts reduced in number.[95]

Differential diagnosis

Early lesions may simulate the brown tumour of hyperparathyroidism, osteosarcoma, myeloma or metastatic deposits. Sclerotic lesions must be distinguished from a wide variety of fibro-osseous conditions and except where the disease is clinically obvious Paget's disease, intraoral or intranasal biopsy is essential.

Treatment

Apart from confirmatory biopsy it is doubtful if surgical reduction is justified unless it is certain that the disease has entered a non-active sclerotic phase. Medical therapy with calcitonin, which, because of its potent antiosteolytic action, has proved to be of value in both Paget's disease and hypercalcinaemia associated with hyperparathyroidism.[96] Buckler et al[97] suggest that the new biphosphate compounds can reduce deformity and 3-aminohydroxy-prophlidene-1,1-biphosphate (APD) was given intravenously in one of the patients reported by Fisher with apparently good short-term results.[89]

Prognosis

Paget's disease involving the upper jaw is invariably part of more extensive disease and consequently the risk of high output cardiac failure from multiple arteriovenous shunts within the diseased bones is high. A risk of secondary osteogenic sarcoma is present in every patient

and progressive facial deformity, orthodontic disruption, nasal obstruction, proptosis and facial neuralgia is inevitable with the passage of time. As yet there is no reliable means of determining the rate of growth nor the expectation of reaching the quiescent stage. Hopefully, this may be expedited by medical means, possibly with the new biphosphate compounds.

OSTEOMA

Definition

A slowly growing, benign bony tumour producing symptoms by deformation.

Historical aspects

There is anecdotal evidence of osteomata occurring within the paranasal sinuses of skulls of ancient Egyptian origin, although the terms osteoma and exostoses have been used interchangeably in the past making surveys open to question.

Incidence and site

Difficulties are encountered when quoting incidence figures since the majority of these slow-growing lesions have no symptoms, being found by chance at radiology. Eickel & Palm after examining 16 000 sinus X-rays found osteomata in 0.4% with 5.1% of these within the maxillary antrum.[101] Childrey reported 15 osteomas amongst 3510 asymptomatic patients (0.42%) based again on sinus X-rays,[102] whilst incidences of 0.1 to 1% have been reported within the Finnish literature.[103] Teed collected 458 cases of sinus osteomata with a maxillary incidence of 8.97%[104] and Boenninghaus examining 234 paranasal sinus osteomata found 11 within the maxillary antrum (4.7%).[105]

Isolated cases of osteomata confined to the maxilla have been reported over many years, each of varying size and symptomatology. Teed[104] said that the first patient recorded in the literature was by Veiga in 1586 but difficulties in clinical interpretation makes this impossible to confirm. There is however, clear evidence that within the paranasal sinuses the frontal is the commonest site, the ethmoid next although the true site of origin is frequently impossible to confirm and many osteomata should more accurately be termed 'fronto-ethmoid'. This is supported by Wilkes et al who reported 16 frontal sinus osteomata, placing 12 in the fronto-ethmoid region.[106]

The exact site of attachment, except in small tumours or those with a clearly defined pedicle, is often impossible to determine with accuracy even utilizing modern radiological technology. Consequently, some of the data presented in publications 1939–1960 by Samy &

Mostafa[107] must be viewed with caution. Their 21 osteo-mata contained six originating within the maxillary antrum (28.5%). A slightly larger series from the Royal National Throat, Nose and Ear Hospital, London had only two definite lesions at this site giving an incidence of only 8.7%.[108]

When considering the upper jaw the maxillary antrum and adjoining ethmoid sinuses can be considered together although both symptoms and management differ between these two sites.

Age, sex and ethnic variation

Available data relate primarily to symptomatic osteomata and although radiological evidence indicates a wide range of age at which these lesions may be found, two being under the age of 10 years,[109] most patients of European origin are diagnosed between the 4th and 6th decades of life.[103] This is also supported by the series of Fu & Perzin of 28 osteomatas but again the site and rate of growth materially influences the age of diagnosis and the absolute age range must be considered as wide.[23]

Most of the published reports quote a male to female ratio of about 2:1 but this must again be viewed in the light of a relatively small number of recorded cases. Apart from the radionuclide bone scan studies of Noyek et al on the growth of sinus osteomata,[110] the growth rate is usually estimated by regular radiological assessment. There are no reports of this being performed on untreated patients in a large trial but the clinical impression exists that amongst the Arab population, age at diagnosis is earlier and growth rate greater than in other races.[107] Handousa in 1940 recorded that osteomata was the commonest benign tumour found within the paranasal sinuses in Egypt, 35 cases in a total of 73 tumours, but it is possible that this reflected his unique position within the country as an authority on tumours rather than any variation in ethnic suscepti-bility.[111]

Aetiology

There is no adequate explanation which covers the development of osteomata in each of the paranasal sinuses. Embryologically, most of the skull base is formed in cartilage whilst the vault ossifies in membrane. Consequently, there is a junctional area in the region of the ethmoid, a common site for osteoma growth. However, many of these tumours arise elsewhere and although embryological origins may offer some explana-tion for differing histological makeup it cannot be the sole aetiological factor.

The face is a common site for trauma and 30% of the cases recorded by Samy & Mostafa had some history of skull or facial injury.[107] Similar arguments will apply to a previous history of sinus infection for both trauma and infection are common and do not usually result in the formation of osteomata.

It is possible that the aetiology is variable and that osteomata should more properly be considered as an osseous hamartoma which, although arising in childhood, grow extremely slowly.

Some consideration must be given to Gardner's syndrome, inherited as an autosomal dominant gene with complete penetration but variable expression.[112] The syndrome is rare with an estimated incidence of one per million population. Endodermal lesions include intestinal polyps; multiple mesodermal osteomata of the skull base and facial region, unerupted teeth and odontoses. The most common ectodermal lesions are epidermoid cysts, fibroma, lipomata, neurofibromata and pigmented skin lesions (Fig. 13.9).

Diagnosis may be difficult because of the considerable variations in clinical presentation but the skin and bony lesions usually predate the intestinal polyposis by about 10 years. The osteomata can appear within the 1st decade of life, most frequently affecting the ramus of the mandible followed by the calvarium and paranasal sinuses. There is some question as to whether growth of the osteomata cease at puberty and this must be considered as a progressive disease.[112]

Clinical features (Figs 13.10 and 13.11)

Most upper jaw osteomata produce few symptoms until large enough to cause facial asymmetry or displacement of the globe. Encroachment on surrounding structures eventually results in bony displacement and resorption with possibly pain from pressure on related nerves such as the infraorbital. Caution is however necessary in offering surgery for small osteomata in expectation of relieving headaches. Obstruction of the maxillary sinus may result in infection but this is uncommon although osteomata are sometimes implicated in the aetiology of fronto-ethmoid mucocoeles when found to be blocking the frontonasal recess. In a series of 80 patients with mucocoeles, osteomata were present in 4%.[114]

Extension into the anterior cranial fossa has been reported to cause leakage of cerebrospinal fluid or pneu-matocoele, and meningitis with brain abscess remains a potential hazard.[115]

Radiology (Figs 13.12–13.14)

Unlike many other bony tumours, osteomata have a characteristic appearance showing a well demarcated rounded area of uniform radio-opacity. This appearance gives little indication of the histological constituents since the outer shell of compact bone effectively shields any inner cellularity. Radiological assessment of the whole

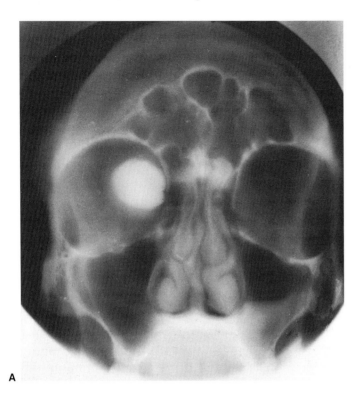

A

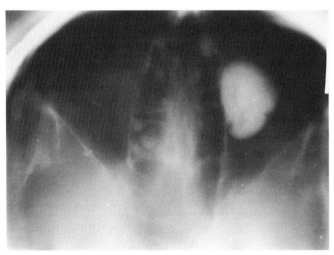

B

Fig. 13.9 **A,** coronal and **B,** axial hypocycloidal tomograms showing multiple osteomata in a case of Gardner's syndrome (Lloyd 1988[113]).

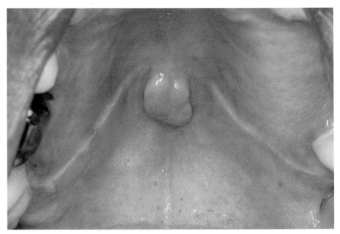

Fig. 13.10 Palatal exostosis.

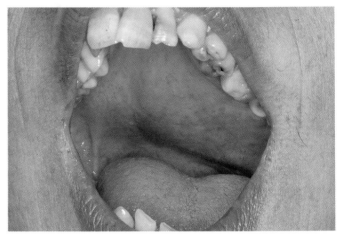

Fig. 13.11 Extensive palatal distortion by an osteoma of the upper jaw.

lesion is vital in planning any surgical removal particularly if it proves possible to demonstrate the site of origin. Polytomography in both the coronal and axial plane has proved valuable but has now been replaced by CT scanning, again in both planes.

Macroscopic and microscopic appearance

Macroscopically, most osteomata are smooth, lobulated hard masses of bone occasionally showing a pedicle marking the point of origin (Fig. 13.15). Acid decalcifica-

tion, which can take many months, allows histological evaluation and most show some fibrous tissue even when described as 'ivory'. These are primarily dense masses of lamellar bone with few marrow spaces, minimal osteoblasts, sparse connective tissue and no evidence of Haversian systems. 'Mature or spongy' osteomata show some lamellated trabeculae, rimmed by active osteoblasts.[23] It has been suggested that the histological nature of an osteoma was in part related to the origin of its forming bone. The maxilla, being developed from both cartilage and membrane would therefore produce 'mature' lesions whilst the frontal sinus, membranous in origin would grow 'ivory' osteomata. Gradual reduction in blood supply of the dense ivory osteoma does occasionally lead to necrosis of a narrow pedicle and the lesion lies free from its origin. Handousa[111] claimed an ability to detect the site of origin by studying these 'free' osteomas after removing them from the nasal cavity. However by this time, although possibly no longer attached to bone, size and surrounding structures ensure that formal excision is required to remove even small tumours safely.

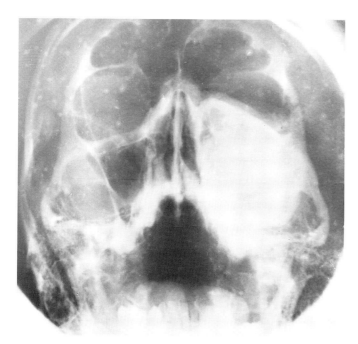

Fig. 13.12 Plain sinus X-ray (occipito-mental view) showing large osteoma arising in maxillary sinus.

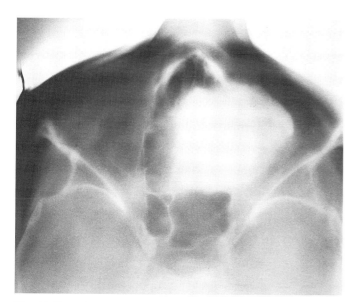

Fig. 13.13 Axial hypocycloidal tomogram showing a large ethmoidal osteoma encroaching on the orbit.

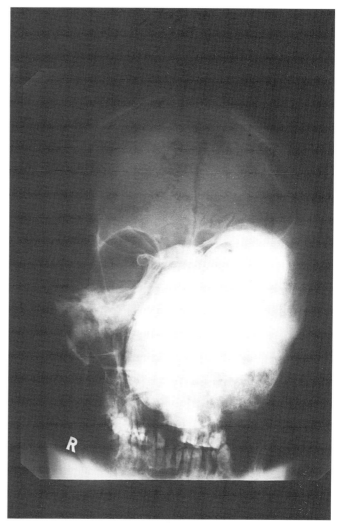

Fig. 13.14 Plain skull X-ray showing enormous osteoma of upper jaw.

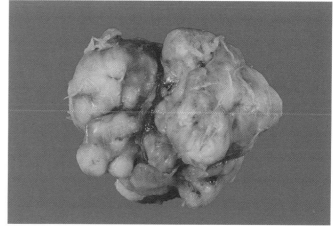

Fig. 13.15 Surgical specimen of osteoma from case shown in Figure 13.13

Natural history

The majority of upper jaw osteomata are asymptomatic and change little in their biological nature over the passing years. Although there has been no formal study of the rate of growth following incomplete removal using radiological assessment, there is clinical evidence that particularly in younger Arabs regrowth may occur relatively quickly. Cases can now be imaged with ^{99m}Tc–methylene disphosphate (^{99m}Tc–MDP) bone scanning in which the radio-actively-tagged phosphate anion is studied semi-quantitatively and then related to clinical or radiological changes.

Noyek et al have reported the use of this technique over a period of 11 years in 13 patients with sinus osteomas.[110] The bone scan in the delayed phase demonstrated the osteoblastic activity of the osteomas, reflecting bone phosphate metabolism as an indicator of growth potential. A 'cold' scan indicated a relatively inert lesion whilst they used a 'hot' scan as indications for surgical removal. This technique was validated by a 4 to 11 year period of non-operative follow-up in the biologically inert osteomata when radiology confirmed cessation of growth.

Differential diagnosis

'Hot' bone scans can occur in many other bony lesions such as metastases, osteoid osteoma, calcifying meningioma, fibrous dysplasia and Paget's disease. A highly sclerosing ossifying fibroma can present considerable problems in radiological differentiation but in all these conditions biopsy is possible with the exception of osteomata where formal removal provides the final diagnosis.

Treatment

Whilst agreeing that only in the presence of symptoms and signs should surgical removal be contemplated, the absence of reliable criteria relating to potential growth rate, together with the technical difficulties of removing large tumours, make identification of general criteria for surgery difficult.

Symptoms of facial pain or headache are subjective, restricting quantitative evaluation of surgical success. Orbital symptoms such as proptosis from ethmoidal osteomas can be relieved although if long-standing their removal may result in diplopia. Indeed, additional iatrogenic disabilities may result from attempts at surgical extirpation in the very large lesions found within the upper jaw.

A 48-year-old male was first seen in 1967 with a history of gradually increasing left-sided facial swelling since the age of 8 years. At the age of 22 years the left external carotid artery had been ligated in India in an attempt at restricting growth but the swelling had continued to increase in size although extremely slowly. There was no nasal obstruction, pain or ocular symptoms and his main complaint was the facial appearance. Skull X-ray's showed hyperostosis in the frontal bone and a bony mass in the left maxillary antrum expanding, and in places eroding its walls. A diagnosis of osteoma was made and partial maxillectomy performed using osteotome, cutting burr and electric saw (Fig. 13.16). Most of the maxilla was removed but the orbital floor remained in situ as did the tuberosity in order to facilitate the fitting of an obturator. The mass was extremely hard and bleeding minimal, the histology confirming the diagnosis of osteoma.

Postoperatively, he developed a right-sided suppurative parotitis and later a small discharging sinus below the left lower eyelid. This was explored later in 1967 with removal of granulations and the underlying abscess cavity curetted. The fistula healed but scar tissue produced a troublesome ectropion

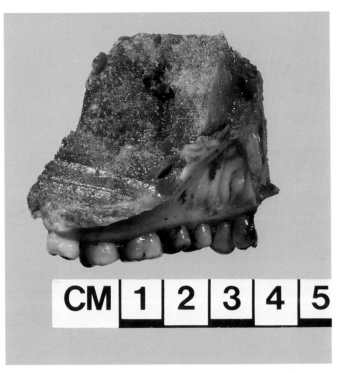

Fig. 13.16 Surgical specimen of osteoma from case shown in Figure 13.12

which despite many attempts at surgical repair has caused distress. In 1971, the remaining orbital floor was removed in the hope of improving his eyelid problems, the bone being soft and cancellous extending posteriorly to the sphenoid but showed no evidence of osteoma. He continues to the present time, 1990 to have problems with this eye although there has been no reformation of the osteomata!

It is quite possible that when seen in 1967 this osteoma had already ceased to grow and could have been left untouched. However, the facial swelling was causing concern and although surgery has resulted in an iatrogenic problem over a period of 21 years the patient remains satisfied.

Apart from small localized osteomata growing from the floor or medial wall of the orbit which can be removed via an external ethmoidectomy incision, most that are large enough to cause symptoms need a more formal procedure if they are to be removed completely and safely. Ethmoidal lesions are invariably lobulated occupying most of the complex and extending into both nasal cavity and orbit. Although distorting and compressing surrounding structures, there is always a fibrous plane and once access is obtained dissection down to the site of origin is feasible. Fragmentation with an osteotome is dangerous, being uncontrolled. However even large lobulated masses can be removed from this region utilizing a lateral rhinotomy approach and a cutting burr.

Greater difficulty is experienced with osteomata reaching or attached to the region of the cribriform plate and here craniofacial resection is the technique of choice.

A 37-year-old male was seen in November 1983 complaining of nasal obstruction, headache and left-sided proptosis for several months. His left frontal sinus had been explored a month previously for 'chronic infection' without relief of symptoms and radiology showed a large ethmoidal osteoma extending into the orbit, nasal cavity and anterior fossa. The mass was removed by a craniofacial approach confirming that the cribriform plate was distorted rather than destroyed. The osteoma together with the whole ethmoidal labyrinth were removed together with complete relief of symptoms and no evidence of recurrence during an 8-year follow-up.

Prognosis

Local recurrence is uncommon even when the base of the osteoma is left in situ because of limited access or broad attachment. However, in young Arabs or where there is suspicion of considerable residual disease, regular radiological assessment together with radionuclide scanning is advisable.

OSTEOBLASTOMA AND OSTEOID OSTEOMA

Definition

Two closely related conditions with similar histological features probably representing different anatomico-clinical expressions of the same osteoblastic process.[116]

Synonyms

Corticoid osteoid, osteoid fibroma, osteoid osteitis, osteogenic fibroma, benign osteoblastoma, giant osteoid osteoma, osteoblastic osteoid tissue forming tumour.

Historical aspects

Osteoid osteoma was first described as a definitive histological entity by Jaffe in 1935[117] but it was not until 1956 that he and Lichtenstein independently suggested that 'benign osteoblastoma' should be used for the larger and clinically different variant of osteoid osteoma.[118,119] Prior to this, such lesions had been called osteogenic fibromas or giant osteoid osteomas.[120] Although clinical differentiation between these two conditions is frequently possible using differences in size and symptoms, variations in histology may cause considerable problems in reaching a diagnosis.

Incidence

Because of confusion in terminology and the preponderance of patients presenting with the more common benign osteoblastoma, most of the more reliable data relates to this condition. Any area of the skeleton may be involved with the greatest incidence being in the vertebral column (34%), appendicular skeleton (30%), small bones of hands and feet (13%) and the skull (15–20%).[121]

By 1980 over 400 cases had been recorded with only 53 being within the skull, two of these involved the paranasal sinuses both affecting the ethmoid labyrinth.[122] By 1983 Osguthorpe & Hungerford,[123] in reporting a case with upper jaw involvement, quoted a small number of other papers with solitary cases of maxillary osteoblastomas giving credit to Freeman for the first publication of this tumour within the upper jaw in 1975.[124] Som et al published the details of an ethmoidal osteoblastoma in 1979 claiming this to be the fourth recorded case.[125] Katsantonis et al emphasized the problems of histological diagnosis in their publication of 1981 'osteoid producing orbital ethmoid tumour'.[126] Occurring in a 4-year-old boy it avoided a definitive diagnostic label although the clinicopathological features were that of an osteoid osteoma-osteoblastoma. Despite these technical 'niceties', benign osteoblastoma although uncommon is a well-recognized clinical entity.

Age and sex variation

In those tumours designated osteoid osteoma, over 75% occurred during the 1st two' decades of life, 80% of patients being below the age of 30 years with a 2:1 male to female ratio.[123] The age range is large with one case, in the tibia, being an infant of 8 months,[127] and one patient 78-years-old.[119]

If the more common and popular term of benign osteoblastoma is analysed then the age incidence is spread wider over the first three decades of life but with most patients diagnosed when under the age of 20 years.[121]

Clinical features

It is the clinical presentation which allows differentiation between osteoid osteoma and benign osteoblastoma. Lesions less than 2 cm in diameter, with no soft tissue mass but causing nocturnal pain promptly relieved by salicylates, are now classified as osteoid osteomata. Schulman & Dorfman[128] found nerve fibres within these tumours which they consider as possibly accounting for the classical nocturnal pain, although these findings have not been found in jaw tumours.

The larger benign osteoblastomata cause symptoms by compression or obstruction. Pain may occur secondary to sinus obstruction and is described as being dull, aching and insidious in nature. There is often a soft tissue swelling with erythema of the overlying skin. When growing within the ethmoid sinuses, nasal obstruction, epiphora and proptosis are common as they are with most other upper jaw tumours. However, although the duration of symptoms may be several years, in some patients the growth rate is rapid with symptoms being present for only a few months. The average delay prior to diagnosis for all sites has been quoted as 17 months but in the head and neck symptoms are usually dramatic and diagnosis, consequently, early.[120]

Radiology (Figs. 13.17 and 13.18)

Radiological examination is essential to delineate the extent of this tumour whilst not necessarily providing an accurate diagnosis. Dahlin & Johnson [120] felt that there were no distinctive radiological features because of the lack of uniformity but others believe that all lesions less than 1.5 cm in diameter are osteoid osteomas, the larger lesions being osteoblastomata.[116,124,129] Pochaczevesky et al say that radiological differentiation is possible, defining benign osteoblastoma as characterized by 'osteolytic expanding lesions with evidence of bone formation or a varying degree of calcification'.[130]

There is general agreement that a soft tissue mass is usually evident in benign osteoblastoma and the tumour is well delimited from normal bone, producing a radiolucency surrounded by a thin shell of new bone. They do not show the new cortical bone formation common to osteoid osteoma and the latter are smaller with a thin central nidus.[121] Neither CT nor MRI is likely to assist in diagnosis except to provide a more precise delineation of the extent of the tumour. Technetium scanning however, may be valuable in confirming increased vascularity and growth potential, useful when planning treatment.[131]

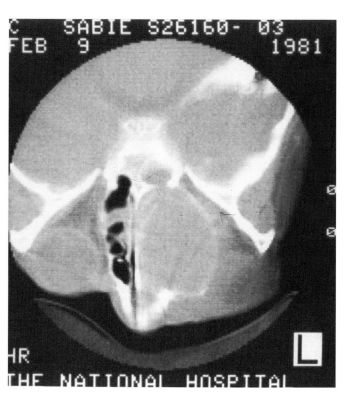

Fig. 13.18 Axial CT scan of extensive benign osteoblastoma of ethmoid region.

Irrespective of size or site both lesions appear to be encapsulated on both radiological and clinical assessment.

Macroscopic and microscopic appearance

The intact specimen shows the tumour to be well circumscribed with a thin shell of cortical bone. The contents are homogeneously granular or gritty as a result of the calcified osteoid and the colour is described as grey or reddish–brown due to the rich vascular component.

Microscopically, there is an abundant fibrous stroma with irregular osteoid deposition and focal calcification. The stroma is often vascular, hence the bleeding after curettage, and the ossified trabeculae are lined with osteoblasts and osteoclasts. The osteoid trabeculae of benign osteoblastoma are said to be broader and the vascular spaces and giant cells, more frequent than in the smaller osteoid osteoma. Mitosis is rare and nuclear atypism absent.[132]

Natural history

Osteoblastoma and its variant is accepted as a benign tumour with malignant transformation only recorded following treatment with irradiation.[133] Even after incomplete removal there is little tendency to recur within the

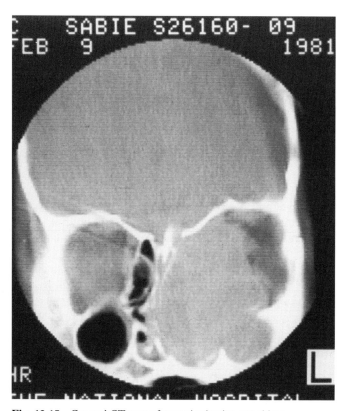

Fig. 13.17 Coronal CT scan of extensive benign osteoblastoma.

postcranial skeleton although this is less certain within the upper jaw. Only a small number of patients have been described with osteoblastomata at this site, some have done well with limited removal whilst others have rapidly recurred and the tumour should be viewed seriously.[134]

Differential diagnosis

It is the larger benign osteoblastoma that must be differentiated from aneurysmal bone cyst, ossifying fibroma, monocystic fibrous dysplasia, giant cell tumour and osteogenic sarcoma. This is not always possible on histological grounds without information provided by the surgeon regarding the appearance of the tumour.

Treatment

Within the upper jaw, radical removal is advised whilst avoiding if possible destruction of normal structures. Curettage or biopsy produces considerable bleeding, Tan et al recording a loss of 1350 ml of blood following the biopsy of a benign maxillary osteoblastoma.[122] Conservation surgery is possible within the maxilla but in the ethmoid a more radical approach is often required.

A 9-year-old girl from Iraq was seen in February 1982 with a 6 month history of increasing left-sided proptosis, periorbital swelling and epiphora. CT confirmed the presence of a soft tissue mass within the ethmoid extending into the orbit and anterior cranial fossa. Intranasal biopsy produced severe bleeding and a provisional diagnosis of an osteoid-producing tumour. The vision in the eye was normal as were the movements but the scans indicated disease close to the optic foramen. A lateral rhinotomy with orbital clearance and removal of ethmoids was combined with a partial maxillectomy. Tumour was present on the roof, medial and lateral walls of the maxillary antrum, orbital periosteum and cribriform plate.

Histological examination showed fibrous tissue, osteoblasts, osteoid and giant cells confirming a diagnosis of benign osteoblastoma. 2 months after this operation a craniofacial resection was performed to remove the disease left around the cribriform plate area and also in the posterior ethmoid. The child was free from disease 1 year later.

A similar case has been reported by Katsantonis et al in 1981 occurring in a 4-year-old boy. This patient had also been treated by lateral rhinotomy and orbital clearance but postoperatively, 4500 cGy in 29 treatments had been given to the orbit because of residual disease around the optic foramen. The patient remained well for the 3-year follow-up.[126]

Another child aged 12 years was treated by primary craniofacial resection but a 22-year-old woman with a well-encapsulated osteoblastoma has been controlled by a lateral rhinotomy excision of the tumour despite having proptosis.

Recurrence has been recorded as developing 9 years after initial removal and long-term follow-up with radiological assessment is advisable in all patients.[132]

Postoperative irradiation (3500 to 6000 cGy) has been used where radical excision is impossible as in the vertebral column. Marsh et al, after reviewing 197 patients of benign osteoblastoma concluded that 'postoperative irradiation does not alter the natural course of this disease and is contraindicated unless there is evidence of continued growth'.[132] Two cases of sarcomatous change following irradiation of an initially benign osteoblastoma have been reported by McLeod et al[129] and Mayer.[135] Even the possibility of a 10% recurrence rate at the less accessible sites does not justify the risk of an irradiation-induced sarcoma[121] and radiotherapy is not recommended routinely.

A suggestion that preoperative embolization would materially affect operative blood loss thus aiding resection is not supported because of the difficulty of identifying the blood supply in these large bony tumours. As with most other upper jaw neoplasms, adequate access is the answer to safe surgery.[122]

OSTEOGENIC SARCOMA

Definition

The commonest and most malignant bony tumour found within the upper jaw.

Synonyms

Osteochondromyxosarcoma, osteochondrosarcoma, osteoid sarcoma and osteosarcoma.

Historical aspects

It has long been recognized that a highly malignant tumour of mesenchymal origin, characterized by the production of osteoid, could develop either primarily or secondarily, within the facial bones. Not until 1938 however, when Ewing separated chondrosarcoma[136] and in 1943 when Budd & McDonald removed fibrosarcoma[137] was osteogenic sarcoma differentiated as a distinct entity. Even then it was appreciated that this tumour could demonstrate a wide variety of histological features, with a predominance of osteoid, chondroid or fibromatous elements occurring in individual tumours.[138]

Incidence

An approximate incidence of one new case per 100 000 population per year is quoted for both plasmacytoma and osteogenic sarcomata within the USA but only 0.07 cases per 100 000 population per year for osteogenic sarcomata arising within the head and neck.[138] This figure varies with different populations, possibly reflecting accuracy of reporting and centralization of data.

Between 0.5 and 6.5% of all osteogenic sarcoma are found within the jaws[139–141] with the mandible more frequently affected than the upper jaw.[142] The largest series of 56 patients collected by Garrington et al in 1967 came from the Armed Forces Institute of Pathology, USA and contained only 17 within the maxilla.[143] Caron et al in their series of 43 jaw osteogenic sarcoma had 15 maxillary lesions[139] and subsequent papers have reported groups of no more than 20 upper jaw tumours.[142,144,145]

Age, sex and ethnic variation (Table 13.2)

In contrast to osteogenic sarcoma occurring elsewhere in the body which develops during the 2nd decade of life, facial lesions are found later with a mean age of 38 years for primary tumours. Secondary osteogenic sarcomata occur later with a mean age of 48 years.[144] Both groups show a range of ages from a low of 6 to a high of 82 years[139] although Singh et al analysing 937 osteogenic sarcomata seen at the Mayo Clinic found only six children under the age of 6 years, all with long bone involvement.[138] Wilimas et al reported two black boys aged 4 months and 3 years with long bone osteogenic sarcoma[146] whilst Singh et al reported an unusual case of a 5-year-old girl with this tumour arising de novo in the nasal bone.[138]

From the small number of patients available in the literature there appears to be no sex variation and non-white patients appear in both the American reports and from our own institution.[145] Only 14 patients were found in 189 cases of osteogenic sarcoma at the Tata Memorial Hospital, Bombay, India (7.4%),[141] and despite the relative frequency of upper jaw neoplasia in Nigeria, Daramola et al recorded only seven osteogenic sarcomata in a period of 14 years, four within the maxilla.[147]

Aetiology

No clearly established cause has been identified for primary osteogenic sarcoma but secondary tumours may develop from pre-existing lesions such as fibrous dysplasia[148] or Paget's disease.[145] Immenkamp identified 52 cases of fibrous dysplasia which underwent malignant change, 30 developed an osteogenic sarcoma in the upper jaw most following irradiation.[148] The average latent period between the diagnosis of the fibrous dysplasia and subsequent malignancy was 13.5 years, most of the patients being then about 35-years-old.[149]

Irradiation-induced osteogenic sarcomata may be from deliberately treating a benign disease, accidental irradiation or following administration of a radionuclide which is then deposited in bone. The latent period can be as short as 3 years or longer than 30 years and a dose of 300 cGy may be sufficient.[149]

Table 13.2 Osteogenic sarcoma of upper jaw (Harrison & Lund)

Sex	Age at diagnosis	Year	Primary condition	Previous radiotherapy	Treatment	Follow-up
F	60	1962	Maxilla	220 kV 5060 cGy (1957)	220 kV & telecaesium 5000 R – radical maxillectomy & orbital clearance. Recurrence 1963 – I.A. chemotherapy	Died 1963 – 1.5 yr
F	69	1966	Pre-maxilla involving antrum		Partial maxillectomy	Died 11/12, local disease
M	30	1970	Maxilla – nasal passage – middle fossa	Co^{60} 5200 cGy (Hyperbaric O_2)	Radical maxillectomy & orbital clearance – cyclophosphamide	Died 3/12 local disease
F	30	1971	Lateral wall nose & antrum	Co^{60} 6100 cGy & lateral rhinotomy		Alive 16 yr
F	58	1972	Paget's disease – maxilla & orbit		Cyclophosphamide I.A.	Died 3/12
M	62	1974	Maxilla		Radical maxillectomy & orbital clearance & adriamycin	Died 1988 (14 yr), trauma
F	45	1976	Maxilla – orbit, middle cranial fossa		Radical maxillectomy & orbital clearance & adriamycin	Alive – 10 yr
F	43	1985	Maxilla – orbit	5250 cGy 4 Mev & vincristine and methotrexate (1984)	Radical maxillectomy & orbital clearance. Recurrence 3/12– cryosurgery	Died 7/12 local disease
M	40	1985	Maxilla	7000 cGy & cis-platinum (1984)	Radical maxillectomy & orbital clearance	Alive with disease 2 yr

I.A., intra-arterial

The prognosis for osteogenic sarcoma arising in Paget's disease or following irradiation is particularly poor with few patients living longer than one year.[144,145]

The atmospheric testing of nuclear devices has been viewed as a potential source of bone-seeking isotopes, e.g. strontium (^{90}Sr), plutonium (^{239}Pu) which could increase the risk of osteogenic sarcomata. To date epidemiological studies have not confirmed this possibility although long-term confirmation is not available.[150]

Of great interest is the relationship of osteogenic sarcoma to retinoblastoma. Most of the latter occur as unilateral lesions but patients with bilateral tumours are possibly genetically predisposed to malignancy and are likely to form other tumours.[151] Most of these occur within the irradiated field and 80% are osteogenic sarcomas. Not all can be attributed to the irradiation however, and it is thought that the retinoblastoma gene predisposes the patient to the formation of a bone malignancy.[138] Abrahamson et al evaluated 2302 patients with retinoblastoma finding secondary neoplasms in 97.5% of patients with bilateral lesions.[152]

Clinical features (Figs. 13.19 and 13.20)

Symptoms and signs will vary with the location, size and rate of growth of individual tumours. The duration of symptoms has been recorded as being as short as 1 month or as long as a year. Most are no more than a few months, the exception being where there is pre-existing pathology such as Paget's disease when growth may be extremely rapid. With secondary neoplasia occurring in fibrous dysplasia diagnosis of malignant change is frequently delayed because of clinical and histological confusion between the benign and co-existing malignant disease. The commonest presentation within the upper jaw is facial swelling, initially painless but becoming painful as bone invasion involves the superior alveolar nerves. Loosening of teeth or the formation of a malignant

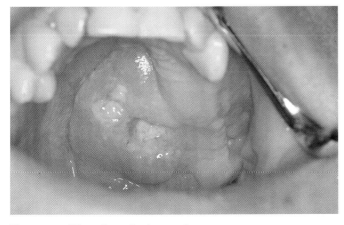

Fig. 13.19   Ulcerating palatal mass of osteosarcoma.

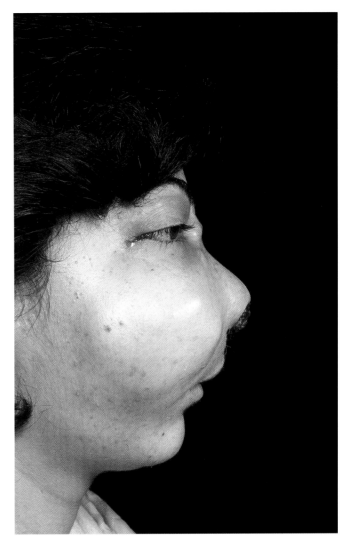

Fig. 13.20   Large maxillary osteosarcoma extending into the cheek.

oro-antral fistula following dental extraction, is common. Proptosis, nasal obstruction and epistaxis is also common as tumour extends into the orbit and nasal cavity.[143–145,153]

Systemic or regional metastases occur late with jaw osteogenic sarcoma and in these cases the serum alkaline phosphatase is elevated in about half of the patients, being related to the degree of bone destruction rather than tumour size.

Radiology

There are no typical radiological appearances that can be considered as diagnostic for osteogenic sarcoma. The features depend largely on the degree of ossification and mineralization within the tumour, ranging from totally lytic to sclerotic with many tumours being a mixture of the two. Penetration of the bony cortex produces a florid periosteal reaction which is characteristically interrupted and multilayered exhibiting either a 'sunburst' or a 'laminated' appearance.

The predominantly fibrosarcomatous tumour will appear lytic whilst osteosclerotic lesions show dense areas of bone with indistinct borders. In the mixed neoplasms, showing both osteolytic and osteosclerotic components there may be a 'ground glass' appearance. Although the 'sunray' effect produced by spicule formation was once considered pathognomonic for osteogenic sarcoma it is seen in other bony tumours such as metastatic carcinoma.

As with other upper jaw tumours CT scanning delineates the neoplasm but it adds little to diagnosis.

Juxtacortical osteogenic sarcoma can be diagnosed with a degree of certainty in the long bones, important since the growth rate of this variant is slow and the prognosis good, only 12 cases involving the jaws have been reported. These were detailed by Millar et al[141] who emphasized that, unlike the long bones, radiological appearances are not characteristic although the prognosis is much better than for other upper jaw bone malignancies.

Macroscopic and microscopic appearance

The macroscopical appearance depends on the degree of osteoblastic, fibroblastic or chondroblastic proliferation within the tumour. Consequently, they are described as being firm, gritty, granular, fleshy or fibrous.[142]

Histologically, there are no important differences between osteogenic sarcoma arising within the upper jaw and the long bones. Osteoblastic, chondroblastic, fibroblastic, cellular and telangiectatic types are all found but tumour osteoid is essential for histological diagnosis. This allows differentiation of the chondroblastic variant from chondrosarcoma, both found in the upper jaw.

Batsakis et al[142] found more vascular and cellular lesions in their series of upper jaw osteogenic sarcomas whilst Huvos et al said that the osteoblastic variant was more common, as it is in associated Paget's disease.[144]

The diagnosis of juxtacortical (periosteal) osteogenic sarcoma is based on both radiological and histological appearances when present in the long bones. It is less clear in the upper jaw but they are well-differentiated neoplasms composed of sheets of osteoid within a spindle-cell stroma. Evidence of malignancy may be difficult to find leading to delay in diagnosis.[147] Nuclear pleomorphism, nucleolar enlargement and mitoses are all present in osteogenic sarcomata together with malignant osteoblasts. Their absence in juxtacortical osteogenic sarcomas may lead to an erroneous diagnosis of osteoma or osteochondroma.[154]

Natural history

Local recurrence is common although systemic metastases are later than in the postcranial lesions. Caron et al reported a local failure rate of 80%, primarily from an inability to resect the primary tumour adequately. This local recurrence invariably occurred within a year of surgery with systemic metastases, in lung or brain, in the 2nd year following treatment.[139]

In the upper jaw 5-year survival figures are about 33%[139] dropping to around zero when the tumour supervenes on existing Paget's disease (Table 13.3).[155] It is unclear as to whether the histological variants materially affect prognosis when staging is taken into account. Anecdotal evidence suggests that chondroblastic osteogenic sarcomata are less aggressive and juxtacortical tumours certainly behave more benignly, Millar et al having no failures in their six patients with maxillary neoplasms.[141]

Differential diagnosis

All the benign and malignant tumours that arise from bone within the upper jaw will enter into the possible diagnosis, and biopsy is essential for confirmation. Ossifying fibroma, osteoblastoma and particularly chondrosarcoma must be excluded, each presenting difficulties in interpretation.

However, frankly sarcomatous stroma with malignant osteoblasts forming osteoid is an essential ingredient for a diagnosis of osteogenic sarcoma.[31]

Treatment (Table 13.2)

Low survival figures for those patients with osteogenic sarcomata of the upper jaw has led to a critical evaluation of treatment philosophies.[155] Radical excision, where technically feasible, is an essential component of all programmes. The use of adjuvant chemotherapy either pre- or post-surgery for long bone sarcoma has attracted interest in using this modality in upper jaw tumours.[156] A wide variety of drugs has been used including methotrexate, adriamycin and cisplatinum. However, the discovery of late metastases in patients receiving post-amputation chemotherapy for limb sarcomata has decreased disease-free survival time when long-term follow-up is employed. Randomized trials are awaited to rationalize the true place of this therapy.

Table 13.3 5-year survival for osteogenic sarcomata of maxilla

Author	No. patients	Survival (%)
Kragh et al 1958[157]	?	19
Garrington et al 1967[143]	17	25
Roca et al 1970[153]	9	30
Caron et al 1971[139]	15	33
LiVolsi 1977[155]	6	0
Harrison & Lund	9	33

Postoperative irradiation with doses of between 5000–6000 cGy using megavoltage have been disappointing in reducing local recurrence or offering realistic palliation. However, some patients, with a favourable histology and a resectable tumour, supplemented with postoperative radiotherapy or chemotherapy do survive and combined therapy still provides the best prospect of cure that is at present available.[156]

A 62-year-old male was seen in late 1974 with a 2 month history of a painless swelling of the right side of his face with some nasal obstruction. Recent extraction of a carious upper molar had been followed by profuse granulations growing in an unhealed socket. A biopsy from this site had confirmed a diagnosis of osteogenic sarcoma.

Examination revealed a large swelling of the anterior wall of the right maxilla with a friable, vascular mass filling the right nasal passage. There was no epiphora or proptosis but tomography showed destruction of the anterior and roof of the maxillary antrum. The histological sections showed areas of spindle cells with atypical features. Osteoid, bone and small amounts of cartilage confirmed the diagnosis of osteogenic sarcoma and a right maxillectomy with orbital clearance was carried out in December 1974.

Postoperative adriamycin, 45 mg daily for 3 days was given by infusion with minimal side effects and this regime was repeated 3 months later. The patient was followed up at regular intervals and died of an unrelated cause without evidence of local or systemic disease in May 1988, 14 years after initial diagnosis.

Prognosis (Table 13.3)

Bentzen et al[158] have examined the survival data of 184 patients with limb osteogenic sarcoma using multivariate regression analysis.

Symptoms of less than 6 months and increasing age carried a bad prognosis, whilst patients aged between 25 and 30 years and tumours dominated by fibroblastic cells had a good prognosis. They calculated a prognostic index which gave an overall 10-year survival figure of $28.6 \pm 3.5\%$ but found that cancer deaths continued after this 10 year period. Even after the 10 years, the hazard rate for osteogenic sarcoma was four times greater than the matched group and eventually most patients might be expected to die from their disease.

REFERENCES

1. Pindborg J J, Kramer I R H 1971 Histological typing of odontogenic tumours, jaw cysts and allied lesions. World Health Organization, Geneva
2. Makek M S 1981 So called 'fibro-osseous lesions' of tumorous origin. Journal of Cranio-Maxillo-Facial Surgery 15: 154–168
3. Harrison D F N 1984 Osseous and fibro-osseous conditions affecting the craniofacial bones. Annals of Otology, Rhinology and Laryngology 93: 199–203
4. Menzel A 1872 Ein fau von osteoforon bes unterkiefers. Archives Klinische Chirurgerie 13: 212–219
5. Montgomery A H 1927 Ossifying fibromas of the jaw. Archives of Surgery 15: 30–44
6. Lichtenstein L, Jaffe H L 1942 Fibrous dysplasia of bone. Archives of Pathology 33: 777–816
7. Schlumberger H G 1946 Fibrous dysplasia (ossifying fibroma) of the maxilla and mandible. American Journal of Orthodontic and Oral Surgery 32: 579–587
8. Eversole L R, Sabes W R, Rovin S 1972 Fibrous dysplasia: a nosologic problem in the diagnosis of fibro-osseous lesions of the jaws. Journal of Oral Pathology 1: 189–220
9. Sherman R S, Glauser O J 1958 Radiological identification of fibrous dysplasia and fibro-osseous neoplastic conditions of the jaws and their treatment. Radiology 71: 553–561
10. Thoma K H 1956 Differential diagnosis of fibrous dysplasia and fibro-osseous neoplastic lesions of the jaws and their treatment. Journal of Oral Surgery 14: 185–194
11. Schmaman A, Smith I, Ackerman L V 1970 Benign fibro-osseous lesions of the mandible and maxilla. Cancer 26: 303–313
12. Coley B L 1960 Neoplasms of bone and related conditions, 2nd edn. Hoeber International, New York, p 16
13. Reed R J, Hagy D M 1965 Benign non-odontogenic fibro-osseous lesions of the skull. Journal of Oral Surgery 19: 214–227
14. Waldron C A 1980 Fibro-osseous lesions of the jaws. Journal of Oral Surgery 28: 58–63
15. Langdon J D, Rapidis A D, Patel M F 1976 Ossifying fibroma – one disease or six. An analysis of 39 fibro-osseous lesions of the jaws. British Journal of Oral Surgery 11: 118–125
16. Williams J L, Faccini J M 1973 Fibrous dysplastic lesions of the jaws in Nigerians. British Journal of Oral Surgery 11: 118–125

17. Adekeye E O, Edwards M B, Goubran G F 1980 Fibro-osseous lesions of the skull, face and jaws in Kaduna, Nigeria. British Journal of Oral Surgery 18: 57–72
18. Dehner L P 1973 Tumors of the mandible and maxilla in children. Cancer 31: 364–384
19. Greer R O, Mierau G W 1980 Tumors of the oral mucosa and jaws in infants and children. University of Colorado Medical Center Press
20. Khanna S, Khanna N N 1979 Primary tumours of the jaws in children. Journal of Oral Surgery 37: 800–805
21. Hamner J E, Scofield H H, Cornyn J 1968 Benign fibro-osseous lesions of periodontal membrane origin. Cancer 22: 861–878
22. Fujimoto Y, Katoh M, Miyata M 1987 Cystic cemento-ossifying fibroma of the ethmoid cells. Journal of Laryngology and Otology 101: 946–952
23. Fu Y, Perzin K H 1974 Non-epithelial tumors of the nasal cavity, paranasal sinuses and nasopharynx. Cancer 33: 1289–1305
24. Sherman R S, Sternbergh W C 1948 The roentgen appearance of fibroma of bone. Radiology 50: 595–609
25. Waldron C A, Giansenti J S 1973 Benign fibro-osseous lesions of the jaws. A clinico-radiologic-histologic review. Oral Surgery 35: 340–350
26. Shanmugaratnam K 1978 Histological typing of the upper respiratory tract tumours, No. 19. World Health Organization, Geneva
27. Lund V J 1982 Ossifying fibroma. Journal of Laryngology and Otology 96: 1141–1147
28. Slow I N, Stern D, Freidman E W 1971 Osteogenic sarcoma arising in pre-existing fibrous dysplasia: report of a case. Journal of Oral Surgery 29: 126–129
29. von Recklinghausen J 1891 Die fibrose oder deformiende osteite. Festchrift R Virchow zei Seinem, Geburtstage, Berlin
30. Lichtenstein L, Jaffe H L 1942 Fibrous dysplasia of bone. Archives of Pathology 33: 901–912
31. Prein J, Remagen W, Spiessl B 1986 Tumours of the facial skeleton. Springer-Verlag, Berlin
32. Albright F, Butler A M, Hamton A O 1937 Syndrome characterized by osteitis fibrosa dissemination, areas of pigmentation and endocrine dysfunction, with precocious puberty in females. Report of a case. New England Journal of Medicine 216: 727–746

33. McCune D S, Bruch H 1937 Osteodystrophia fibrosa: report of a case in which the condition was combined with precocious puberty, pathologic pigmentation and hyperthyroidism. American Journal of Diseases of Childhood 54: 806–848
34. Lichtenstein L (1938) Polyostotic fibrous dysplasia. Archives of Surgery 36: 874–898
35. Vehlinger E 1940 Osteofibrosis deformans juvenilis. Archives of Pathological Anatomy 306: 355–299
36. Pritchard J E 1952 Fibrous dysplasia: review of 35 cases. American Journal of Medical Science 222: 313–332
37. Hunter D, Turnbull H M 1931 Fibrous dysplasia. British Journal of Surgery 19: 203–284
38. Albright F 1947 Polyostotic fibrous dysplasia. Journal of Clinical Endocrinology 71: 307–324
39. Jaffe H L 1953 Giant-cell reparative granuloma, traumatic bone cyst and fibrous dysplasia of bone. Oral Surgery 6: 159–175
40. Kramer I R H 1973 The histopathology of some central non-odontogenic tumours and tumour-like conditions of the jaws. Transactions of the International Conference of Oral Surgery 4: 28–32
41. Langdon J D, Rapidis A D, Patel M F 1976 Ossifying fibroma – one disease or six? British Journal of Oral Surgery 14: 1–11
42. Smith J F 1965 Fibrous dysplasia of the jaws. Archives of Otolaryngology 54: 507–527
43. Zimmerman D C, Dahlin D C, Stafne E 1958 Fibrous dysplasia of the maxilla and mandible. Oral Surgery 11: 55–68
44. Powell S P, Liu W Y, Rabuzzi D D 1980 Fibrous dysplasia of the ethmoid bone. Head and Neck Surgery 88: 22–24
45. Firat D, Stutzman L 1968 Fibrous dysplasia of bone, review of 24 cases. Annals of the Journal of Medicine 44: 421–430
46. Ehrig U, Wilson D R 1972 Two cases of fibrous dysplasia associated with primary hyperparathyroidism. Annals of Internal Medicine 77: 234–238
47. Schlumberger H G 1946 Fibrous dysplasia of single bones. Military Surgery 99: 504–527
48. Changus G W 1957 Osteoblastic hyperplasia of bone: histochemical appraisal of fibrous dysplasia of bone. Cancer 10: 1157–1165
49. Edgerton M T, Persing J A, Jane J A 1985 The surgical treatment of fibrous dysplasia. Annals of Surgery 202: 459–479
50. Viljoen D L, Versfeld G, Losken W 1988 Polyostotic fibrous dysplasia with cranial hyperostosis. American Journal of Medical Genetics 29: 661–667
51. Camilleri A E 1991 Craniofacial fibrous dysplasia. Journal of Laryngology and Otology 105: 662–666
52. Boysen M E, Olving J W, Vatne K 1979 Fibro-osseous lesions of the craniofacial bones. Journal of Laryngology and Otology 93: 793–807
53. Fries J W 1957 The roentgen features of fibrous dysplasia of the skull and facial bones: a critical analysis of 39 pathologically proved cases. American Journal of Roentgenology 77: 71–88
54. Reed R S 1963 Fibrous dysplasia of bone. Archives of Pathology 75: 480–495
55. Kwee T H 1964 Fibreuze osteodysplastie. Academisch Proefschrif, Camsen, Amsterdam
56. Mock D, Rosen I B 1986 Osteosarcoma in irradiated fibrous dysplasia. Journal of Oral Pathology 15: 1–4
57. Williams D M L, Thomas R S A 1975 Fibrous dysplasia. Journal of Laryngology and Otology 88: 359–374
58. Schwartz D R, Alpert M A 1964 Malignant transformation of fibrous dysplasia. American Journal of Medical Science 274: 1–20
59. Schofield I D F 1974 An aggressive fibrous dysplasia. Oral Surgery 38: 29–35
60. Jackson I T, Hilde A H, Gomuwka P K 1982 Treatment of cranio-orbital fibrous dysplasia. Journal of Cranio-Maxillo-Facial Surgery 10: 138–141
61. Ewing J 1928 Neoplastic diseases: a treatise on tumours. Saunders, Philadelphia, p 312
62. Albright F, Aub J, Bauer W 1934 Hyperparathyroidism: a common and pleomorphic condition as illustrated by 17 previous cases from one clinic. Journal of the American Medical Association 102: 1276–1287
63. Jaffe H L 1953 Giant cell tumour (ostoeclastoma) of bone. Annals of the Royal College of Surgeons of England 12: 343–355
64. Lichtenstein L 1959 Bone tumours. Mosby Co, St. Louis, p 119
65. Austin L T, Dahlin D C, Royer R Q 1959 Giant cell reparative granuloma and related conditions affecting the jaw bones. Oral Surgery 12: 1285–1291
66. Dahlin D C 1978 Bone tumours, 3rd edn. C C Thomas, Illinois, p 99
67. Quick C A, Anderson R, Stool S 1980 Giant cell tumours of the maxilla in children. Laryngoscope 90: 784–791
68. Burnam J A, Benson J, Cohen I 1979 Giant cell tumour of the ethmoid sinuses: diagnostic dilemma. Laryngoscope 89: 1415–1423
69. Waldron C A, Schafer W C 1966 The central giant cell reparative granuloma of the jaws. American Journal of Clinical Pathology 45: 437–440
70. Batsakis J J 1979 Tumours of the head and neck, clinical and pathological considerations, 2nd edn. Williams & Wilkins, Philadelphia
71. Geschickter C F, Copeland M M 1949 Tumours of bone, 3rd edn. Lippincott, Philadelphia
72. Peiner R 1954 Benign giant cell tumours of skull and nasal sinuses. Archives of Otolaryngology 60: 186–193
73. Bullock W K, Luck J V 1957 Giant cell tumour-like lesions of bone and preliminary report of a pathological entity. Medicine 87: 32–36
74. Hiyeda H, Friedmann B, Mack R P 1970 Ultrastructure and histogenesis of giant cell tumour of bone. Cancer 25: 1408–1423
75. Steiner G C, Ghosh L 1972 Ultrastructure of giant cell tumours of bone. Human Pathology 3: 569–572
76. Hamylin W B, Lund P K 1967 Giant cell tumours of the mandible and facial bones. Archives of Otolaryngology 86: 658–665
77. Sabantos A O, Dahlin D C, Childs D S 1972 Postradiation sarcoma of bone. Cancer 9: 528–532
78. Albright F 1948 A page out of the history of parathyroidism. Journal of Clinical Endocrinological Medicine 8: 637–642
79. Friedman W, Nafees P, Swartz J 1974 Brown tumour of the maxilla in secondary hyperparathyroidism. Annals of Internal Medicine 63: 468–474
80. Broadus A E 1981 Mineral metabolism. In: Baxter P, Broadus A E (eds) Endocrinology and metabolism. McGraw Hill, p 1019
81. Black B K, Ackermann I V 1950 Tumours of the parathyroid. A review of 23 cases. Cancer 3: 415–444
82. Robinson P J, Woodhead P 1988 Primary hyperparathyroidism presenting with a maxillary tumour and hydrocephalus. Journal of Laryngology and Otology 162: 1164–1167
83. Broadus A E 1982 Primary hyperparathyroidism viewed as a hormonal disease process. Minor Electrolyte Metabolism 8: 199–206
84. Hellquist H B 1990 Pathology of the nose and paranasal sinuses. Cambridge University Press, Cambridge
85. Leppla D C, Northcutt C, Snyder W 1982 Sequential changes in bone density before and after parathyroidectomy in primary hyperparathyroidism. Investigative Radiology 17: 604–607
86. Lloyd H M 1968 Primary hyperparathyroidism. Medicine 47: 53–56
87. Paget J 1877 On a form of chronic inflammation of the bone (osteitis deformans). Medical Chirurgical Transactions 60: 37–42
88. Nager G T 1975 Paget's disease of the temporal bone. Annals of Otology, Rhinology and Laryngology (Suppl. 22) 3–32
89. Fisher E W 1990 Rhinological manifestations of Paget's disease of bone. Journal of Cranio-Maxillo-Facial Surgery 18: 169–172
90. Stafne E C, Austin L J 1938 A study of dental roentgenograms in cases of Paget's disease, oseitis fibrosis cystica and osteoma. Journal of the American Dental Association 25: 1202–1210
91. Harvey L 1984 Viral aetiology of Paget's disease of bone: a review. Journal Royal Society of Medicine 77: 943–948
92. Fuller A P 1961 Paget's disease of the ethmoids. Journal of Laryngology and Otology 75: 860–863
93. Harrison D F N 1949 A case of Paget's disease of bone. Guy's Hospital Reports 948: 168–172
94. Smith G S, Eveson J W 1981 Paget's disease of bone with particular reference to dentistry. Journal of Oral Pathology 10: 233–235
95. Batsakis J J 1974 Tumours of the head and neck. Non-odontogenic tumours of the jaws. Williams & Wilkins, Baltimore

96. Potts J T, Defros L S 1974 Parathyroid hormone, calcitonin, vitamin D and bone mineral metabolism. In: Bondy P K, Rosenberg L E (eds) Duncan's diseases of metabolism, Vol. 2, 7th edn. W B Saunders, Philadelphia

97. Buckler H M, Cantrill J A, Klimiuk P S 1987 Paget's disease of the orbit: before and after APD. British Medical Journal 295: 1655–1657

98. Knaggs R L 1923 Leontiasis ossea. British Journal of Surgery 11: 347–348

99. Harris C L 1948 A case of leontiasis ossea. British Dental Journal 84: 193–195

100. Drury B J 1962 Paget's disease of the skull and facial bones. Journal of Bone and Joint Surgery (American) 44: 174–178

101. Eickel W, Palm D 1959 Statistische unde rastgenologische untersuchungen einiges stagen des nebenhohlenostema. Archives fur Ohren Nasen Kehlkopfheilkunde 120: 147–440

102. Childrey J H 1939 Osteomas of the sinuses, of the face and sphenoid bone. Archives of Otolaryngology 30: 63–66

103. Hallberg O E, Bagley J W 1950 Origin and treatment of osteomas of the paranasal sinuses. Archives of Otolaryngology 51: 750–756

104. Teed W R 1941 Primary osteoma of the frontal sinus. Archives of Otolaryngology 33: 255–259

105. Boenninghaus K 1923 Blumenfeld's handbuch d. speziellen. Chirurgie der Ohres 3: 372–373

106. Wilkes S R, Trantmann J C, DeSanto L W 1979 Osteoma. An unusual case of amaurosis fugax. Mayo Clinic Proceedings 54: 258–260

107. Samy L L, Mostafa H 1971 Osteoma of the nose and paranasal sinuses with a report of twenty one cases. Journal of Laryngology and Otology 85:449–469

108. Atallah N, Say M M 1981Osteomas of the paranasal sinuses. Journal of Laryngology and Otology 95: 291–304

109. Gardner E J, Richards R C 1953 Multiple cutaneous and subcutaneous lesions occurring simultaneously with hereditary polyposis and osteomatas. American Journal of Human Genetics 5: 139–142

110. Noyek A M, Chapnik J S, Kirsh J C 1989 Radionuclide bone scan in frontal sinus osteoma. Australian and New Zealand Journal of Surgery 59: 127–132

111. Handousa A J 1940 Nasal osteomata. Journal of Laryngology and Otology 55: 197–224

112. Jones K, Korzcak P 1990 The diagnostic significance and management of Gardner's syndrome. British Journal of Oral and Maxillofacial Surgery 28: 80–84

113. Lloyd G A S 1988 Diagnostic imaging of the nose and paranasal sinuses. Springer Verlag, Berlin

114. Lund V J 1987 Anatomical considerations in the aetiology of fronto-ethmoid mucocoeles. Rhinology 25: 83–88

115. Blitzer A, Post K D, Conley J 1989 Craniofacial resection of ossifying fibromas and osteomas of the sinuses. Archives of Otolaryngology 115: 1112–1115

116. Byers P B 1968 Solitary benign osteoblastic lesions of bone. Cancer 22: 43–57

117. Jaffe H L 1935 Osteoid osteoma: a benign osteoblastic tumour composed of osteoid and atypical bone. Archives of Surgery 31: 709–728

118. Jaffe H L 1956 Benign osteoblastoma. Bulletin of the Hospital for Joint Diseases, Orthopaedic Institute 17: 141–151

119. Lichtenstein L 1956 Benign osteoblastoma. Cancer 9: 1044–1052

120. Dahlin D C, Johnson E W 1954 Giant osteoid osteoma. Journal of Bone and Joint Surgery (American) 36: 569–572

121. Clutter D J, Leopold D A, Gould L V 1984 Benign osteoblastoma. Archives of Otolaryngology 110: 334–336

122. Tan L W C, Lowry L D, Quinn-Bogard A 1980 Benign osteoblastoma of the maxillary sinus. Otolaryngology, Head and Neck Surgery 88: 397–402

123. Osguthorpe J D, Hungerford G D 1983 Benign osteoblastoma of the maxillary sinus. Head and Neck Surgery 6: 605–609

124. Freeman S R 1975 Benign osteoblastoma of ethmoid bone. American Journal of Clinical Pathology 63: 391–396

125. Som P M, Bellot P. Blitzer A 1979 Osteoblastoma of the ethmoid sinus. Archives of Otolaryngology 105: 623–625

126. Katsantonis G, Friedman W H, Smith K 1981 Osteoid producing orbital ethmoid tumour. Otolaryngology, Head and Neck Surgery 89: 717–722

127. Habermann E T, Stern R E 1974 Osteoid osteoma in the tibia of an eight month old boy. Journal of Bone and Joint Surgery (American) 56: 633–636

128. Schulman L, Dorfman H D 1970 Nerve fibres in osteoid osteoma. Journal of Bone and Joint Surgery (American) 52: 1351–1356

129. McLeod R A, Dahlin D C, Beabout J W 1976 The spectrum of osteoblastoma. American Journal of Roentgenology 126: 321–335

130. Pochaczevsky R, Ten Y M, Sherman R S 1960 The roentgen appearance of benign osteoblastoma. Radiology 75: 429–437

131. Williams R N, Boop W C 1974 Benign osteoblastoma of the skull. Journal of Neurosurgery 41: 769–772

132. Marsh B W, Bonfiglo M, Brady L P 1975 Benign osteoblastoma; range of manifestations. Journal of Bone and Joint Surgery 57: 1–9

133. Schasowicz F 1981 Tumours and tumourlike lesions of bones and joints. Springer, Berlin

134. Remagen W, Prein J 1975 Benign osteoblastoma. Oral Surgery 39: 279–283

135. Mayer L 1967 Malignant degeneration of so-called benign osteoblastoma. Bulletin of the Hospital for Joint Diseases, Orthopaedic Institute 28: 4–13

136. Ewing J 1939 A review of classification of tumours. Surgery of Gynaecology and Obstetrics 68: 971–976

137. Budd J W, McDonald J 1943 Osteogenic sarcoma. A modified nomenclature and a review of 118 five-year cures. Surgery of Gynaecology and Obstetrics 77: 413–421

138. Singh J, Gluckman J L, Kaufman R A 1982 Osteosarcoma of the nasal bone in a child. Head and Neck Surgery 4: 246–250

139. Caron A S, Hasdu S I, Kaufman R A 1971 Osteogenic sarcoma of the face and cranial bones. American Journal of Surgery 122: 506–512

140. De Fries C H, Perlin C E, Liebel S A 1979 Treatment of osteogenic sarcoma of the mandible. Archives of Otolaryngology 105: 358–359

141. Millar B G, Browne R M, Flood T R 1990 Juxtacortical osteosarcoma of the jaws. British Journal of Oral and Maxillofacial Surgery 28: 73–79

142. Batsakis J J, Solomon A R, Rice D H 1971 Pathology of the head and neck: neoplasms of cartilage, bone and notochord. Part 7. Head and Neck Surgery 3: 43–47

143. Garrington G E, Scofield H H, Corwyn J 1967 Osteogenic sarcoma of the jaws. Analysis of 56 cases. Cancer 20: 377–391

144. Huvos A G, Sundarbsan N, Bretsky S 1985 Osteogenic sarcoma of the skull. Cancer 56: 1214–1221

145. Windle-Taylor P C 1977 Osteosarcoma of the upper jaw. Journal of Maxillofacial Surgery 5: 62–68

146. Wilimas J, Barrett G, Pratt C 1977 Osteosarcoma in two very young children. Clinical Paediatrics 16: 548–551

147. Daramola J C, Aghadiuno P U, Ajabbe A 1976 Osteogenic sarcoma of the jaws in Ibadan, Nigeria. British Journal of Oral Surgery 14: 23–30

148. Immenkamp M 1975 Die mahne enfartung bei fibroser dysplasle. Zeitschrift fur Orthopadie und ihre Grenzgebiete (Stuttgart) 113: 331–342

149. Remagen W, Morscher E, Rosli A 1980 Primare und sckundere tumeren der knochen. In: Kuhlencordt F, Barhelheimer H (eds) Springer, Berlin

150. Glass A G, Fraumeni J F 1970 Epidemiology of bone cancer in children. Journal of the National Cancer Institute 44: 187–199

151. Sorby A 1972 Bilateral retinoblastoma – a dominantly inherited affliction. British Medical Journal 2: 580–583

152. Abrahamson D H, Ellisworth R W, Zimmerman L F 1976 Non-ocular cancer in retinoblastoma survivors. Transactions of the American Academy of Ophthalmology and Otorhinology 81: 454–457

153. Roca A N, Smith J A, Jung B 1970 Osteosarcoma and parosteal osteogenic sarcoma of the maxilla and mandible. American Journal of Clinical Pathology 54: 194–203

154. Newland J R, Ayala A G 1977 Parosteal osteosarcoma of the maxilla. Oral Surgery 43: 727–733
155. LiVolsi V 1977 Osteogenic sarcoma of the maxilla. Archives of Otolaryngology 103: 485–488
156. Gooran A M, Abelson H, Frie E 1985 Osteosarcoma: Twelve years later. New England Journal of Medicine 313: 1637–1639
157. Kragh L V, Dahlin D C, Erich J B 1958 Osteogenic sarcoma of the jaws and facial bones. American Journal of Surgery 96: 496–505
158. Bentzen S M, Poulsen H S, Kaae S et al 1988 Prognostic factors in osteosarcoma. Cancer 62: 194–202
159. Yalowitz D L, Brett A S, Earl J M 1984 Far advanced primary hyperparathyroidism in an 18-year-old young man. American Journal of Medicine 77: 545–548

14. Chordoma

Definition

A chordoma is a malignant dysontogenetic neoplasm, arising in residual or vestigial remnants of embryonic notochord.

Historical aspects

In 1857 Virchow[1] and Luschka[2] independently described this lesion which it was suggested originated in cartilage. The notochordal origin was first recognized by Muller[3] who used the term 'ecchordosis physaliphoria'. The term 'chordoma' was first applied by Ribbert in 1895.[4] A chordoma in the nasopharynx was first reported in 1909.[5]

Incidence

The lesion is relatively uncommon, constituting less than 1% of all central nervous system neoplasms.[6] Although a third affect the cranial region, there are few large series and the sinonasal tract is infrequently involved. In a series of 20 cases reported by Perzin & Pushparaj, seven affected the sinonasal region, mainly from the sphenoid.[7]

Age, sex and ethnic variation

Any age can be affected but the cranial lesions tend to occur in younger patients (range 20–40 years, average 38 years) when compared with the sacro-coccygeal area (range 40–60 years, average 58 years).[8] Men are more commonly affected than women (3:1).

Site

Chondromas can be divided into three main groups depending upon site of origin: cranial (36–39%), sacro-coccygeal (45–49%) or vertebral (8–15%).[9,10] The cranial lesions can be further anatomically divided into those affecting the superior nasopharynx, involving the spheno-occipital area, upper nasal cavity, ethmoid, maxilla, pterygoid area, periorbital bone, clivus, dorsum sellae, mastoid, petrous pyramids and middle cranial fossa and those involving predominantly the inferior nasopharynx and pharynx.[7] A fourth subgroup arises primarily in the maxillary and mandibular regions and is rarely encountered (Table 14.1).[7,11–16]

Lesions in the clivus region can extend into the nasopharynx and thence occasionally into the antro-nasal region. The few cases reported in the literature, including those from the Institute of Laryngology and Otology are shown in Table 14.1.[7,11–16]

Binkhorst indicated seven points of origin in the craniocervical region:

Dorsum sellae
Clivus
Retropharyngeal notochord vestiges
Remnants in the apical ligament of the dens
Nucleus pulposus of cervical vertebra
Vestiges in the squama occipitalis
Ectopic tissue in the mandible, maxilla and frontal sinus.

Aetiology

The notochord is an axial structure characterizing the phylum of Chordata. In higher animals, it is replaced by the vertebral column and part of the skull and can be seen in the bodies of the primitive vertebrae by the 5th intrauterine week. Considerable rearrangement in this region may result in small ectopic rests and the distribution of these parallels the distribution of chordoma. The fact that 90% occur at the top and bottom of the vertebral column supports this origin rather than the alternative suggestion from remnants of the nucleus pulposus in the intervertebral discs.[17]

Clinical features

With clival lesions, presentation is usually late after intracranial extension has occurred. Thus neuro-ophthal-

Table 14.1   Chordoma: in the literature

Author	Male	Female	Age (yr)	Site	Treatment	Outcome
Adams 1948[11]		1	64	Frontal sinus	DXT	A&W 1 yr
Pastore et al 1949[13]		1	21	Maxilla, nasopharynx	Local surgery	DOD 16/12
Berdal & Myhre 1964[12]		1	46	Ethmoid	Transantral & external ethmoidectomy, × 2, 8 yr apart	A&W 10 yr
	1		49	Nasopharynx, maxilla (Previous lesions in soft palate, pharyngeal wall)	DXT All treated DXT	A&W 20 yr from diagnosis No FU after sinus lesion
		1	51	Palate, septum	DXT Sublabial transmaxillary resection DXT 6 yr later multiple recurrence, local surgery	AWR 25 yr
	1		18	Nasopharynx	DXT	A&W 2 yr
		1	10	Antro-ethmoid	External approach	A&W 14/12
		1	40	Alveolar ridge	DXT Recurrence 8 yr – maxillectomy Recurrence 4 yr – radical surgery	AWR 14 yr
Wright 1967[15]	1		16	Nasopharynx	Transpalatal approach	AWR 14/12
		1	26	Nasopharynx	Transpalatal approach	A&W 2 yr
		1	53	Nasopharynx, middle cranial fossa	DXT	AWR 6 yr
	1		52	Sphenoid, ethmoid	External ethmoidectomy, DXT	MCF recurrence at 4 yr DOD 4.5 yr, meningitis
Zizmor & Noyek 1968[16]		1	60	Nasopharynx, antrum, orbit	Multiple excision	–
Shugar et al 1980[14]		1	30	Maxilla	Radical maxillectomy	A&W 19/12
Perzin & Pushparaj 1986[7]	1		68	Nasopharynx, maxilla, sphenoid	DXT	DOD 4.5 yr
	1		60	Nasopharynx, sphenoid	DXT, craniotomy	DOD 1 yr 4/12
	1		48	Sphenoid, clivus	DXT, Craniotomy DXT	AWR 6 yr 3/12
	1		46	Nasopharynx, sphenoid	DXT	AWR 10/12
	1		14	Nasopharynx, middle cranial fossa	DXT	No FU
	1		59	Sphenoid, ethmoid	Craniotomy, DXT	AWR 5 yr
		1	15	Nasopharynx, sphenoid	Craniotomy	No FU
Harrison & Lund	1		70	Anthro-ethmoid and orbit	Maxillectomy & orbit	AWR 4 yr
	1		70	Nasopharynx	DXT	No FU
	1		16	Nasopharynx	Transpalatal approach	DOD 5.5 yr
		1	49	Nasopharynx	Transpalatal approach, DXT	A&W 13 yr
	1		70	Nasopharynx	DXT	No FU

A&W, alive and well; AWR, alive with recurrence; DOD, dead of disease; No FU, no follow-up; DXT, radiotherapy mological symptoms predominate, with associated cranial nerve symptoms in up to half the cases. The majority present with visual problems such as decreased visual acuity, diplopia due to occulomotor, trochlear and abducent nerve involvement, limitation of visual fields, paralysis of eye muscles and ptosis.[7] The trigeminal, facial and vestibulocochlear nerves may also be affected. Fronto-orbital headaches affect half the patients and intracranial extension may produce hypophyseal and bulbar-pontine signs. The duration of symptoms ranges from 2 weeks to 14 years, though the majority complain of symptoms for 6 months to 3 years.

Anterior extension commonly produces nasal symptoms (92%) such as obstruction, anosmia, mucopurulent discharge and epistaxis.[18,19] Serous otitis media can also result from nasopharyngeal involvement and inferior extension may affect the pharynx and larynx.

Radiology

The chordoma produces an expansile osteolytic lesion which may be calcified due to sequestration of bone fragments. A plain submento-vertical view and CT will show a soft-tissue mass in the nasopharynx with destruction of the basisphenoid and clivus. Chordomas are best shown on MR with a characteristic high signal on T2 weighted sequences and strong enhancement on T1 weighted post-gadolinium scans.

Macroscopic and microscopic appearance

The tumour is usually a lobulated, partially translucent, gelatinous lesion which readily invades bone. It frequently has a pseudocapsule.

The histology can be quite variable though some features are constant.[20]

1. Overall lobular arrangement
2. Tendency for the cells to form strands
3. Abundant intercellular mucinous matrix
4. Large vacuolated or 'bubble' cells. This last feature increases with age to produce characteristic physaliophorous cells.

Stains for mucus and glycogen are positive.[7] Immuno-chemistry for cytokeratins and S100 protein are positive, though negative for lysozyme distinguishing chordoma from chondrosarcoma.[21]

Natural history

The lesion is usually midline and can invade bone and dura, ensheathing structures such as the spinal column and spreading from the clivus into the body of the sphenoid and nasopharynx. Metastases are unusual.[22] An incidence of 10% has been reported in a series of 155 cases from all sites,[9,23] but are more frequently associated with the sacro-coccygeal region.

Differential diagnosis

A diagnosis of chordoma can sometimes be difficult and it must be distinguished from chondroma, chondrosarcoma, a mucinous-forming adenocarcinoma, mixed salivary tumours and benign processes such as a mucocoele. A deep biopsy through the pseudocapsule is important to obtain representative tissue.

Treatment

The position of the tumour usually compromises complete surgical excision. The gelatinous portions can be suctioned away but total removal is rarely possible. Consequently, although chordoma is radioresistant, a course of high-dose postoperative radiotherapy is frequently given.[8,24-26]

The surgical approach depends upon the position and extent of the lesion but generally a lateral rhinotomy or craniofacial approach is employed. The transpalatal approach has also been described but has been superseded by the midfacial degloving and maxillary swing approaches.

Prognosis

Location is the most important determinant of prognosis.[7] There are few large series of cranial chordomas but the majority of cases are extensive at presentation, precluding complete excision. Thus with inevitable recurrence, overall prognosis is generally poor, though because the lesion may be slow-growing, patients can survive for many years. However, the majority of patients (80%)[27] with cranial lesions are dead within 5 years and in Dahlin & MacCarty's series only two out of 15 cases survived longer than this.[8]

CHONDROID CHORDOMA

A variant lesion has been described by Heffelfinger et al[9] and Richter et al[19] which represents a merging of these two histologies which must be distinguished from chondrosarcoma. The tumour which is commoner in women, occurs in the base of the skull and generally has a better prognosis than its non-chondroid counterpart. Heffelfinger et al[9] reported 22 cases, 19 affecting the spheno-occipital region, who survived an average of 15.8 years compared with an average of 4.1 years in 36 patients with non-chondroid chordomas. Management was the same for both groups, relying on extensive surgical excision combined with irradiation.

REFERENCES

1. Virchow R 1857 Untersuchungen uber die entwickelung des Schadelgrundes. Berlin
   Cited by Windeyer B W 1959 Proceedings of the Royal Society of Medicine 52: 1088–1100
2. Luschka H 1857 Chordoma malignum. Virchows Archives of Pathological Anatomy and Histopathology 11:8
   Cited by Windeyer B W 1959 Proceedings of the Royal Society of Medicine 52: 1088–1100
3. Muller H 1858 Chordoma malignum. Zeitschrift ration Medizinische 2:202
   Cited by Windeyer B W 1959 Proceedings of the Royal Society of Medicine 52: 1088–1100
4. Ribbert H 1895 Zentralblatt fur Allgemeine Pathologie und Pathologische Anatomie 6: 268
   Cited by Windeyer B W 1959 Proceedings of the Royal Society of Medicine 52: 1088–1100
5. Linck A 1909 Chordoma malignum, ein Beitrag fur Kenntnis der Geschwulste un der Schadelbas. Beitrage Pathologische Anatomie 46: 573–585
6. Poppen J L, King A B 1952 Chordoma: experience with thirteen cases. Journal of Neurosurgery 9: 139–163
7. Perzin K H, Pushparaj N 1986 Nonepithelial tumors of the nasal cavity, paranasal sinuses, and nasopharynx. A clinicopathologic study. XIV: chordomas. Cancer 57: 784–796
8. Dahlin D C, MacCarty C S 1952 Chordoma: a study of fifty-nine cases. Cancer 5: 1170–1178
9. Heffelfinger M J, Dahlin D C, MacCarty C S, Beabout J W 1973 Chordomas and cartilaginous tumors at the skull base. Cancer 32: 410–420
10. Utne J R, Pugh D G 1955 The roentgenologic aspects of chordoma. American Journal of Roentgenology 74: 593–608
11. Adams W S 1948 A case of chordoma of the right frontal sinus. Journal of Laryngology and Otology 62: 93–95
12. Berdal P, Myhre E 1964 Cranial chordomas involving the paranasal sinuses. Journal of Laryngology and Otology 78: 906–919
13. Pastore P N, Sahyoun P F, Mandeville F B 1949 Chordoma of the maxillary antrum and nares. Archives of Otolaryngology 50: 647–658
14. Shugar J M A, Som P M, Krespi Y P, Arnold L M, Som M L 1980 Primary chordoma of the maxillary sinus. Laryngoscope 90: 1825–1830
15. Wright D 1967 Nasopharyngeal and cervical chordoma - some aspects of their development and treatment. Journal of Laryngology and Otology 81: 1337–1355
16. Zizmor J, Noyek A M 1968 Cysts and benign tumors of the paranasal sinuses. Seminars in Roentgenology 3: 172–202
17. Binkhorst C D, Schierbeek P, Petten G J W 1957 Neoplasms of the notochord. Acta Otolaryngologica 47: 10–20
18. Campbell W M, McDonald T J, Unni K K, Laws E R 1980 Nasal and paranasal presentations of chordomas. Laryngoscope 90: 612–618
19. Richter H J, Batsakis J G, Boles R 1975 Chordomas: nasopharyngeal presentation and atypical long survival. Annals of Otology, Rhinology and Laryngology 84: 327–332
20. Batsakis J G 1980 Tumors of the head and neck. Williams and Wilkins, Baltimore, pp. 350–354
21. Salisbury J R, Isaacson P G 1984 Application of immunohistochemistry and histochemistry to the differential diagnosis of chordomas. Journal of Pathology (abstr) 143: 330A
22. Batsakis J G, Kittleson A C 1963 Chordomas: Otorhinolaryngologic presentation and diagnosis. Archives of Otology and Laryngology 78: 168–175
23. Gentil F, Coley B L 1948 Saccrococcygeal chordoma. Annals of Surgery 127: 432–455
24. Higinbotham N L, Phillips R F, Farr H W, Hustu H O 1967 Chordoma: thirty-five year study at the Memorial Hospital. Cancer 20: 1841–1850
25. Pearlman A W, Friedman M 1970 Radical radiation therapy of chordoma. American Journal of Roentgenology 108: 333–341
26. Tewfik H H, McGinnis W L, Nordstrom D G, Latourette H B 1977 Chordoma: evaluation of clinical behaviour and treatment modalities. International Journal of Radiation and Oncology 2: 959–962
27. Hyams V J, Batsakis J G, Michaels L 1988 Tumors of the upper respiratory tract and ear. Armed Forces Institute of Pathology, Washington, pp 192–196

15. Eosinophilic granuloma

Definition

This non-neoplastic condition of unknown aetiology is characterized by an intense proliferation of eosinophils, lymphocytes, plasma cells and multinucleated giant cells.

Synonyms

There is some debate as to whether eosinophilic granuloma is a separate entity or represents a localized manifestation of histiocytosis X which also includes Hand–Schuller–Christian (characterized by the triad of diabetes insipidus, exophthalmos and lytic lesions of the skull) and Letterer–Siwe disease (hepatosplenomegaly, lymphadenopathy, lytic lesions of bone and cutaneous eruptions).

Historical aspects

In 1929 Finzi[1] reported an eosinophilic lesion in the frontal bone of a 15-year-old boy which was diagnosed as myeloma. A similar case was published a year later by Mignon.[2] A link between the three conditions of eosinophilic granuloma, Hand–Schuller–Christian and Letterer–Siwe was first suggested by Farber in 1941[3] and supported by Lichtenstein[4] who drew them together as 'histiocytosis X'. This common origin from the Langerhans-type histiocyte has been supported by subsequent studies.[5]

Incidence

Eosinophilic granuloma is uncommon and though there is a tendency for lesions to occur in the skull, the sino-nasal tract is rarely affected.

Age, sex and ethnic variation

Although any age from 1 to 80 years can be affected, over two-thirds are under 10 years old at presentation.[6]

It is twice as common in males than females[6] and one American series suggested that Caucasians were more often affected than Negroes.[7]

Site

The lesions predominantly occur in bones though other sites such as skin and the gastro-intestinal tract have been recorded. 40% of these bony lesions are found in the skull,[8] affecting the temporal, frontal and parietal bones. The orbit is involved in about one-fifth of cases[9] and lesions have been reported in the maxilla, lateral nasal wall and mandible.[10] However, in 12 cases presenting with symptoms in the head and neck, none were sited in the sinonasal region.[7]

Aetiology

The aetiology is unknown although the basic pathological process for all three conditions in histiocytosis X is a non-neoplastic hyperplasia of Langerhans' cells.[11] Genetic factors have been suggested in Letterer–Siwe but there is no evidence for this in eosinophilic granuloma.[12]

Clinical features

Cases of eosinophilic granuloma frequently manifest otolaryngologic symptoms (85%)[7] which are the presenting complaint in 75% of cases. The patient typically presents with a painful swelling over the affected bone of a few weeks' duration. If the alveolus is involved there may be displacement of teeth, ulceration and pain. Cervical lymphadenopathy is often present.

The condition has been divided into two main groups:

Type I, an acute progressive disease, with hepatosplenomegaly, lymphadenopathy, skin lesions and pituitary insufficiency (diabetes insipidus) in addition to osseous lesions.

Type II, characterized by a single osseous lesion. Approximately one-quarter of cases present in this way.[7]

In 1975 a 7-year-old girl presented with swelling of the right cheek and lower lid which had failed to resolve with antibiotics. There was evidence of bone erosion and, via a Caldwell–Luc approach, a large quantity of haemorrhagic tissue was removed from the maxilla. This was diagnosed as eosinophilic granuloma and a course of radiotherapy was given.

No recurrence or other lesions occurred after 5 years' follow-up.

Radiology

The osseous lesion has a 'punched-out' appearance due to localized bone destruction. In the flat bones of the skull these produce a map-like design which has been termed 'geographic skull'.[7] In the alveolus the radio-opaque tooth root surrounded by radiolucent bone gives the tooth the appearance of floating in soft tissue.[13]

Macroscopic and microscopic appearance

The lesions are a yellowish to red–brown colour and microscopically are composed of numerous histiocytic cells and eosinophils with associated fibrosis. The number of eosinophils can vary considerably, the greater the number being associated with an improved prognosis.

On electron microscopy, all forms of histiocytosis X demonstrate a rod-shaped inclusion in the cytoplasm of histiocytes known as a Birbeck granule.[14] It is identified as similar to structures seen in the cytoplasm of Langerhans' cells in the epidermis.

Differential diagnosis

The differential diagnosis includes any condition of destructive inflammation such as syphilis, TB, Wegeners, sarcoid and osteomyelitis. Other osseous tumours and conditions such as ameloblastoma, osteogenic sarcoma and fibrous dysplasia must be excluded. Both deposits of multiple myeloma and Hodgkin's must also be differentiated.

Treatment

For unifocal disease, a combination of curettage and radiotherapy is usually curative and evidence of the bone

defects usually resolve within a few years. Local injections of steroid into the lesions have also been suggested.[15]

In the Type I systemic disease, chemotherapy has been used in addition to these other modalities. The most effective chemotherapy regimes are vinblastine–corticosteroids and etoposide–corticosteroids given for 3 to 12 months dependent upon response.[16] Other treatments, including low-dose cytosine, alpha-interferon or even autologous or allogeneic bone marrow transplantation have also yielded promising results but need to be confirmed by larger series.

Natural history and prognosis

The acute Type I patients with generalized disease have a short course and poor prognosis. Those with localized lesions in the Type II group generally do better. In Appling's series of 25 cases, 22 presented with unifocal disease, which became multifocal within 5 months in one-third.[6] If no new osseous lesions appear within 1 year, it is likely that the individual will remain in remission.[17] Generally in multifocal disease, survival is better if the age of onset is older, there is no visceral involvement and the number of eosinophils in the lesions is high. Overall mortality rates vary, but have been reported as high as 50% in patients less than 2 years of age.[18] When the disease begins in neonates the mortality may be as high as 77%.[19]

A third group has been defined of unifocal eosinophilic granulomas which sometimes recur after treatment but whose long-term prognosis is excellent. In addition proven lesions have been reported as undergoing spontaneous remission.[20]

In histiocytosis X, attempts at predicting prognosis and response to therapy have led to several staging systems. Lahey[21,22] proposed a scoring system based on age at presentation and the number of organs involved placing a significant emphasis on organ dysfunction. Using this staging system, Nezelof et al[23] reported an apparent linear association between the number of organs involved and mortality (25% mortality for two organs involved, 33% for three or four organs, 72% for five organs and 100% for six or more organs).

REFERENCES

1. Finzi O 1929 Mieloma con prevalenza delle cellule eosinofile circoscritto all osso frontale in un giovane di 15 anni. Minerva Medica 91: 239–241
2. Mignon F 1930 Ein Granulations tumour des Stirnbeins. Fortschritte auf dem Gebiete der Rontgenstrahlen 42: 749–751
3. Farber S 1941 The nature of solitary or eosinophilic granuloma of bone. American Journal of Pathology 17: 625–626
4. Lichtenstein L 1953 Histiocytosis X. Archives of Pathology 56: 84–102
5. Wright D H, Isaacson P G 1983 Biopsy pathology of the lymphoreticular system. Chapman and Hall, London
6. Appling D, Jenkins H A, Patton G A 1983 Eosinophilic granuloma in the temporal bone and skull. Otolaryngology, Head and Neck Surgery 91: 358–365
7. Cinberg J Z 1978 Eosinophilic granuloma in the head and neck: a five year review with report of an instructive case. Laryngoscope 88: 1281–1289
8. Oschner S F 1966 Eosinophilic granuloma of bone. American Journal of Roentgenology 97: 719–726
9. Enriquez P, Dahlin D C, Hayles A B, Henderson E D 1967 Histiocytosis X, a clinical study. Mayo Clinic Proceedings 42: 88–99

10. Gondalia V, Jyrwa J, Bahadur S, Prakash H, Chopra P 1984 Eosinophilic granuloma with bilateral maxillary and mandibular involvement. Journal of Laryngology and Otology 98: 1143–1145

11. Hellquist H B 1990 Pathology of the nose and paranasal sinuses. Butterworths, London, pp. 76

12. Zinkham W H 1976 Multifocal eosinophilic granuloma: natural history, etiology and management. American Journal of Medicine 60: 457–463

13. Standish S M, Gorlin R J 1970 Thomas's oral pathology, Ch. 12. CV Mosby, St Louis

14. Michaels L 1987 Ear, nose and throat histopathology. Springer-Verlag, Berlin, pp. 230

15. Cohen M, Zornoza A, Cangir A, Murray J A, Wallace S 1980 Direct injection of methyl prednisolone sodium succinate in the treatment of solitary eosinophilic granuloma of bone: a report of 9 cases. Radiology 136: 289–293

16. Benz-Lemoine E 1989 Prognostic factors in histiocytosis X. Annales de Pediatrie (Paris) 36: 499–503

17. Schajowicz F, Stullitel J 1973 Eosinophilic granuloma of bone and its relationship to Hand-Schuller-Christian and Letterer-Siwe syndromes. Journal of Bone and Joint Surgery 55: 545–565

18. Greenberger J S, Crocher A C, Vawler G, Jaffe N, Cassidy J 1981 Results of treatment of 127 patients with systemic histiocytosis (Letterer-Siwe syndrome, Schuller-Christian syndrome and multifocal eosinophilic granuloma). Medicine 60: 311–338

19. Lucaya J 1971 Histiocytosis X. American Journal of Diseases of Childhood 121: 289–295

20. Platt J L, Eisenberg R B 1948 Eosinophilc granuloma of bone. Journal of Bone and Joint Surgery 30A: 761–768

21. Lahey M E 1975 Histiocytosis X: An analysis of prognostic factors. Journal of Pediatrics 87: 184–198

22. Lahey M E 1975 Comparison of three treatment regimens. Journal of Pediatrics 87: 179–183

23. Nezelof C, Frileux-Herbert F, Cronier-Sachet J 1979 Disseminated histiocytosis X, analysis of prognostic factors based on a retrospective study of 50 cases. Cancer 44: 1824–1838

16. Hamartomas, teratomas and dermoid cysts

Definition

The terms hamartoma, teratoma and dermoid are applied to a variety of lesions representing a spectrum of growth from embryological malformations to true neoplasia and their usage is sometimes confused in the literature.

A hamartoma is a developmental anomaly characterized by an accumulation of tissue which is normally present in this particular location.[1] A hamartoma (derived from 'hamartia' or error) may thus be derived from any of the three germinal layers and can be composed of one or more tissue types such as vessels, fibroblasts and smooth muscle.[2] They are sometimes encountered in the sinonasal region of children and young adults (Table 16.1). Lesions such as haemangiomas may be included in this definition.

Another term, *choristoma*, is applied to new growths from misplaced tissue such as ectopic glial masses occasionally encountered in the nasal cavity.

A dermoid has been regarded as an inclusion error during embryogenesis or may represent a spontaneous autonomous new growth from pluripotential tissue. Both mechanisms for development probably exist.[3] The lesion is composed of two germinal layers, ecto- and mesodermal and is usually cystic.

A teratoma also arises as a spontaneous autonomous new growth from pluripotential tissue but contains elements of all three germinal layers; ecto-, endo- and mesodermal. It is thus a true neoplasm composed of multiple tissues foreign to the part of the body in which it arises. Benign and malignant forms can exist.

Thus in considering cysts in this region three varieties may be distinguished determined by their origin:

Epidermoid. A cyst lined by simple squamous epithelium with fibrous walls and no adnexal structures.

Dermoid. An epithelial-lined cavity containing variable numbers of skin appendages.

Teratoid. An epithelial cyst, often of mixed types of epithelium, which may contain skin appendages in addition to mesodermal and endodermal derivatives.

TERATOMAS

Incidence

These lesions are extremely rare in the sinonasal region. Benign teratoma occasionally occur in infants and children, predominating in girls(6:1).[4] Malignant teratomas (teratocarcinosarcomas) affect the young or middle-aged adult (18–79 years) and mainly occur in men (4:1) (Table 16.2).[5] There does not seem to be any ethnic predilection.

Site and aetiology

Teratomas mainly arise within the nasopharynx and cervical regions from whence they may produce nasal

Table 16.1 Hamartomas of nasal cavity and paranasal sinuses: in the literature

Author	Sex	Age (yr)	Site	Presentation	Histologic type
Kacker & Das Gupta 1973[25]			Nasal cavity	Bleeding polyp	Angiomatous
Majumder et al 1977[26]	M	19	Hard palate Nasopharynx	Nasal obstruction Secretory otitis media	Angiomatous
Mahindra et al 1978[27]	F	10	Nasal cavity	Bleeding	Angiomatous
	F	26	Nasal cavity	Bleeding, nasal obstruction	Angiomatous
	–	2 mth	Nasal cavity	Nasal obstruction	Lipomatous
Chisin et al 1987[2]			Nasal cavity		

Table 16.2   Malignant teratomas of upper jaw: in the literature

Author	Male	Female	Age (yr)	Site	Treatment	Outcome
Patchefsky et al 1968[28]	1		39	Nasal cavity Ethmoid	Caldwell–Luc	Massive recurrence DOD 2/12
Abt & Toker 1970[29]	1		49	Nasal cavity Antro-ethmoid	DXT (Initially surgery refused)	Rapid recurrence 3/52 – radical maxillectomy & orbital clearance A&W 6 yr
Dicke & Gates 1970[30]	1		44	Nasal cavity Ethmoid	Total ethmoidectomy	Rapid recurrence 3/12 – surgery Recurrence – C DOD 1.2 yr
Meinecke et al 1976[31]	1		62	Nasopharynx	Radical surgery & DXT	DOD 3 yr
Devgan et al 1978[32]		1	60	Nasal cavity Ethmoid Sphenoid	Surgical debulking, DXT	Recurrence 6/12 – maxillectomy, orbital clearance. C A&W 1.8 yr
Patterson & Ballard 1980[33]		1	38	Nasal cavity	Surgery DXT	A&W 1.5 yr
Heffner & Hyams 1984[5]	16	4	18–79 (av. 60)	Nasal cavity (16) Nasopharynx (2) Ethmoid (9) Maxilla (11)	Surgery (5) DXT (3) DXT/C (1) Surgery/DXT (11)	DOD (9) 0.6–2.7 yr DICD (1) 6.5 yr AWD (1) 1 yr A&W (5) 3–9 yr Lost (4)

A&W, alive and well; AWD, alive with disease; DOD, dead of disease; DICD, dead of intercurrent disease; DXT, radiotherapy; C, chemotherapy

obstruction and epistaxis in some cases. The malignant teratomas generally have a short history of a few weeks and produce radiological evidence of a soft tissue mass and bone destruction.

Macroscopic and microscopic appearance

The benign teratoma is histologically well-differentiated, composed largely of neural derivatives both mature and immature. The malignant variety contains a bizarre collection of epithelial and connective tissue elements of every and any sort from neural elements, cartilage and bone, to liver, muscle and glands.

Treatment and prognosis

The benign teratoma can be readily excised surgically and rarely recurs. The teratocarcinosarcoma by contrast infiltrates locally in a most aggressive fashion usually producing the demise of the patient by intracranial extension before manifesting any metastatic spread. One series[5] did report cervical metastases in six out of 20 cases of sinonasal teratocarcinosarcoma. The few cases in the literature have been treated with radical surgery, radiotherapy and in some cases, chemotherapy. In Heffner & Hyams' series 60% of patients succumbed in under 3 years (average survival 1.7 years) regardless of therapy but in those treated aggressively with surgery and radiotherapy, 40% survived 3 years or longer (average follow-up 6.1 years).

DERMOID CYSTS

Historical aspects

The first nasal dermoid was described by Dieffenbach in 1829[6] and Lawrence reported the first case in the English literature in 1838.[7]

Incidence

Dermoids in the head and neck account for 7% of all cases[8] and those of the nose 1–3%.[9,10] Up to the early 1980s around 150 cases of median nasal dermoids had been reported but this almost certainly underestimates the true incidence as many go unrecognized or un-reported. Bradley reported a series of 74 cases treated during a 22-year period which represented 0.02% of admissions to two children's hospitals.[11]

Age, sex and ethnic variation

The age range varies from 3 months to 59 years but the majority are recognized in childhood. The median age at presentation in Bradley's series was 5.5 years.[11] Males are more often affected(2:1).[12,13]

Site

The median nasal lesions can be found in a variety of positions: glabellar, dorsum of nose, tip of nose between alar cartilages, or columella. The lesion can be superficial or may communicate with a deeper component like an 'hour-glass' through a tract between the nasal bones. The 'simple' variety accounts for two-thirds of cases[11] but the location of the dermal manifestation does not indicate the underlying tissue penetration.

It should also be remembered that other dermoids such as those arising in the orbit can occasionally impinge on the sinuses.

Aetiology

Of the several suggested theories for median nasal dermoids, two hypotheses prevail. The cranial theory postulates that as the dura mater recedes from the prenasal space, it pulls the nasal ectoderm forming a sinus. If the sinus is pinched off, a cyst is formed. The superficial theory suggests that the ectoderm of the fusing right and left medial nasal process is pulled in to form a sinus tract or is trapped submucosally to form a cyst.[14,15] In either case, the dermoid could be 'simple' confined to the skin alone or 'complex' extending to the nasal septum, fronto-ethmoid region and up to or through the cribriform plate[8,16] and the tract may be found opening on the skin anywhere along the midline of the nose.

Several instances of familial cases have been reported, first by New & Erich in 1937[17] and more recently by Khan et al in which four members of a family were affected.[9]

Clinical features

These range from a small dimple to a pit which may have hairs protuding or discharges from time to time. If there is a 'dumb-bell' lesion beneath the nasal bones, broadening of the nasal bridge and nasal obstruction can result.

Radiology

Radiological assessment is most important to differentiate the lesion from encephalocoeles and gliomas and to establish any intracranial connection. On plain X-rays a broadened or bifid nasal septum may be seen with separation of the nasal bones but a CT scan and more recently MRI better demonstrate the situation. Two-thirds of dermoids have characteristic areas of low attenuation on CT due to the presence of fat within the cyst.[18]

Differential diagnosis[19]

It is primarily encephalocoeles and gliomas which must be distinguished from this lesion but many other lesions including sebaceous cysts can cause clinical confusion.

Treatment and prognosis

Complete surgical excision is important to avoid recurrence which is estimated to occur in up to half of cases[8,20] and this should be undertaken as soon as possible to prevent deformity of the growing nose[21] and to reduce the risk of infection and subsequent meningitis.[22,23]

The position of the cyst may make excision difficult but the fistula tract must be excised and if necessary a neurosurgical approach used to deal safely with any intracranial connection. The surgical approach will thus be determined by the position and extent of the cyst and may range from craniofacial resection, osteoplastic flap via a spectacle incision, external ethmoidectomy, lateral rhinotomy or external rhinoplasty. After dissection of the dermoid, any residual structural defect should be repaired primarily but parents should be warned that further cosmetic surgery is often required.[22]

'HAIRY POLYP'

A lesion which is variably described as a choristoma, dermoid or teratoma is sometimes encountered in the nasopharynx.[24] This pedunculated lesion can be attached to the hard or soft palate and may fill the nares or oral cavity, reaching up to 6 cm in diameter. It mainly occurs in males and is composed of fibroadipose tissue, cartilage, bone and skeletal muscle. It is cured by surgical excision.

REFERENCES

1. Albrecht E 1904 Hamartoma. Verhandlungen der Deutschen pathologischen Gesellschaft 7: 153
2. Chisin R M, Ragazzino M W, Flexon P B 1987 MR assessment of a hamartoma of the nasal cavity. American Journal of Roentgenology 149: 1083–1084
3. McAvoy J M, Zuckerbraun L 1976 Dermoid cysts of the head and neck in children. Archives of Otolaryngology 102: 529–531
4. Foxwell P B, Kelham B H 1958 Teratoid tumors of the nasopharynx. Journal of Laryngology and Otology 72: 647–657
5. Heffner D K, Hyams V J 1984 Teratocarcinosarcoma (malignant teratoma?) of the nasal cavity and paranasal sinuses. Cancer 53: 2140–2154
6. Dieffenbach 1829 Quoted by Bramann F 1890 Langenbecks Archiv fur Klinische Chirurgie 40: 101–108
7. Lawrence W 1838 Nasal midline cyst. London Medical Gazette 21: 471–474
8. Taylor B W, Erich J B 1967 Dermoid cysts of the nose. Mayo Clinic Proceedings 42: 488–494
9. Khan M A, Gibb A G 1970 Median dermoid cysts of the nose familial occurrence. Journal of Laryngology and Otology 84: 709–718
10. Skolnik E M, Campbell J M, Meyers R D 1971 Laryngoscope 81: 1632–1637
11. Bradley P J 1983 The complex nasal dermoid. Head and Neck Surgery 5: 469–473
12. Horton C E, Adamson J E, Crawford H C, Brown L H 1967 Dermoid cysts of the nose in children. Virginia Medical Monthly 94: 274–278
13. Ryan A J 1948 Dermoid cyst of the bridge of the nose. Connecticut State Medical Journal 12: 218–221

14. Littlewood A H M 1961 Congenital nasal dermoid cysts and fistulae. Plastic and Reconstructive Surgery 27: 471–488
15. Pratt L W 1965 Midline cysts of the nasal dorsum: embryologic origin and treatment. Laryngoscope 75: 968–980
16. McCaffrey T V, McDonald T J, Gorenstein A 1979 Dermoid cysts of the nose. Otolaryngology, Head and Neck Surgery 87: 52–59
17. New G B, Erich J B 1937 Dermoid cysts of the head and neck. Surgery, Gynecology and Obstetrics 65: 48–55
18. Lloyd G A S 1988 Diagnostic imaging of the nose and paranasal sinuses. Springer-Verlag, London, p 54
19. Hughes G B, Sharpino G, Hunt W, Tucker H M 1980 Management of the congenital midline nasal mass: a review. Head and Neck Surgery 2: 222–233
20. Nydell C C, Masson J K 1959 Dermoid cysts of the nose. Annals of Surgery 150: 1007–1016
21. Masing H, Gunther H 1979 Some clinical considerations on congenital anomalies of the nose. Rhinology 17: 143–153
22. Jaffe B F 1981 Classification and management of anomalies of the nose. Otolaryngological Clinics of North America 14: 989–1004
23. Matson D D, Ingraham F D 1951 Intracranial complications of congenital dermal sinuses. Paediatrics 8: 463–474
24. Michaels L 1987 Ear, nose and throat histopathology. Springer-Verlag, Berlin
25. Kacker S K, Das Gupta G 1973 Hamartomas of the ear and nose. Journal of Laryngology and Otology 81: 801–805
26. Majumder N K, Venkataramaniah N K, Gupta K R, Gopalakrishen S 1977 Hamartoma of nasopharynx. Journal of Laryngology and Otology 91: 723–727
27. Mahindra S, Daljit R, Sohail M A, Malik G B 1978 Hamartomas of the nose. Journal of Laryngology and Otology 92: 57–60
28. Patchefsky A, Sundmaker W, Marden P A 1968 Malignant teratoma of the ethmoid sinus. Cancer 21: 714–721
29. Abt A B, Toker C 1970 Malignant teratoma of the paranasal sinuses. Archives of Pathology 90: 176–180
30. Dicke T E, Gates G 1970 Malignant teratoma of the paranasal sinuses. Archives of Otolaryngology 91: 391–394
31. Meinecke R, Bauer F, Skouras J, Mottu F 1976 Blastomatous tumors of the respiratory tract. Cancer 38: 818–823
32. Devgan B K, Devgan M, Gross C W 1978 Teratocarcinoma of the ethmoid sinus: review of literature plus a new case report. Otolaryngology, Head and Neck Surgery 86: 689–695
33. Patterson S D, Ballard R W 1980 Nasal blastoma: a light and electron microscopic study. Ultrastructural Pathology 1: 487–494

17. Lymphoreticular tissue neoplasia and destructive lesions

The conditions included in this section have been amongst the greatest sources of confusion and diagnostic contention in the sinonasal region. Fortunately, this situation has been improved by a greater understanding of the natural history of these pathologies, considerably enhanced by advances in histopathology techniques. The realization that many midline destructive lesions are T-cell lymphomas leading to appropriate treatment has considerably improved prognosis. However, the results of a detailed clinical history, thorough physical examination, X-rays and blood tests are essential to the diagnosis and a meticulous search both microbiologically and histologically must be made to exclude the many infectious conditions which can sometimes mimic the destructive lesions. The conditions covered are:

1. Burkitt's lymphoma
2. Non-Hodgkin's lymphoma
3. Extramedullary plasmacytoma
4. Midline destructive granuloma.

BURKITT'S LYMPHOMA

Definition

A tumour of childhood particularly affecting the maxilla of males living within specific African territories and composed of malignant lymphoid cells.

Historical aspects

In 1958 Denis Burkitt, a surgeon practising in Uganda, published an account of a highly malignant tumour of the jaws which affected young children within a defined 'geographical belt' in Africa.[1] These boundaries were defined by Burkitt in his paper of 1961[2] and it was evident that this tumour, which primarily affected the maxilla, occurred across Africa with cases being found in Kenya, Ghana, Nigeria as well as Uganda. As a result of his meticulous observations it was concluded that if areas over 5000 feet (1524 m) in altitude, where the mean

rainfall was below 20 inches per year (50.8 cm) and the mean temperature less than 60°F (15.5°C) were excluded, the residual area was identical with a map of tumour distribution. The similarity between a map showing tumour incidence and climatic conditions favouring the growth of certain mosquitoes, suggested that an arthropod vector might play some part in the development of this tumour, and would go some way in explaining the localization of areas of high incidence.

Histologically, the tumour was a malignant lymphoma, eventually shown to be developed from B-cell lymphocytes and associated with the presence of the Epstein-Barr (EB) virus.

Incidence

The suggestion that an endemic malignant lymphoma affecting the jaws of young African children and confined within specific environmental conditions excited great interest, particularly when it proved to be highly sensitive to chemotherapy. Burkitt & Wright, the latter being the pathologist who had originally described the morphology of this tumour, published their account of the 'geographical and tribal distribution of the African lymphoma in Uganda' in 1966.[3] This was a detailed analysis of 450 histologically proven cases seen over a period of 8 years and showed a 20-fold difference in incidence rates between the lowland areas along the Nile, where the tumour was common, and the low incidence in the mountainous areas of south-western Uganda.

Khan reported his experience in Kenya of 140 patients treated between 1958–1962.[4] One patient was a pure-blooded Arab child from Zanzibar but his series included no European or Indian children. The geographical distribution of the patients was similar to that recorded by Burkitt in Uganda, except that several patients came from the highlands of Kenya, over 5000 feet in altitude.

Clifford et al[5] later analysed in considerable detail 65 patients with Burkitt's lymphoma treated in Nairobi from 1963–1967. None of these were in Masai children or from the Nilo-Hamitic Kenyan tribes and they confirmed a high incidence of this tumour in both Malaysia and New Guinea. All their cases were from indigenous African rural stock and from families living in poor socio-economic circumstances. Nkrumah & Perkins (1976) reported the findings in 110 patients from Ghana treated under the auspices of the Burkitt Lymphoma Research Unit, a collaborative project between the Ghana Medical School and the National Cancer Institute, Bethesda, USA. Every patient was seen between 1968 and 1972 but this paper is primarily concerned with the effects of chemotherapy rather than confirming the geographical locations of their patients.[6] However, in 1977 Kummona published his account of six patients with jaw lymphoma occurring in Middle East children whose histological and radiological appearances were suggestive of Burkitt's tumour. All failed to respond to chemotherapy[7] and Wright had previously recognized that non-African cases did occur elsewhere which although morphologically similar to Burkitt's lymphoma were probably not aetiologically similar.[8]

It is now apparent that although this tumour is endemic in certain clearly defined geographical, and possibly ethnic populations in Africa, nonendemic cases occur throughout the world. In countries where the climatic conditions are similar to the high endemic areas within Africa, Burkitt's lymphoma may be common or rare, as in Singapore.[9,10] It is now clear that this tumour cannot be regarded as exclusively an African disease since it has a worldwide incidence. However, specific geographical conditions can be identified where the tumour is endemic, elsewhere cases are rare and sporadic. Within the endemic areas, incidence rates are at least 50% of all malignant tumours of childhood[11] whereas this falls to around 15% elsewhere.[12]

Age, sex and ethnic variation

Within endemic populations the maximum incidence is between the ages of 5 and 9 years depending upon differing publications.[3–5,13] The range has been reported as between 2 and 16 years, although in the immigrant population of Uganda half the cases were over the age of 15 years with a quarter of these older than 30 years.[3]

Whilst jaw tumours most commonly occur in the very young, around 3 years of age, abdominal Burkitt's lymphoma occurs in a slightly older group and this is reflected in the varying sex ratios that appear in the literature. This is quoted as between 2 and 2.5:1 with a distinct male preference.[3–5] Older patients are most commonly found in nonendemic areas where in North America the mean age is 11 to 12 years. These cases tend to present with abdominal rather than jaw tumours and the latter are unusual after the age of 15 years.[14]

Within the larger African reports there appears to be no tribal variations in incidence rates. Burkitt &

Wright's cases came from 373 different tribes within Uganda and surrounding countries. Any variations in incidence within Uganda were primarily related to geographical and socio-economic factors rather than ethnic differences.[3] A similar situation was found by Clifford et al in Kenya[5] who included an ethnographic distribution of 23 tribes in their analysis of Burkitt's lymphoma. Further studies of nonendemic cases throughout the world have failed to show a specific ethnic susceptibility but the numbers are too small for valid conclusions to be drawn except to support the view that black populations appear to be more susceptible.[12]

Site

The condition as originally described by Burkitt primarily affects the non-lymphoid tissues, particularly the jaws and face and on occasions may be multicentric. Isolated orbital tumours without involvement of the related maxilla have been recognized and over 40% of the patients discussed by Nkrumah & Perkins also had associated abdominal tumours.[6] These cases usually have multiple lesions with malignant ascites and involvement of kidneys, liver, ovaries and retroperitoneal lymph nodes. The cervical lymph nodes are rarely involved even in advanced disease.

A serious complication of systemic spread is paraplegia from spinal cord invasion or vascular compression, and invasion of the central nervous system is now recognized as a usually fatal complication of this disease.

Although many of the clinical features of the endemic variety of Burkitt's lymphoma are characteristic, only the jaw lesions can be considered as pathognomonic. Massive growth in children between the age of 3 and 6 years is typical. Although initially developing in the molar–premolar region with loosening of deciduous teeth or premature eruption of permanent teeth, death from renal failure may take place before diagnosis is made. Kinetic studies have shown that Burkitt's lymphoma is the fastest growing human tumour with a cell doubling time of 24 hours.[6] The jaw tumour originates around developing odontogenic tissue, attacking the lamina dura of tooth sockets, surrounding bone and soft tissues. The teeth become displaced, mobile and then dislodged, being finally embedded within the tumour. Destruction of the maxilla can take place within a few days with tumour visible intraorally in the palate or extending into the orbit, nasal cavity or infratemporal fossa.[7]

Isolated lesions in the thyroid and parotid gland, long bones, skin, breasts and ovaries (usually bilaterally) have been reported, usually from nonendemic areas where growth may be less rapid. Although the jaw lesions are the most characteristic feature they are rare after the age of 15 years and in nonendemic areas it is the systemic manifestations that may be the presenting symptoms.

Aetiology

Haddow in 1964 showed that the cumulative age incidence curve for the Burkitt lymphoma was similar to that of yellow fever antibodies in Uganda.[15] This was consistent with the hypothesis that this tumour might be induced by an insect vectored virus. The absence of cases younger than 2 years of age could then be explained by protection by maternal antibodies. The almost complete absence of cases in adults indigenous to the high risk lowland areas of Uganda was then explained by the proposition that initial exposure to potential environmental carcinogens always occurred before the age of 15 years. Almost half of these tumours developing in immigrants to the high risk regions were in patients older than 15 years and one-fifth were over 30 years of age.[3]

However, cases bearing clinical and pathological similarities to the endemic form of Burkitt's lymphoma do occur in regions where the climate is neither hot nor humid, suggesting that all cases are not due to an insect-born virus. Mycoplasmas, vaccinia virus and herpes simplex have all been found in association with Burkitt's lymphoma tissue and Bell et al isolated reovirus 3 (CAN 230) from a culture of tumour tissue taken from four cases with this lesion in 1964.[16] Clinical studies showed that cases of this lymphoma had a higher incidence of neutralizing antibody to this virus than in the sera from normal controls (4:1) and in mice this virus has induced tumours that resemble Burkitt's lymphoma and contain reovirus 3 antigen.[14,17]

Epstein–Barr virus (EBV), the causative agent of infectious mononucleosis, has been implicated as a possible factor in the genesis of Burkitt's lymphoma as well as nasopharyngeal cancer. EB virus nuclear antigen and virus DNA have both been identified in tumour tissue from these neoplasms but not from other jaw tumours within high risk regions of Africa.[18] Although high titres to EB virus occur in most Burkitt's lymphoma this virus is not vectored and is present in all parts of the world.[19–22]

There is no evidence to support the hypothesis that persistent malarial infection produces lymphoreticular hyperplasia thus allowing the EB virus to become oncogenic, but in the presence of immunosuppression this virus might well be potentially oncogenic. Perhaps the most plausible explanation for endemic Burkitt's lymphoma is that an insect-born agent, possibly one of several viruses, acts co-carcinogenetically by stimulating the proliferation of lymphoid cells already transformed into a neoplasm by an unknown agent.[10]

Ziegler in his comprehensive review of this tumour includes not only the EB virus but genetic factors manifested by a t(8:14q) chromosomal translocation as well as malaria as possible causes in what is now recognized as a neoplasm of B-lymphocytes.[12]

Clinical features

One of the most striking features of the endemic form of Burkitt's lymphoma is its predilection for the bones of the jaws and facial tissues. This varies with the age of the patient being greatest at 3 years and thereafter gradually decreasing up to 15 years of age.[3] In those patients with nonendemic disease, abdominal involvement is more common, with jaw tumours a rarity[7] and this may be a reflection of a greater susceptibility of the African jaw to tumour formation. The mandible may be the seat of a primary tumour or a part of multifocal disease and isolated orbital tumours without maxillary involvement have been described by Nkrumah & Perkins in their studies of 110 cases.[6] Over half of these patients had abdominal organ tumours at diagnosis when they presented with swelling of the maxilla. Central nervous system disease was discovered on cerebrospinal fluid examination in 10% of all their patients.

Their classification was based upon the presence or absence of spread outside the face and CNS involvement.[5]

Stage 1. Single facial tumour
Stage 2. Multiple facial tumours with involvement of any other site except the CNS or abdomen
Stage 3. Intra-abdominal or intrathoracic spread without CNS involvement
Stage 4. CNS involvement.

The kidneys, liver, breasts and ovaries are frequently affected with bilateral gonadal tumour a characteristic feature of this disease. There is usually sparing of the peripheral lymph nodes, spleen and Waldeyer's ring in endemic Burkitt's lymphoma.

Since prognosis is directly related to tumour mass at presentation, early diagnosis, accurate assessment of the extent of the disease and rapid institution of therapy is essential and must take president over prolonged elaborate investigations.

Radiology

Although the largest series of patients has come from endemic areas of Africa where rapid tumour growth combined with limited medical and radiological facilities limits early diagnosis, diagnostic radiology can play an important role in differential diagnosis. Burkitt's lymphoma is osteolytic in nature destroying the maxilla within several days. This can be recognized by radiological rarefaction, usually in the molar–premolar area and may be visible before the clinical appearance of tumour in surrounding soft tissues. One of the first radiographic signs is loss or breakage of the lamina dura around deciduous or permanent teeth, leading eventually to loosening or tooth loss.[7] Convential tomography or CT scanning are valuable in showing the extent of maxillary destruction or orbital invasion but with such a rapidly growing neoplasm, radiology has little prognostic value. Intravenous pyelography is important to detect renal invasion and radiology may be helpful in detecting retroperitoneal or ovarian masses, for ultimately prognosis is related to some extent by the extent of abdominal disease.[23]

Macroscopic and microscopic appearance

Lennert's classification of non-Hodgkin's lymphomata[24] places Burkitt's lymphoma in the high grade B type of lymphoblastic lesions and it is accepted that histologically there is no difference between the African endemic lesion and that found elsewhere in the world. The lymphoblasts are primitive lymphoid precursors and do not correspond to a cell with a recognizable counterpart in normal postnatal life.[25a] The tumour is described as composed of sheets of undifferentiated lymphoreticular cells with little variation in size or shape of the nuclei. Nucleoli are prominent and mitotic activity, as might be expected in such a rapidly growing neoplasm, is high. Non-neoplastic macrophages containing tumour cells or cellular debris, break up the uniform pattern producing a 'starry sky' effect which, although not diagnostic, points towards Burkitt's lymphoma as a possible diagnosis.

The neoplastic cells are monoclonal with distinguishing markers, some of which carry a chromosome 8 to 14g translocation, and the monomorphism of the dominant cells ultramicroscopically are said to be diagnostic.[11,26]

However, tissue biopsy with imprint preparations are said by Batsakis to be the method of choice for rapid diagnosis, essential for early treatment.[14]

Natural history

The rapid growth and high malignancy of the endemic form of Burkitt's lymphoma ensures that without urgent treatment, complications from obstruction or systemic spread to kidneys or central nervous system will lead to death in most patients. However, this is one of the few neoplasms that responds dramatically to chemotherapy and even a short course of cytotoxic drugs can produce long remissions in at least 20% of patients.[14] Relapse is however common and this may be associated with the development of systemic disease which, when affecting the CNS, is frequently fatal.

Differential diagnosis

When the lesion is confined to the upper jaw this will include other lymphoreticular neoplasms, sarcomas, neuroblastomas, benign lymphoid hyperplasia, Ewing's sarcoma, leukaemic infiltration and undifferentiated carcinoma. The socio-ethnic specificity when considered with the clinical history, age, appearance of the tumour and histology will in most cases lead to accurate diagnosis in the endemic disease.

Treatment

The frequency with which Burkitt's lymphoma occurred in those countries initially lacking in modern radiotherapy facilities provided a unique opportunity for the investigation of the value of cytotoxic agents in this disease.

Clifford et al's paper of 1967 reported the long-term survival of 65 patients treated solely with various combinations of 15 agents during the period 1963–1967.[5] They used a staging system similar to that accepted for Hodgkin's disease and concluded that prognosis was related to staging rather than age, sex, site or tumour size. Previous reports from the same centre based upon 47 patients treated with methotrexate, melphalan or cyclophosphamide had resulted in a 100% mortality, although there had been some short-lived responses.[4]

53% of Clifford et al's Stage 1 tumours had a long-term response (duration unrecorded) but this dropped to 25% for Stage 2 tumours and the overall survival rate was 17%. They concluded that large single doses of endoxana (cyclophosphamide) 40 mg/kg or orthomelphalan 1–2 mg/kg was the most effective means of treatment and showed that patients who remained free from disease for more than 270 days might be classified as long-term survivors.[27] They also concluded that since each patient and his tumour presented as a distinct problem, treatment should be individually planned particularly with reference to the choice of cytotoxic drugs. Endoxana and vincristine have remained popular and complete remission for up to 6 years has been reported. There is evidence, some of which is anecdotal, that more than 20% of Burkitt's lymphoma will survive for long periods of time if treated adequately at initial diagnosis.[28] However, the chemotherapy must be adequate, for failure to respond initially invariably leads to early death from renal failure or CNS invasion. The latter indicates a need for intrathecal chemotherapy or cranial irradiation.

During the treatment of large intra-abdominal masses there is a potential risk of renal failure from the high uric acid load from tumour destruction. Allopurinol promotes urinary excretion of uric acid but dialysis may be required.

Reliable data from large series of Burkitt's lymphoma treated with a planned regime and with adequate long-term follow-up is lacking but 5-year survival for lymphomata in general is quoted by McClatchey as 23% with a median survival time of 0.7 years.[29] The median age of these patients was 29.8 years and included patients with both endemic and nonendemic Burkitt's lymphoma.

Prognosis

Burkitt himself thought that the natural history of patients presenting with jaw lesions was more favourable than those with involvement of the abdomen, although the high incidence of the latter in upper jaw lesions made it difficult to separate the groups.[1] Central nervous system invasion is a serious prognostic sign with few patients surviving more than a short time and surgical reduction of tumour bulk by bilateral oopherectomy was soon abandoned.[27] When dealing with such young patients only actuarial survival rates can realistically reflect ultimate prognosis and this information is not available. However, there does appear to be some evidence that in early Stage 1 tumours, high dose chemotherapy can be expected to produce a rapid reduction in tumour size and long-term remission.

NON-HODGKIN'S LYMPHOMA

Definition

Non-Hodgkin's lymphoma exists in both nodal and extra-nodal forms. Within the head and neck region the extranodal form is more common owing to the lymphoid tissue found within Waldeyer's ring. About 50% of these lymphomata occur within the nasal cavity and paranasal sinuses.[30]

Synonyms

Malignant lymphoma, lymphosarcoma.

Incidence

Data published for the United States in 1978 reported that about 25 000 individuals each year developed a malignant lymphoma and that this disease was the 7th most common cause of death in that country.[31] Of all the patients with non-Hodgkin's lymphoma within the head and neck, less than 5% arise within the nose and sinuses, most being found in the cervical lymph nodes and lymphoid tissue of Waldeyer's ring.[32] Freeman et al in 1972 found only 33 of 1467 cases were primarily within the upper jaw.[33] Gall & Mallory had two patients in their total series of 618 extranodal lymphomata[34] and Catlin 16 in his 249 head and neck lymphomata.[35] Most other reports confirm the rareness of lymphoma within the upper jaw and are summarized by Wilder et al in 1983 when they reported their account of 37 patients seen within an 18-year period.[31] Duncavage et al in the same year published their experience of 15 cases treated in 7 years[36] whilst Kapadia et al had 17 patients between 1963 and 1979.[37]

The largest published series is by Robbins et al in 1985 based upon 38 patients with non-Hodgkin's lymphoma confined to the nasal cavity and paranasal sinuses and treated between 1947 and 1983, with an overall 5-year survival rate of 56%.[38]

Neither polymorphic reticulosis or NACE (necrosis with atypical cellular exudate) is included in any of these reports, despite increasing awareness that both are probably T-cell lymphoma.[39]

Age, sex and ethnic variation

Whilst the mean age at diagnosis appears to be about 55 years, as with most other uncommon tumours, the range varies considerably from a low of 11 years to over 80 years.[31,37,39,40,41]

Most series show a clear male predominance of 3:1 but with such small numbers this may not be significant. There is no reliable data relating to racial susceptibility.

Site

Paranasal sinus and nasal cavity lymphoma probably arise from lymphoid cells situated within the sinus bone marrow or submucosa.[39] This neoplasm usually grows from the maxillary or ethmoid sinuses, lateral nasal wall or occasionally the nasal septum. However, non-Hodgkin's lymphoma has the propensity to destroy bone and invade adjacent tissue, so that considerable local extension at initial diagnosis makes the primary site of origin difficult to determine.

Kapadia et al[37] evolved a clinical classification based not upon the American Joint Committee (AJC) lymphoma staging system,[42] which is primarily related to nodal involvement, but one more suited to extra-nodal lymphoma arising within the upper jaw.[37]

1. Involvement limited to the nose and paranasal sinuses (with extension to soft tissues of the face)
2. Cervical node and sinonasal involvement (with extension to the soft tissues of the face)
3. Nodal involvement of regions above and below the diaphragm (together with sinonasal involvement)
4. Disseminated involvement of one or more extralymphatic organs or tissue, in addition to sinonasal involvement.

Robbins et al[38] adapted the AJC classification for sinus carcinoma to stage their upper jaw lymphoma.[43] Although this appears to be poorly suited to this neoplasm it is far superior for prognostic evaluation to the Ann Arbor staging system which is primarily concerned with lymph node disease.[44,45]

Within the upper jaw it is often difficult to differentiate those lesions that originate within the sinuses. Reimer et al suggest that primary bone lymphoma account for only 5% of all extranodal lymphomas but clinically it is doubtful if this differentiation has any prognostic or therapeutic significance.[46]

Clinical features and radiology

When discussing the varied symptoms observed at presentation in 37 patients with lymphoma of the nose and paranasal sinuses, Wilder et al[31] divided them into three categories. Within the first group were common rhinological complaints such as nasal obstruction, rhinorrhoea and epistaxis. Extension of the tumour from the nasal cavity and sinuses to adjacent structures produced the macroscopically obvious disease (Fig. 17.1) and occasional pain of group two, whilst systemic spread resulted in weight loss, fever and nocturnal sweating, constituting group three.

The commonest finding is a bleeding tumour within the nasal cavity but in half of patients there is also facial swelling. Rapid extension to related structures produces proptosis, epiphora, palatal swelling, cranial nerve involvement and cervical lymph node invasion (Fig. 17.2).

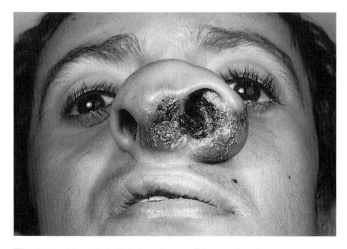

Fig. 17.1 Non-Hodgkin's lymphoma of the nasal cavity.

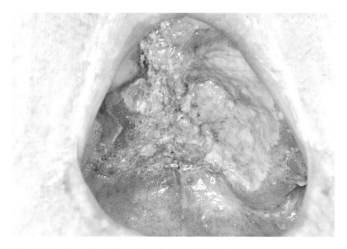

Fig. 17.2 Non-Hodgkin's lymphoma of the palate.

Plain X-ray and tomography will show any maxillary sinus opacity or bony destruction of the lateral nasal wall. Evidence of a soft tissue mass within the nasal cavity or facial tissues confirms the frequency with which several sites within the upper jaw may be involved at initial presentation. CT scanning is useful in establishing the true extent of the primary lesion and essential in examining the mediastinum, retroperitoneal lymph nodes and liver and spleen.

Lymphangiography has been recommended by Duncavage et al[36] on patients with a negative abdominal CT scan because it can detect abnormal distribution of contrast material in an otherwise normal sized lymph node. However, this technique is not widely used in pretherapy staging for sinonasal lymphoma, nor is laparotomy. Greater reliance is now placed on CT scanning and marrow examination to detect dissemination.

In most patients, tissue for biopsy and subsequent diagnosis is readily available transnasally, although Wilder et al[31] have reported a wide variety of more extensive operations designed to obtain tissue from less accessible sites.

Macroscopic and microscopic appearance

Non-Hodgkin's lymphoma form a large and varied group that differ in natural history, response to treatment and prognosis. The classification introduced in 1966 by Rappaport[47] has been widely used although now criticized for failure to recognize newly identified types of lymphoid cells and for retaining descriptive terminology no longer considered to be accurate.[48] Tindle in his publication on malignant lymphomata said 'Classification of tumours in order to be useful, must have relevance to the clinical approach to the patient's treatment, must be easily reproducible amongst various diagnosticians to allow for universal acceptance and use of the terminology, and should be scientifically correct as related to current concepts of pathogenesis and aetiology'.[41]

Recent years have seen an evolution of classifications based upon increased knowledge of the pathogenesis of lymphoreticular neoplasms particularly in relation to specific monoclonicity. The identification of two major lymphocytic subclasses, bursial- and thymic-derived, as shown by immunomarkers, has provided insight into both lymphoid physiology and neoplastic expression. For example, cell marker studies have demonstrated that the cells of non-Hodgkin's lymphoma with a nodular pattern are bursial-derived lymphocytes.[49] These findings have been incorporated into an International Working Formulation sponsored by the American National Cancer Institute in order to standardize the nomenclature for non-Hodgkin's lymphomata (Table 17.1).[50]

Follicular refers to the aggregation of neoplastic cells resembling normal lymphoid follicles. *Diffuse* describes

Table 17.1 Working formulation for classification of non-Hodgkin's lymphomas

Low-grade
    Small lymphocyte
    Follicular, small cleaved cell (SCC)
    Follicular, mixed SCC and large cell

Intermediate-grade
    Follicular, large cell
    Diffuse, SCC
    Diffuse, mixed small and large cell
    Diffuse, large cell, cleaved and transformed

High-grade
    Large cell, immunoblastic
    Lymphoblastic
    Burkitt's and Burkitt's-like

From Burres et al[49]

the histological appearance of tissue invaded by lymphoma without follicular formation. Most lymphoma found in the upper jaw are diffuse although there is a considerable range of types within any tumour.

Lymphomas of low-grade are said to be associated with a relatively good prognosis whilst high-grade tumours do poorly. However, this morphological classification is not entirely satisfactory because of subjectivity in interpretation. With the use of automated flow cytometry, DNA analysis can recognize aneuploid populations of cells, a good indication of malignancy; whilst monoclonal antibodies allow differentiation of B and T-cell subgroups. However, the complexity of sites, variable rates of growth of the differing histological types, and limited data has prevented accurate evaluation of both clinical stage and the various classification systems.

Natural history

Kapadia et al have said that the clinical stage at diagnosis has little effect on ultimate prognosis, quoting survival times of 9 months for Stage 1 and 11 months in their patients staged 3 or 4.[37] However, Wilder et al said that prognosis was better with unicentric Stage 1 lymphomas, providing they were limited to the sinonasal region.[31] As a group, non-Hodgkin's lymphoma are usually disseminated at the time of diagnosis and Portlock & Glastein found that with thorough examination, 70% of their patients had Stage 3 or 4 disease.[45] Since lymphoid cells exist within the bone marrow, biopsy is needed to eliminate involvement and realistic staging is therefore dependent not only on local and histological assessment but also on the presence of distant disease.

Local control is usually possible, although in Eichel et al's series of 22 patients, 69% died eventually from disseminated disease but with no obvious local neoplasm.[51] Half of the Stage 1 upper jaw lymphomata

cases reported by Harrison[39] also died with disseminated disease suggesting that many patients presenting with apparently localized sinonasal lymphoma have undetected systemic spread.

Differential diagnosis

Problems with differential diagnosis arise even with sophisticated immunochemical techniques, particularly with small, crushed, poorly fixed or unrepresentative biopsies.

Confusion exists with small round-cell malignancies such as anaplastic carcinoma, melanoma, olfactory neuroblastoma, Ewing's sarcoma, embryonal rhabdomyosarcoma, plasmacytoma. Wegener's granulomata and polymorphic reticulosis (destructive midline granuloma) have been diagnosed in error in the past. Non-Hodgkin's lymphoma is a clone of lymphocytes carrying a monoclonal surface marker pattern which can be identified and then typed as being B- or T-cell in origin. Hodgkin's disease carries no such marker pattern, allowing clear differentiation.

Kapadia et al have discussed many of the problems of differential histological diagnosis in non-Hodgkin's lymphoma emphasizing the need for accurate histomorphic classification of each lymphoma into one of the ten major subtypes within the three subgroups.[37]

Treatment

Once the histological diagnosis of a non-Hodgkin's lymphoma has been made, further investigations are needed to assess the presence of disseminated disease. Whilst irradiation alone has been shown to be effective in controlling local neoplasm, addition of chemotherapy is required in more advanced cases. A history of fever, weight loss or night sweats may provide concern for undetected dissemination. Complete physical examination supported by abdominal CT scans is essential to detect nodular or hepato-splenic enlargement, whilst lymphangiography or bone scans are less helpful. Laboratory investigations include haematological surveys and bone marrow smears although formal staging laparotomy is now unusual.

With upper jaw lymphomata there is support for treating even advanced tumours 'curatively' in order to produce realistic palliation. Indeed, many authors consider that lymphoma is only a local manifestation of a systemic defect in immunoregulation and suggest that ALL patients should receive systemic chemotherapy 'prophylactically'.[30,52] Cabanillas et al used combinations of irradiation and chemotherapy for both Stage 1 and 2 non-Hodgkin's lymphoma achieving 85% long-term remissions.[53] A wide variety of cytotoxic agents have been used including cyclophosphamide, vincristine, doxorubicin, procarbazine and prednisolone – all with variable success!

Before 1960 patients were treated primarily with orthovoltage irradiation now superseded by Co^{60} giving doses of between 4000–6000 rad within 4 to 6 weeks.[33]

A 72-year-old nun was first seen in October 1987 with pain and right-sided proptosis, tenderness and swelling of the right face, and nasal obstruction occurring for over 3 months. Symptoms had increased over the last 2 weeks and CT scan elsewhere had shown destruction of the right lateral nasal wall. There was also an enhancing mass extending from the ethmoid into the adjoining orbit. MRI with gadolinium confirmed the non-enhancing lesion (Fig. 17.3) which was about 2 cm in diameter and was also in the maxillary sinus. Part of the orbital floor had been destroyed.

Transnasal biopsy of a polypoidal nasal tumour localized to the region of the middle meatus was reported as being, 'a large cell, anaplastic B-cell lymphoma positive for KI-I antigen, suggesting a high-grade lesion'.

There was no evidence of lymphadenopathy or other spread and she was treated with 5500 rad on the 5 Mev Linear Accelerator to the upper jaw and remains well 4 years post-treatment.

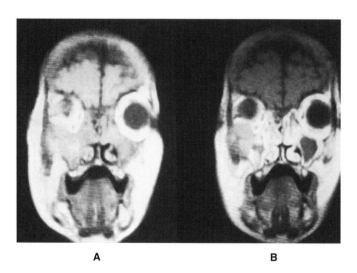

A   **B**

Fig. 17.3 **A**, coronal MR scan, T1 weighted sequence showing abnormal tissue throughout sinus system in a case of non-Hodgkin's lymphoma. **B**, coronal MR scan, T1 weighted sequence with gadolinium showing lymphoma of maxillary sinus (arrowed) delinated against high signal from inflamed mucosa.

Prognosis

Variations in both clinical and histological classifications used in publications over the past decade makes it almost impossible to evaluate the sparse data relating to long-term stage-related survival. Conley et al reviewing 287 patients with non-Hodgkin's lymphoma presenting within the head and neck, gave a figure of 50% total 5-year survivals for all stages with this figure then decreasing secondary to late dissemination.[48] Similar experiences have been recorded by others (Table 17.2) but many other publications give no detailed survival data or combine the upper jaw with the nasopharynx. Harrison[39] found that despite the absence of detectable regional or systemic disease at initial diagnosis, dissemination appeared within 3 to 7 months after completion of irradiation. Despite chemotherapy, all these patients died. He suggests that every patient with non-Hodgkin's lymphoma affecting the upper jaw irrespective of stage, should be treated with both radiotherapy and chemotherapy. Hopefully, this would improve long-term survival figures.

EXTRAMEDULLARY PLASMACYTOMA

Definition

A neoplasm of cells recognizable as plasma cells.[25b]

Historical aspects

Booth et al[54] say that the first reported case of extramedullary plasmacytoma within the upper respiratory tract was by Schriddle in 1905 and that by 1973 over 250 further cases had appeared in the world literature.

Incidence

Extramedullary plasmacytoma may arise in any structure containing reticulo-endothelial tissue and these tumours can be isolated as the initial lesion of generalized disease. There is good evidence to support the predominance of extramedullary lesions for the head and neck area,

Table 17.2 Results of treatment for non-Hodgkin's lymphoma of the upper jaw (all stages)

Author	No. cases	Sex M	Sex F	Treatment Radiotherapy	Treatment Radiotherapy & chemotherapy	Dead of disease at 5 yr No. (%)
Kapadia et al 1981[37]	17	14	3	8	9	11 (69%)
Duncavage et al[36]	15	9	6	0	15	8 (55%) at 1 yr
Robbins et al[38]	38	28	10	28	10	(56%)
Harrison & Lund	23	18	5	17	6	13 (56%)

particularly the nasal cavity and paranasal sinuses[55,56] with incidence rates varying from 75%[57] to 90%.[54]

Although at least two-thirds of these lesions present primarily in the nose, nasopharynx or sinuses, they form only 0.5% of all malignancies within the upper respiratory tract and must therefore be considered as exceedingly rare.[58]

Michaels[25b] analysed 53 patients with extramedullary plasmacytoma of the upper air and food passages recorded at the Armed Forces Institute of Pathology Tumor Registry, USA between 1940–1980. 44% were localized to the nose, nasopharynx or sinuses with the remainder in tonsil or vallecula.

Pahor[59] using data gathered from the cancer registry of a large city in the United Kingdom with a population of over five million, found an average of two new cases per year of extramedullary plasmacytoma during the period 1963–1972. This gave a crude annual incidence of 0.04 per 100 000 people compared with 1.9 per 100 000 people for medullary tumours. Expressed differently, the incidence of extramedullary plasmacytoma as compared with multiple myeloma was 1:40.

Most personal experience of this condition is limited to small numbers of patients, Helmus in 1964[60] after reviewing the literature added 24 cases, including three of his own, to the 126 previously recorded by Dolin & Dewar in 1956.[61] Castro et al reviewed 24 patients seen at the Memorial Hospital, New York over a 40-year period[55] and the nine patients discussed by Booth et al[54] were treated at the Royal National Throat, Nose and Ear, Hospital, London between 1949 and 1969.

Age, sex and ethnic variation

There is general agreement in the published series that extramedullary plasmacytoma show a definite male predominance of between 2 and 2.5:1. Pahor however, whilst agreeing that the overall ratio of males and females was around 2.5:1 found that it rose in single tumours to 14:1, being less than unity with multiple-site lesions. These figures were based upon a total series of 943 plasmacytoma which included both medullary and extramedullary, single and multiple lesions.[59]

Age distribution is wide with patients as young as

7 years being reported (plasmacytoma of the bronchus) to as old as 76 years.[62] This gives an average age at diagnosis of 50 years, younger than is usual for most upper jaw malignancies. Medullary plasmacytoma occur in an older group which averages about 65 years for those patients with multiple lesions.[59,63]

There appear to be no data supporting an ethnic variation in incidence but with such an uncommon condition this is not surprising.

Site

Cases affecting the nose and paranasal sinuses are more numerous than the total of all other sites within the head and neck. Nasal septum, lateral nasal wall and maxillary antrum are the common locations for single lesions, with Castro et al quoting published figures of 72 patients with sinonasal tumours, 14 in the nasopharynx, 26 in tonsil and pharynx and other sites 19.[55]

Table 17.3 shows the site figures from the largest published series available, confirming the frequency of the nasal cavity and sinuses for solitary extramedullary phasmacytoma.

Aetiology

Multiple myeloma remains a disease of unknown aetiology usually beginning within the bone marrow and after an insidious start is diagnosed at an advanced stage. Occasionally it may present as a solitary bone lesion or as an extramedullary soft tissue mass. Previously it had been thought that these solitary extramedullary lesions were areas of plasmacytic dysplasia with only a proportion ultimately developing generalized disease. Some patients would die from local invasion whilst others appeared to be cured after control of the local disease.

Wiltshaw, analysing the long-term histories of published cases, computed a 10-year survival rate of more than 50%[57] and survivals of over 15 years for localized extramedullary plasmacytoma were not uncommon. However, Carson et al[64] say that eventually all patients with solitary lesions will develop disseminated disease and Pahor reported local recurrence 7 years after apparently successful control of a maxillary sinus tumour.[59]

Table 17.3 Site of presentation of extramedullary plasmacytoma in the upper air and food passages: in the literature

Author	No. cases	Nose, sinuses	Nasopharynx	Tonsil	Other sites
Booth et al 1973[54]	11	7	–	1	3
Castro et al 1973[55]	24	19	4	–	1
Pahor 1977[59]	14	3	4	4	3
Michaels 1987[25b]	53	28	10	3	12

Clinical features and radiology

The commonest symptoms are those that are secondary to a mass within the nasal cavity or paranasal sinus. Obstruction, intermittent epistaxis, proptosis from orbital involvement, pain when associated with infection and palpable cervical lymph nodes have all been recorded. The duration of symptoms range from less than 3 months up to a year or more although the average is about 6 months. As with other jaw malignancies, diagnosis is related to the site and duration of severe symptoms, with pain, epistaxis and proptosis causing more concern than nasal obstruction.

Willis presented a useful clinical and pathological classification into three groups which is suitable for all plasmacytoma.[65]

Group 1. Characterized by generalized bone involvement and with classical X-ray findings with frequently, abnormal serum protein and Bence–Jones proteinuria

Group 2. Solitary plasmacytoma of bone which can be single or multiple

Group 3. Primary plasmacytoma of the soft tissues which can be single or multiple.

Since the non-specific triad of epistaxis, nasal obstruction and a visible mass is the most frequent presenting symptom, biopsy is essential for diagnosis. Cervical node involvement is variable with incidence rates changing with the primary site but probably between 15 and 25%.[58] The most important aspect of clinical diagnosis is the determination of local extent of the tumour and the presence or absence of generalized disease. Elevation of serum immunoglobulin or the presence of Bence–Jones protein is rarely found initially and Wiltshaw found that no more than 10% of patients with extramedullary plasmacytoma subsequently developed paraproteinuria. Even then there was always advanced disease with large masses of immunoglobulin-secreting tumour. Consequently, most of the patients fall into Willis Group 3.[65]

Haematological, serological, radiological and bone marrow examinations are essential but are expected to be within normal limits unless the patient already has generalized disease. Skeletal surveys to exclude unsuspected bone disease are important for Ewing & Foote in 1952 found that one-third of their patients with upper respiratory tract plasmacytoma already had unsuspected multiple myeloma.[56] However, this may be a reflection of their special experience as a secondary oncologic referral centre, for most other publications have not shared this experience with extramedullary plasmacytoma being a solitary lesion at diagnosis. Apart from the identification of bony lesions or tumour masses within the lungs, radiology will show soft tissue changes within the nasal cavity or sinuses together with any associated bone erosion.[66] The patient reported by Chaudhuri et al[67] had destruction of the skull base from a nasopharyngeal plasmacytoma and radiological assessment of the tumour extent is essential prior to irradiation.

Macroscopic and microscopic appearance

The gross appearances of plasmacytoma vary from yellow–grey to dark red in colour whilst being generally smooth and rubbery in consistency.

Microscopically, plasma cells are a common feature of many tumours and the histological recognition of malignancy must satisfy the criteria of large sheets of plasma cells lying alone and replacing tissue structures with local invasion. Sometimes these tumours may appear to be supported by blood vessels producing an alveolar pattern. Michaels found Russell bodies in 13% of plasmacytoma and in 20% of cases deposition of amyloid.[25b] This has the same chemical composition as Bence–Jones protein and it is suggested that the association of myelomatosis with amyloidosis can be explained by the accumulation of light chain products of catabolism of the specific immunoglobulin produced by the monoclonal plasma cell proliferation.[68] The development of amyloid deposits within the tumour is likely therefore in view of the concentration of monoclonal antibodies in close proximity to the tumour cell. Little is known of the immunochemical activity of upper respiratory tract plasmacytoma but the structure of Russell bodies is gamma-globulin and, despite contrary opinions,[63] these bodies have been found by Michaels & Hyams in some of their cases.[69]

The classical histological appearances of plasmacytoma were described by Rawson et al in 1950 when they confirmed that locally malignant extramedullary disease was identical to the medullary form.[70] The presence of amyloid gives no indication of the malignant potential of the lesion although it is only present in primary plasmacytoma, not in metastases. Michaels & Hyams however, found that lesions with a mean nuclear diameter of more than 6 μm tended to behave in an aggressive fashion with a poor prognosis.[69]

Natural history

One of the most comprehensive accounts of the natural history of extramedullary plasmacytoma has been recorded by Wiltshaw based upon extensive personal experience and an analysis of the literature.[57] Single bone secondaries were found in 19% of patients but marrow involvement was uncommon. In 18% of all cases there was spread to at least one cervical lymph node but in one-third of these there was no further extension to other nodes in the neck. Spread also occurred to the skin, liver, lungs and the gastro-intestinal tract and the 10-year survival rate was estimated as greater than 50%.

Local recurrence or dissemination can occur many years after treatment of the primary lesion but lack of long-term follow-up data in patients uniformly treated prevents rationalization of treatment policies. Radio-therapy with surgery for residual or recurrent disease is favoured and 5-year survival figures of over 50% can be expected although many of these may fail with longer follow-up.

Differential diagnosis

Clinical diagnosis is unlikely and histologically, extra-medullary solitary plasmacytoma must be differentiated from the other conditions within the upper jaw with an abundance of plasma cells. Yaws, sarcoidosis, neuroblast-oma and reticulosarcoma as well as infections have all presented difficulties in the past although the availability of modern immunohistochemical techniques have markedly increased the facility of early, accurate identification of plasmacytoma.

Treatment

Many of the older publications included primary maxil-lectomy with orbital clearance as well as irradiation as the treatment of choice, all with variable short- and long-term success.[54,55] Survival appeared to correlate with duration of follow-up and the extent of the primary disease, with deaths most frequently associated with local extension or generalized disease. Small numbers of patients however, survived for long periods. Booth et al quote periods of between 3 and 22 years,[54] following irradiation. Poole & Marchetta in 1968 advocated primary radiotherapy for all localized disease with doses of between 5500 and 6000 rad given over 5 to 7 weeks.[71]

A 38-year-old woman was seen in February 1974 with swelling of the left face, numbness and slight proptosis, all for the past 3 months. There was a friable mass obscuring the left lateral nasal wall and radiologically the left maxillary antrum was opaque without bone erosion. Biopsy of the nasal mass was reported as typical of a plasmacytoma.

A skeletal survey, haematological and biochemical tests were all within normal limits and electrophoresis showed IgG 1090 mg/100 ml (normal 700–1800), IgA 165 mg/100 ml (normal 80–400) and IgM 395 mg/100 ml (normal 40–300). She was given 4947 rad of Co^{60} to the upper jaw and left neck over 50 days finishing April 1974.

Apart from recurrent attacks of bilateral maxillary sinusitis, treated conservatively with antral wash-outs and antibiotics, the patient has remained free of disease up to her last visit, May 1991 – 17 years post-irradiation.

Generalized disease requires systemic chemotherapy, possibly with Melphalan (Alkeran) or cyclophosphamide (Endoxan) and some success has been claimed over a short period of time.[67]

Prognosis

Long-term survival appears possible in at least half of all patients presenting with solitary extramedullary plasma-cytoma and treated with adequate dosage of irradiation with surgery for residual disease or recurrence. However, recurrence may occur many years later apparently after a good initial response and permanent follow-up is necessary. An increase in the number of marrow plasma cells by up to 6 to 8% with increased levels of serum immunoglobulins (especially IgA and IgG) has been suggested as an early indication of developing multiple myeloma.[59] The borderline between extramedullary plas-macytoma and multiple myeloma is difficult to define and some authors believe that both are in fact phases of the same condition.[56,61] The mean age at diagnosis is greater for multiple myeloma but increasingly lengthy follow-up of patients with controlled extramedullary plasmacytoma shows an increasing frequency of late-developing multiple myeloma; Carson et al reporting a patient 36 years after initial therapy.[64]

Long-term prognosis must therefore be guarded.

MIDLINE DESTRUCTIVE GRANULOMA

Definition

A slowly progressive, unrelenting ulceration and necrosis of the midline facial tissues.[72]

Synonyms

Stewart's granuloma, non-healing granuloma, granuloma gangrenescens, lethal midline granuloma, midline malig-nant reticulosis, polymorphic reticulosis, sacrolupus pernio, granulomatous ulcer of the nose and face, osteomyelitis necroticans and mutilating granuloma.[73]

Historical aspects

At the meeting of the Laryngological Society of London on 9 December 1896, Dr Peter McBride showed some photographs of a 28-year-old house painter with progres-sive destruction of the nose and face. The man had scratched his nose one year previously and this eventually had led to ulceration within the left nostril followed by destruction of the nose and upper lip.[74] He died 18 months after the initial consultation and since the patho-logists had failed to find evidence of malignancy, syphilis or tuberculosis at autopsy this case was presented as 'unusual'.

A more detailed account of a similar clinical condition was published by Sir Robert Woods in 1921 based upon two patients who he described as having 'a wave of granulation tissue advancing irregularly into healthy parts, breaking down behind as it advanced in front, so that there was never any great depth of pathological growth present'. The term 'malignant granuloma' was then suggested for this condition by his Dublin colleague Dr O'Sullivan.[75]

Woods described these lesions as disconcerting and enigmatic for both the pathologist and clinician, which aptly expresses the concept for many years of 'malignant granuloma' as a progressively destructive ulcerating lesion of the oronasal region without clearly defined pathological appearances.[76]

It is generally accepted that the first comprehensive account of the clinical and histological features of this condition was published by Stewart in 1933.[72] Ten cases with severe nasal ulceration were described in detail, although only two appeared to have been personally observed. The remainder came from other publications,

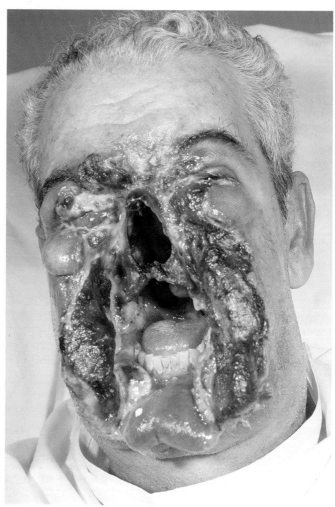

Fig. 17.5 Massive destruction of face in midfacial destructive granuloma.

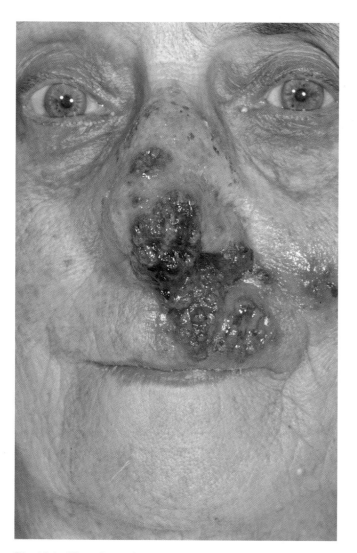

Fig. 17.4 Ulceration and crusting of midfacial destructive granuloma.

one going back over 35 years! Whilst admitting that the condition was rare, he wisely cited the many diseases that must be excluded before reaching a diagnosis of lethal granulomatous ulceration. One of these was an underlying malignancy, yet in three of his 10 patients quoted, pathologists had diagnosed 'atypical carcinoma, sarcoma and Hodgkin's lymphoma'. However, his clinical classification provided an accurate description of the manifestations of the disease being divided into three stages.

1. Prodromal. This may last for many years with the patient complaining of persistent nasal obstruction and rhinorrhoea. Minor nasal surgery to relieve these symptoms is common, as has been described by Harrison in his account of 36 patients with midline destructive granuloma.[39]

2. Period of activity. Areas of necrosis develop on and around the nasal cavity resulting in purulent discharge, crusting and tissue loss (Fig. 17.4). Expansion with involvement of the nasal framework, palate, pharynx or

orbit may occur together with an associated pyrexia secondary to infection.

3. Terminal stage. Exhaustion, haemorrhage, gross mutilation of the face but without pain leads eventually to death, usually after many years and fruitless attempts to establish a definitive diagnosis (Fig. 17.5).

As more cases were published however, it became clear that many patients did not fit this classical description with instances where patients died from metastases to lymph nodes or lungs. Variations in the histological appearances suggested in some patients a neoplasm, and the detailed autopsy report of Spears & Walker in 1956 suggested that the lesion was a lymphoma.[77] Unfortunately, limited personal experience resulted in some authors failing to appreciate the wide variations in the natural history and histological appearances of this condition. Walton in 1959 studied only five cases and then stated confidently that dissemination never occurred. Those that did so, he said, had been wrongly diagnosed being almost certainly sarcomata.[78]

This controversy was not helped by Friedmann who in 1963, whilst accepting that malignant granuloma could disseminate suggested that there was a definite relationship with Wegener's granulomatosis.[79]

In recent years attention has been drawn to the difficulty of differentiating histologically nasal lymphoma from chronic inflammation. Eichel et al (1966) reported seven patients diagnosed clinically as having lethal midline granuloma but who, after repeated biopsies, proved to have malignant lymphoma.[51] They also drew attention to the histological similarity between pleomorphic reticulosis and lethal granuloma. Michaels & Gregory reexamining tissue from 30 patients diagnosed as midline granuloma or Wegener's granuloma found that 10 cases selected on the basis of widespread necrosis with atypical cellular exudate, which they named as NACE, represented a malignant neoplasm of histiocytic lymphoma type.[80] Erythrophagocytic activity was marked and infiltration within the marrow indicated a more generalized activity and it is now recognized that some of these patients have T-cell type lymphomas.[81]

Incidence

Inconsistency in terminology and histopathological criteria, together with reliance on small collective series for clinical descriptions and natural history, has resulted in an absence of reliable data relating to world-wide incidence rates. Figures of 1 per 25 000 population probably include patients who later prove to have been wrongly diagnosed but some guidance may be obtained from the publications of Harrison based upon 27 years working in a specialized ear, nose and throat hospital and known for his interest and experience in both midline destructive

lesions of the face and Wegener's granuloma.[39,82] 42 patients were diagnosed as having a midline destructive granuloma and although six of these were eventually shown to have a T-cell lymphoma he suggested that all were probably manifestations of this tumour. Distinction between polymorphic reticulosis, NACE or other neoplasms with necrosis and inflammation may be dependent on the use of monoclonal antibodies. Increasing use of these techniques is leading to greater diagnosis of lymphoma in these cases.[83]

Age, sex and ethnic variation

Batsakis & Luna in their clear account of the differential diagnosis of midfacial necrotizing lesions[84] give a 2:1 female preponderance with a median age incidence of 41 years (range 9 to 59 years). No data are given for the basis on which these figures are produced but Harrison's series of 36 patients had a range of 23 to 72 years without a definite sex or ethnic variation.[85] This probably accurately reflects the data for this uncommon condition, although more accurate diagnosis may eventually present a picture closer to classical extranodal nasal lymphoma.

Site

Initially most patients present with what appears to be non-specific rhinitis which gradually progresses to crusting on the nasal mucosa with some bleeding after crust removal. Extension of crusting, ulceration with some discomfort and involvement of surrounding skin is followed by tissue loss. The ulceration extends both superficially and deeply to involve bone or cartilage and is eventually followed by massive destruction of the face (Fig. 17.5). Slow progression combined with difficulties in determining the exact amount of tissue loss makes localization of the site of origin difficult to determine. In most cases the septum is involved early in the disease.

Aetiology

Despite the common histological features of necrosis and non-specific inflammation, no causal organism has been found. Early authors sought a relationship with syphilis and other conditions familiar at that time, whilst confusion with Wegener's granuloma inevitably raised the possibility of an immunological reaction. Walton[78] commented that midline facial tissues had the capacity for localizing antigens and this may be of some significance in the aetiology of Wegener's granuloma but not with destructive granulomas.

The availability of monoclonal antibodies and immunochemical techniques has increasingly confirmed that many (if not all) of midline destructive granulomata are T-cell lymphoma, with varying degrees of necrosis and activity.[86] The aetiology of lymphoreticular neoplasms is still undecided as is the role of exogenous carcinogens and viral infections. However, the development of sarcomata following immunosuppression is well recognized and Duvall et al described two patients who developed midline granulomata following renal transplantation with prolonged immunosuppression.[87]

Clinical features

In 1974 Kornblut & Fauci[88] gave one of the earliest accounts of patients with progressive lethal facial destruction and these bear some similarity to the active lesions seen today. However, the absence of reliable clinical and histological data from most early reports makes it almost impossible to exclude the many common conditions of past years which could have caused confusion and misdiagnosis. A typical case history was published by Friedmann et al[89] in 1978.

A 63-year-old woman suffered from repeated nasal obstruction and sinusitis leading eventually to nasal polypectomy in 1959. She remained trouble-free until 1963 when her persistent nasal stuffiness, rhinorrhoea and alar swelling led to a further nasal polypectomy and septal surgery. This was followed within 6 months by some facial pain, fever and purulent rhinorrhoea. Examination showed loss of the whole septum with crusting in both nasal passages. Biopsy showed gross necrosis with pleomorphic granulation tissue but without giant cells or periarteritis. There was no evidence of any systemic abnormality and she was given 1000 rad of Co^{60} irradiation together with 60 mg prednisolone. There was local improvement but 4 months later there was evidence of further tissue loss and she died from pneumonia with middle fossa invasion, 6 years after the onset of symptoms. Autopsy confirmed the diagnosis of 'lethal midline granuloma' with destruction of nasal septum, maxillary and ethmoid sinuses together with the palate. There was extension into the orbit and middle fossa but the kidneys, lungs and other organs remained unaffected.

A more dramatic case was described by Harrison where the complete midface had been destroyed over a period of 6 years. Active granulation tissue was still macroscopically present at the margins of the defect and were reported as showing 'the non-specific' features of a Stewart's granuloma. The erythrocytic sedimentation rate (ESR) was 90 mm in 1 hour but there was no evidence of disease elsewhere.[82] This patient illustrated in Harrison's paper of 1987[39] is perhaps more typical of the clinical presentation seen today. With a 1 year history of nasal obstruction, epistaxis and crusting over the dorsum of the nose, multiple biopsies eventually produced a diagnosis of NACE. Separation of the crusts revealed a large defect of skin and underlying bone. 2 years after irradiation of 2500 rad of Co^{60} a T-cell lymphoma developed which has been controlled with additional radiotherapy.

Characteristically, these patients have a long history of nasal obstruction for which minor nasal surgery has been performed unsuccessfully. There is usually a history of frequent attacks of sinusitis and eventually crusting followed by ulceration appears within the nasal cavity. Nasal septum, turbinates, ethmoids and the palate are involved.[90] Extension into the orbit or skull base occurs in the untreated or late case and the end result is gross facial destruction.

Radiology

There are no specific features of midline destructive granuloma although the consistent features of soft tissue and bone destruction without a gross tumour mass may arouse suspicion (Fig. 17.6). Computerized tomography will show the extent of the disease whilst the T2 weighted tissue response may be helpful in differential diagnosis.

Macroscopic and microscopic appearance

The problems of both clinical and histological identification of necrotizing lesions affecting the upper airway have been identified by Batsakis in 1982.[92] Although the clinical

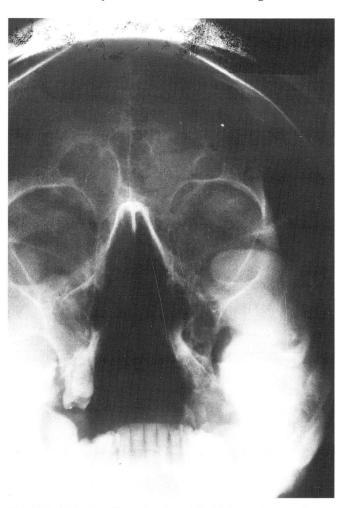

Fig. 17.6 Plain sinus X-ray showing midfacial destructive granuloma with central loss of hard palate, nasal bones and ethmoid labyrinths (Lloyd 1988[91]).

history and behaviour of destructive midline granulomata is in many cases characteristic, there has been a failure by histopathologists to identify a lesion, whose local (and occasionally systemic) behaviour is neoplastic. The consistent features of non-specific inflammation and necrosis has previously led to a diagnosis 'by exclusion'. Indeed, cases still exist where even the most diligent search with repeated biopsies fails to detect any cellular areas. Granulomas and giant cells are rare as is the intense arteritis found in Wegener's granuloma. In recent years attention has been drawn to the difficulty of distinguishing lymphomata from chronic inflammation when the nasal tissues are involved. Eichel et al[51] found that seven patients diagnosed as malignant granuloma were in fact malignant lymphoma and this was also the experience of Michaels & Gregory in 10 of 30 cases re-examined.[80] However, in their paper of 1966, Eichel et al gave the name of polymorphic reticulosis to their non-lymphoma cases[51] and Gauland et al[81] have confirmed that this is a variant of 'angiocentric T-cell lymphoma'. This view is shared by Jaffe[83] who proposes that all patients with lethal midline granuloma should be investigated for the presence of a T-cell clone and then staged as for other lymphomata.

It appears that there is a marked similarity between polymorphic reticulosis and NACE, although the cytological features of the cells may not always suggest malignancy. The atypical cells are described by Michaels & Gregory as arranged in broad groups with a fine reticulum pattern surrounding individual cells. They are frequently accompanied by areas of necrosis and may be seen to infiltrate nerve, bone, muscle or arterial wall providing evidence of an invasive destructive neoplasm.[80]

Aozasa described the biopsy findings in 19 patients diagnosed clinically as lethal midline granuloma. 11 showed pleomorphic reticulosis which subsequently changed to a monoclonal pattern. These cells showed cytochemical evidence of a non-specific esterase suggesting a histiocystic origin and the autopsy findings in 10 of these patients indicated death from a malignant histiocytosis.[93] However, Chan et al (1987) using monoclonal antibodies and immunochemistry, have confirmed that the lesion is of T-cell type[94] and their findings have been confirmed by Yamanaka et al in 1985[95] and by Ramsay et al in 1988.[86] Thus there is now clear evidence that in patients with progressive midline destructive granuloma there is an underlying T-cell lymphoma. Only by repeated biopsies (avoiding if possible areas of gross necrosis) and employing modern immunohistochemical techniques will the correct diagnosis be supported.

Natural history

Untreated, slow destruction of the midfacial region can be expected to progress with death eventually occurring from infection, haemorrhage, local extension or inanition. This was the usual outcome prior to the appreciation that, like other lymphomata, irradiation would control the local disease. However, Harrison in his analysis of 36 patients treated personally over many years, found that despite effective local control some patients died from disseminated lymphoma, particularly after non-curative dosage radiotherapy.[39] Many of these patients on histological review proved to have NACE, whilst others showing only necrosis and inflammation were cured by low doses of irradiation.[85] It appears therefore that those lesions which show cellular exudate (called either NACE or polymorphic reticulosis) and which might now be expected to be confirmed as a T-cell lymphoma, require full oncologic dose irradiation and are at risk of developing lymphomatosis.

Differential diagnosis

It now appears unlikely that midline destructive granuloma exists as a distinct pathological entity, although cases clearly exist where clinical evidence of midfacial destruction is accompanied by histological evidence of no more than gross necrosis and non-specific inflammation. Persistent search for cellular areas together with the use of immunohistochemistry will undoubtedly lead to a reduction in the 'undiagnosed' cases.

All patients with nasal ulceration must be investigated routinely to exclude the wide range of more common conditions which present at this site. These have been tabulated by Michaels[25c] and include rhinoscleroma, tuberculosis, syphilis, sarcoid, carcinoma and Wegener's granuloma. The latter has been misdiagnosed in the past because of occasional histological similarities. However, it is a systemic disease, rarely localized only to the nose and never producing the gross destruction which is the major feature of a midline destructive granuloma.

Treatment

There is no reliable evidence to support the localized cure of a midline granuloma (NACE or polymorphic reticulosis) using antibiotics, surgery or steroids. In 1960 Dickson & Cantab reported successful local control with irradiation[85] and it has now been accepted that this is the most effective treatment of the local condition. Initially, dosage varied with individual radiotherapists many of whom were reluctant to use a cancerocidal regime for what was then considered to be a non-neoplastic disease. Many of Harrison's patients were treated in the early 1960s with between 1000 and 4000 rad.[39] However, some of those receiving no more than 3000 rad developed local or disseminated lymphoma 6 months to 3 years later and it is now accepted that doses of at least 5000 rad of supervoltage irradiation with wide field coverage including the nose, sinuses and palate is essential for successful long-term control.

Tsokos et al reported 11 patients with NACE, treated with 4000–6000 rad of Co^{60} with good response lasting between 6 months and 18 years.[96] Harrison's patients showed survivals ranging from 2 to 19 years following irradiation.[39]

Prognosis

The well recognized dramatic response of an occasional patient with a midline destructive granuloma to doses as low as 800 rad of irradiation illustrates the varied malignant potential seen within the full spectrum of this disease. The absence of detectable NACE or polymorphic reticulosis supports the concept that the most 'benign' variety of this condition might be expected to respond favourably to low doses of irradiation. However, immuno-chemistry can be expected to detect the underlying T-cell lymphoma more frequently and most patients must be treated with full dose radiotherapy. Late development of local or disseminated lymphoma worsens the prognosis, as it does in primary extra-nodal nasal lymphoma. Since it is unlikely that every patient presenting with a destructive midfacial granuloma will be confirmed as a T-cell lymphoma the term 'middle destructive granuloma' appears to serve as an adequate initial diagnostic title.

REFERENCES

1. Burkitt D 1958 A sarcoma involving jaws in African children. British Journal of Surgery 46: 218–223
2. Burkitt D 1961 Observations of the geography of malignant lymphoma. East African Medical Journal 38: 511–514
3. Burkitt D, Wright D 1966 Geographical and tribal distribution of the African lymphoma in Uganda. British Medical Journal 1: 569–573
4. Khan A G 1964 The multifocal lymphoma syndrome in African children in Kenya. Journal of Laryngology and Otology 78: 480–498
5. Clifford P, Singh S, Sternsward J 1967 Longterm survival of patients with Burkitt's lymphoma. An assessment of treatment and other factors which may relate to survival. Cancer Research 27: 2578–2615
6. Nkrumah F K, Perkins I V 1976 Burkitt's lymphoma. A clinical study of 110 patients. Cancer 37: 671–676
7. Kummona R 1977 Jaw lymphoma in Middle East children. British Journal of Oral Surgery 15: 153–159
8. Wright D H 1970 Burkitt's lymphoma. E & S Livingstone, Edinburgh, p. 83
9. Hoogstraten J 1967 Burkitt's lymphoma. International Journal of Cancer 2: 566–569
10. Leader article 1968 Reappraisal of Burkitt's lymphoma. British Medical Journal Feb. 10
11. Dodge O G 1965 Pathology of the African lymphoma. Journal of Laryngology and Otology 79: 940–946
12. Ziegler J L 1981 Burkitt's lymphoma. New England Journal of Medicine 305: 735–749
13. Berry C G 1964 Lymphoma syndrome in Northern Nigeria. British Medical Journal 2: 668–670
14. Batsakis J J 1979 Tumours of the head and neck, 2nd edn. Williams & Wilkins, Baltimore, p 360.
15. Haddow A J 1964 Relations between the incidence of Burkitt's lymphoma and yellow fever. East African Medical Journal 41: 1–6
16. Bell T M, Massie A, Williams M C 1964 Isolation of a reovirus from a case of Burkitt's lymphoma. British Medical Journal 1: 1212–1213
17. Keast D, Stanley N F 1966 Production of Burkitt's lymphoma in mice with reovirus 3. Proceedings of the Society for Experimental Biology (NY) 122: 1091–1097
18. Shepherd J, Woodward C G, Turnbull L 1987 Epstein-Barr virus and jaw tumours in Northern Nigeria. Cancer 59: 1150–1153
19. Adatia A K 1978 Significance of jaw tumours in Burkitt's lymphoma. British Dental Journal 145: 263–266
20. Henle G, Henle W, Clifford P, et al 1969 Antibodies to EBV in Burkitt's lymphoma and control groups. Journal of the National Cancer Institute 43: 263-266
21. Nonayama M, Huang C H, Pagano J S 1973 DNA of Epstein-Barr virus detected in tissues of Burkitt's lymphoma and nasopharyngeal cancer. Proceedings of the National Academy of Sciences USA 70: 3205–3268
22. Old L J, Boyse E A, Oettgen H F et al 1966 Precipitating antibody in human serum to an antigen present in cultured Burkitt's lymphoma. Proceedings of the National Academy of Science USA 56: 1699–1704
23. Whittaker L R 1973 Burkitt's lymphoma. Clinical Radiology 24: 339–342
24. Lennert K 1981 Histopathology of non-Hodgkin's lymphoma (based on the Kiel classification). Springer-Verlag, Berlin
25. Michaels L 1987 Ear, nose and throat histopathology. Springer-Verlag, Berlin, a: p 280; b: Ch. 22; c: p 163
26. Katayama I, Uehara H, Gleser R A 1974 The value of the electron microscope in the diagnosis of Burkitt's lymphoma. American Journal of Clinical Pathology 61: 540–546
27. Clifford P 1968 Treatment of Burkitt's lymphoma. Lancet, March 16, p. 599
28. Leader article 1966 Chemotherapy of Burkitt's lymphoma, Lancet Oct. 8, p 788
29. McClatchey K D (ed) 1987 Comprehensive management of head and neck tumours, Ch. 71. Lymphoreticular disorders of the head and neck. Saunders, Philadelphia
30. Rosenberg S A, Diamond H D, Jaskowitz B 1961 Lymphosarcoma: a review of 1269 cases. Medicine 40: 31–46
31. Wilder W H, Harner J G, Banks P M 1983 Lymphoma of the nose and paranasal sinuses. Archives of Otolaryngology 109: 310–312
32. McNelis C L, Pai V T 1969 Malignant lymphoma of the head and neck. Laryngoscope 79: 1076–1087
33. Freeman C, Berg J W, Cutler C S 1972 Occurrence and prognosis of extranodal lymphoma. Cancer 29: 252–260
34. Gall E A, Mallory T B 1942 Malignant lymphoma: a clinicopathological survey of 618 cases. American Journal of Pathology 18: 381–429
35. Catlin D 1966 Surgery for head and neck lymphoma. Surgery 60: 1160–1166
36. Duncavage J A, Campbell B H, Hanson G A et al 1983 Diagnosis of malignant lymphomas of the nasal cavity, paranasal sinuses and nasopharynx. Laryngoscope 93: 1276–1280
37. Kapadia J B, Barnes L, Deutsch M 1981 Non-Hodgkin's lymphoma of the nose and paranasal sinuses. A study of 17 cases. Head and Neck Surgery 3: 490–499
38. Robbins K T, Fuller L M, Osborne B 1985 Primary lymphoma of the nasal cavity and paranasal sinuses. Cancer 56: 814–819
39. Harrison D F N 1987 Midline destructive granuloma. Laryngoscope 97: 1049–1053
40. Steg R F, Dahlin D C, Gores R J 1959 Malignant lymphoma of the mandible and maxilla. Oral Surgery 12: 128–141
41. Tindle B H 1984 Malignant lymphoma. American Journal of Pathology 116: 119–124
42. Manual of Staging of Cancer 1978 American Joint Committee for Cancer Staging and End-Results Whiting Press, Chicago

43. Manual for Staging of Cancer 1983 American Joint Committee for Cancer Staging and End-Results. J B Lippincott, Philadelphia
44. Aisenberg A C 1973 Malignant lymphoma. New England Journal of Medicine 288: 883–890
45. Portlock C S, Glatstein E 1978 The non-Hodgkin's lymphoma - current concepts and management. Annual Review of Medicine 29: 81–91
46. Reimer D R, Chabner B A, Young R C 1977 Lymphomas presenting in bone. Annals of Internal Medicine 87: 50–56
47. Rappaport H 1966 Tumours of the haematopoietic system. Armed Forces Institute of Pathology. Fascicle 8
48. Conley J F, Staszak C, Clamon G H 1987 Non-Hodgkin's lymphoma of the head and neck: the University of Iowa experience. Laryngoscope 97: 291–300
49. Burres S A, Crissman J D, McKenna J 1984 Lymphoma of the frontal sinus. Archives of Otolarynlogy 110: 270–273
50. Rosenberg S A, Berard C W, Brown B W 1982 National Cancer Institute sponsored study of classification of non-Hodgkin's lymphoma. Cancer 49: 2112–2135
51. Eichel B S, Harrison E G, Devine K D 1966 Primary lymphoma of the nose including a relationship to lethal midline granuloma. American Journal of Surgery 112: 597–605
52. Berard C W 1981 A multidisciplinary approach to non-Hodgkin's lymphoma. Annals of Internal Medicine 94: 218–235
53. Cabanillas F, Bodney G P, Freireich E J 1980 Management with chemotherapy of stage 1 and 2 malignant lymphomas of aggressive histologic type. Cancer 46: 2356–2359
54. Booth J B, Cheesman A D, Vincenti N H 1973 Extramedullary plasmacytoma of the upper respiratory tract. Annals of Otology, Rhinology and Laryngology 82: 709–715
55. Castro E B, Lewis J S, Strong E W 1973 Plasmacytoma of paranasal sinuses and nasal cavity. Archives of Otolaryngology 97: 326–329
56. Ewing M R, Foote F W 1952 Plasma cell tumours of the mouth and air passages. Cancer 5: 499–513
57. Wiltshaw E 1976 The natural history of extramedullary plasmacytoma and its relation to solitary myeloma of bone and myelomatosis. Medicine 55: 217–238
58. Webb H E, Harrison E G, Masson J K 1962 Solitary extramedullary plasmacytoma of the upper part of the respiratory tract and oropharynx. Cancer 15: 1142–1155
59. Pahor A L 1977 Extramedullary plasmacytoma of the head and neck, parotid and submandibular gland. Journal of Laryngology and Otology 91: 241–257
60. Helmus C 1964 Extramedullary plasmacytoma of the head and neck. Laryngoscope 74: 553–559
61. Dolin J, Dewar J P 1956 Extramedullary plasmacytoma. American Journal of Pathology 32: 83–103
62. Youssef B, Touma L 1971 Extramedullary plasmacytoma of the head and neck. Journal of Laryngology and Otology 85: 125–128
63. Stout A P, Kenny F R 1949 Primary plasma cell tumours of the upper air passages and oral cavity. Cancer 2: 261–278
64. Carson C P, Ackerman L V, Maltby J D 1955 Late dissemination of extramedullary plasmacytoma. American Journal of Clinical Pathology 25: 849–852
65. Willis R A 1967 Pathology of tumours, 4th edn. Butterworths, London, p 795
66. Schabel S I, Rogers C L, Rittenberg G M 1978 Extramedullary plasmacytoma. Radiology 128: 625–630
67. Chaudhuri J N, Khatri B B, Chattersi P 1988 Plasmacytoma of the nose with intracranial spread. Journal of Laryngology and Otology 102: 538–539
68. Osserman E F, Takatsuki K, Talal N 1964 The pathogenesis of amyloidosis. Seminar of Haematology 1: 3–10
69. Michaels L, Hyams V J 1978 Amyloid in localised deposits and plasmacytomas of the respiratory tract. Journal of Pathology 128: 29–38
70. Rawson A J, Eyler P W, Horn R 1950 Plasma cell tumours of the upper respiratory tract: clinicopathological study with emphasis on criteria for histological diagnosis. American Journal of Pathology 26: 445–461
71. Poole A G, Marchetta F C 1968 Extramedullary plasmacytoma of the head and neck. Cancer 22: 14–21
72. Stewart J P 1933 Progressive lethal granulomatous ulceration of the nose. Journal of Laryngology and Otology 48: 657–701
73. Butler D S, Thompson H 1972 Malignant granuloma. British Journal of Oral Surgery 11: 128–132
74. McBride P 1897 Photographs of a case of rapid destruction of the nose and face. Journal of Laryngology and Otology 12: 64–65
75. Woods R 1921 Malignant granuloma of the nose. British Medical Journal 2: 65–68
76. Walton E W 1933 Non-healing granulomata of the nose. Journal of Laryngology and Otology 73: 4–7
77. Spears G S, Walker W G 1956 Lethal midline granuloma (granuloma gangraenescens). Bulletin of the Johns Hopkins Hospital 99: 313–332
78. Walton E W 1959 More thoughts on non-healing nasal granulomata. Journal of Laryngology and Otology 73: 242–246
79. Friedmann I 1963 The pathology of midline granuloma. Proceedings of the Royal Society of Medicine 57: 289–297
80. Michaels L, Gregory M M 1977 Pathology of non-healing midline granuloma. Journal of Clinical Pathology 30: 317–327
81. Gauland P, Henni T, Haioun C 1988 Lethal midline granuloma (polymorphic reticulosis) and lymphomatoid granulomatosis. Cancer 62: 705–710
82. Harrison D F N 1974 Non-healing granulomata of the upper respiratory tract. British Medical Journal 4: 205–209
83. Jaffe E S 1984 Pathology and spectrum of post-thymic T-cell malignancies. Cancer Investigations 2: 413–426
84. Batsakis J G, Luna M A 1987 Midfacial necrotizing lesions. Seminars in Diagnostic Pathology 4: 90–116
85. Dickson R, Cantab D 1960 Radiotherapy of lethal midline granuloma. Journal of Chronic Diseases 12: 417–421
86. Ramsay A D, Michaels L, Harrison D F N 1988 Lethal midline granuloma - a T-cell lymphoma. Journal of Pathology 154: 56A
87. Duvall A J, Nelms C R, Williams H L 1969 Midline granuloma in patients with immunosuppression. Transactions of the American Academy of Ophthalmology and Otolaryngology 73: 1187–1189
88. Kornblut A D, Fauci A 1974 Non-healing granulomata of the upper respiratory tract. Otolaryngologic Clinics of North America 15: 685–692
89. Friedmann I, Sando I, Balkany T 1978 Idiopathic pleomorphic midfacial granuloma. Journal of Laryngology and Otology 92: 601–611
90. Butler D S 1972 Malignant granuloma. British Journal of Oral Surgery 9: 208–221
91. Lloyd G A S 1988 Diagnostic imaging of the nose and paranasal sinuses. Springer Verlag, Berlin
92. Batsakis J G 1982 Midfacial necrotizing diseases. Annals of Otology, Rhinology and Laryngology 91: 541–542
93. Aozasa K 1982 Biopsy findings in malignant histiocytosis presenting as lethal midline granuloma. Journal of Clinical Pathology 35: 599–605
94. Chan J K, Ng S, Lau W H 1987 Most nasal lymphomas are peripheral T-cell neoplasms. American Journal of Surgical Pathology 11: 418–429
95. Yamanaka N, Kataura A, Sambe S 1985 Midfacial T-cell lymphoma. Characterization by monoclonal antibodies. Annals of Otology, Rhinology and Laryngology 94: 207–211
96. Tsokos M, Fauci A S, Costa J 1982 Idiopathic midline destructive disease, a subgroup of patients with midline granuloma. American Journal of Clinical Pathology 77: 162–168

18. Wegener's granulomatosis

Definition

Characterized by necrotizing granulomas, vasculitis of the upper respiratory tract and systemic vasculitis.

Synonyms

There are none, only confusion in terminology and errors in diagnosis.

Historical aspects

In 1931 Heinz Klinger at the University of Berlin reported post-mortem studies on two patients who had died of prolonged sepsis with disseminated vasculitis.[1] He believed that this was an untypical form of polyarteritis nodosa. 5 years later, Frederick Wegener in Breslau described a syndrome comprising of necrotizing granulomas of the respiratory tract, generalized arteritis and renal changes similar to those found in toxic glomerulonephritis in patients dying from sepsis.[2] He published a more detailed account of the natural history of this condition in 1939 under the name of 'rhinogenic granulomatosis'.[3] All the patients died between 4 and 7 months after diagnosis from irreversible renal disease.

In 1954, detailed reviews by Fahey et al[4] and Goodman & Churg[5] describing a total of seven patients, established definitive criteria for the diagnosis of what is now termed 'Wegener's granulomatosis'. They described the pathological changes of disseminating necrotizing vasculitis involving both arteries and veins of the upper respiratory tract, together with glomerulonephritis, although they appreciated that this was a generalized condition in which any organ could be involved.

Carrington & Liebow in 1966[6] recognized that a more limited form of Wegener's granulomatosis could occur describing 16 patients with pulmonary lesions identical to those seen in this disease but initially without evidence of disease elsewhere. Some of these cases survived for years without other clinical 'manifestations'

or glomerulonephritis, although six died quite rapidly from widespread Wegener's granulomatosis. The basis for concluding that limited forms of the disease could exist appears to be founded on the seven patients who remained alive for more than 6 months, some of whom had received no treatment, the others varying doses of steroids! This view was supported by Cassan et al in 1970 although they also found that some patients initially presenting with just pulmonary lesions soon developed disease elsewhere.[7]

DeRemee et al[8] have shown that interest in systemic vasculitis started with Kussman & Maier's paper on periarteritis nodosa in 1866; they described how all vasculitides were called periarteritis nodosa until the late 1930s. Then Klinger in 1931[1] and later Wegener[2] described patients whose 'vasculitis' differed from periarteritis nodosa and eventually by general convention Wegener's granulomatosis was the name given to these patients. Wegener's description of this condition was unique since he correlated histological criteria with clinical observation emphasizing that no granulomas are found in periarteritis nodosa.[9] Later accounts did little more than confirm these pathological findings, confirming that although initially localized, this is a systemic disease with protean manifestations.

Incidence

The clinical incidence is difficult to determine, for inconsistency in terminology and the occasional error in applying accepted diagnostic criteria, have resulted in a possible degree of underreporting. The classical description emphasizes renal involvement but many patients present without this and the nose and sinuses are the commonest site for initial presentation. However, any organ can be involved and in unusual sites this may lead to delay in diagnosis due to inexperience with this uncommon condition.

Age and sex variation

The age distribution shows a broad spectrum ranging from adolescence to the 7th decade of life. McDonald & DeRemee have published a series of 108 patients showing equal sex incidence and an age range of between 8 and 75 years.[9] This is similar to our own unpublished experience of 48 patients. Halstead et al[10] in their series of 50 patients found that 10 (20%) were under the age of 25 years, varying from 13 to 23 years of age. They concluded that, contrary to current opinion, Wegener's granulomatosis occurs quite frequently in young people, usually in a generalized form.

Site

Most publications confirm that this disease predominates within the respiratory tract and kidneys. However diagnosis depends to some extent upon the site of the presenting symptoms, although in active cases other organs may be rapidly involved. Consequently, the frequency with which individual sites are involved, both initially and subsequently vary within published reports reflecting the author's speciality and interest. In many it is unclear as to whether the author is differentiating between symptoms at diagnosis or late involvement but Table 18.1 summarizes data from the larger and more reliable publications. These figures emphasize variations in system involvement but confirm that in most patients the respiratory tract and kidneys will be affected at some stage of the disease. However, Batsakis has emphasized that diagnosis cannot be made solely on renal involvement since necrotizing glomerulitis is non-specific.[11]

This disease may evolve from a single presenting focus then rapidly progressing to affect other systems, or remain stationary within the respiratory tract without renal involvement. This possibly represents interpatient differ-ences within the natural history of the disease or for some as yet unknown reason, local control. Neither can be anticipated with our present state of knowledge.

Aetiology

The pathogenesis is unknown although the histological resemblance to polyarteritis nodosa has suggested a hypersensitivity reaction based upon a misdirected immune response to an unknown stimulus. Many attempts have been made to implicate an antigen, particularly inhaled bacteria, to explain the frequency with which the respiratory tract is involved. Shillitoe et al[12] studied 10 patients with Wegener's granulomatosis, finding some association between an intact macrophage migration-inhibition function and impaired skin delayed hypersensitivity and lymphocyte transformation to a number of antigens. They suggested that Wegener's granulomatosis might be associated with a partial cell-mediated immunodeficiency. However, all except two of their patients were already receiving immunosuppressive drugs.

The deposition of immune complexes is thought to be responsible for vasculitis in other conditions, although they have only been demonstrated in a small proportion of patients with Wegener's granulomatosis.[13,14] It has been suggested that following deposition of these complexes in the vessel wall, inflammation and leucocyte destruction lead to platelet aggregation and fibrin deposition, producing further vascular obstruction and necrosis. However, McDonald & DeRemee reported that the results of immunofluorescence microscopy of renal biopsies in this condition rarely show deposition of immunoglobulin and complement.[9] Occasionally, scattered deposits of IgG and C3 are seen forming an irregular linear pattern not typical of the smooth linear pattern seen in established auto-immune diseases. Their findings of

Table 18.1 Sites of involvement of Wegener's granulomatosis: cited in the literature

System involved (% of patients)	Kornblut et al 1980[40]	Illum & Thorling 1981[23]	McDonald & DeRemee 1982[9]	Harrison & Lund
Nose – paranasal sinuses	90	82	96	100
Lungs	100	88	61	65
Larynx – trachea	6	24	13	6
Ears	36	47	21	18
Kidneys	85	35	45	30
CNS	15	29	12	14
Eye	55	24	24	16
Joints – muscle	48	41	–	5
Skin	37	29	15	20
Cardiovascular system	17	12	–	–
Mouth etc.	–	18	2	4
Total no. patients in study	47	17	108	48

impaired delayed hypersensitivity and lymphocytic transformation to non-specific antigens does support the conception of Shillitoe et al that this is an auto-immune disease.[12]

Acute Wegener's granulomatosis is characterized by widespread inflammation, cell necrosis and infection which are all associated with elevation of IgA, IgE and IgD, as well as C-reactive protein. This may explain the discrepancies between authors when reporting this data since the degree of tissue damage varies with the acuteness and extent of the disease in individual patients.

Of considerable aetiological and diagnostic importance is the finding of antibodies reacting with the cytoplasm of ethanol-fixed granulocytes and monocytes in 25 patients with Wegener's granulomatosis, reported by der Woude et al in 1985.[15] Although this finding was initially questioned by Hinde & Pepys[16] who suggested that elevation of the C-reactive protein was a constant feature of this disease and simpler to estimate, Lockwood et al[17] have now shown that patients with microscopic polyarteritis (MP) also have circulating autoantibodies to neutrophil cytoplasmic antigens (ANCA). They suggest that these autoantibodies may be fundamental to the development of systemic vasculitides being directed towards at least one epitope of the enzyme alkaline phosphatase. In general patients with Wegener's granulomatosis have cytoplasmic or C-ANCA whereas those with MP may show perinuclear (P-ANCA) or C-ANCA. The antigenic targets of ANCA have been defined, with most C-ANCA recognizing a 29 kD serine proteinase in neutrophil primary granules now identified as proteinase-3. A cDNA clone encoding it has been isolated.[18]

Although the pathogenicity of ANCA has not been proven, there is evidence for their role in disease. ANCA are more readily detected in patients with active Wegener's granulomatosis and titres of ANCA have been found to correlate with disease activity.[19,20] Cohen-Tervaert et al[21] showed that a four-fold rise in titre of ANCA predicted a clinical relapse, and proceeded to a trial of treatment response to rising titres. Patients with a four-fold rise in titres were randomized to receive treatment or await evidence of disease. Not surprisingly, the treated group showed no relapses in contradistinction to the untreated patients. However, it is known that ANCA can be found without overt disease and it remains controversial whether immunosuppression should be based on serological grounds alone.

There is some evidence for the pathogenic role of ANCA from in vitro experiments. Incubation of C- and P-ANCA, or their F(ab)2 fragments with normal neutrophils (primed with TNF) leads to degranulation and to a respiratory burst.[22] There is also some evidence that ANCA can stimulate primed neutrophils to cause endothelial cell injury.

How can the autoantibody present in these vasculitides induce tissue injury? One possibility is a combination with the antigen in the fluid phase with formation of soluble immune complexes. These retain enzymatic activity, and if deposited in tissue would produce local damage.

Clinical features

The classical presentation of Wegener's granulomatosis with vasculitis of the respiratory tract together with fulminating glomerulonephritis and systemic vasculitis, is well recognized and frequently fatal. Fortunately, this is now a distorted impression of the patients most usually seen by the ear, nose and throat surgeon, although subacute or chronic cases whilst offering greater possibility of control, do pose problems in diagnosis. This is of great importance since rapid progression with a fatal outcome can occur within 48 hours.

The duration of significant symptoms before diagnosis is variable, being related to both site and severity of the disease. Anecdotal evidence suggests an average of 4 months, but the range may be as short as 24 hours or as long as a year in the most 'chronic' cases.[23] Most patients present with a short history of progressive malaise, pyrexia, weight loss and a disproportionate feeling of 'unwellness', in relation to what at this time is often fairly non-specific physical findings. This may result in delay whilst investigations are carried out, although an ESR (erythrocyte sedimentation test) of over 80 mm/hour, a constant finding in acute cases, should arouse suspicion. In more than 80% of patients, the nose and sinuses will be involved with complaints of nasal obstruction, rhinorrhoea and vague pain. This is usually followed by crusting and slight bleeding with friable granulation tissue and septal perforation, although this may be iatrogenic following enthusiastic biopsies. The perforation rarely involves the bony septum in contradistinction to more malignant conditions. However, subsequent infection often leads to collapse of the nasal bridge (Fig. 18.1).

Ostial obstruction with pansinusitis may result in permanent mucosal damage requiring sinus surgery following control of the primary disease, although Wegener's granulomatosis does itself affect the mucosal lining resulting eventually in destruction.

Problems in diagnosis occur in those patients whose disease remains localized to the nose or sinuses. Failure to consider Wegener's granulomatosis, or at worse make a misdiagnosis of midline granuloma, may lead to the use of irradiation. This results in severe irreversible fibrosis, which in the orbit can produce blindness (Figs 18.2 and 18.3) and in the nose, severe crusting or impairment of lachrymal drainage (see case report p.291). In addition this delay may be followed by extension of the underlying disease.

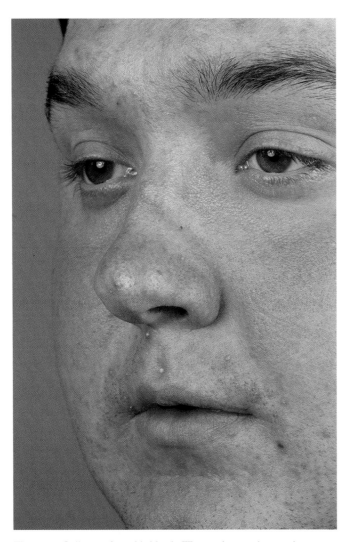

Fig. 18.1 Collapse of nasal bridge in Wegener's granulomatosis.

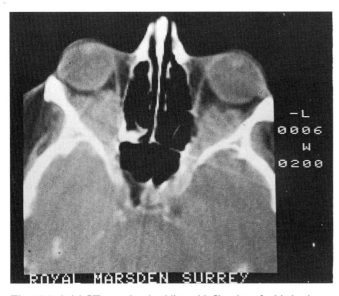

Fig. 18.2 Axial CT scan showing bilateral infiltration of orbital apices in Wegener's granulomatosis.

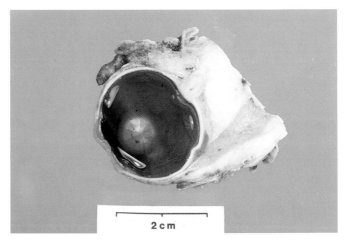

Fig. 18.3 Surgical specimen of orbital clearance performed in a case of Wegener's granulomatosis. Extensive fibrosis following active disease had rendered the eye blind, proptosed and painful.

Pulmonary symptoms

Most patients with active disease can be expected to have some pulmonary symptoms with cough, haemoptysis or pleuritic pain. Infiltrations, which can be well-defined and diffuse (Fig. 18.4) or sometimes cavitating (Fig. 18.5) will be seen radiologically in most of these patients. Occasionally, this will be the presenting symptom with diagnosis being then made by bronchoscopy. Necrotic lung tissue may be coughed up followed by fibrosis or if this does not occur, it may form an encapsulated lung abscess.

Renal symptoms

The organs most seriously affected are the kidneys and although they may be spared in the more limited forms of this disease, they are involved in between 30 and 85% of more generalized cases. Clinically, obvious renal damage is uncommon except in the more fulminating cases where death from renal failure can take place within 24 hours. However, every patient with suspected Wegener's granulomatosis must have their urine examined for protein, red blood cells and casts. Asymptomatic microscopical haematuria, which can be detected by 'stick test' even in as few as 5×10^6 red cells per litre, must be fully investigated in all patients over the age of 40 years after exclusion of possible sources of contamination.[24] However, microscopy for casts is more useful for detecting early or chronic renal disease and in these cases, plasma urea or creatinine assays are essential. Both casts and red cells may appear in the urine of subacute cases of Wegener's granulomatosis possibly heralding early renal involvement. Early treatment is vital, since once renal dysfunction has taken place, residual damage will occur even after effective control of the underlying disease. This

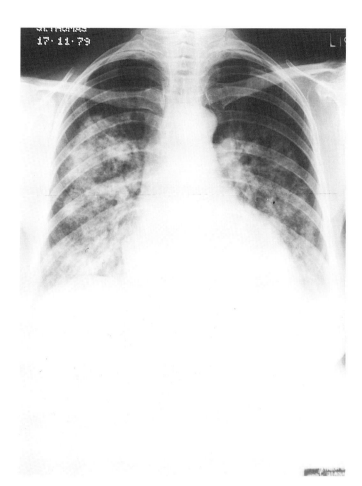

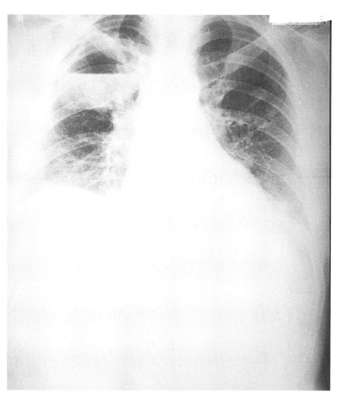

Fig. 18.5 Chest X-ray showing a large cavitating pulmonary lesion in Wegener's granulomatosis.

Fig. 18.4 Chest X-ray showing diffuse pulmonary lesions in Wegener's granulomatosis.

leaves the patient with a risk of future renal failure from ascending pyleonephritis.

Otological symptoms

Between 20 and 40% of patients can expect to develop otological symptoms at some time during their disease. These will fail to respond to conventional measures unless the underlying condition is controlled and even then, some residual damage will remain. Friedmann & Bauer[25] have comprehensively reviewed earlier historical accounts of otological involvement, stating that Druss & Maybaum in 1934 described a case of periarteritis nodosa of the temporal bone that probably represented Wegener's granulomatosis. They noted vascular changes in the bone marrow of the petrous bone together with subendothelial proliferation and vascular necrosis.[26] Fahey et al[4] and Goodman & Chung[5] in 1954 reviewed a total of 29 patients with Wegener's granulomatosis, describing otological complaints as the presenting symptom in two patients. In 1960, Brown & Woolner reporting six patients, found that four had otitis media, three of whom also had sensorineural deafness.[27]

The first account of the pathological changes found in the temporal bone is by Blatt & Lawrence in 1961.[28] Two specimens were examined, only one of which showed bony obliteration of the scala tympani of the basal turn of the cochlea. Friedmann & Bauer[25] reported the temporal bone findings in a 45-year-old woman dying from renal failure from uncontrolled Wegener's granulomatosis. They found necrotizing granulation tissue filling the tympanic cavity and generalized vasculitis. Many other reports have now been published describing the otological manifestations of this disease which may cause serous otitis or chronic media, and conductive or sensorineural deafness.[29]

Serous otitis, which can be uni- or bilateral, is usually secondary to nasopharyngeal ulceration or obstruction to the mouth of the Eustachian tube. Involvement of the tympanic membrane or the middle ear produces pain, suppuration, deafness, and in some patients facial nerve paralysis.[23] Sensorineural hearing loss, invariably associated with conductive deafness from middle ear involvement, was found in 43% of the 21 patients with otological disease described by McCaffrey et al.[30] Response to treatment was variable, although eventually five of their patients had complete or partial recovery of hearing. Malcomson[31] reported one case of Wegener's granulomatosis presenting with otorrhoea and facial paralysis, stressing that when this is the first symptom diagnosis is invariably delayed until failure to control the infection or extension of the disease causes concern. It is essential to consider Wegener's granulomatosis in all cases of long-standing and atypical inflammatory conditions affecting the middle ear.

Ocular symptoms

Although the commonest ocular manifestation of Wegener's granulomatosis is orbital involvement, conjunctivitis, dacrocystitis, episcleritis, corneal ulceration, optic neuritis and retinal artery occlusion also occur (see case report p. 291).[32] Proptosis from an orbital mass or extension from surrounding sinuses can be expected in about 20% of patients, presenting diagnostic problems if occurring as a solitary symptom. As with many other sites, the frequency with which this occurs is primarily related to the speciality concerned and inexperience, with subsequent delay in treatment, is responsible for failure to control many of the orbital symptoms and the eventual loss of vision (Figs 18.2 and 18.3).

Payton & Boulton Jones[33] published a case of cortical blindness in a 35-year-old woman with generalized Wegener's granulomatosis. This was thought to be secondary to thrombosis of the posterior cerebral arteries with bilateral infarction within the occipital cortex. Although cortical blindness has been described in association with hypertension secondary to glomerulonephritis, vision recovered and the blindness was thought to be due to vascular spasm.[34] In the patient reported by Payton & Boulton Jones, vision did not improve and they advised the use of antiplatelet agents to minimize this risk in patients with this disease.

Oral symptoms

A wide variety of oral lesions have been described, the most common of which is a distinctive hyperplastic gingivitis originating in the area of the interdental papillae. The gingiva are usually described as granular and if extensive may cause tooth mobility or loss.[35] Once a tooth is lost the socket fails to heal and this may be the first sign of this disease.[36,37] Extensive ulcerative stomatitis has also been reported and in most cases the prognosis for patients presenting initially with disease within the oral cavity has been poor with a mean duration of life of less than 6 months (Fig. 18.6).[35]

Larynx and tracheal symptoms

Laryngitis is not uncommon in Wegener's granulomatosis secondary to postnasal infection, though actual laryngeal involvement is unusual. When present however, the subglottis or upper trachea are most commonly affected and Arauz & Fonsera described 10 patients, all females

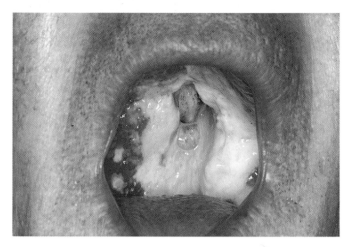

Fig. 18.6 Extensive ulceration of the palate in Wegener's granulomatosis.

with a mean age of 30 years, who presented with laryngotracheal obstruction. Although all biopsies were reported as showing only non-specific changes, every patient already had lesions consistent with Wegener's granulomatosis elsewhere.[38] Surgical dilatation or resection proved unsuccessful but there was a good response to steroid-cytotoxic therapy. Active granulomatous lesions are sometimes visible within the larynx or trachea but the ANCA test has now shown that some cases of 'idiopathic' subglottic stenosis are positive, suggesting that a benign, localized form of Wegener's granulomatosis may exist within the larynx.[39]

Other symptoms

Skin involvement with vasculitic changes, with or without granulomas, are typically seen on the extremities and can cause ulceration. Arthralgia is common but appears to be unrelated to the overall activity of this disease and may be self-limiting. Nervous system involvement is said to be present in about 15% of patients[40] being caused by granulomatous invasion of neural tissues, intercerebral or meningeal granulomas as well as neuritic vasculitis. Facial paralysis is one of the commonest neurological signs but any cranial nerve can be involved.

Case reports are available describing solitary examples of the involvement of most of the bodies' organs in Wegener's granulomatosis making it a possible diagnosis in a wide range of obscure, even bizarre clinical conditions. Although uncommon, it must always enter the differential diagnosis of inflammatory, vasculitic diseases.

Classification

DeRemee et al proposed that Wegener's granulomatosis should be classified according to the anatomical region involved which would allow changes to be made during the progression of the disease.[8] This has been called the ELK system, the E for upper respiratory tract and ear, L for lungs and K for the kidneys. This does not allow for other organ system involvement and has proved to be of little prognostic value.

Radiology

The most significant changes are to be found in the lungs where single or multiple nodular densities or infiltration are seen (Fig. 18.4); this may be followed by unilocular and multilocular cavitation (Fig. 18.5). Both lung fields are usually involved although infiltration may be short-lived in adequately treated cases showing a good response.

Radiology of the sinuses shows opacity or fluid levels, whilst CT scans can reveal unsuspected bone erosion. Within the orbit, granulomatous masses at the apex are often associated with proptosis or visual loss (Figs 18.2 and 18.3). Tomography of the temporal bones will show changes varying from clouding of the mastoid air cells suggestive of mastoiditis, to extensive destruction of the petrous bone.[23]

However, none of these radiological changes can be considered diagnostic although they do assist in confirming organ involvement and possibly, response to therapy.

Macroscopic and microscopic appearance

Given an adequate tissue sample, Hellquist considers that three histological features are needed to substantiate a diagnosis of Wegener's granulomatosis.[41]

1. Pyogenic granulation tissue with fibrin and inflammatory cells
2. Granulomas of epithelioid cell type which tend to be large, irregular and lined with histiocytes, multinucleated giant cells are invariably present
3. Vasculitis is mandatory with fibrinoid vascular necrosis a common finding.

Close to the granulomas it is usual to see vasculitis with thrombosis and fibrous obliteration of small arteries. The characteristic multinucleated giant cells contain compact hyperchromatic nuclei forming bizarre patterns; the cytoplasm is pale and eosinophilic being wider round the nuclei than in the Langerhans' type giant cell. These have been called 'Wegener-type giant cell'.

Although the essential component of the histological diagnosis of Wegener's granulomatosis is vasculitis, the vasculitides represent a wide spectrum of clinical diseases ranging from acute necrotizing vasculitis to chronic indolent vascular inflammation and benign granulomata.[9]

They may however, be separated by the organ affected, size and type of blood vessel involved as well as other histological features. The lung has proved a good source of diagnostic biopsy tissue whereas nasal biopsies present problems because of gross crusting and infection. Superficial biopsies are frequently reported as showing only acute or chronic nonspecific inflammatory changes and repeated deep tissue must be taken to substantiate clinical suspicion.

Renal biopsies are rarely needed except to confirm a suspicion of kidney involvement in the absence of definitive urinary evidence.

Natural history

Before the availability of the glucocorticoids in the 1950s, patients with 'classic' Wegener's granulomatosis invariably died within months from renal failure. This is still true for those cases with fulminating renal disease, but the use of glucocorticoid therapy, by reducing constitutional symptoms and vasculitis, did produce some regression of granulomas within the respiratory tract without materially affecting renal involvement or eventual prognosis. In 1954, Fahey et al[4] reported some success with the addition of nitrogen mustard to the steroids and subsequently, many other less toxic chemotherapeutic agents were shown to halt the progression of this disease.[42–46] The precise mechanism by which these drugs succeed in suppressing progression of Wegener's granulomatosis is unknown although it is possible that it is by steroid-sparing immunosuppression rather than any direct attack upon the organ itself. There can be no doubt however, that adequate medication introduced early in the disease, often without waiting for histological confirmation, can halt progression thus avoiding potentially fatal renal involvement. This dramatic change in disease management has however, brought with it considerable problems in maintaining individual patient control, for both steroids and cytotoxic agents have severe long-term side effects. Although discontinuation of treatment has been the aim of treatment regimes, the disease is not cured and our own personal follow-up of 48 patients for, in some cases, over 20 years has shown that late recurrences in apparently 'cured' patients may occur at any time despite many years without treatment (see case report, p. 291).

Differential diagnosis

Wegener's granulomatosis can now be defined as a clinical and pathological entity but the similarity of many of its clinicopathological features can create significant diagnostic difficulties. Batsakis[11] has tabulated some of the commoner conditions that must enter into the differential diagnosis, grouping them under the headings of vasculitic, specific and non-specific granulomatous, bacterial and neoplastic diseases. Even with the localized forms of this 'systemic' disease, diagnosis can be made but only if the condition is considered. Previous confusion, particularly with polymorphic reticulosis (lethal midline destructive granuloma) has now been eliminated by our better understanding of both conditions, whilst routine use of the ANCA test may prove to be of diagnostic value. Preliminary assessment on a sample takes 2 days with indirect immunofluorescence but only 4 hours with radioimmunoassay.[47] Sensitivity for active Wegener's granulomatosis has been quoted as 100%[48] but this is probably also related to the extent of the disease and the amount of tissue damage. Consequently, a negative ANCA test does not invalidate a clinical diagnosis of Wegener's granulomatosis. Since the titres appear to be related to disease activity, falling after effective therapy, it is expected that this test will be of value not only diagnostically but for detecting early relapse. However as experience has shown that there are many false positive results and the test rapidly becomes negative once treatment is started, care is needed in interpretation.

Treatment

For many years patients were treated empirically in the hope of arresting progression of the disease. Despite all attempts, most patients died of secondary infection, haemorrhage or more frequently, end-stage renal failure. Survival was rarely longer than 12 to 24 months following initial diagnosis, depending upon the degree of renal damage. Errors in diagnosis resulted in some patients receiving radiotherapy which was not only ineffective but produced iatrogenic fibrosis. The corticosteroids by reducing inflammatory reactions produced some objective improvement but had little effect on existing renal disease or on the progression of the disease. The realization by Fahey et al that combination of corticosteroids and a variety of cytotoxic drugs could materially improve short-term prognosis has resulted in over 90% of patients with Wegener's granulomatosis obtaining some remission.[4] However, any renal damage prior to beginning treatment is unlikely to be reversed and avoidance is only possible if therapy is begun as soon as the diagnosis is suspected rather than waiting for histological verification.

Most patients during the active stage feel extremely ill even in the absence of physical or radiological changes. Local tissue damage invokes a systemic response that includes fever, leucocytosis and an increase in plasma proteins. This response is mediated by cytokines released by macrophages at the site of the tissue damage. Since 1921 the erythrocyte sedimentation rate (ESR) has been the most useful method for assessing the protein component of this response (Fig. 18.7).[49] Advocates of this test cite its usefulness and reliability in monitoring the progress of inflammatory disease, although admitting its

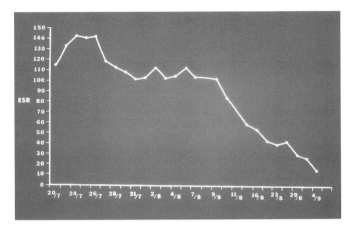

Fig. 18.7 The use of ESR in monitoring clinical improvement in response to treatment in Wegener's granulomatosis.

non-specific role. Critics emphasize its lack of quality control and the inability to correct for anaemia. Quantitative assay of C-reactive protein is thought to be more reliable with changes detectable within 10 hours of tissue damage. In acute Wegener's granulomatosis the ESR is always raised, usually around 80 mm/hour, and despite its limitations this test is generally used to titrate levels of medication.

The earliest sign of renal involvement is the presence of red blood cells, protein and casts in an uncontaminated specimen of urine and this test should be carried out regularly. It is also important to establish levels of renal function early in the disease, both to determine eventual prognosis and also to detect any future change or involvement. Glomerular filtration rate is usually estimated by creatine clearance although there is some doubt as to whether plasma creatinine concentration alone is more reliable.[50] A simple guide to renal function is the plasma urea concentration although this does depend on other factors, such as dietary protein intake and the rate of tissue catabolism. Unfortunately, both plasma urea and creatinine levels are susceptible to rapid changes in renal function though serving as useful base lines.

Sharpstone has also shown that the excretion of both the cytotoxic drugs commonly used to treat Wegener's granulomatosis, cyclophosphamide and azathioprine, is only minimally affected by renal clearance rates greater than 10 ml/min, or plasma urea levels of less than 2.5 g/litre. This enhances their value in patients with severe renal disease.[51]

It is now accepted that the titre of antibody to neutrophil cytoplasmic antigen should be measured at diagnosis, since it is not only helpful in substantiating histological evidence but serves as a baseline for monitoring therapeutic response or detecting early recurrence. As yet however, there are no prospective reports as to the real value of this test in patient management nor its sensitivity with regard to the early detection of remission failure.

Despite many encouraging reports of good initial control of Wegener's granulomatosis using a combination of prednisolone and either cyclophosphamide or azathioprine, there are few long-term studies, which emphasizes the inherent problems in managing patients during remission. In patients with acute, potentially fulminating disease, treatment should aim at immediate control to minimize renal damage. Prednisolone, 60 to 80 mg/day with cyclophosphamide 2 mg/kg or azathioprine 200 mg/day should produce a dramatic improvement in the patient's subjective feeling of well-being despite no objective change in the disease parameters. Lowering of the ESR occurs slowly and gradual reduction of both drugs has to be based on clinical and laboratory assessment and cannot be generalized. With the exception of the fulminating, progressive cases, initial control can now be confidently expected and the principle problems lie in long-term care. The side effects of continued steroid therapy are well recognized but little attention has been paid to the side effects of cytotoxic drugs given for non-neoplastic disease.

A major complication of cyclophosphamide is leucopenia and dosage should be adjusted to prevent the WBC falling below 3000 cells per ml. Alopecia can occur even with low doses but of more significance is the possible development of haemorrhagic cystitis. Over 40% of patients taking this drug may have some bladder bleeding which will be exacerbated if there is an associated marrow depression. Since even the presence of red blood cells may signify early renal involvement in Wegener's granulomatosis, this is a considerable disadvantage in patient management.[52] However, routine use of folate reduces this although not the possibility of red blood cells being found microscopically.

Azathioprine however, has none of these side effects when given at maximum dosage of 200 mg/day even though there is some evidence of a synergistic effect when given with prednisolone. In our own series of patients, all of whom received azathioprine with prednisolone, there was 100% immediate control and over a 20-year follow-up in some cases, no patient had alopecia, leucopenia or iatrogenic haemorrhage cystitis.

Many young fertile women treated for neoplasia can now expect to be long-term survivors. Concern that as a result of 'cure' they may be sterile due to chemotherapeutic gonadal destruction, applies equally to young patients with Wegener's granulomatosis. This is certainly not so with azathioprine and two of my patients have been safely delivered of normal babies despite several years of high dose chemotherapy. Patients should however be made aware of the possibility of gonadal failure although ozoospermia can be reversible after some cytotoxic regimes.[53]

In view of the unavoidable side effects of continued steroid and cytotoxic therapy there is a natural desire by both patient and doctor to reduce or stop treatment as soon as possible. Although the ESR and possibly the ANCA test are of value in monitoring disease resolution or progression, change can occur suddenly. The patient is often aware of variations in well-being which herald a worsening of their condition and in my experience are particularly sensitive to changes in dosage. They should be listened to even after many years of apparent control, particularly after immunological challenges such as influenza or during pregnancy. Clinical 'flare ups', can usually be controlled by raising of drug dosage but carry a recurring penalty of fibrous reaction. This swing between remission and recurrence results in considerable tissue reaction and subsequent fibrosis which in the orbit can result in painful proptosis, visual defect or blindness and in the lung, in pulmonary fibrosis with consequent severe dyspnoea.

The following case history clearly illustrates the management problems that are inherent in the long-term care of a young patient initially diagnosed as an 'early' case of Wegener's granulomatosis.

During 1971, a young girl aged 16 years developed granular lesions within the left nose and on the tongue base. Although diagnosed histologically as Wegener's granulomatosis she was given an unspecified dosage of irradiation which had no immediate effect upon the lesions but eventually produced intranasal fibrosis. In January 1972 she was started on prednisolone 30 mg daily together with azathioprine 200 mg daily. At this time there was no evidence of disease in either lungs or kidneys but the ESR was 60 mm/hour.

There was a gradual disappearance of the lingual lesion but considerable intranasal crusting and this encouraging response, together with a falling of the ESR to 20 mm/hour continued until March 1972. Her increase in weight and general good health led to a decrease in the daily prednisolone to 10 mg daily whilst maintaining the azathioprine at 200 mg daily. Despite fluctuations in the ESR related to mild upper respiratory tract infections she remained on this regime and in March 1973 had a left dacrocystorhinotomy for persistent epiphora. This was secondary to the postradiotherapeutic scarring and persistent intranasal crusting obliterating the nasolacrimal duct. Despite several further operations this iatrogenic problem was never solved.

By this time a large septal perforation was present together with some depression of the nasal bridge which caused considerable cosmetic disability in this young woman. The dosage of prednisolone was varied in relation to the patient's subjective impression of her health together with estimations of WBC and ESR. Azathioprine had been reduced to 100 mg daily and in December 1975 she had an uncomplicated appendicectomy and in April 1977 drainage of a left-sided periorbital abscess. By now the azathioprine had been stopped and she was taking a maintenance dose of 10 mg prednisolone daily to keep the serum cortisol levels normal. In January 1980 a silastic implant was used to correct the nasal deformity and several months later she became pregnant.

Despite intermittent elevation of the ESR and the introduction of bilateral T-tubes for serous otitis media, the pregnancy was uneventful with delivery of a normal baby. The following year she had another normal child and although in subsequent years there were fluctuations in her general health causing concern, she remained well though troubled by persistent nasal crusting and epiphora.

Early in 1980 she became pregnant once more but when 14 weeks became seriously ill with 'fulminating' pulmonary Wegener's granulomatosis, ESR of 90 mm/hour, joint pains and haemoptysis but fortunately no renal involvement. The pregnancy was terminated, the patient sterilized and full steroid–azathioprine therapy commenced. She continued on this regime with slow reduction in dosage until August 1989 when she developed pain in the right face with anaesthesia in the 2nd division of the right Vth nerve. Despite extensive neurological and radiological investigations no explanation was found for this but in October 1989 she developed a right orbital apex syndrome losing vision in the right eye. Once again a full regime of therapy was started, the ESR gradually falling from a high of 51 to 19 mm/hour within a month. Full ocular movements returned but not the vision and in March 1990 whilst taking prednisolone 15 mg and azathioprine 100 mg daily she developed dysphagia but not hoarseness. However, a left recurrent nerve paresis was found and an MRI showed extensive bony destruction of the paranasal sinuses and medial skull base with a high signal from either inflammatory tissue or Wegener's granulomatosis. No neoplasm was found to account

for these changes and at this time the ANCA was negative, ESR 30 mm/hour with creatinine clearance 78 ml/min.

Prednisolone 60 mg and azathioprine 200 mg daily produced recovery of swallowing but in July 1990 she had a large right lung abscess which resolved with conservative therapy. She remains well when last seen September 1991, 19 years post-diagnosis.

Prognosis

The patient in the case report clearly illustrates the need for long-term follow-up of large series of patients in order to quantify prognosis. It is impossible to predict the likelihood of any individual patient suffering late recurrence, especially after immunological challenges such as influenza or pregnancy. The severe side effects of all the drugs which have dramatically changed the immediate prospects of survival, necessitate reduction in dosage when possible. This requires a balance between the intrinsic risks of a potentially hazardous relapse against the surety of drug toxicity. As yet this cannot be quantified but permanent follow-up is essential.

REFERENCES

1. Klinger H 1931 Grenzformen der periarteritis nodosa. Frankfurt Journal of Pathology 42: 455–480
2. Wegener F 1936 Uber generaliserle, septische geffasserkrankugen. Verhandlungen der Deutschen Gesselschaft fur Pathologie 29: 202–210
3. Wegener F 1939 Uber eine eigenartige rhinogene granulomatese mit besonderer beteilgung des arteriensystems und der mieren. Beitrage zur Pathologie 102: 36–68
4. Fahey J, Leonard E, Churg J 1954 Wegener's granulomatosis. American Journal of Medicine 17: 168–170
5. Goodman G C, Churg J 1954 Wegener's granulomatosis: pathology and review of the literature. Archives of Pathology 58: 533–553
6. Carrington C B, Liebow A A 1966 Limited forms of angiitis and granulomatosis of Wegener's type. American Journal of Medicine 41: 497–527
7. Cassan J M, Coles D T, Harrison E G 1970 The concept of a limited form of Wegener's granulomatosis. American Journal of Medicine 49: 366–379
8. DeRemee R A, Weiland L H, McDonald T J 1980 Respiratory vasculitis. Mayo Clinic Proceedings 55: 492–498
9. McDonald T J, DeRemee R A 1983 Wegener's granulomatosis. Laryngoscope 93: 220–231
10. Halstead L A, Karmody C S, Wolff S M 1986 Presentation of Wegener's granulomatosis in young patients. Otolaryngology, Head and Neck Surgery 94: 368–371
11. Batsakis J G 1979 Wegener's granulomatosis and midline (non-healing) granuloma. Head and Neck Surgery 1: 213–222
12. Shillitoe E J, Lehner T, Lessof M H 1974 Immunological features of Wegener's granulomatosis. Lancet 1: 281–285
13. Howell J, Epstein W 1976 Circulating immunoglobulin complexes in Wegener's granulomatosis. American Journal of Medicine 60: 259–268
14. Ronco P, Verroust P, Mignon F 1983 Immunological studies of polyarteritis nodosa and Wegener's granulomatosis. Quarterly Journal of Medicine 206: 213–223
15. der Woude F J, Rasmussen N, Wilk A 1985 Autoantibodies against neutrophils and monocytes: tool for diagnosis and marker of disease activity in Wegener's granulomatosis. Lancet 23 Feb: 425–429
16. Hinde C P K, Pepys M B 1985 Anticytoplasmic antibodies in Wegener's granulomatosis. Lancet 8 June: 1336
17. Lockwood C M, Bakes D, Jones J 1987 Association of alkaline phosphatase with an autoantigen recognized by circulating anti-neutrophil antibodies in systemic vasculitis. Lancet 28 March: 716–719
18. Campanelli D 1990 Cloning of cDNA for proteinase 3: a serine protease, antibiotic and autoantigen from human neutrophils. Journal of Experimental Medicine 172: 1709–1715
19. Nolle B, Specks U, Ludermann J 1989 Anticytoplasmic autoantibodies: their immunodiagnostic value in Wegener's granulomatosis. Annals of Internal Medicine 111: 28–40
20. Specks U, Wheatley C L, McDonald T J 1989 Anticytoplasmic autoantibodies in the diagnosis and follow-up of Wegener's granulomatosis. Mayo Clinic Proceedings 64: 28–36
21. Cohen-Tervaert J W et al 1989 Association between active Wegener's granulomatosis and anticytoplasmic antibodies. Lancet 336: 709–711
22. Falk R J 1990 ANCA-associated renal disease. Kidney International 38: 998–1010
23. Illum P, Thorling K 1981 Wegener's granulomatosis, longterm results of treatment. Annals of Otology, Rhinology and Laryngology 90: 231–235
24. Bullock N 1986 Asymptomatic microscopical haematuria. British Medical Journal 292: 645
25. Friedmann I, Bauer F 1973 Wegener's granulomatosis causing deafness. Journal of Laryngology and Otology 87: 449–464
26. Druss J G, Maybaum R 1934 Periarteritis nodosa of the temporal bone. Archives of Otolaryngology 19: 502–507
27. Brown H A, Woolner L B 1960 Findings referable to the upper part of the respiratory tract in Wegener's granulomatosis. Annals of Otology, Rhinology and Laryngology 69: 810–829
28. Blatt I M, Lawrence M 1961 Otological manifestations of fatal granulomatosis of respiratory tract in Wegener's granulomatosis. Archives of Otolaryngology 73: 639–643
29. Bradley P 1983 Wegener's granulomatosis of the ear. Journal of Laryngology and Otology 97: 623–626
30. McCaffrey T V, McDonald T J, Facer G W 1980 Otologic manifestations of Wegener's granulomatosis. Otolaryngology, Head and Neck Surgery 88: 586–593
31. Malcolmson K G 1966 Wegener's giant cell granuloma treated with steroids. Journal of Laryngology and Otology 80: 640–645
32. Koornneff L, Melief J M, Peterse H L 1982 Wegener's granulomatosis of the orbit. Orbit 2: 1–10

33. Payton C D, Boulton Jones J M 1985 Cortical blindness complicating Wegener's granulomatosis. British Medical Journal 290: 676

34. Huber M, Poon C, Buchanan N 1981 Acute glomerulonephritis presenting with acute blindness. Medical Journal of Australia 1: 595–598

35. Hanlers J P, Waterman J, Abrahams A M 1985 Oral features of Wegener's granulomatosis. Archives of Otolaryngology 111: 267–270

36. Israelson H, Binnie W H, Hurt W C 1981 The hyperplastic gingivitis of Wegener's granulomatosis. Journal of Peridontology 52: 81–87

37. Scott J, Finch L D 1972 Wegener's granulomatosis presenting as gingivitis. Oral Surgery 34: 920–933

38. Arauz J C, Fonsera R 1982 Wegener's granulomatosis appearing initially in the trachea. Annals of Otology, Rhinology and Laryngology 91: 593–594

39. Hoare T J, Jayne D, Evans P R, Howard D J 1989 Wegener's granulomatosis, subglottic stenosis and anti-neutrophil cytoplasm antibodies. Journal of Laryngology and Otology 103: 1187–1191

40. Kornblut A D, Wolff S M, DeFries H O 1980 Wegener's granulomatosis. Laryngoscope 90: 1453–1465

41. Hellquist H B 1990 Pathology of the nose and sinuses. Granulomatous lesions of the nose and sinuses. Butterworths, London, p 62

42. Aungst C W, Lessman E M 1962 Wegener's granulomatosis treated with nitrogen mustard. New York State Journal of Medicine 62: 3302–3310

43. Bouroncle B A, Smith E S, Cuppage F E 1967 Treatment of Wegener's granulomatosis with imuran. American Journal of Medicine 42: 314–318

44. Choy D S, Gould W S, Gearhart R P 1969 Remission of Wegener's granulomatosis with steroids and azathioprine. New York State Journal of Medicine 69: 1205–1209

45. Novac S N, Pearson C M 1971 Cyclophosphamide therapy in Wegener's granulomatosis. New England Journal of Medicine 284: 938–942

46. Capizzi R L, Bertino J R 1971 Methotrexate therapy in Wegener's granulomatosis. American Journal of Internal Medicine 74: 74–79

47. Savage C O S, Winearls C G, Jones S 1987 Prospective study of radioimmunoassay for antibodies against neutrophil cytoplasm in diagnosis of systemic vasculitis. Lancet 20 June: 1389–1393

48. Venning M C, Arfeen S, Bird A G 1987 Antibodies to neutrophil cytoplasmic antigen in systemic vasculitis. Lancet 10 Oct: 850

49. Stuart J, Lewis S M 1988 Monitoring the acute phase response. British Medical Journal 297: 1143–1144

50. Grabiel R 1986 Time to scrap creatinine clearance. British Medical Journal 293: 1119–1120

51. Sharpstone P 1977 Disease of the urinary system. British Medical Journal 2: 36–37

52. Rubin J J, Robin R T 1966 Cyclophosphamide haemorrhagic cystitis. Journal of Urology 96: 313–316

53. Mills J F 1985 Cancer, chemotherapy and fertility. British Medical Journal 290: 1096–1097

19. Neuroectodermal lesions

Primary neurogenic tumours of the sinonasal tract are rare. In the series presented by Friedmann & Osborn[1a] there were only 11 neurogenic tumours out of 1043 tumours in this region (1.5%). However, they cover a range of activity and can pose special problems of management where once again the concept of 'benign' disease is called into question by the consequences of intracranial spread. Malignant melanoma is included in this section to reflect its origin from neural crest tissue.

1. Nasal encephalocoele and glioma
2. Schwannoma
3. Neurofibroma (benign and malignant)
4. Extracranial meningioma
5. Neuroendocrine carcinoma
6. Olfactory neuroblastoma
7. Malignant melanoma
8. Melanotic neuroectodermal tumour of infancy.

NASAL ENCEPHALOCOELE AND GLIOMA

Definition

Nasal encephalocoeles are protrusions of brain contents through a congenitally deficient defect in the skull, if no defect is present then the mass is termed a glioma.

Synonym

Vestigial encephalocoele, glial ectopia, foetal glial migration, encephaloma.[2]

Historical aspects

In 1890 Berger used the term 'encephaloma' with reference to a young person with a nasal glioma[3] but the first comprehensive description of this lesion is usually credited to Schmidt in 1900.[4] Black & Smith published the case histories of two patients with nasal gliomas in 1950[5] and in 1963 Walker & Resler reviewed a further 65 cases

which had been published between 1950 and 1963.[6] Karma et al in 1977 found another 71 patients in the literature making a total of about 150 patients with nasal glioma which had by then become a well-recognized condition.[2]

Incidence

Although an established clinical entity, nasal gliomas and encephalocoeles remain uncommon. During a 10-year period (1970–79) at a major children's hospital in the United Kingdom, only five cases were diagnosed[7] whilst a similar number were reported by Gorenstein et al from the Mayo Clinic, USA over a 40-year period.[8] In their review of the literature Karma et al found that in a total of 71 patients the largest single experience was the six patients reported by Agarwal et al in India.[2,9]

Age, sex and ethnic variation

Nasal gliomas are usually diagnosed or suspected at birth although Karma et al in their comprehensive review found two adults, aged 51 and 54 years old whose gliomas had only recently been diagnosed. No explanation was given for these late growths but Ogura & Schenck also found several adult patients in their series,[10] and Pollard & Carter reported a patient aged 25 years with von Recklinghausen's neurofibromatosis and a nasal glioma.[11]

Nasal glioma are not familial nor is there any sex predilection. There is not usually an association with other developmental abnormalities and cases have been found in most countries and ethnic groups.

Site and Aetiology (Figs 19.1–19.4)

Gorenstein et al concluded from their literature review that 60% of nasal gliomas are external, 30% intranasal and the remainder have both intra- and extranasal components.[8] External lesions may be found over the dorsum,

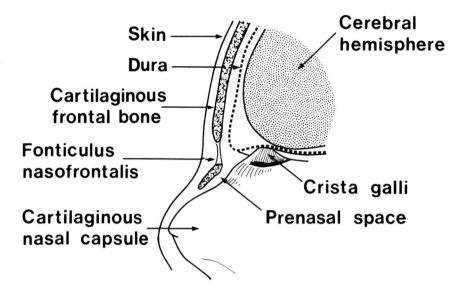

Fig. 19.1   The normal situation during development of anterior cranial fossa and glabellar region.

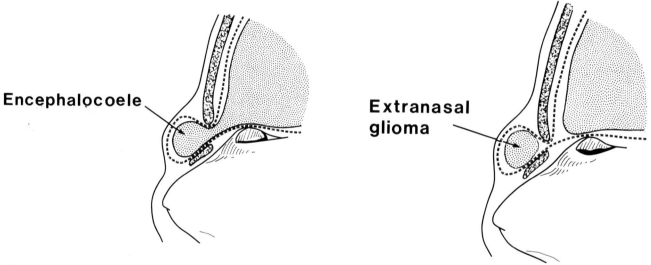

Fig. 19.2   Formation of an encephalocoele.

Fig. 19.3   Formation of extranasal glioma.

to one side, at the junction of the bony and cartilaginous parts of the nose, near the medial canthus or between the nasal, ethmoid, frontal or lacrimal bones.[6,12] Intranasal gliomas are usually situated in the nasal or nasopharyngeal cavities, in the mouth or even the pterygopalatine fossa.[13–16] The attachment within the nasal fossa may be high although more usually it is to the middle turbinate in adults. Communication with the intracranial contents is usually through the cribriform plate but intranasal lesions may communicate with an extranasal glioma through a defect in the nasal bone.

There is general agreement that nasal encephalocoeles and gliomas are developmental in origin rather than neoplasms. Embryologically, a nasal encephalocoele must be associated with a defect in the anterior cranial fossa with herniation of the intracranial contents. The frontal and nasal bones develop anterior to their cartilaginous precursors by intramembranous ossification. A space is present between the newly formed bone and the cartilage and in the early stages this is occupied by a dural protrusion through a bony foramen, the foramen caecum. This

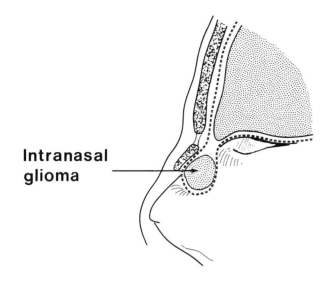

Intranasal glioma

A

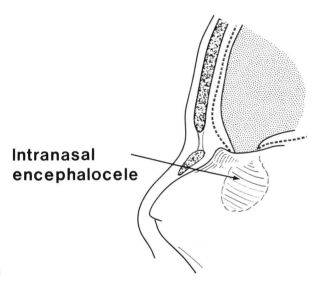

Intranasal encephalocele

B

Fig. 19.4 **A**, formation of intranasal glioma and **B**, intranasal encephalocoele.

becomes sealed with further development but it has been suggested that nasal encephalocoeles, and possibly gliomas, result from failure of the foramen caecum to close thus permitting the brain to extrude.[17a] Nasal gliomas therefore could have a similar aetiology to encephalocoeles but have lost their intracranial connection.[18] However, other proposals have been advanced regarding pathogenesis of nasal gliomata.

1. They are areas of brain isolated during embryological development by closure of cranial sutures[4,19,20]

2. They are isolated in early foetal life then occur later as separate embryonal neuroglia that differentiate into mature glioma[2]

3. Intranasal glioma arise from neurological cells surrounding the olfactory bulb growing into the nose via the cribriform plate or externally through a separation in the fronto-ethmoid suture.[21]

It has also been suggested by Strauss that these congenital benign lesions have a multiple mode of origin.[22] Despite the variety of aetiological explanations, Macomber & Wang's analysis confirmed that the only difference between gliomas and encephalocoeles lies in the severity of the basic error in development and gliomas might be best regarded as 'vestigial encephalocoeles'.[23]

Clinical features

Nasofrontal encephalocoeles are compressible, fluctuating, pulsating and bluish in colour. The swelling may increase in size on crying or straining as a result of an increase in cerebrospinal pressure. Intranasal encephalocoeles always protrude through a defect in the cribriform plate area and can be mistaken for a nasal polyp. However, the encephalocoele develops alongside the nasal septum and although a probe can be passed lateral to the mass there is no plane medially. This lesion is not pedunculated and the overlying mucosa is a continuation of the septal lining.[24]

Extranasal glioma are usually found on the dorsum of the nose with covering skin varying in colour from normality to a faint bluish tinge. The size and shape does not vary with crying or straining since there is no intracranial connection. Most of these gliomata are diagnosed at or soon after birth because of cosmetic deformity.

Intranasal gliomas are firm, pale or grey in colour and obstruct the nasal passage. They are not compressible and show no impulse on crying. They have a high attachment within the nasal vault and the nose may be broadened with a polypoidal mass visible at the anterior nares causing confusion with nasal polypi although the latter are rare in children under the age of 5 years.[25] Nasal obstruction can interfere with feeding and intranasal glioma possess the potential for producing substantial deformity by displacement of the nasal skeleton, septum or orbital bones, although the rate of growth appears to be variable.[6]

Radiology (Fig. 19.5)

A complete radiological evaluation is necessary in all patients presenting with a swelling in the frontonasal region although in the case of nasal encephalocoeles and gliomata, it may not always be conclusive.[26] Although a diagnosis can often be made on clinical grounds the main

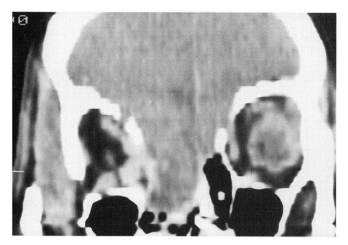

Fig. 19.5 Coronal CT scan showing large encephalocoele.

problem in management is confirmation of an existing intracranial connection, present in 15 to 20% of all nasal gliomas according to Lowe et al.[27] However, Smith et al when reviewing 93 patients with proven nasal gliomas only found an intracranial connection in 14 cases, all of whom had transnasal biopsies.[12]

Radiology shows the soft tissue mass, bony changes and any septal deviation whereas a small defect in the cribriform plate may be difficult to identify, particularly in a baby. Pneumoencephalography may be useful in demonstrating a communication with the subarachnoid space or ventricular system[28] but even the most sophisticated radiological investigation may fail to demonstrate very small defects or intracranial connections.

Macroscopic and microscopic appearance

The term glioma implies a true neoplasm and this term is therefore a misnomer although in constant usage. The lesion is uncapsulated and composed of fibrillary neuroglial cells mainly astrocytes of the plump gemistocytic type. These are interlaced with a variable amount of fibrous and vascular connective tissue with occasional nerve cells, although the last may be difficult to identify because of distortion. Characteristically, mitosis is scanty

or absent and the tumour stalk is usually fibrous with glial elements.[28] Extranasal lesions are covered with dermis and appendicular structures whilst intranasal gliomas are surrounded by fibrovascular tissue.

The term 'facial glioma' has been suggested to encompass all extracranial glial lesions found in the head region since histologically identical lesions have been found in the tongue and face as well as the nose. These rare ectopic glial lesions have been said to arise from blastomous rests arising within tissues with limited powers of differentiation.[29]

In contrast to gliomas, encephalocoeles contain brain, meningeal tissue and in some even parts of the intracranial ventricular system.[17a]

Differential diagnosis

This must include all the congenital nasal tumours classified by Macomber & Wang in their comprehensive monograph of 1953.[23] Although the most important differentiation is between gliomas and encephalocoele (or meningocoele) the last two have meningeal envelopes and a connection with the subarachnoid space which carries the risk of meningitis or CSF leakage. With older patients nasal polypi must be considered and extranasal gliomata must be differentiated from a dermoid cyst (Table 19.1).

Treatment

In those instances where an intranasal glioma can be shown to have an intranasal connection, a neurosurgical approach through a frontal craniotomy is needed, particularly when there is an associated CSF rhinorrhoea or previous meningitis.[19]

At craniotomy, the cribriform plate is explored and the bony defect and intracranial connection identified. Since there is rarely a definite demarcation of abnormal glial tissue from related brain, a wide excision is required to avoid recurrence and the resulting bony and dural defect repaired. The intranasal portion of the glioma or encephalocoele is removed at a further operation to minimize morbidity. These operations should be carried out

Table 19.1 Differential diagnosis of nasal glioma (after Bradley & Singh[7])

	Glioma	Encephalocoele	Dermoid	Polyp
Patients' age (yr)	<5	<5	Any age	>5
Pulsation	No	Yes	No	No
Variable size	No	Yes	No	No
CSF aspirated	?Rare	Yes	No	No
Cranial defect	Rare	Yes	Rare	No
Texture	Hard	Cystic	Variable	Soft

in early childhood to reduce subsequent deformity in the developing facial bones.[30] However, an identifiable intracranial connection is in practice uncommon, Alexander in 1978 when reviewing 50 cases found only three requiring craniotomy[30] and since craniotomy in the young carries a considerable morbidity, most authors advise a conservative surgical approach in those patients with no clinical or radiological evidence of an intracranial connection.

An extranasal surgical approach allows identification of the posterior and inferior limits of an intranasal glioma so that any connection with the cribriform plate can be identified and occluded. Snaring or avulsion is not acceptable because of the intrinsic risk of incomplete removal and CSF leakage.[8] Lateral rhinotomy is most frequently used for access, although the dorsal rhinotomy recommended by Mallen & Kudryk in 1974 is useful for purely extranasal gliomata.[31] Other variations of extranasal procedures have been suggested by Hage in 1960[32] and O'Brien in 1970[20] but all these operations appear to be safe when performed under antibiotic cover.

Since nasal gliomata are benign lesions with a low recurrence rate, the most cosmetically conservative surgical procedure should be used unless an intracranial connection can be identified when complete neurosurgical removal is indicated.

SCHWANNOMA

Definition

A tumour of nerve sheath origin being derived from the Schwann cells surrounding the neural tissue.

Synonym

Neurilemmoma, neuromas or peripheral fibromatosis. Malignant schwannomas are also known as malignant neurilommas, malignant nerve sheath tumours, neurogenic tumours, neurogenic sarcomas and neurosarcomas.

Historical aspects

Verocay described a nerve sheath tumour in 1908 which he believed was derived from the Schwann cell and possibly of ectodermal origin. In 1910 he called it a neurinoma.[33] Elucidation of the histology was reported by Antoni in 1920 when he described two characteristic forms, later to be known as Antoni A and B.[34] In 1926 Terplan & Rudofsky reported the first documented neuroma involving the nasal cavity and ethmoid sinuses[35] and in 1935 Stout gave this lesion the name 'neurilemmoma' thereby recognizing its cell of origin.[36] In 1942, Del Rio-Hortega proposed that Schwannoma was a more accurate term and this has now been universally accepted.[37]

Incidence

Schwannomas are tumours originating from the neuroectodermal Schwann cell of cranial, intraspinal, peripheral and autonomic nerve sheaths and are the most common neurogenic tumour found within the sinonasal region. Although between 25%[38] and 45%[39] of schwannomas occur within the head and neck region no more than 4% involve the nasal cavity and paranasal sinuses.[40] Kragh et al reported 152 peripheral nerve tumours of the head and neck seen at the Mayo Clinic, finding only five which originated within the nose or maxillary sinus.[41]

Robitaille et al reviewing the world literature in 1975 found only 12 patients acceptable as schwannomas arising within the sinonasal region although they excluded lesions confined to the nasal cavity.[42] Friedmann & Osborn when reporting their specialist experience in head and neck pathology found that four of their five sinonasal schwannomas were sited in the nose[1a] and Perzin and colleagues identified six further cases amongst 430 000 patients with head and neck tumours.[43] Small numbers of patients have been published by Dutt in 1969,[44] Kaufman & Conrad 1976,[45] Thomas 1977,[46] Pasic & Makielski 1990,[47] and Younis et al in 1991.[40] No case has been reported as arising from the frontal sinus nor from the olfactory or optic nerves which have no schwann cells.

Even less common is a malignant change with Ghosh et al finding 16 malignant tumours within the head and neck in a total of 115 malignant schwannomas. 30% of all these cases were associated with von Recklinghausen's disease.[48] Multiple schwannomas are usually found with neurofibromatosis and were termed schwannomatosis by Purcell & Dixon.[49] However Hellquist, whilst recognizing a malignant variant, feels that neurogenic sarcoma is a better term. He contends that malignant lesions may be more common than is at present thought, and that modern immunohistochemistry will lead to a reclassification of some sinonasal fibrosarcomata. He reported five cases of confirmed malignancy.[50] This view has been supported by Maroun et al[51] although doubt remains as to whether schwannomas ever become malignant.

Age, sex and ethnic variation

There appears to be no association with race or sex and most cases are diagnosed between the ages of 20 and 60 years.[42]

Site

With the exception of the olfactory and optic nerves, schwannomas have been reported in relation to all the cranial nerves. The scalp, face, oral cavity, larynx, pharynx, parotid, paranasal sinuses, middle ear and nasal cavity have all been reported as sites of origin.[47] However, it is not always possible to identify the precise nerve of origin at the time of surgical removal but within the upper jaw it is usually branches of the ophthalmic and maxillary divisions of the trigeminal nerve which are most affected. An autonomic source originating within the pterygopalatine fossa has also been found.[52] Published reports suggest that in descending order of frequency the sites for sinonasal schwannomas are the naso-ethmoid area, maxillary sinus, nasal septum and sphenoid sinus although in larger tumours more than one area may be involved.[53]

The difficulties inherent in identifying the source of this tumour are well illustrated by a lesion arising from the nasal septum. There are three possible sources:

1. Sympathetic nerves to the septal blood vessels reaching the septum via the greater palatine nerve. (Cell bodies of these axons are in the stellate ganglion.)

2. Parasympathetic innervation to the septal mucous glands which also reach the septum via the greater palatine nerve. (Cell bodies of these axons lie in the sphenopalatine ganglion.)

3. Finally, the sensory innervation of the septum which includes the nasopalatine nerve and the anterior and posterior branches of the nasociliary nerve.[47]

Clinical features

Clinical presentation is similar to other tumours affecting the upper jaw, being primarily dependent upon location and size of the tumour. Nasal obstruction, rhinorrhoea, epistaxis, facial swelling, anosmia and proptosis can all occur with epistaxis said to be more likely with naso-ethmoidal lesions and pain when the maxillary antrum is involved.[42,54] Growth of sphenoid sinus tumours can involve the 3rd, 4th and 6th cranial nerves but non-specific clinical symptoms can be caused by tumour necrosis or pressure exerted by the tumour mass.[55]

Naso-ethmoidal schwannomas spread locally producing nasal blockage and epistaxis from necrosis. Extension may occur superiorly through the roof of the nose into the anterior cranial fossa. Enion et al reported such a patient where no obvious nasal symptoms occurred until the intracranial lesion had reached a large size, olfaction remained normal both pre- and postoperatively.[56] In such cases hypopituitarism may be evident if there is posterior extension and this has been reported in sphenoid sinus schwannomas. Deep retro-orbital pain was a feature in the case reported by Calcaterra et al.[57]

Radiology (Figs 19.6 and 19.7)

Characteristically, schwannomas expand and thin the bony surroundings of cavities or foramina within the

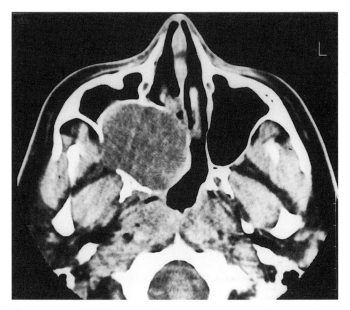

Fig. 19.6 Axial CT scan showing schwannoma encroaching on right maxillary sinus and nasal cavity.

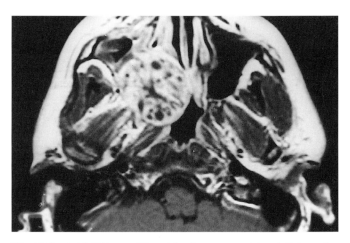

Fig. 19.7 Axial MR scan, T1 weighted sequence with gadolinium of case in Figure 19.6 showing enhancing lesion with signal voids from large vascular components.

upper jaw due to their slow growth. These changes may be seen on routine plain views but high resolution CT with contrast is the best means of identifying the location and extent of intraorbital, intracranial or soft tissue mass. Computed tomography delineates an image of the soft tissue tumour whilst outlining the bony margins to detect any erosion.[55] Schwannomas usually show a mottled central lucency with peripheral enhancement, probably due to variations in vascularity and non-enhancing cystic or necrotic areas. Magnetic resonance imaging may be superior in defining the vascular soft tissue mass but not any bone loss which is common with larger schwannomas.[53]

Macroscopic and microscopic appearance

These tumours are well encapsulated, usually solitary, rarely if ever undergo malignant change, do not have nerve fibres of the affected nerve incorporated within its structure and are not usually associated with von Recklinghausen's disease.[54] Histologically, upper jaw schwannomas do not differ from similar tumours found elsewhere in the body. Two distinct histological patterns occur. Antoni A has areas composed of spindle-shaped cells arranged in compact bundles or interlacing fascicles with nuclei arranged in palisades whose spaces form 'Verocay' bodies. In Antoni B areas, the spindle-shaped cells are more loosely arranged in a fibrillar myxoid-like stroma. However, the distinction between Antoni A and B although of academic interest appears to be of no clinical importance. Schwannomas are usually S-100 positive although this is also true for melanocytes and occasionally melanin pigment may be seen demonstrating the capability of the Schwann cell to store this pigment.[58] In older tumours hyalization is common and the multinucleated Schwann cell, the 'pleomorphic schwannoma' may cause problems in diagnosis.

The typical appearance of the neurogenic sarcoma (malignant schwannoma) is a dense fibrosarcomatous pattern with occasional neurogenic features such as palisading nuclei alternating with poorly cellular areas. Immunohistochemistry shows a strong positive reaction to S-100 in many of the neoplastic cells.[50] However, doubt remains as to whether benign schwannomas ever become malignant[59] and the true origin of the 'malignant schwannoma' is possibly a change in an existing neurofibroma. Neurogenic sarcoma or malignant peripheral nerve sheath tumour are less confusing terms for this lesion.[60]

Natural history

Schwannomas slowly grow in size producing symptoms by impinging on related structures or obstruction. Bone resorption leads to extension into the orbit or intracranially and where feasible the lesion should be removed by enucleation with minimal prospect of recurrence. Unless irradiated, malignant change appears unlikely although the true origin of the neurogenic sarcoma is not yet clear.

Differential diagnosis

A wide variety of conditions must be excluded in differentiating a schwannoma within the upper jaw. Glioma, papilloma, olfactory neuroblastoma, sarcoma, lymphoma, carcinoma and even a mucocoele, although the last may be secondary to obstruction from an undiagnosed tumour as in the following case report.

A 51-year-old man was seen in July 1985 with a swelling in the region of the superior medial quadrant of the left orbit, present for 6 months. There was some lateral displacement of the globe producing diplopia and a clinical and radiological diagnosis of fronto-ethmoid mucocoele was made. A left fronto-ethmoidectomy confirmed this diagnosis but also revealed blockage of the frontonasal recess by a small mass. The histological report read: 'A tumour composed of spindle cells which are cellular in places with a hint of palisading together with Verocay bodies. Typical Antoni A and B areas are present but no nerve tissue identified.' The patient has remained free of symptoms 2 years postoperatively.

The pathologist must differentiate schwannomas from neurofibroma, fibromatosis, fibrosarcoma, fibrous histiocytoma, fibrous dysplasia and osteosarcoma. This is only possible by examination of biopsy material which may be difficult to obtain because of intense vascularization.[40]

Development of neurogenic sarcoma from peripheral nerve sheath tumours is said to occur in 2.4 to 16.5% of cases.[61] This malignancy represents less than 2% of all malignant upper jaw tumours and few cases have been recorded. Maroun et al in 1986 reviewed the literature finding only six patients, including one of their own.[51] However, increasing use of immunohistochemistry may result in more diagnoses, for fibrosarcomata are not positive to S-100 and antigens may be detected in neurosarcomas such as myelin basic proteins and possibly Leu-7 which might assist more accurate diagnosis.[58]

Neurosarcomata are highly malignant and must be differentiated from rhabdomyosarcoma, chondrosarcoma or amelanotic melanoma.

Treatment

The definitive treatment of upper jaw schwannomas is complete surgical removal or at least, decompression for these tumours are slow growing. The operative approach must provide wide exposure enabling identification and preservation of adjacent structures. Lesions within the nasal cavity are suitable for lateral rhinotomy preserving the lacrimal sac and infraorbital nerve. Tumours involving or arising within the maxillary antrum can be approached via a sublabial incision or a formal midfacial approach although invasion of the pterygopalatine fossa requires more radical surgery.

Invasion of the anterior cranial fossa necessitates a craniofacial technique[56] as illustrated by the following case report.

A 37-year-old woman was first seen in March 1985 with a 2 month history of right-sided epistaxis. There was no obvious intranasal lesion but radiology of the sinuses had shown opacity of the right ethmoids and maxillary antrum. However, antral washout had produced severe bleeding and examination under anaesthesia showed a mass at the roof of the posterior nares extending into the nasopharynx. Biopsy from this area was reported as showing, 'a schwannoma of predominantly Antoni A type which stained positively to S-100. This tumour is rather cellular with some mitosis.'

CT scans showed a mass in the right nasal cavity extending into the antrum, ethmoids and posteriorly the nasopharynx.

The sphenoid appeared involved on the right side and there was a definite area of erosion in the cribriform plate.

Removal was carried out by a right craniofacial approach which confirmed the defect in the cribriform plate and absence of dural invasion. The sphenoid sinus was filled with mucopus but without tumour. Removal was complete and the patient is free from tumour 6 years postoperatively.

Schwannomas have been considered as radioresistant[55] but Younis et al believe that this is incorrect and based upon the use of orthovoltage at inadequate dosage.[40] They report good results with external irradiation and radon seed implantation and this technique is certainly necessary with neurogenic sarcomas and possibly where remnants have been left in situ following removal of a schwannoma not associated with malignant change.[43]

NEUROFIBROMA (BENIGN AND MALIGNANT)

Definition

A non-encapsulated tumour of Schwann cells differing from a schwannoma in its structure and clinical behaviour.

Synonyms

Neurilemmoma, plexiform neurofibroma, von Recklinghausen's disease.

Historical aspects

Von Recklinghausen described neurofibromatosis over 100 years ago,[62] although this condition, an autosomal dominant disorder due to a lesion on chromosome 17,[63] is usually associated with multiple neurofibromata. However, Kragh et al found that of 328 patients with von Recklinghausen's disease seen at the Mayo Clinic, 47 had solitary neurofibromata removed from the head and neck. During this time only 21 patients without von Recklinghausen's disease had neurofibroma within the head and neck region.[64]

Incidence

Neurofibromas are rare tumours within the upper jaw and a review of the European and American literature up to 1975 by Robitaille et al could find only four neurofibromas but 12 neurilemmoma.[42] A review of 430 000 pathology specimens by Perzin et al in 1982 revealed six neurofibromas and two neurilemmomas involving the nasal cavity and paranasal sinuses[43] whilst Harrison reviewing 639 cases of upper jaw tumours found seven neurofibromas.[65] Many authors however make little distinction between neurilemmomas and neurofibromas and the true incidence of these two conditions remains uncertain although undoubtedly uncommon within the upper jaw.

Solitary neurofibromas by definition occur in patients who do not have von Recklinghausen's disease.

Geschickter in 1935[66] found that 90% of all reported neurofibromata were in fact solitary occurring anywhere within the head and neck region; nasopharynx, paranasal sinuses, hypopharynx, larynx, tongue, floor of mouth, salivary glands and buccal cavity.[15,43,67,68] Individual series however, remain small and in Kragh et al's review of 152 benign and malignant nerve tumours only five were within the nasal cavity or paranasal sinuses,[64] whilst New & Devine found 19 neurofibromas of the upper respiratory tract five of which were situated in this region.[14] Conley & Janecka in their review of 90 patients with Schwann cell tumours of the head and neck located six within the upper jaw.[69]

Age, sex and ethnic variation

The evidence suggests that neurofibroma tend to occur earlier than neurilemmoma being found between the ages of 20 and 40 years or younger when associated with von Recklinghausen's disease, and with an equal sex incidence.[70]

Isolated cases have been recorded from most countries suggesting that there is no obvious ethnic variation.

Although growing from a peripheral nerve sheath it is rarely possible to determine the site of origin with accuracy since by the time of diagnosis there has usually been expansion or destruction of surrounding structures hindering identification.

Aetiology

Both Schwann and perineural cells are thought to be derived from neuroectoderm although these cells are located in different positions within the nerve sheath; otherwise they are indistinguishable. Both give rise to neoplasms included in the general group of Schwann cell tumours which are uncommon within the upper jaw despite the frequency with which these lesions occur within the body.[71] Some guidance as to aetiological factors may be gained from the genetic studies reported by Constantino et al on acoustic neurofibromatosis.[63] They have emphasized that von Recklinghausen's disease and recurrent neurofibromatosis are two genetically distinct disorders that should more correctly be referred to as 'neurofibromatosis'. Von Recklinghausen's disease results from an abnormal gene on chromosome 17 whilst acoustic neuroma (more accurately called schwannoma) is due to a lesion on chromosome 22q. Both forms show autosomal dominant inheritance with variable penetration. It is the acoustic lesion which is more frequently associated with neurofibromas and 90% of these patients with the abnormal gene will develop bilateral acoustic tumours. The significance of an abnormal gene on chromosome 17 may account for the other associated defects recognized with von Recklinghausen's disease, cerebral aqueduct stenosis, lambdoidal suture and sphenoid bone defects and nasal glioma as reported by Pollard & Carter.[11]

Clinical features

Neurofibromas occurring within the nose and paranasal sinuses may be solitary or multiple whilst the plexiform type is usually associated with von Recklinghausen's disease and most commonly found within the orbit.

Solitary lesions are slow growing, non-tender and although non-encapsulated are frequently well circumscribed. Multiple tumours, frequently associated with von Recklinghausen's disease, are often painful. Symptoms are produced by the progressive expansion upon surrounding tissues and obstruction of sinus openings. The cases reported by Stevens & Kirkham had nasal obstruction, proptosis and headaches,[70] all common to slow-growing neoplasms within this region and no symptom can be considered as pathognomonic of neurofibroma.

Radiology

A soft-tissue mass with a characteristic irregular patchy appearance after contrast may be seen on CT.[72] Displacement of soft tissues and bony walls or erosion, although non-specific, assists in determining the tumour extent.

Macroscopic and microscopic appearance

In most instances there is little difficulty in distinguishing neurofibromas from neurilemmomas because of their distinctive histological appearances. However, in small non-representative biopsies or when a neurofibroma shows areas resembling neurilemmoma, a clear distinction may be impossible.[71]

On gross examination neurofibromas tend to be soft with a grey, glistening cut surface suggesting a myxoma. When associated with a large nerve the trunk may be seen to be integrated into the tumour preventing free dissection.

Histologically, neurofibromas are characterized by a mixture of cells lying in a mucinous or collagenous stroma. These cells are fibroblasts, neurites and Schwann cells, some being S100 positive. Scattered lymphocytes and mast cells are common and neurites are situated within the tumour substance. The myxoid stroma tends to be more fibrillar than when seen in myxomas and plexiform neurofibromata may contain large amounts of normal nerve lying within the mucoid matrix. Despite these characteristics, overlapping features between neuro-

fibroma and neurilemmoma do occur although malignant changes are found only in the former. Malignant transformation is uncommon in solitary neurofibromata but more common with multiple lesions. Malignant tumours of peripheral nerves have been called erroneously 'malignant schwannomas' although this tumour virtually never undergoes malignant change. These malignant nerve tumours tend to be undifferentiated with little to suggest a Schwann cell origin and should more accurately be called 'neurosarcoma'. They may be difficult to distinguish from fibrosarcoma for S-100 can be demonstrated in many lesions but neurogenous sarcoma usually have areas of palisading nuclei alternating with poorly cellular areas. To avoid confusion, many pathologists restrict the diagnosis of neurosarcoma to tumours clearly arising from a nerve, containing areas of neurofibroma or developing in patients with von Recklinghausen's disease. These make up approximately 5 to 10% of all sarcomas and in the series of malignant nerve sheath neoplasms reported by Trojanowski et al, there were 24 patients with neurosarcoma in a total of 607 cases of neurofibroma or neurilemmoma seen between 1962 and 1979.[73] Kragh et al found only four malignant neurogenous tumours in 148 cases of neurilemmomas situated within the head and neck[64] whilst in Conley & Janecka's 90 neural head and neck lesions, 14 were said to be malignant.[69] However, many authors fail to detail the criteria on which a diagnosis of von Recklinghausen's disease or even malignancy was made and malignant degeneration, in the absence of previous irradiation, is uncommon. A real incidence of less than 10% of all neurosarcomata are found within the head and neck region making the upper jaw a rare site.[69,74]

Natural history

Neurofibromas are slow growing expansive tumours producing symptoms by pressure as well as local infiltration. Bone erosion does not necessarily indicate malignant change although if not removed completely, neurofibroma can behave aggressively with local recurrences. Neurosarcoma are highly aggressive and if incompletely removed recur rapidly with death occurring from intracranial invasion or pulmonary metastases. Spread to regional lymph nodes is uncommon and there appears to be a 'low-grade' variety with few mitotic figures (less than 5 to 50 per high power field) which may have an unexpected protracted course despite failure to gain local tumour control.[74]

Rapid growth in an existing neurofibroma, especially in a patient with von Recklinghausen's disease, is highly suspicious of malignant change although rare within the nasal cavity or paranasal sinuses. Hellquist says that within this region neurogenic sarcoma is as likely to arise de novo as from malignant change in an existing neurofibroma although there are few publications supporting this opinion.[75]

Differential diagnosis

Schwann cell tumours may be difficult to distinguish from neoplasms derived from fibroblasts especially when the biopsy is small. Neurofibromas can usually be separated from neurilemmomas, but when myxoid changes are present confusion with myxoma is possible although the tumour cells in the latter have stellate-shaped fibrocytic cells with enlarged nuclei.[67]

Highly cellular neurosarcomata may resemble fibrosarcomas and the identification of a nervous origin or the presence of existing areas of neurofibroma may be needed to verify diagnosis (Table 19.2).

Treatment

If not removed completely, neurofibromata may recur locally requiring further surgery. Kragh et al reported the successful management of two patients in whom further surgery produced control for more than 14 years.[64] Radical resection with a functional or cosmetic disability however, can only be justified for extensive, progressing lesions and the two patients reported by Stevens & Kirkham were successfully managed by tumour removal via a lateral rhinotomy despite orbital involvement.[70] Solitary neurofibroma in the nasal cavity or paranasal sinuses have a low rate of local recurrence even when small amounts of tumour remain in situ.[76]

Neurosarcoma however, are highly malignant especially when associated with von Recklinghausen's disease. Recurrence following local excision is recorded as being as high as 80% with a 5-year survival rate of between 15 and 30%.[77] Metastases may occur as late as 5 to 10 years following treatment despite good local control.

In the absence of concurrent von Recklinghausen's disease however, cure rates may rise to 50% although in the patients reported by Conley & Janecka, 12 of the 14 patients with neurogenic sarcoma died within 3 years and evidence suggests that the prognosis for this neoplasm within the head and neck is inferior to that for those situated elsewhere in the body, possibly because of the limitations of radical excision.[64]

There is no evidence that combination with radiotherapy or chemotherapy materially affects the incidence of local control or long-term prognosis and at present the emphasis should be on effective local excision.

EXTRACRANIAL MENINGIOMA

Definition

Tumours of the central nervous system which are believed to originate in arachnoid villous structures of the meninges.

Incidence and site (Table 19.3)

Because of the rarity of extracranial meningioma and the difficulties of differentiating extensions of an intracranial lesion from meningioma presenting primarily in the upper jaw, discussions of incidence cannot be considered separately from the site of origin. Meningiomas constitute about 12 to 15% of all intracranial tumours with about 20% of these having an extracranial component.[78–81] In descending order the sites of these extensions are: orbit, outer tables of the cranium and soft tissues of the scalp, upper airway (nasal cavity, nasopharynx, paranasal sinuses) and the pterygoid region.[82] Far less frequently, extracranial meningiomas arise without any apparent association with an intracranial lesion and within the upper jaw this may be from three sources.

1. Extracranial extension from an undetected intracranial tumour
2. Involvement from an orbital tumour
3. In-situ.

Table 19.2 Pathological differences between fibroblastic and Schwann cell tumours (after Perzin et al[43])

	Fibrosarcoma	Neurilemmoma	Neurofibroma	Neurogenic sarcoma
Border	Infiltrative	Encapsulated	Infiltrative	Infiltrative
Low power appearance	Moderate cellularity	Highly cellular (Antoni A)	Moderate cellularity	Highly cellular
Fibrous tissue	Decreasing with increased cellularity	Variable	Small amounts	Small amounts
Myxoid tissue	Unusual	Focally (Antoni B)	Prominent	?
Nuclear appearance	Spindle-shaped	Tapered	Tapered	Spindle-shaped
Nuclear pleomorphism	Minimal	Bizarre	Bizarre	Minimal
Mitotic activity	Moderate	Few	Few	Numerous

Table 19.3 Meningiomas (Harrison & Lund)

Male	Female	Age (yr)	Site	Treatment	Outcome
1		38	Frontal bone	(×2) Frontal craniotomy External ethmoidectomy Acrylic obturator Radiotherapy Craniofacial resection	AWR 12 yr
	1	68	Orbit	(L) Orbital clearance, craniofacial resection (R) Orbital decompression – completely blind	DOD 8 yr
1		14	Orbit	Orbital explorations (×6) Bifrontal craniotomy Craniofacial resection & orbital clearance	9 yr FU AWR then lost
1		54	Sphenoid	Orbital explorations (×2) Radiotherapy Craniofacial resection – bilateral visual loss	3 yr FU then lost
1		17	Septum	Lateral rhinotomy Craniofacial resection Decompression – L orbital apex Orbital clearance	DOD 9.5 yr
1		64	Nasal septum	Lateral rhinotomy 285 Craniofacial resection	A&W 6 yr (FU – CT scans normal)

A&W, alive and well; AWR, alive with recurrence; DOD, dead of disease; FU, follow-up

3% of the cases discussed by Farr et al had upper airway involvement by direct extension of an olfactory groove or middle fossa meningioma.[79] However, Lopez et al when reviewing the literature in 1974 found 140 cases of extracranial meningioma, 90 (64%) of which were diagnosed as primary extensions and 50 (36%) secondary extensions from an existing intracranial tumour.[83] In 1980, Ho also reviewed the literature finding 18 cases of nasal and paranasal meningiomata adding one additional patient[84] and 5 years later, Atherino et al had increased this to 21 cases.[78]

Isolated cases of 'primary' nasal or sinus meningioma have been published for more than 20 years but lack of adequate radiological evaluation and minimal follow-up fails to establish the absence of an unsuspected intracranial tumour in many of these papers.[85–92] This criticism applies particularly to some of the very early papers such as Shahen in 1931 who was one of the first to report a meningioma thought to originate within the maxillary sinus.[93] Many of these papers described ectopic meningioma as arising within the frontal sinuses although the limitations of radiological assessment may have failed to detect a small intracranial tumour extending through the posterior sinus wall. The real incidence of these extracranial meningioma is therefore in doubt although there is general agreement that this is a rare condition and only by thorough radiological assessment supported by pathological evidence obtained at excision will reliable data be forthcoming.

Age, sex and ethnic variation

Age at diagnosis ranges from late childhood to over 80 years with no obvious sex discrimination nor ethnic susceptibility. Cushing & Eisenhardt's classical review of meningiomas provides little assistance since only one patient was reported in which an intracranial meningioma had eroded through the posterior wall of the frontal sinus to present in the nasal cavity![94]

Aetiology

Secondary extension from an intracranial meningioma is the commonest means by which this tumour presents within the upper jaw. Although occasionally associated with an iatrogenic, surgically-produced defect, this is not a prerequisite since tumour may readily pass through foramina in the skull base, enter the orbit via the supra-orbital fissure, nasopharynx and nasal cavity through existing holes in the cribriform plate and reach the pterygoid region through the floor of the middle fossa or suture lines.[82] Tumour can also reach the nasal cavity and less commonly the maxillary antrum, via the orbit where it may also arise as a primary tumour or secondary extension.[95]

The histogenesis of primary extracranial meningioma remains uncertain although it is recognized that intracranial meningiomata have several foci of predilection and are commonly found in association with arachnoid granulations. The cells of origin are meningocytes, and it has been suggested that groups of heterotopic meningocytes dislocated during the closure of midline structures during foetal life could be the site of origin of some extracranial meningiomata.[81,82,96] Other authors believe that ectopic lesions come from meningocytic cellular rests, including the perineural sheaths accompanying the nerves passing through foramina in the skull or inter-vertebral foramen.[92] Craig & Gogela have found clusters of meningocytes within the sheath of the optic nerve and these authors described 17 patients with orbital meningiomata concluding that the most likely origin was from arachnoid tufts which had grown into and through the dural layer of the optic nerve sheath.[97]

Despite enthusiasm for the 'cell rest' theory it fails to explain how tumours distant from the optic or other nerves develop. Differentiation of Schwann cells into meningocytes has been suggested by Bain & Shnitka because of the similarity between cells within meningocytic meningioma and cells considered to be derived from the Schwann cell.[98] Meningocytes are however, not the only cells found in meningiomata. Occasionally mesenchymal cells such as fibroblasts are present and Shuangshoti et al believe that meningiomata may arise directly from meningocytes, fibroblasts, Schwann cells or a combination of these cells, classifying this tumour as a mesenchymal neoplasm.[99] Certainly, a pluripotential mesenchymal origin would explain patients with a meningioma apparently unassociated with the more obvious sites of origin, although the possibility in such instances of a small plaque of meningioma on the surface of the dura cannot be discounted unless this region is visualized surgically.[84]

The relationship between radiotherapy and subsequent development of a meningioma is well recognized.[100,101] Zirkin et al[102] reported the case of a 49-year-old woman successfully treated by lateral rhinotomy and 2000 rad of irradiation for an olfactory neuroblastoma who 10 years later developed a transitional type meningioma above the cribriform plate at the site of the original neoplasm. Development of meningiomas at irradiated sites within the head and neck have been documented in 38 cases by Iacona et al.[100] A delay of several years occurred before the development of this second pathology and in one patient the initial therapy was for tinea capitis.[103]

Clinical features

Although Lopez et al have said that a cutaneous mass is the commonest clinical presentation of an extracranial meningioma;[83] nasal obstruction, epistaxis, anosmia and proptosis are most likely to occur when an olfactory groove meningioma enters the nasal cavity.[81] When the original tumour is sited within the orbit, then nasal symptoms may be associated with severe proptosis or visual loss. As with chondrosarcomata in this region, uncontrolled disease may lead to bilateral blindness particularly in children.

Sadar et al found that half of their 21 paranasal sinus meningiomas were located in the frontal sinus presenting with frontal swelling and proptosis. The remainder were sited within the ethmoids, maxillary sinus and nasal

cavity.[91] Nasal obstruction, facial swelling, proptosis and epistaxis were all common but are non-specific and clinically it is usually impossible to differentiate between ectopic lesions and an extension from an un-diagnosed intracranial tumour. However, Kjeldsberg & Minckler have divided extracranial meningiomas into four 'theoretical' groups for the purpose of clinical presentation and subsequent analysis.[89]

1. Meningioma representing an extension from a primary intracranial tumour
2. Meningioma arising from arachnoid cell rests of cranial sheaths
3. Extracranial meningioma without any connection with foramina or cranial nerves
4. Metastases from an intracranial meningioma.

This last group is of some importance since despite its usual benign histological appearance, meningiomas occasionally demonstrate invasive properties. Direct extension by bony invasion to the calvaria, sinuses, nasal cavity or middle ear have all been described[104] although a true metastasis from an intracranial meningioma must remain the least likely reason for an extracranial lesion within the upper jaw.[99]

Radiology (Fig. 19.8)

In the absence of intracranial abnormalities, the radiological picture of extracranial meningioma involving the

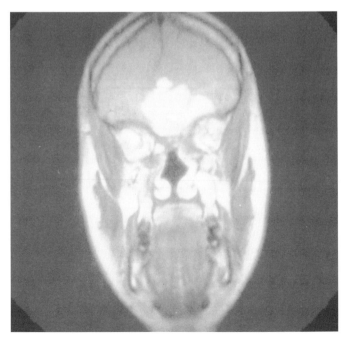

Fig. 19.8 Coronal MR scan, T1 weighted sequence with gadolinium showing large intracranial extension of recurrent meningioma.

upper jaw may show on CT a minimal hyperdense, well circumscribed soft tissue mass with uniform enhancement. In addition there are frequently areas of calcification. MRI shows a high signal with a low density rim but none of this can be considered as specific for meningioma. Papavasiliou et al[105] have discussed the associated facial skeletal changes that can occur with both intra- and extracranial meningioma, the most common being bony hyperostosis which Cushing found to be present in 25% of his patients.[106] Tucker et al in 1959 found these changes in half of meningiomas affecting the tuberculum sellae[107] and Persky & Som considered hyperostosis of the planum sphenoidale to be a characteristic finding in most olfactory groove meningiomata.[81] These bony changes may be overgrowths or osteomas without active tumour invasion or tissue spread through the Haversian system. Hyperostotic changes are also known to result from meningiomatous cellular invasion but can be found some distance from the primary tumour suggesting an aetiological hormonal factor. Shuangshoti et al consider this bony response to be indicative of the mesenchymal origin of meningioma with the multipotential cell differentiating into bone.[99] However, hyperostosis when present, must be considered as highly indicative of an associated meningioma situated either intra- or extracranially. Pneumosinus dilatans, an abnormal dilatation of the paranasal sinuses can also be associated with meningioma. First described by Benjamins in 1918[108] this condition has been found in the frontal, ethmoid and sphenoid sinuses. Lombardi et al reported 13 (38%) cases with pneumosinus dilatans in 34 meningiomas of the tuberculum sellae; eight (20%) of 40 meningiomas affecting the olfactory groove also had this condition.[109] However, Lloyd emphasizes that pneumosinus dilatans is not pathognomonic of meningioma and can occur in fibro-osseous disease.[110]

Macroscopic and microscopic appearance

It is generally accepted that meningiomas arise from the same cells that give origin to the arachnoid villi and epithelium. Arachnoid villi may be found in abundance close to the glial-schwannian junction (Obersteiner-Redlich zone) which is an unstable transitional zone where meninges change into endoneurium. It is thought that meningiomata may develop from arachnoid-producing cells in this region. The meningo-endothelial regions of the olfactory nerves passing through the cribriform plate are less defined but this could also be the site for a primary extracranial tumour.[89] Courville & Abbott demonstrated this transition between the meningocytic clusters of an arachnoid villi and a symptomless prefrontal meningioma found accidentally at autopsy.[111]

Macroscopically, many nasal meningioma present as nasal polypi with a firm consistency and a friable or granular appearance on their cut surface.[17a]

Histological variation is common and may present some difficulty in diagnosis. Four major variants are described:

1. Syncytial, composed of sheets of polygonal cells
2. Transitional, with a whorled pattern of spindle cells and psammoma bodies
3. Fibrous, with less cellularity but more collagen
4. Angioblastic

Batsakis[82] believes that the syncytial and transitional forms comprise the majority of extracranial lesions with the classical appearance of concentric whorls of cells and laminated calcified (psammoma) bodies. However, the latter can be found in other tumours, notably being papillary thyroid carcinoma and serous tumours of the ovary.[87]

There appears to be no biological or prognostic difference between these varying histological sub-groups, indeed several types may be found in the same tumour. A major exception is the angioblastic meningioma which resembles a haemopericytoma and has a more aggressive natural history. It has been suggested that this variant is a meningeal haemopericytoma rather than a meningioma.[112] Although meningiomata expand by infiltration of surrounding structures such as bone or fibrous tissue, they are considered to be benign tumours. Rarely, meningiomas behave aggressively recurring locally or even metastasizing. Histological features which might indicate this behaviour include hypercellularity, increased mitosis, a papillary pattern and invasion of brain tissue.[87] However, failure to eradicate completely the primary lesion may lead to local recurrence in any meningioma and even 'benign' lesions have been reported as metastasizing, possibly from involvement of adjoining vascular spaces.

Natural history

The small number of fully documented cases of extracranial meningiomata together with the limited data on long-term follow-up, seriously restricts our knowledge of the natural history of this tumour. It is possible that every patient has a small undetected intracranial component which in time will manifest itself on routine radiological examination. Most meningiomas are slow growing, and when the extracranial component is radically removed the prognosis is considered as good, particularly in the older patient. In the young patient or where complete excision is not feasible, it is essential that CT scanning is carried out at all follow-up visits in order that early detection of recurrence or regrowth of tumour may be possible. In those cases where the extracranial meningioma is an extension of a detectable intracranial lesion then the natural history will be influenced by the control of the primary lesion.

Treatment (Table 19.3)

Although the preferred treatment for all extracranial meningiomata is surgical excision, preoperative assessment with CT and MRI is essential for surgical planning. A detectable intracranial component will necessitate a craniofacial approach although evidence is now accumulating that suggests that this approach should be used for most, if not all, nasal or fronto-ethmoid meningioma. Adequate resection of the cribriform plate and associated dura is not possible by an inferior approach and operative specimens indicate that some of these patients have an undetected plaque of meningioma on the associated dura.

Routine CT evaluation is essential for at least 5 years postoperatively and in histologically aggressive lesions this should include a search for systemic metastases.

Involvement of the ethmoid by an optic nerve sheath or orbital extradural meningioma necessitates a multidisciplinary approach as discussed by Wright et al.[113] Orbital clearance may be combined with a craniofacial resection but in some instances local dissection within the orbit may preserve vision although leaving tumour in situ.

NEUROENDOCRINE CARCINOMA

Definition

A neoplasm derived from cells belonging to the widely dispersed neuroendocrine system which share the ability to synthesize, store and in some instances, secrete a variety of biogenic amines and peptides.[114]

Synonyms

Carcinoid tumour, atypical carcinoid, large and small cell neuroendocrine tumour, apudomata.

Historical aspects

The APUD (amine precursors uptake and decarboxylation) or neuroendocrine system is composed of cells derived from endothelial epithelium and neuroendothelial cells derived from neuroepithelium. There is doubt as to the embryogenesis of these cells which have the potential for hormone production being present in the adrenal medulla, thyroid C-cells, gastrointestinal tract, paraganglia, larynx, etc. The nasal neuroepithelium, whilst not derived from neuroectoderm but from the olfactory placode, produces nerve fibres and may therefore produce neoplasms with characteristics similar to those of ectoderm origin.[17b] Olfactory neuroblastomata have morphological and biochemical similarities to neuroecto-

dermal tumours and in 1980 Kameya et al described four cases of neuroectodermal carcinomata of the nose and paranasal sinuses.[115] Although neuroectodermal neoplasms have been described in many sites, dilemmas over histological terminology has caused confusion, particularly in the separation of neuroendocrine (glandular) tumours from neuroblastomata (neurofibril).[17b] Within the larynx however, a clear separation of paragangliomas from neuroendocrine neoplasms has been reported by Milroy et al.[116]

Incidence

Although clearly recognized as a neuroblastoma or phaeochromocytoma in the adrenal medulla, medullary carcinoma in the thyroid or carcinoid in the appendix, there have only been a small number of neuroendocrine tumours reported originating in the upper jaw. Neuroendocrine carcinomas are even less common with Kameya et al finding four cases[115] and Silva et al, analysing 29 nasal tumours originally described as neuroblastomas, reclassifying 20 as neuroendocrine carcinomata.[117] The mean age of this group was 50 years compared with 20 years for their neuroblastoma patients. Silva et al also considered patients with nasal lesions reported by Chaudhry et al,[118] Friedmann & Osborn[119] and Kahn[120] concluding that these were also probably neuroendocrine carcinomas. There was an equal sex distribution and the series included a small number of black patients.

Clinical features

From the scanty evidence available there appears to be no discernible aetiological factor causing nasal neuroendocrine carcinoma, which present as a proliferative mass within the nasal passage and appear to be located on the lateral nasal wall. Epistaxis is common and extension to related structures such as the maxillary sinus or orbit is common to most malignant upper jaw neoplasms. In 14 of the patients discussed by Silva et al, no site of origin could be determined.[117]

Radiology

Apart from demonstrating a soft tissue mass, radiology is of most use in identifying bone destruction or intracranial extension. No data are available regarding specific changes in neuroendocrine carcinoma of the upper jaw except its siting in the lateral nasal wall rather than the cribriform plate.

Macroscopic and microscopic appearance

In differentiating neuroendocrine carcinomas within the nasal cavity Silva et al[117] emphasized the importance of the presence of uniform cells growing in connection within glandular structures which were usually Grimelius-positive although, unlike these tumours in the larynx, rarely secreted calcitonin.

Histologically, these small cells with atypia tend to be arranged in nests and spheres but there are always areas with glandular structures.

Immunohistochemistry demonstrating ACTH and other peptide hormones in combination with positive immunoreactivity for chromogranin is said by Hellquist to strongly support a diagnosis of neuroendocrine carcinoma.[75]

When discussing these tumours within the larynx, Milroy et al consider that there is a spectrum between the well-differentiated carcinoid as seen in the gastrointestinal tract, and the poorly differentiated small cell carcinoma. The large cell neuroendocrine carcinoma as seen in the larynx represents a position within these two extremes.[116] They comment that these neoplasms may arise from uncommitted cells in the basal layer of the epithelium which differentiate along an epithelial or neuroendocrine pathway according to microenvironmental conditions and supporting evidence for this is provided by tumours with both epithelial and neuroendocrine differentiation.[121,122]

Unfortunately, nasal neuroendocrine carcinoma has not received the same attention as laryngeal neuroendocrine carcinoma although Hellquist[75] has summarized the main histological differences between olfactory neuroblastoma and neuroendocrine carcinoma as being:

1. Neuroendocrine carcinoma have greater numbers of epitheloid cells containing more cytoplasm and with different immunohistochemical reactions
2. There are no rosettes or neurofibrils in neuroendocrine carcinomata.

However, both Silva et al[117] and Michaels[17b] admit that tumours characterized as neuroectodermal may be derived from olfactory epithelium and like neuroblastoma may show interlobular neurofibrillary changes as well as glandular differentiation in the same tumour.

Natural history (Fig. 19.9)

Although neuroendocrine neoplasms are a heterogeneous group of tumours with site variations in their biological behaviour, Silva et al found differences in natural history between patients with an olfactory neuroblastoma and neuroendocrine carcinoma. The latter showed a greater tendency for local recurrence, 54% to 25%, and with neuroendocrine recurrences or metastases not occurring until after the 3rd year following therapy. They also found a 100% survival at 5 years, 88% at 7 years and 77% at 10 years for the carcinoma. Only three patients died in their group of 20 patients, two from intracranial extension and one with metastases.[117] Long-term experi-

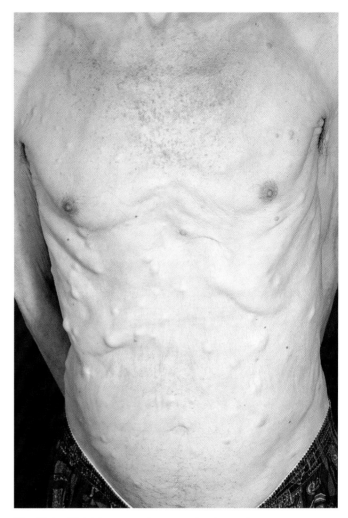

Fig. 19.9 Multiple metastatic neuroendocrine carcinoma.

ence of this uncommon neoplasm is not yet available but many pathologists, whilst maintaining some reservation regarding the acceptance of neuroendocrine carcinoma as a distinct entity, recognize the possibility that the histological features described by Silva et al may be related to subsequent biological behaviour with this lesion being less malignant than the olfactory neuroblastoma.

Differential diagnosis

Apart from the major difficulty of differentiating neuroectodermal carcinoma from olfactory neuroblastoma; undifferentiated carcinoma, Ewing's sarcoma, lymphoma and poorly differentiated adenocarcinoma can all present difficulties in diagnosis. Table 19.4 shows the principal differences between neuroendocrine carcinoma and poorly differentiated adenocarcinoma and these characteristics can serve to assist in all differential diagnoses for this tumour.

Table 19.4 Differential diagnosis between poorly differentiated adenocarcinoma and neuroendocrine carcinoma[117]

	Poorly differentiated adenocarcinoma	Neuroendocrine carcinoma
Pattern	Variable	Well circumscribed group of cells (basement membrane can be present)
	Malignant glands	Malignant cells growing from glands, which are neither malignant nor dysplastic
	Glands can be present in metastases	Glands absent in metastases
Cellular characteristics	Moderate to marked variation in cell size and shape Scanty cytoplasm	Monotonous uniformity Abundant
	High NC ratio	Low
	Usually high mitotic rate	Usually low
Grimelius stain	Negative, can be positive in mucinous carcinoma	Positive
Nuclei	Marked variation in size	Predominantly round or oval, same spindle, similar size
	Irregular distribution of chromatin	Even chromatin
	Atypical mitoses	No

NC, nuclear cytoplasmic

Treatment

Insufficient data are available to support a definitive treatment regime but there appears to be good anecdotal evidence to suggest that these tumours should be managed in a similar manner to olfactory neuroblastomas. Where technically feasible and following radiological assessment, radical resection should be combined with oncologic dosage irradiation. However despite the encouraging results reported by Silva et al, which were based upon patients pathologically reclassified, it is likely that unless primary control is obtained, the incidence of late recurrence and metastases will be compatible with those obtained for olfactory neuroblastoma. There is no good reason for expecting neuroendocrine carcinoma to behave in a biologically more benign manner although the localization of the tumour in the region of the middle turbinate rather than the cribriform plate may assist radical resection.

OLFACTORY NEUROBLASTOMA

Definition

A malignant neoplasm arising from the olfactory epithelium and comprised of undifferentiated neuroectodermal tissue.

Synonyms

Esthesioneuroblastoma, olfactory neuroepithelioma, esthesioneuroma, olfactory esthesioneuroepithelioma, esthesioneurocytoma, esthesioneuroepithelioma and olfactory neuroepithelial tumour.

Historical aspects

The description by Berger et al in 1924[123] of a nasal tumour with histological evidence of olfactory differentiation was the first of several attempts to define the unique morphological characteristics of neuroblastomas arising within this location. The original description featured a prominent rosette pattern resembling retinal neuroblastomas but a later account by Berger & Coutard in 1926[124] found neurofibrils rather than rosettes which was considered as a mature variant of the original tumour. On this basis they assumed that this neoplasm arose from the sensory cells of the olfactory mucosa. However, the preparatory term 'esthesio' refers non-specifically to sensory or sensory perception and its previous use in the terminology of this tumour represents a derivation from the original French description of l'esthesio-neuroepithelioma rather than any semantic accuracy. For many years lack of consensus regarding terminology existed, based upon variations in the presence or not of different types of rosettes, e.g. esthesioneuroepithelioma – esthesioneuroblastoma – esthesioneurocytoma. The nomenclature proved confusing since no relationship has been found with subsequent biological behaviour and these terms have now been generally replaced by the descriptive and generic terms 'olfactory neuroblastoma'.[75]

Incidence

O'Connor et al in 1989 estimated that less than 300 cases had been published and that this tumour represented between 1 and 5% of all malignant tumours within the nasal cavity.[125] When Skolnik et al reviewed the available literature in 1966 they found only 97 cases in a total of

42 publications in the English language, only one author having treated more than 15 patients. Indeed, the majority had experience of only two or three cases some of whom had been treated 20 years previously emphasizing the limitations of this type of literature search.[126]

Within the last decade this neoplasm has been reported more frequently although this appears to reflect an increasing awareness and improvements in pathological recognition rather than any real increase in incidence.[127] However, personal experience continues to be limited to small numbers of patients. Levine et al, 26 cases in 25 years,[128] O'Connor et al, 15 cases in 17 years,[125] Beitler et al, 14 cases in 10 years,[129] Shah & Feghali, 31 cases in 26 years,[130] and our own experience of 20 patients treated over a period of 14 years.[131]

Age, sex and ethnic variation (Table 19.5)

Most of the larger series report a bi-modal age distribution with peaks in the 2nd and 3rd decades and later in the 6th and 7th decades of life. Schwabb et al had a patient aged 8 years[132] whilst Ijaduola et al reported an olfactory neuroblastoma in a 5.5 month-old Nigerian baby.[133] There appears to be a slight male preponderance but few patients have been diagnosed in black individuals in North America or elsewhere.[134,135]

Site

Olfactory neuroblastoma arise exclusively in the nasal roof corresponding to the anatomical distribution of the specialized neuroepithelial cells of the olfactory mucosa. This covers the superior turbinals, varying amounts of the upper nasal septum and the least accessible area being the cribriform plate. Evaluation of clinical, radiological and serially sectioned anatomical material by Harrison[136] has emphasized the importance of the cribriform plate in relation to the spread of the tumour intracranially. The floor of the olfactory fossa is formed by the cribriform plate which in the adult has an average length of 21 mm with a breadth increasing evenly (anteriorly to posteriorly) from 4 to 5.4 mm. Schmidt has differentiated five morphological types of cribriform plate each varying in both breadth and length.[137] These variations are of clinical importance since the dural-lined olfactory fossa is considerably smaller than the cribriform plate. Within

Table 19.5 Olfactory neuroblastomas (Harrison & Lund)

Patient	Age (yr)	Sex	Surgery	Radiotherapy	Follow-up (mth)	Outcome
1	20	F	LR	Postoperative	180	A&W
2	59	M	LR	Postoperative	Lost	–
3	45	M	LR	Preoperative	156	A&W
4	17	M	LR	Postoperative	10	DOD
5	23	M	None	To primary & neck	Lost	–
6	54	M	CF	Preoperative	102	DOD
7	62	M	CF	None	89	A&W
8	57	F	CF	Preoperative	120	DOD
9	26	F	CF	None	27	A&W
10	47	F	CF	None	44	A&W
11	67	F	CF	None	43	A&W
12	61	F	CF	None	39	A&W
13	14	M	CF	Preoperative	31	DICD
14	57	M	CF	None	30	DOD
15	57	F	CF	Preoperative	70	A&W
16	38	M	CF	Postoperative	48	A&W
17	37	M	CF	Preoperative	4	A&W
18	47	M	CF	None	28	A&W
19	64	M	CF	None	36	A&W
20	52	F	CF	None	55	AWR

LR, lateral rhinotomy; CF, craniofacial resection; A&W, alive and well; AWR, alive with recurrence; DOD, dead of disease; DICD, dead of intercurrent disease this fossa lies the kidney-shaped, or oval olfactory bulb and the central processes of the olfactory cells within these bulbs are gathered together as fibres which pass through dural openings and accompanied by arachnoid sheaths enter the nose via pre-existing holes in the cribriform plate. Normal channels thus exist whereby tumour may pass from the upper nasal cavity to olfactory bulb without eroding the cribriform plate. It could well be assumed that every olfactory neuroblastoma in the cribriform plate area has an intracranial component.

The staging system suggested by Kadish et al in 1976[138] which has been extensively used in publishing survival data, ignores this essential aspect of surgical pathology.

Stage 1 are lesions confined to the nasal cavity

Stage 2 show involvement of nasal cavity plus one or more of the paranasal sinuses

Stage 3 have involvement beyond the nasal cavity including the orbit, skull base, intracranial cavity, cervical lymph nodes or systemic metastases.

Kadish et al used this system to analyse 17 patients retrospectively and with the aid of clinical and radiological assessment placed half the patients in Stage 1. All survived for more than 3 years following treatment with limited surgery (lateral rhinotomy or ethmoidectomy) plus irradiation![138]

The availability of CT scanning and MRI, together with the greater usage of craniofacial resection, has resulted in more accurate assessment of the real extent of this tumour and many now question both the validity and usefulness of this classification which at best can only offer a general estimate of tumour extent.[117,136]

Aetiology

Embryological sites of origin have included the olfactory placode, sphenopalatine ganglion, vomeronasal organ and ectopic olfactory epithelium within the paranasal sinuses.[139] The olfactory placode, an embryonic progenitor of the olfactory membrane, does not persist into postembryonic life[140] whilst the vomeronasal organ disappears in man about the 20th embryonic week. The sphenopalatine ganglion is also an unlikely source since its position is inconsistent with the usual site of olfactory neuroblastoma.

Herrold has shown that in the Syrian hamster it is possible to produce tumours looking and behaving like olfactory neuroblastoma by administering diethylnitrosamine.[141] This can be given by a variety of routes (intragastric, intratracheal, intradermal, intraperitoneal or even subcutaneous injections in the interscapular region) each of which produces an invasive malignant neuroepithelial tumour. However, this appears to bear no

relevance to the human condition the aetiology of which remains unknown.

Clinical features (Fig. 19.10)

The presenting symptoms, as with most upper jaw malignancies, remain non-specific with nasal obstruction and epistaxis predominant. Symptoms reflect the areas of neoplastic involvement, although with such a vascular tumour bleeding is common in most instances. Despite the frequency of nasal obstruction anosmia is rarely recorded although this may simply be the result of inadequate questioning. In 25% of the patients reported by Schwabb et al[132] the predominant symptoms were ocular whilst Levine et al[128] found pain from sinus obstruction was the commonest presenting symptom with 5 to 10% of their patients also having neurological deficiencies. As with cervical lymphadenopathy any evidence of extension from the nasal cavity is significant of late disease carrying a poor prognosis.

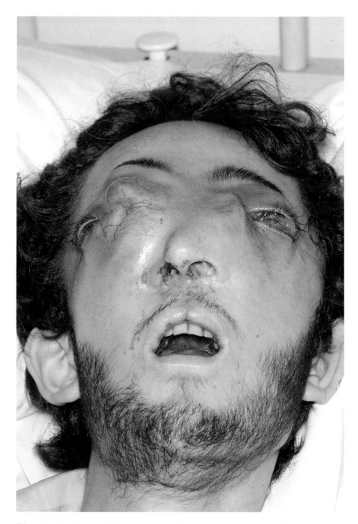

Fig. 19.10 Large olfactory neuroblastoma causing dramatic splaying of nasal bones.

Schwabb et al analysing 40 cases treated between 1956 and 1987 found that 40% had symptoms for more than 3 months prior to diagnosis but 24% had significant symptoms for more than a year.[132] In most cases this malignancy is slow growing and despite its vascularity and concurrent nasal obstruction, considerable delay in seeking attention is quite common. Obert et al[142] reported that two of their eight patients had nasal obstruction for more than 7 years although the possibility of other benign pathology, such as polypi was not excluded in their patients!

Radiology (Fig. 19.11)

Although the final diagnosis of olfactory neuroblastoma is established by histological examination of biopsy material, the staging of the tumour is determined by clinical and radiological assessment. Initially, there is unilateral involvement of the cribriform plate area but tumour may extend to the ethmoid labyrinths and bone erosion is a common radiological finding at initial diagnosis. However, as Harrison has emphasized, its absence cannot be taken as an indication of absence of intracranial extension since traversion of existing holes in the cribriform plate remains an undetectable possibility in every patient.[136]

Woodhead & Lloyd[144] evaluated the role of radiology in 24 patients with histologically confirmed olfactory neuroblastoma seen since 1975 at the Royal National Throat, Nose and Ear Hospital, London. The imaging characteristics on plain films, CT and MRI combined with intravenous gadolinium were considered, with a conclusion that no features could be considered as wholly specific. However, a tumour within the ethmoid and upper nasal airway expanding into the orbit and eroding the roof of the fronto-ethmoid complex or cribriform plate unilaterally in a young patient, is highly significant of olfactory neuroblastoma.

Typical features are those of an intense signal on pre-contrast T2 weighted spin echo sequences and strong enhancement after gadolinium on T1 weighted sequences. A characteristic feature of the response to gadolinium is tumour enhancement greater than the turbinals on inverse recovery but less when T1 weighted spin echo sequences are used.

Extension of tumour within the paranasal sinuses can be shown on CT but is probably best seen after MRI with intravenous gadolinium, a technique now essential prior to craniofacial surgery.[145] The role of the radiologist is to map as accurately as possible tumour extent prior to consideration of treatment, particularly when irradiation precedes surgery. The degree of surgical exposure is largely influenced by the amount of tumour within the anterior cranial fossa, although this is limited to macroscopical evaluation whereas success is measured by tumour-free margins. The other area requiring accurate

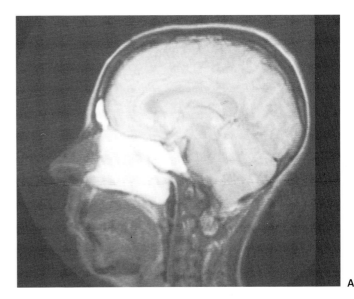

A

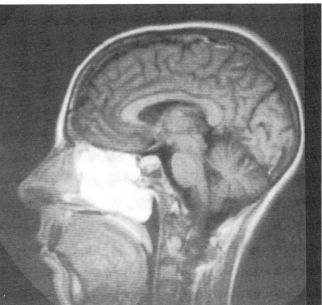

B

Fig. 19.11 Olfactory neuroblastoma. **A**, sagittal MR scan, T2 weighted spin echo sequence. There is poor discrimination between tumour and retained secretion in the frontal and sphenoid sinuses. **B**, T1 inversion recovery sequence with gadolinium. Enhancement of the tumour now allows discrimination between tumour and retained secretion (Lloyd 1988[143]).

preoperative assessment is the degree of orbital involvement since this will influence the need for orbital clearance.

Macroscopic and microscopic appearance

Grossly, this tumour is usually described as a polypoidal mass, reddish–grey in colour and highly vascular. The consistency varies from very soft to firm in different tumours or in parts of the same lesion but diagnosis is not possible on macroscopic examination alone. Prior to the development of specialized histopathological techniques, differentiation of this 'difficult to diagnose' member of the round-cell group of tumours presented considerable problems.[146]

Olfactory neuroblastomata arise from the basal cells of the olfactory neuroepithelium which itself is derived from the olfactory placode. Although formed from ectoderm this forms nerve fibres and therefore the basal cells within the mature olfactory neuroepithelium differ from the primitive sympathetic cells which give rise to sympathetic neuroblastoma. Microscopically, clusters of cells slightly larger than lymphocytes and arranged in patterns which vary from small nests surrounded by a fibrillary stroma to diffuse areas separated by fibrovascular septa, are usually seen. Locally, cells appear to palisade around blood vessels which are themselves numerous accounting for the well recognized vascularity of this tumour.[146] Occasionally, true rosettes can be seen consisting of columnar-like cells arranged to define a lumen – in other cases perivascular rosettes are visible with the neuroblasts arranged around a vessel. It had been suggested that by recognizing various histological patterns guidance as to biological behaviour and prognosis might be possible. Experience has shown that such correlation does not exist.[147] Catecholamines are present, both adrenaline and noradrenaline, but not to the same extent as in sympathetic neuroblastoma. The presence of catecholamines within the tumour can be demonstrated by fume-induced fluorescence as described by Judge et al.[148] This is a modification of the original technique of Falck et al[149] and proves simple, inexpensive, quick and sensitive, being suitable for frozen section specimens. Combined with information provided by electron microscopy, which shows the membrane-bound dense granules 100 nm to 150 nm in diameter, it is possible to establish accurate diagnosis in difficult cases.

Olfactory neuroblastoma has been studied extensively at the ultrastructural level[1a,150] but today diagnosis is largely centralized by a combination of light microscopy and immunohistochemistry. This has proved of value either in confirming a suspected diagnosis or when light microscopy is equivocal. A number of publications have evaluated the immunohistochemical features of olfactory neuroblastoma and the results of staining with the main antibodies that have been used are summarized in Table 19.6. These data are taken from a paper by Lund & Milroy[131] who concluded that diagnosis is best made by using a panel of antibodies, although general neuroendocrine markers such as NSE and PGP 9.5 are usually positive. Synaptophysin and chromogranin are reliable markers of neuroendocrine differentiation although not always positive in olfactory neuroblastomas. Positive staining for S100 protein is frequently found within cells at the periphery of lobules these being sustenticular cells which are modified Schwann cells. Similar cells are found at the periphery of the lobules of paragangliomas and phaechromocytoma. In the former these cells also stain with GFAP but not in olfactory neuroblastoma. Application of these new histopathological modalities has undoubtedly led to increased accuracy in the diagnosis of neuroendocrine tumours and an apparent increase in the frequency with which olfactory neuroblastoma is now diagnosed.

Natural history

Literature reports, admittedly only of small numbers of patients, suggest that the natural history of this malignancy is both variable and unpredictable. There is no

Table 19.6 Olfactory neuroblastoma: immunohistochemistry findings from published series

Authors	NSE	Synaptophysin	Chromogranin	Leu7	Antibodies Cytokeratin	S100	GFAP	Neurofilament	EMA
Choi & Anderson 1985[153]	10/10	–	–	–	1/10	0/10	–	–	–
Taxy et al 1986[154]	20/27	–	–	–	10/25	15/27	–	4/27	–
Axe & Kuhajda 1987[155]	6/8	–	1/8	–	0/8	5/8	0/8	1/8	0/8
Wick et al 1988[58]	–	5/5	–	–	0/5	0/5	–	–	0/5
Durham 1989[156]	10/14	–	6/10	8/10	4/10	10/14	–	–	–
Frierson et al 1990[157]	11/11	7/11	1/11	–	4/11	8/11	1/11	7/11	0/11
Schmidt et al 1990[158]	4/4	4/4	1/4	–	0/4	4/4	0/4	0/4	–
Lund & Milroy 1992[131]	10/10	6/10	5/10	3/10	2/10	6/10	0/10	–	0/10*

*HMFG2 and AUA1
NSE, neurone-specific enolase; GFAP, glial fibrillary acid protein; EMA, epithelial membrane antigen

evidence to suggest that this tumour possesses any specifically lethal characteristics except for its anatomical location which makes wide-field resection on occasions impossible. The high local recurrence rate of 62% recorded by Appelblatt & McClatchey[146] can now be reduced by more radical resection although, as with many other head and neck neoplasms, it may then be associated with an increased incidence of late metastases. A high rate of cervical lymph node metastases has been reported by Beitler et al[129] and 10-year survival figures are invariably worse than those found at 3 or 5 years, due to late local recurrence. Although often slow growing, olfactory neuroblastoma must be considered as a highly malignant neoplasm requiring radical initial treatment.

Differential diagnosis

Neuroblastomas of olfactory origin are undoubtedly uncommon making up between 2 and 3% of all true nasal tumours. They resemble those of the adrenal gland and retina although differing in their biological behaviour. Prior to the use of the electron microscope and now immunohistochemistry, histological diagnosis was often difficult. Differential diagnosis includes undifferentiated adenocarcinoma, adenocarcinoma, lymphoma, malignant melanoma, transitional cell carcinoma, anaplastic carcinoma, plasmacytoma, rhabdomyosarcoma and neuroendocrine carcinoma. However, the lengthy survival time and relatively slow growth of olfactory neuroblastomata is unusual in other nasal malignancies and the last decade has witnessed a considerable increase in the diagnosis of this lesion. This undoubtedly represents an increasing awareness rather than a change in prevalence.

Treatment (Table 19.5)

Limited personal experience, together with variations in intrinsic biological behaviour has resulted in a variety of therapies being advocated and practised over the past 30 years. The most constant feature appearing in the literature has been a high incidence of local recurrence, largely due to failure to determine the true extent of the neoplasm together with inadequate excision. A propensity for intracranial spread is implicit in the surgical pathology of this tumour as described by Harrison[136] but even with a relatively short follow-up of 4 years, Levine et al found an improvement in survival of 37.5% to 82% when limited resection was replaced by craniofacial surgery.[128]

Despite its limitations and failure to appreciate the significance of the normal holes in the cribriform plate in the intracranial spread of olfactory neuroblastoma, the staging system of Kadish et al has been used in most of the papers concerning treatment success.[138] Although Elkcon et al[151] concluded from their review of 97 patients previously reported in the world literature, that a single

modality such as radiotherapy or limited surgery, gave as good results as combined treatment in Stage 1 and 2 lesions, this paper suffered from the intrinsic inaccuracies and variations common to all such analyses. Levine et al in 1986[128] more effectively evaluated present day attitudes by advising that surgically resectable tumours should be given preoperative radiotherapy (5000 cGy) to the area of primary disease followed by craniofacial resection. Preoperative irradiation is preferred since a delay of several months is necessary following craniofacial resection before radiotherapy can be safely given in oncological dosage and this delay is unacceptable when excisional margins are doubtful.

Combination of lateral rhinotomy and radiotherapy in selected cases has given good results and a 20-year-old woman treated in this manner with 6000 cGy of CO^{60} in 1975 remains free of disease in 1992.

Although preoperative radiotherapy is now considered advisable in most patients, radical excision alone has also given good results as illustrated in the following case report.

A 62-year-old man with a 3 year history of unilateral nasal obstruction, epistaxis and intermittent facial pain was diagnosed as having an olfactory neuroblastoma in October 1983. A vascular tumour filled the right nasal airway and CT showed bony erosion of both ethmoids and the cribriform plate. Preoperative urinary VMA per day was 41 μmol which fell to 24.0 μmol per day following surgical removal. Craniofacial resection with removal of both ethmoids, cribriform plate, anterior fossa dura and associated olfactory bulbs was carried out and the histological report read, 'large deposits of tumour showing the features of an olfactory neuroblastoma was present in each bulb (Fig. 19.12). In several serial sections neoplasm is seen to be penetrating through the dura along the pathway of the olfactory nerves. Neoplasm is also seen in tissue removed from the frontonasal duct, both ethmoids and the right inferior turbinate'. This patient received no irradiation and remains free of disease 9 years postoperatively. Follow-up has been at 6 monthly intervals extended to yearly and evaluation carried out by MRI with gadolinium enhancement.

Berger et al[123] have evaluated the incidence of neck node failure in patients treated for cure without evidence of regional metastases at initial presentation. 110 patients from 16 institutions were identified, 21 (19%) of whom developed late neck disease. Six of these died from their disease. 18 of these failures occurred within 60 months of the initial diagnosis of the primary tumour and they calculated from these data that 9% of patients with olfactory neuroblastoma would be potentially cured if an elective neck dissection was combined with initial resection of the primary lesion. However, only two patients could be identified in the literature who had been treated in this manner and its value remains unproven.

As with most other head and neck neoplasms, systemic metastases are uncommon at initial diagnosis but common with local recurrence. Appelblatt & McClatchey quote a general figure of 28%, the commonest sites being

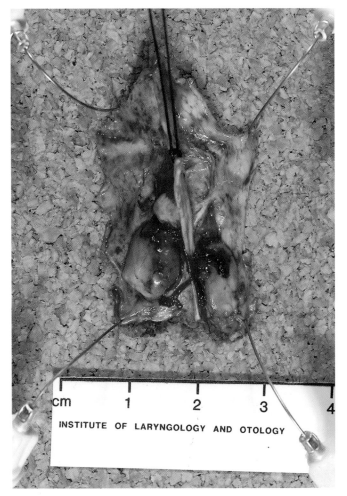

Fig. 19.12 Surgical specimen from craniofacial resection showing swollen olfactory bulbs due to infiltration with olfactory neuroblastoma[135] (courtesy of A.D. Cheesman).

the lung, vertebra, brain and liver.[146] The success of chemotherapy in the treatment of childhood neuroblastoma has encouraged a similar regime to be used in patients with advanced olfactory neuroblastoma or as adjuvant treatment to reduce the risk of late metastases. Levine et al[128] gave cyclophosphamide and vincristine both pre- and postoperatively in patients with late disease. 80% were alive and well but for an unspecified period of time! Schwabb et al used varying amounts of adriamycin, vincristine and cyclophosphamide for patients with metastases or as adjuvant therapy and concluded that, 'the role of chemotherapy seems interesting but more information is needed'.[132]

Weiden et al[152] described one patient given cisplatinum and fluorouracil followed by radiotherapy who remained free of tumour for 3 years. Undoubtedly, more information will slowly become available regarding the value of chemotherapy but with such small numbers of available patients these drugs will probably be limited to the management of advanced cases.

Prognosis

From available evidence it is not possible to determine with any accuracy the prospects of long-term cure in individual patients. Surgically accessible lesions treated with combinations of radiotherapy and radical excision can expect a 60% prospect of surviving at least 3 years, at 5 years this will have fallen to 40% disease-free. Survival rates in excess of this have been reported by some authors (Table 19.7) although absence of data regarding tumour extent and verification of histology must cast some doubt over exceptionally good results. Cervical or systemic metastases drastically reduce the prospect of survival and follow-up longer than 10 years confirms that even in apparently controlled cases late recurrence may occur.

MALIGNANT MELANOMA OF THE NASAL CAVITY AND PARANASAL SINUSES

Definition and aetiology

Melanocytes are derivations of neural crest and are widely distributed throughout cutaneous and mucosal surfaces.

Table 19.7 Olfactory neuroblastoma: survival data from literature

Author	No. cases	Disease free – all stages (%) at		
		3 yr	5 yr	10 yr
Bailey & Barton 1975[147]	50 (from literature)	–	18	–
Kadish et al 1976[138]	17	76	–	–
Shah & Feghali 1981[130]	31	–	33	–
Appelblatt & McClatchey 1982[146]	21	70	40	–
Levine et al 1986[128]	16	82	–	–
Schwabb et al 1988[132]	36	–	60	21
O'Connor et al 1989[125]	15	73	–	–
Beitler et al 1991[129]	14	–	57	41
Lund & Milroy 1992[131]	20	50	35	–

They are present in nasal mucosa, in the glands, superficial and deep stroma of the septum and turbinates, being particularly common in the supporting cells of the olfactory epithelium though they appear to be absent in fetal and neonatal nasal mucosa.[159] The observation of junctional activity which is of such interest in cutaneous melanoma is not directly applicable to nasal mucosa though it has been suggested that dormant cells may be present which have the potential for transformation into melanocytes.[1b]

In the oral cavity, melanin deposition is common on the buccal mucosa, gingiva, hard and soft palate as well as the lips and tongue. However, 0.5–30% of all oral mucosal melanoma are preceded by hyperpigmented lesions.[160–162] In the Japanese, 66% have associated mucosal melanosis[163] and benign pigmentation has been reported in 87% of Negroes.[164]

An aetiological study on 50 surviving patients with malignancy of the upper jaw revealed that three of the eight individuals with malignant melanoma had had extensive exposure to formaldehyde.[165,166] A subsequent survey of British ear, nose and throat surgeons revealed an additional 181 cases who had not been referred to the Institute of Laryngology and Otology (ILO), averaging one case/10 years. The study further revealed that 26% of these cases (one case/2 years) had occurred in a particular geographical area: Leicestershire, Nottinghamshire and the West Midlands. There are many distorting factors in a study of this sort but the clustering of cases in one of the industrial areas of Great Britain warrants further investigation. Of these 181 patients, 20 were available for interview regarding possible carcinogen contact but only one individual who had worked in a tyre-factory could be said to have been potentially at risk.

Formaldehyde is a known carcinogen in animal experiments, with 50% of rats exposed for long periods to doses greater than 15 ppm developing tumours (squamous cell carcinoma).[167] It is known to have a significant damaging effect on the physiology and histology of the upper respiratory tract in occupationally-exposed workers with dose-related decreases in mucociliary clearance and olfaction.[168,169] It produces cilial loss, metaplasia and occasional dysplasia and is both cytotoxic and teratogenic.[170] In the literature, cases have been made for and against a carcinogenic role in sinonasal malignancy. There have been reports of a positive association in the textile industry but a large study of 26 000 occupationally-exposed workers by Blair et al found no cases.[171] Walrath & Fraumeni investigated embalmers who have arguably the highest exposure to formaldehyde and found an increased incidence of colonic carcinoma and cutaneous melanoma but not mucosal melanoma.[172] Thus at present the case is unproven but worthy of further investigation.

Synonyms

Malignant melanoma, melanocarcinoma, melanosarcoma.

Historical aspects

The first mention of a nasal melanoma was by Lucke in 1869[173] and the first reported case in Great Britain was in 1912 by Wilkinson.[174]

Incidence

Mucosal melanoma is fortunately a rare condition and does not appear to be increasing unlike cutaneous melanoma where there has been a 95% increase in incidence in the United States since 1930 compared to an 11% increase in population.[175] It has been estimated that between 15 and 20% of all malignant melanomas arise in the head and neck[176,177] but that only 0.5–2% occur in the mucous membrane[178,179] of which the majority affect the oral cavity.[17a] The risk of developing mucosal disease is one-sixth that of cutaneous melanoma.[175] Shah et al[162] found 74 patients between 1943 and 1977 with mucosal disease of which only 39 affected the nasal cavity. Malignant melanoma affecting the nasal cavity accounts for less than 1% of all malignant melanoma[161,180,181] where they constitute about 3.5% of all sinonasal neoplasia.[162,182–184]

Age, sex and ethnic variation

In a personal series of 60 patients who have been treated between 1961–1990 at the ILO, the ages range from 16–90 years with the majority (44) presenting in the 6th to 7th decades, maximally between 60–69 years (Fig. 19.13). 92% were over 50 at initial diagnosis. This is in keeping with the findings in the few other large series.[183,186]

The ratio of men to women is roughly equal with a slight male preponderance[183,187] which is more marked in palatal lesions.[160,185]

The disease predominantly affects Caucasians though it has been reported in Negroes who constituted 16% in the Armed Forces Institute of Pathology series[183] and indeed one series found it to constitute 2.6% of all malignant melanomas affecting Ugandan Negroes.[164] Mucosal melanoma is also relatively common in Japan with the oral cavity being a favoured site constituting 7.5% of all malignant melanomas and 34.4% of all mucosal melanomas.[163]

Site

The commonest site of origin is from the lateral wall and in particular from the middle and inferior turbinates,

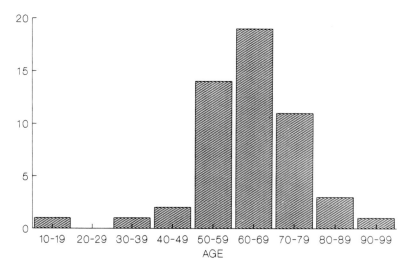

Fig. 19.13 Distribution of malignant melanoma patients by age in our series.

followed by the nasal septum (Table 19.8) (Fig. 19.9). However patients may also have disease arising from the maxilla and ethmoids. Although the frequency of the sites of origin is said to correlate with areas of pigmentation in the noses of normal Ugandan Africans[164] it is of interest that tumours do not arise from the olfactory region where pigmentation is greatest. In addition disease may be too extensive to determine the exact site of origin. Malignant melanoma in the nose is almost always a primary lesion. It is an unusual site for secondary deposits but Allen & Spitz[180] have suggested that patients with malignant melanoma have an increased liability to develop a second primary tumour in another site.

The oral cavity is a somewhat more common site than the upper airway for malignant mucosal melanoma, with the palate and upper alveolar gingivae most frequently affected.[162,163,184,185,188] Consequently nearly 80% arise in the mucosa of the upper jaw.[160]

Table 19.8 Malignant melanoma of the upper jaw: recorded site of origin in our series

Site of tumour	No. of cases
Lateral wall	31
(Middle & inferior turbinates −17)	
Nasal septum	16
Nasal vestibule & floor of nose	4
Maxilla	4
Nasal polyps	3
Ethmoids	2
Total	60

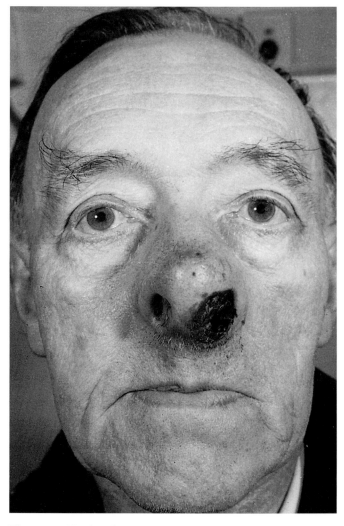

Fig. 19.14 Nasal malignant melanoma appearing at the vestibule.

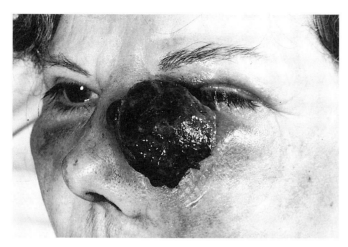

Fig. 19.15   Pigmented mass arising in ethmoids which has broken through skin.

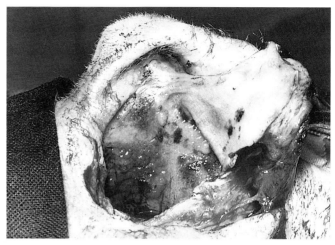

Fig. 19.17   Intra-operative photograph showing appearances of malignant melanoma on nasal mucosa with satellite lesions via a lateral rhinotomy incision.

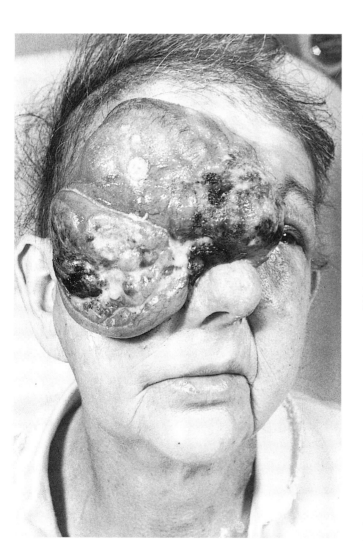

Fig. 19.16   Massive malignant melanoma.

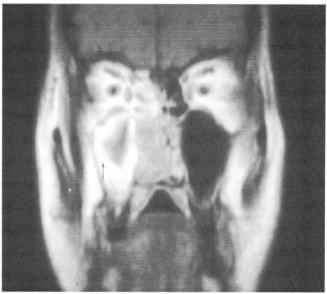

Fig. 19.18   Coronal MR scan, T1 weighted sequence showing satellite lesion in maxillary sinus (arrow).

Clinical features

The majority of patients present with either unilateral nasal obstruction (46%), epistaxis (19%) or a combination of the two (23%). Few complain of pain (4%). Occasionally patients may notice proptosis (2%) in addition to other symptoms and sometimes swelling of the nose or an actual mass is visible at the vestibule (6%) (Figs 19.14–19.17).

The delay in presentation from the onset of symptoms is difficult to assess accurately but varies from 1 month to 2 years, the average being 4 months. This is probably due to fairly innocuous symptoms and if patients have had benign polyps in the past, they are not alarmed by a recurrence of similar symptoms. There is however, no association of malignant melanoma and nasal polyps.

On the palate, a lump which frequently ulcerates and bleeds is the commonest presentation. As the disease progresses bone destruction may result and with alveolar lesions, loosening of the teeth. However, the symptoms may be minimal for some time and pain is rarely a feature, so a history of 1–7 years is not unusual.

A 63-year-old man presented with nasal obstruction and epistaxis due to a pigmented lesion on the left septum. This was removed via a lateral rhinotomy (Fig. 19.17). 18 months later a single node was removed from the left side of the neck and over the next 2.5 years a further five nodes were removed, containing metastatic disease. 4 months later a deposit was found in a rib and this was followed by widespread cutaneous secondaries co-incident with the patient developing a viral upper respiratory tract infection. The patient died shortly after, 5 years from initial diagnosis.

This case illustrates a typical history characterized by multiple nodal recurrence and systemic metastases potentiated by a change in the host–tumour immunological balance.

Radiology

No specific features are associated with malignant melanoma. On plain X-ray a soft tissue mass may be seen in the nasal cavity (25%) and there may be evidence of bone destruction in 50% of cases. The extent of this can be better defined with CT scanning when orbital and anterior cranial fossa involvement can be demonstrated in half the cases. MRI characteristics are non-specific with variable enhancement after intravenous gadolinium-DTPA depending on tumour vascularity. Relatively avascular tumour may be outlined against strongly enhancing inflamed mucosa (Fig. 19.18).

Macroscopic and microscopic appearance

The macroscopic appearances are variable. The tumour may be polypoid and friable, bleeding easily on touch, with evidence of infiltration and bone destruction, or the lesions can be firmer and more sessile. It can look deceptively benign. A brownish-black coloration is apparent in 75% of cases but the unwary should beware of amelanotic areas and satellite lesions. Indeed up to 10% of tumours may be completely amelanotic.[189]

Microscopic appearance

Diagnosis can often be difficult as the tumour is composed of polygonal or spindle-shaped cells with many mitotic figures. The identification of melanin pigment in tumour cells is an important part of light microscopy and diagnosis can be made with confidence if the following 3 staining criteria are satisfied:[190]

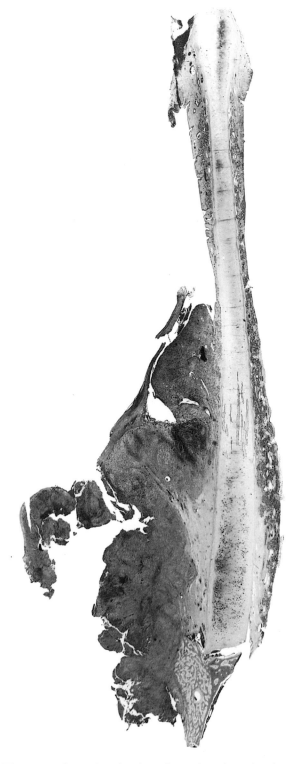

Fig. 19.19 Coronal section through septal specimen showing mucosal origin of malignant melanoma.

1. The Fontana stain for melanin should be positive
2. The pigment should be bleached by potassium permanganate oxalate
3. A stain for hemosiderin should be negative.

To some extent this has been superseded by the immuno-cytochemical identification of protein S100, VIM and HMB-45 which are particularly helpful in the absence of melanin pigment. In addition electron microscopy can occasionally confirm diagnosis in difficult cases by the demonstration of melanosomes, ovoid structures in the cytoplasm which are the precursors of melanin.

It is often possible to detect melanogens in the urine particularly in the presence of large tumour bulk or disseminated metastases.

Assessment of morphology and proliferative activity in conjunction with ploidy status may be of value in predicting prognosis in the future. Recent ploidy analysis suggests that tumour survival times are longer in patients with diploid tumours and showing spindle cell morphology. Proliferating cell nucleus antigen (PCNA) expression was more marked in hyperdiploid and tetraploid tumours and lowest in diploid neoplasms. The mitotic rate appeared unrelated to ploidy status or PCNA expression.[191]

Natural history

Mucosal melanoma is always a malignant condition and no 'benign' variants have so far been described. Clark et al's technique[192] of correlating depth of invasion and junctional activity with prognosis are not applicable to mucosal melanoma and no satisfactory staging system exists.

Between 10 and 18% of patients will present with cervical lymphadenopathy[182,187] and 4% with lung metastases.[187] Local recurrence, cervical lymphadenopathy and metastatic disease can occur at any time[193] though Gallagher[190] reported that 55% of patients manifested this within 1 year of diagnosis. Systemic metastases are found in the lung, liver, brain and skin and the vast majority of patients will die of or with such secondary disease.

Differential diagnosis

'Anaplastic' tumours are often revealed as malignant melanomas on closer inspection. However, melanomas may also be confused with other small-cell tumours such as lymphoma and olfactory neuroblastoma and immuno-cytochemistry is mandatory in these cases.

Treatment (Table 19.9)

Radical local surgery alone or in combination with other modalities has been the treatment of choice.[187] Total excision is often compromised by the presence of amelanotic areas and satellite lesions. The majority of our patients have undergone lateral rhinotomy (79%). In addition total rhinectomy (8%), craniofacial resection (6%) and total maxillectomy (4%) have also been performed though invasion of the anterior cranial fossa is associated with a uniformly bad prognosis. Initial surgery can be followed by repeated excision, as local recurrence occurs, with cryosurgery or laser.

The role of elective neck dissection is unclear. In Conley's series of 660 melanomas of the head and neck,[194] which included a small but unknown number of nasal mucosal cases, 5-year survival figures suggested that elective neck dissection was of benefit but it has also been argued that formal neck dissection in the clinically-negative neck is of no benefit and may even be detrimental. As the incidence of micrometastases is unknown, neck dissection or even removal of individual nodes when palpable may be more appropriate to the natural history of the disease.

Radiotherapy has also been used in treatment but only in combination with surgery and/or chemotherapy. Although the tumour is said to be radioresistant, it may rather be that the cells have a great capacity to repair after subtotal radiation damage[178] resulting in interest in sensitizers such as ICRFI59.[195] Single and multiple agent chemotherapy has been used alone or in combination with radiotherapy, immunotherapy or surgery though no single agent has proved of great benefit with duration of response limited in most cases to a few months.[196] Interest in the immune balance between host and tumour led to the use of topical BCG (Bacille Calmette–Guérin vaccine) injected in tissue adjacent to the tumour in some early series. More recently interferon and monoclonal

Table 19.9 Malignant melanoma of the upper jaw: results of treatment in our patients with >5 years follow-up

	Surgery	Surgery/DXT	Surgery/DXT/C	Surgery/C	C
Total no. of patients (52)	26	10	6	9	1
Dead <1 yr	7	–	3	2	–
Survival(yr)					
1–3	13	3	2	3	1
3–5	4	–	1	2	–
5–10	2	2	–	1	–
10+	–	5	–	1	–

DXT, radiotherapy; C, chemotherapy

antibodies such as interleukin 2 and lymphokine-activated-killer cells have been used for metastatic cutaneous melanoma. Whilst initial responses are sometimes promising (though not without side effects), the long-term results are unknown and no data are available for mucosal disease.[197-199] Melanoma vaccines to prevent disease progression may have a role in the future.

Prognosis (Table 19.10)

Looking at our 52 patients and those of others,[200] the age and sex of the patients do not affect the outcome and histological features such as quantity of pigmentation and mitoses do not correlate with prognosis, though as already noted assessment of morphology, proliferative activity and ploidy status may be of value in the future.

Despite the relative lack of radiosensitivity, some of the longest survivors are those receiving surgery and radiotherapy. In our series of patients with greater than 5-year survival, the time from presentation to death varied from 4 months to 20 years and the average survival time was 3 years and 7 months compared with 2.3 years reported by Gallagher.[190] It is an undisputed fact that the prognosis with this tumour is poor with more than 50% dead within 3 years and just over 66% dead within 5 years (and half of those alive have residual disease). 5-year survival rates of 6.5–31% have been quoted,[162,182,183,186,193,201] but the natural history of the disease makes 5-year survival meaningless and the patient is constantly at risk of death from this condition from which virtually all will succumb eventually (Fig. 19.20). The palatal lesions have an even worse prognosis with the majority dead within 1 to 2 years from presentation. The cause of death in the majority of patients is

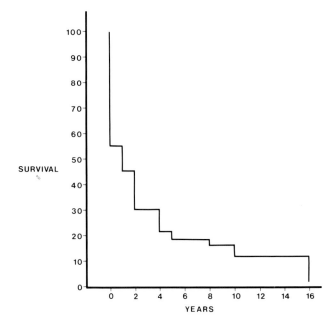

Fig. 19.20   Kaplan–Meier survival curve for malignant melanoma.

melanomatosis.

Clearly this is much worse than for cutaneous melanoma where 77% can expect to be alive at 5 years if there is no nodal involvement.[202] Our personal experience with a relatively large number of patients suggests that they may be broadly divided into three clinical groups which are related to the individual's host-tumour relationship. Some patients die within a few weeks or months of presentation with rapidly disseminating disease despite surgery. Others have a long expectation of many years with no recurrence until some event disturbs the

Table 19.10   Malignant melanoma of the upper jaw: 5-year survival reported in the literature

Author		No. of cases	Female : Male	Age range (yr)	5-year survival (%)
Moore & Martin 1955[161]	Nose/sinuses	9	–	–	0
	Upper alveolus	7	–	–	8
Chaudhry et al 1958[160]	Upper alveolus	75	1:1.9	22–90	3
Holdcraft & Gallagher 1969[183]	Nose/sinuses	39	15:24	17–84	11
Trodahl & Sprague 1970[185]	Upper alveolus	42	36:6	24–79	22
Freedman et al 1973[182]	Nose/sinuses	56	23:33	–	31
Eneroth & Lundberg 1975[186]	Nose/sinuses	24	–	34–80	17
	Oral cavity	17			
Shah et al 1977[162]	Nose/sinuses	45	–	–	20
	Upper alveolus	12			17
Panje & Moran 1986[203]	Upper alveolus	15	8:7	30–85	13
Trapp et al 1987[204]	Nose/Sinuses	17	10:7	44–88	25
Harrison & Lund	Nose/sinuses	52	24:28	16–90	34

immunological balance such as an infection and promotes dramatic recurrence. The rest may survive for reasonable periods punctuated by frequent local recurrences and cervical lymphadenopathy which can be controlled surgically. However, evidence suggests that prophylactic neck dissection may actually promote lymphatic dissemination by encouraging more distant drainage. It is the unpredictability of the immunological balance which led to the use, albeit in vain, of nonspecific immunotherapy such as topical BCG in the past and which may offer some hope for this most capricious of sinonasal tumours in the future.

MELANOTIC NEUROECTODERMAL TUMOUR OF INFANCY

Definition

A benign neuroectodermally-derived tumour with a predilection for the anterior maxilla of children under the age of 1 year.

Synonyms

Pigmented ameloblastoma, melanotic ameloblastic odontoma, melanotic pronoma, retinal anlage tumour, congenital melanocarcinoma, pigmented congenital epulis and retinoblastic teratoma.

Incidence and site

Variations in terminology which Batsakis says reflects the various histological theories of an odontogenic, neural crest or germ cell origin, makes it impossible to determine the real incidence of this tumour.[205] 100 cases were collected from two publications, Johnson et al[206] and Hupp et al[207] and several small series published by Cutler et al,[208] Williams[209] and Brekke & Gorlin.[210] The majority of the tumours were diagnosed within the 1st year of life, within the upper jaw almost always before 9 months of age although Slootweg et al reported a 'primitive neuroectodermal tumour of the maxilla' in a 10-year-old boy.[211] Occasionally, sites of origin are in the skull bones and oropharynx but 80% of all reported cases occur within the premaxilla.[206,207] Rarely, tumours have been found in the epididymis, thigh, femur and mediastinum[206,212] although no sex predilection has been shown for any specific site.

Aetiology

Ultrastructurally, there is good evidence of a neuroectodermal origin for the cell junctions are of the close (zonal adherens) or modified-type (zonal occludens). In addition, there are cytoplasmic filaments as seen in melanocytes and melanin granule formation. The neuroblasts show secretary granules with eccentric cores suggesting noradrenaline and Dehner et al have reported an elevated urinary VMA in some patients[213] adding further support to a neural crest derivation.

Although other theories of histogenesis have been proposed, melanocarcinoma derived from enclosed epithelial rests or from an odontogenic origin, there is agreement that this tumour originates from the neural crest. An odontogenic origin is only supported in the sense that there is a common origin of tumour melanocytes and dental lamina melanocytes also from the neural crest.[214]

Clinical features

A firm painless mass covered by normal mucosa but of a blue-black appearance, which is situated in the region of the premaxilla is the commonest form of presentation. Growth is rapid with the lesion extending into the adjoining alveolar-buccal sulcus which may seriously affect the baby feeding. The baby is otherwise well and ulceration of the overlying mucosa only occurs after biopsy. Invasion of cancellous bone with expansion of the cortical plates may occur with displacement of the partially formed deciduous teeth. This tumour varies in size from about 0.5 to more than 3.0 cm in diameter.

Radiology

It appears as a cystic, lytic, poorly demarcated lesion typically located in the premaxilla although the mandible may also be involved. Destruction of the alveolus is common as is displacement of the teeth.

Macroscopic and microscopic appearance

The tumour may appear to be encapsulated showing a pigmented surface. Microscopically, it is composed of a prominent fibrous connective tissue stroma containing two cell populations. Cuboidal cells containing melanin granules lining numerous alveolar spaces, and small dark cells arranged in an alveolar pattern. The stroma exhibits varying degrees of hyalinization and contains these smaller cells arranged in groups, cords or singly.[205] Less frequently, there is odontogenic epithelium or focal areas of osteogenesis.[209]

Natural history

Melanotic neuroectodermal tumours of infancy are considered as being essentially benign with a local recurrence rate following removal of between 10% and 15% for lesions within the head and neck.[208,210] The multifocal nature of this condition accounts for a proportion of recurrences but a small number of these tumours have been considered as malignant because of rapid growth or metastases. Stowens & Lin in 1974 described a malignant melanotic neuroectodermal tumour with metastases in a stillborn infant,[215] but Cutler et al found only eight patients in their review of 160 published cases of melanotic neuroectodermal tumours. Three of the five extragnathic lesions were suspected of misclassification and they considered the true malignancy rate to be 3%.[208]

Treatment

This has varied in the past from simple curettage with excision of the soft tissue mass without clear margins around the tumour, to wide resection. The latter is associated with dental deformity and most authors recommend local excision for both primary and recurrent lesions.[216] Hupp et al attribute the success of this approach to tumour reduction allowing host immune response to destroy any remaining tumour cells.[207] However, although histologically benign, the occasional documented malignancy suggests that careful consideration should be paid to the management of each case. Radiotherapy and chemotherapy are never indicated.

REFERENCES

1. Friedmann I, Osborn D A 1982 Tumours of the nose and sinuses – material and classification. In: Pathology of granulomas and neoplasms of the nose and paranasal sinuses. Churchill Livingstone, Edinburgh, a: pp 100–102; b: 162–172
2. Karma P, Rasanen O, Karja J 1977 Nasal glioma: a review and report of two cases. Laryngoscope 87: 1169–1179
3. Berger P 1890 Considerations sur l'origine le mode de la development et le traietment de certaines encephalocoeles. Revue Chirurgie 10: 269–321
4. Schmidt M B 1900 Uber seltese Spaltildungen im Bereiche des mittleren Strenfortsatze Virchows Archiv fur Pathologie, Anatomie, Physiologie 162: 614–630
5. Black B K, Smith D E 1950 Nasal glioma: two cases with recurrences. Archives of Neurology and Psychiatry 64: 614–630
6. Walker E A, Resler D R 1963 Nasal glioma. Laryngoscope 76: 93–107
7. Bradley P J, Singh S D 1985 Nasal glioma. Journal of Laryngology and Otology 99: 247–252
8. Gorenstein A, Kern E B, Facer G W 1980 Nasal glioma. Archives of Otolaryngology 106: 536–540
9. Agarwal S, Gandagule V N, Chouhan S S 1968 Neurogenic tumours of the nose. Indian Journal of Cancer 5: 127–131
10. Ogura J H, Schenck N 1973 Unusual nasal tumours. Otolaryngological Clinics of North America 6: 813–837
11. Pollard K, Carter D A 1987 A case of nasal glioma and neurofibromatosis. Journal of Laryngology and Otology 101: 497–499
12. Smith K R, Schwartz H G, Lusa J E 1963 Neurogenic tumours of the nose and throat. Archives of Otolaryngology 46: 163–179
13. Katz A, Lewis J S 1971 Nasal gliomas. Archives of Otolaryngology 94: 351–355
14. Muller H, Slootweg P J, Troust J 1981 An encephalocoele of the sphenomaxillary type. Journal of Maxillofacial Surgery 9: 180–184
15. New G B, Devine K D 1947 Neurogenic tumours of the nose and throat. Archives of Otolaryngology 46: 163–179
16. Zarem H A, Gray G F, Morehead D 1967 Heterotopic brain in the nasopharynx and soft palate. Surgery 61: 483–486
17. Michaels L 1987 Ear, nose and throat histopathology. Encephalocoeles. a: pp 189–192; b: p 498. Springer-Verlag, London
18. Mazzola R F 1976 Congenital malformations in the frontonasal duct area; pathogenesis and classification. Clinical Plastic Surgery 3: 573–609
19. Bratton A B, Robinson P 1946 Gliomata of the nose and oral cavity. Journal of Pathology and Bacteriology 58: 643–648
20. O'Brien P 1970 Surgical approach to nasal glioma. British Journal of Plastic Surgery 23: 30–35
21. Anglade P 1920 Le gliome des fosses nasales. Presse Medicale 2: 464–465
22. Strauss R B 1966 Intranasal neuroglial herotypia. American Journal of Diseases of Children 111: 317–320
23. Macomber W B, Wang M K H 1953 Congenital neoplasms of the nose. Journal of Plastic and Reconstructive Surgery 11: 215–229
24. Luyenduk W 1969 Intranasal encephalocoele. Psychiatry, Neurology and Neurosurgery 72: 77–87
25. Bradley P J 1982 Nasal polyps in children. Irish Medical Journal 75: 154
26. Sessions R B 1982 Nasal dermoid sinuses - a new concept and explanations. Laryngoscope 92: suppl. 29 (2)
27. Lowe R S, Robinson D W, Ketchum L D 1971 Nasal gliomata. Journal of Plastic and Reconstructive Surgery 47: 1–5
28. Ross D E 1966 Nasal glioma. Laryngoscope 76: 1602–1611
29. Dawson R L G, Muir I F R 1955 Frontonasal glioma. British Journal of Plastic Surgery 8: 136–143
30. Alexander T A 1978 Nasal glioma. Journal of Paediatric Surgery 13: 512–524
31. Mallen R W, Kudryk W H 1974 A dorsal rhinotomy approach to nasal glioma. Canadian Journal of Otolaryngology 3: 187–193
32. Hage J 1960 Surgical approach to the external and internal nose. British Journal of Plastic Surgery 12: 327–339
33. Verocay J 1910 Zur kennetnis der neurofibrome. Beitrage Pathologische Anatomy Allergy 48: 1–6
34. Antoni N R E 1920 Uber Ruckenmarkstumoven und Neurofibrome. Bergmann-Verlag, 413–423
35. Terplan K, Rudofsky F 1926 Uber zwei neurogene tumoren in der nasen und mundhohle. Zeitschrift, Hals-Nasen-Ohrenheilkunde 14: 260–268
36. Stout A P 1935 Peripheral manifestations of specific nerve sheath tumours. American Journal of Cancer 24: 751–796
37. Del Rio-Hortega P 1942 Characteres einterpretation de las celulas especificas de los neurinomas. Archives Society Argentine Anatomy 4: 103–105
38. Katz A D, Passy V, Kaplan L 1971 Neurogenous neoplasms of various nerves of face and neck. Archives of Surgery 103: 51–58
39. Hawkins D B, Luxford W M 1980 Schwannoma of the head and neck in children. Laryngoscope 12: 1921–1926
40. Younis R T, Gross C W, Lazar R H 1991 Schwannomas of the paranasal sinuses. Archives of Otolaryngology 117: 677–680
41. Kragh L V, Soule E H, Masson J K 1960 Benign and malignant neurilemmomas of the head and neck. Surgery, Gynecology and Obstetrics 3: 211–215
42. Robitaille Y, Seemayer T A, Eldeiry A 1975 Peripheral nerve tumours involving paranasal sinuses. Cancer 35: 1254–1258
43. Perzin K H, Panyu H, Wechter J 1982 Nonepithelial tumours of the nasal cavity, paranasal sinuses and nasopharynx. XII.Schwann cell tumours, malignant schwannomas. Cancer 50: 2193–2202
44. Dutt P K 1969 A case of nasal neurilemmoma. Journal of Laryngology and Otology 83: 1209–1213
45. Kaufman J M, Conrad L P 1976 Schwannoma presenting as a nasal polyp. Laryngoscope 86: 595–597

46. Thomas J N 1977 Massive schwannoma arising from the nasal septum. Journal of Laryngology and Otology 91: 63–68
47. Pasic T R, Makielski K 1990 Nasal schwannoma. Otolaryngology, Head and Neck Surgery 103: 943–946
48. Ghosh B C, Ghosh L, Huvos A G 1973 Malignant schwannomas, a clinicopathologic study. Cancer 31: 184–190
49. Purcell S M, Dixon S L 1989 Schwannomatosis, an unusual variant of neurofibromatosis or a distinct entity? Archives of Dermatology 125: 390–393
50. Hellquist H B 1991 Neurogenic sarcoma of the sinonasal tract. Journal of Laryngology and Otology 105: 186–190
51. Maroun F B, Sadler M, Murray G P 1986 Primary malignant tumours of the trigeminal nerve. Canadian Journal of Neurology 13: 146–148
52. Williams P L, Warwick R 1980 Gray's Anatomy, 36th edn. Churchill Livingstone, Edinburgh, pp 1064–1149
53. Schugar J M A, Som P M, Biller H F 1981 Peripheral nerve sheath tumours of the paranasal sinuses. Head and Neck Surgery 4: 72–76
54. Yusuf H, Fajemsin O A, McWilliam L S 1989 Neurilemmoma involving the maxillary sinus, a case report. British Journal of Oral and Maxillofacial Surgery 27: 506–511
55. Ross C, Wright E, Moseley J 1988 Massive schwannoma of the nose and paranasal sinuses. Southern Medical Journal 81: 1588–1591
56. Enion D S, Jenkins A, Miles J B 1991 Intracranial extension of a naso-ethmoidal schwannoma. Journal of Laryngology and Otology 105: 578–581
57. Calcaterra T C, Rich R, Ward P W 1974 Neurilemmoma of the sphenoid sinus. Archives of Otolaryngology 100: 383–385
58. Wick M R, Stanley J, Swanson P E 1988 Immunohistochemical diagnosis of sinonasal melanoma, carcinoma, and neuroblastoma with monoclonal antibodies, HMB-45. Archives of Pathology and Laboratory Medicine 112: 616–620
59. Enzinger F M, Weiss S W 1988 Benign tumours of the peripheral nerves. In: Soft tissue tumours, 2nd edn. Mosby, St. Louis, pp. 719–815
60. Erlandson R A, Woodruff J M 1982 Peripheral nerve sheath tumours: an electron microscopic study of 43 cases. Cancer 49: 273–287
61. Leslie M D, Cheung K Y P 1987 Malignant transformation of neurofibroma at multiple sites in a case of neurofibromatosis. Postgraduate Medical Journal 63: 131–133
62. Von Recklinghausen J 1981 Die fibrose oder deformiende osteite. Festschrift R Virchow zei Seinem, Geburstage, Berlin
63. Constantino P D, Friedman C D, Pelzer H J 1989 Neurofibromatosis Type 2 of the head and neck. Archives of Otolaryngology 115: 380–383
64. Kragh L V, Soule E H, Masson J K 1960 Neurofibromatosis of the head and neck – cosmetic and reconstructive aspects. Plastic and Reconstructive Surgery 25: 565–571
65. Harrison D F N 1971 In: Scott-Brown's diseases of the ear, nose and throat, 3rd edn. Butterworths, London, p 300
66. Geschickter C F 1935 Tumours of the peripheral nerves. American Journal of Cancer 25: 377–410
67. Fu Y S, Perzin K H 1977 Non-epithelial tumours of the nasal cavity and paranasal sinuses. VII Myxomas. Cancer 39: 195–203
68. Oberman H A, Sullenger G 1967 Neurogenous tumours of the head and neck. Cancer 20: 1992–2003
69. Conley J J, Janecka I P 1975 Neurilemmoma of the head and neck. Transactions of the American Academy of Ophthalmology and Otolaryngology 80: 459–464
70. Stevens D J, Kirkham N 1988 Neurofibromas of the paranasal sinuses. Journal of Laryngology and Otology 102: 256–259
71. Harkin J C, Reed R J 1969 Tumours of the peripheral nervous system. Atlas of Tumour Pathology, 2nd Series, Fascicle 3. Armed Forces Institute of Pathology, Washington DC, pp 1–150
72. Mancuso A A J, Hanafee W N 1982 Paranasal sinuses, normal anatomy and pathology. In: Computed tomography of the head and neck. Williams and Wilkins, Baltimore
73. Trojanowski J Q, Kleinman G M, Proppe K H 1980 Malignant tumours of nerve sheath origin. Cancer 46: 1202–1208
74. Das Gupta T K, Brasfield R D 1970 Solitary malignant schwannoma. Annals of Surgery 171: 419–421
75. Hellquist H B 1990 Pathology of the nose and paranasal sinuses. Butterworths, London, pp. 99–104
76. Das Gupta T K, Brasfield R D, Strong E W 1969 Benign solitary neurilemmomas. Cancer 24: 355–359
77. D'Agostino A N, Soule E H, Miller R H 1963 Malignant neurilemmomas in patients with von Recklinghausen's disease. Cancer 16: 1003–1102
78. Atherino C C T, Garcia R, Lopez J 1985 Ectopic meningioma of the nose and paranasal sinuses. Journal of Laryngology and Otology 99: 1161–1166
79. Farr H W, Gray G F, Vrana M 1973 Extracranial meningioma. Journal of Surgical Oncology 5: 411–420
80. Majoros M 1970 Meningiomas of the paranasal sinuses. Laryngoscope 80: 640–645
81. Persky M S, Som M L 1978 Olfactory groove meningioma with nasal and paranasal extension. Annals of Otology, Rhinology and Laryngology 86: 714–720
82. Batsakis J J 1984 Extracranial meningioma. Annals of Otology, Rhinology and Laryngology 93: 282–283
83. Lopez D A, Silvers D N, Helwig E B 1974 Cutaneous meningiomas: a clinicopathological study. Cancer 34: 728–744
84. Ho K L 1980 Primary meningioma of the nasal cavity and paranasal sinuses. Cancer 46: 1442–1447
85. De S K, Chatterjee A K, Misra A K 1986 An unusual presentation of meningioma in the frontal sinus. Head and Neck Surgery 5: 319–328
86. Godel V, Samuel Y, Shanon E 1981 Maxillary meningioma appearing as exophthalmos. Archives of Otolaryngology 107: 626–628
87. Granich M S, Pilch B Z, Goodman M L 1983 Meningiomas presenting in the paranasal sinuses and temporal bone. Head and Neck Surgery 5: 319–328
88. Hill C L 1962 Meningioma of the maxillary sinus. Archives of Otolaryngology 78: 547–549
89. Kjeldsberg C R, Minckler J 1972 Meningiomas presenting as nasal polyps. Cancer 32: 153–156
90. Papini M, Chiantelli A, Cantani R 1988 Nasal meningioma: report of a case. Acta Otolaryngologica Belgium 42: 40–44
91. Sadar E S, Conomy J P, Benjamin S P 1979 Meningiomas of the paranasal sinuses, benign and malignant. Neurosurgery 4: 227–232
92. Shuangshoti S, Panayathanya R 1973 Ectopic meningiomas. Archives of Otolaryngology 948: 102–105
93. Shahen H B 1931 Psammoma in the maxillary sinus. Journal of Laryngology and Otology 46: 117–120
94. Cushing H, Eisenhardt L 1969 Meningioma – their classification, regional behaviour and life history. Hapner Publishing, New York
95. Lloyd G A S 1982 Primary orbital meningioma: a review of 41 patients investigated radiologically. Clinical Radiology 33: 181–187
96. Belal A 1955 Meningiomas infiltrating the nasal cavity, sinuses and orbit. Journal of Laryngology and Otology 69: 59–69
97. Craig W M, Gogela L S 1949 Intraorbital meningioma. American Journal of Ophthalmology 32: 1663–1680
98. Bain G O, Shnitka T K 1956 Cutaneous meningioma (psammoma). Archives of Dermatology 74: 590–594
99. Shuangshoti S, Hongsaprabhas C, Netsky M G 1970 Metastatizing meningioma. Cancer 26: 832–841
100. Iacona R P, Appuzzo M L J, Davis R L 1981 Meningiomas following radiation therapy for medulloblastoma. Journal of Neurosurgery 55: 282–286
101. Watts C 1976 Meningioma following irradiation. Cancer 38: 1939–1940
102. Zirkin H J, Puterman M, Tovi F 1985 Olfactory groove meningioma following radiation therapy for esthesioneuroblastoma. Journal of Laryngology and Otology 99: 1025–1028
103. Beller A J, Feinsool M, Sohar A 1972 The possible relationship between irradiation to the scalp and intracranial meningioma. Neurochirurgia 15: 135–143

104. Anglein T J, Hermann G A 1961 Meningioma presenting as an antral cancer. Archives of Otolaryngology 874: 549–555
105. Papavasiliou A, Sawyer R, Lund V 1982 Effects of meningiomas on the facial skeleton. Archives of Otolaryngology 18: 255–257
106. Cushing H 1922 The cranial hyperostosis produced by meningeal endotheliomas. Archives of Neurology 8: 139–154
107. Tucker R L, Holman C B, MacCarth C S 1959 The roentgenology manifestations of meningioma in the region of the tuberculum sellae. Radiology 72: 348–355
108. Benjamins C E 1918 Pneumosinus frontalis dilatans. Acta Otolaryngologica 1: 412–422
109. Lombardi G, Passerini A, Cecchni A 1968 Pneumosinus dilatans. Acta Radiologica Diagnostica 7: 535–542
110. Lloyd G A S 1985 Orbital pneumosinus dilatans. Clinical Radiology 36: 381–386
111. Courville C B, Abbott K H 1942 The histogenesis of meningioma with particular reference to the meningoepithelial variety. Journal of Neuropathology and Experimental Neurology 1: 337–343
112. Goellner J R, Laws E R, Soule E H 1978 Haemopericytoma of the meninges. American Journal of Clinical Pathology 70: 375–380
113. Wright J E, Call M B, Liaricos S 1980 Primary optic nerve meningioma. British Journal of Ophthalmology 64: 553–558
114. Pearse A G E 1974 The APUD cell concept and its implications in pathology. Pathology Annual 9: 27–41
115. Kameya T, Shimojato Y, Adachi I 1980 Neuroendocrine carcinoma of the paranasal sinuses. A morphological and endocrinological study. Cancer 45: 330–339
116. Milroy C M, Rode J, Moss E 1991 Laryngeal paraganglioma and neuroendocrine carcinoma. Histopathology 18: 201–209
117. Silva E G, Butler J J, Mackay B 1982 Neuroblastomas and neuroendocrine carcinomas of the nasal cavity. Cancer 50: 2388–2405
118. Chaudhry A P, Haar J G, Koul A 1979 Olfactory neuroblastoma. Cancer 44: 564–579
119. Friedmann I, Osborn D A 1974 The ultrastructure of olfactory neuroblastoma. Minerva Otorhinolaryngology 24: 66–74
120. Kahn L B 1974 Esthesioneuroblastoma: a light and electron microscopic study. Human Pathology 5: 364–367
121. Gneep D R, Ferlito A, Hyams V 1983 Primary small cell carcinoma of the larynx: a report of 18 cases. Cancer 51: 1731–1745
122. Milroy C M, Robinson P J, Grant H R 1989 Primary composite large cell neuroendocrine carcinoma and squamous carcinoma of the hypopharynx. Journal of Laryngology and Otology 103: 1093–1096
123. Berger L, Luc G, Richard D 1924 L'esthesioneuroepitheliome olfactif. Bulletin Association French Studies of Cancer 13: 410–421
124. Berger L, Coutard H 1926 L'esthesioneurocytoma olfactif. Bulletin Association French Studies of Cancer 15: 404–414
125. O'Connor T A, McLean P, Juillard G S 1989 Olfactory neuroblastoma. Cancer 63: 2426–2428
126. Skolnik E M, Massari F S, Tenta L T 1966 Olfactory neuroepithelioma. Archives of Otolaryngology 84: 644–653
127. Oberman H A, Rice D H 1976 Olfactory neuroblastomas, a clinicopathological study. Cancer 38:2494–2502
128. Levine P A, McLean W C, Cantrell R W 1986 Esthesioneuroblastoma: the University of Virginia experience. Laryngoscope 96: 742–746
129. Beitler J J, Fass D E, Brenner H A 1991 Esthesioneuroblastoma: is there a role for elective neck dissection? Head and Neck Surgery 13: 321–326
130. Shah J P, Feghali J 1981 Esthesioneuroblastoma. American Journal of Surgery 142: 456–458
131. Lund V J, Milroy C 1992 Olfactory neuroblastoma: chemical and pathological aspects. Rhinology: In press.
132. Schwabb G, Michean C, Le Guillou C 1988 Olfactory esthesioneuroma: a report of 40 cases. Laryngoscope 98: 872–876
133. Ijaduola G T A, Olude I O, Okeowo P A 1982 Olfactory neuroblastoma in a 5½ month old Nigerian baby. Clinical Oncology 8: 159–162
134. Aghadiuno P V, Thomas J M, Ogan O 1983 Olfactory neuroblastoma – a case report in an African child. Journal of Laryngology and Otology 97: 261–265
135. Ejecham G C, Sidigui N, Mukherjee D K 1980 Esthesioneuroblastoma: a report of two cases in Nigeria. Journal of Laryngology and Otology 94: 1081–1085
136. Harrison D F N 1984 Surgical pathology of olfactory neuroblastoma. Head and Neck Surgery 7: 60–64
137. Schmidt H M 1973 Uber grobe, form und lage von bulbus and tractus olfactorus des inenschen. Gegenbaur Morphologisches Jahrbuch 119: 227–237
138. Kadish S, Goodman M, Wang C C 1976 Olfactory neuroblastoma – a clinical analysis of 17 cases. Cancer 37: 1571–1576
139. Baker D C, Perzin K H, Conley J J 1979 Olfactory neuroblastoma. Otolaryngology, Head and Neck Surgery 87: 279–283
140. Joachims H Z, Altman M M, Mayer J W 1975 Olfactory neuroblastoma. Journal of Laryngology and Otology 89: 335–343
141. Herrold K 1964 Induction of olfactory neuroepithelial tumours in Syrian hamsters by diethylnitrosamine. Cancer 17: 205–215
142. Obert G J, Devine K D, McDonald J R 1960 Olfactory neuroblastoma. Cancer 13: 205–215
143. Lloyd G A S 1988 Diagnostic imaging of the nose and paranasal sinuses. Springer Verlag, Berlin
144. Woodhead P, Lloyd G A S 1988 Olfactory neuroblastoma, imaging by Magnetic Resonance, CT and conventional techniques. Clinical Otolaryngology 13: 387–394
145. Lund V J, Lloyd G A S, Cheesman A D 1989 Magnetic resonance imaging of paranasal sinus tumours for craniofacial resection. Head and Neck 11: 279–283
146. Appelblatt N H, McClatchey K D 1982 Olfactory neuroblastoma: a retrospective clinicopathological study. Head and Neck Surgery 5: 108–113
147. Bailey B J, Barton S 1975 Olfactory neuroblastoma. Archives of Otolaryngology 101: 1–5
148. Judge D M, McGavran M M, Trapukdi S 1976 Fume-induced fluorescence in diagnosis of nasal neuroblastoma. Archives of Otolaryngology 101: 1–5
149. Falck B, Hillarp N, Thieme G 1962 Fluorescence of catecholamines and related compounds. Journal of Histochemistry and Cytochemistry 10: 348–354
150. Takahashi H, Ohara J, Yamada M 1987 Esthesioneuroepithelioma, a tumour of olfactory epithelial origin. Ultrastructural and immunohistochemical study. Acta Neuropathol (Berlin) 75: 147–155
151. Elkcon D, Hightower S, Lim M L 1979 Esthesioneuroblastoma. Cancer 44: 1087–1094
152. Weiden L, Yarrington C T, Richardson R G 1984 Olfactory neuroblastoma, chemotherapy and radiotherapy for extensive disease. Archives of Otolaryngology 110: 759–760
153. Choi H H, Anderson P J 1985 Immunohistochemical diagnosis of olfactory neuroblastoma. Journal of Neuropathology and Experimental Neurology 44: 18–31
154. Taxy J B, Bharani N K, Mills J E 1986 The spectrum of olfactory neuroblastoma. American Journal of Clinical Pathology 10:687–695
155. Axe S, Kuhajda F P 1987 Esthesioneuroblastoma, intermediate filaments – neuroendocrine and tissue specific antigens. American Journal of Clinical Pathology 88: 139–145
156. Durham J C 1989 Olfactory neuroblastoma. Ear Nose and Throat Journal 68: 185–204
157. Frierson H P, Ross G W, Mills J E 1990 Olfactory neuroblastoma. American Journal of Clinical Pathology 94: 547–553
158. Schmidt J L, Zarbo R S, Clark J L 1990 Olfactory neuroblastoma: clinicopathological and immunohistochemical characterization of four cases. Laryngoscope 100: 1052–1058
159. Zak F G, Lawson W 1974 The presence of melanocytes in the nasal cavity. Annals of Otology, Rhinology and Laryngology 83: 515–519

160. Chaudhry A P, Hampel A, Gorlin R J 1958 Primary melanoma of the oral cavity. Cancer 11: 923–928
161. Moore E S, Martin H 1955 Melanoma of the upper respiratory tract and oral cavity. Cancer 8: 1167–1176
162. Shah J P, Huvos A G, Strong E W 1977 Mucosal melanomas of the head and neck. American Journal of Surgery 134: 531–535
163. Takagi M, Ishikawa G, Mori W 1974 Primary malignant melanoma of the oral cavity in Japan. Cancer 34: 358–370
164. Lewis M G, Martin J A M 1967 Malignant melanoma of the nasal cavity in Ugandan Africans. Cancer 20: 1699–1705
165. Holmstrom M, Lund V J 1991 Malignant melanoma of the nasal cavity following occupational exposure to formaldehyde. British Journal of Industrial Disease 48: 9–11
166. Lund V J 1991 Malignancy of the nose and sinuses: epidemiological and aetiological considerations. Rhinology 29: 57–68
167. Kerns W D, Pavkov K L, Donofrio D J, Gralla E J, Swenberg J A 1983 Carcinogenicity of formaldehyde in rats and mice after long-term inhalation exposure. Cancer Research 43: 4382–4392
168. Andersen I, Molhave L 1983 Controlled human studies with formaldehyde. In: Gibson J E, (ed.) Formaldehyde toxicity. Hemisphere Publishing Corporation, Washington DC, pp 154–165
169. Holmstrom M, Wilhelmsson B 1988 Respiratory symptoms and pathophysiological effects of occupational exposure to formaldehyde and wood dust. Scandinavian Journal of Work and Environmental Health 14: 306–311
170. Holmstrom M, Wilhelmsson B, Hellquist H 1989 Histological changes in the nasal mucosa in rats after long-term exposure to formaldehyde and wood dust. Acta Otolaryngologica (Stockholm) 18: 274–284
171. Blair A, Stewart P, O'Berg M 1986 Mortality among industrial workers exposed to formaldehyde. Journal of the National Cancer Institute 76: 1071–184
172. Walrath J, Fraumeni J F Jr 1983 Mortality patterns among embalmers. International Journal of Cancer 31: 407–411
173. Lucke A 1869 Die melanotischen Geschwulste. Die Lehre von de Geschwulsten in anatomischer und klinische Beziehung. In: Pitha F, Billroth T (eds) Handbuch der allgemeinen und speziellen Chirurgie, Erlangen, Band 2, Abteil 1, Seite 244
174. Wilkinson G 1912 A case of melanotic sarcoma of the nose. Journal of Laryngology and Otology 27: 1–9
175. Garbe C 1991 Epidemiologie des malignen Melanoms. In: Waclawiczek H W, Gebhart W, Manfreda D, Schlag P (eds) Das Maligne Melanom. Springer Verlag, Berlin, pp 1–14
176. Conley J, Pack G T 1974 Melanoma of the mucous membranes of the head and neck. Archives of Otolaryngology 99: 315–319
177. Hyams V J, Batsakis J G, Michaels L 1988 Tumors of the upper respiratory tract and ear. Armed Forces Institute of Pathology, Washington. 2nd Series Fascicle 25
178. Harwood A R 1984 Melanoma of the head and neck. In: Million R R, Cassisi N J (eds) Management of head and neck cancer. Lippincott, Philadelphia, pp 513–528
179. Iversen K, Robins R E 1980 Mucosal malignant melanomas. American Journal of Surgery 139: 660–664
180. Allen A C, Spitz S 1953 Malignant melanoma. Cancer 6: 1–45
181. Mesara B W, Burton W D 1968 Primary malignant melanoma of the upper respiratory tract. Cancer 21: 217-225
182. Freedman H M, DeSanto L W, Devine K D, Weiland L H 1973 Malignant melanomas of the nasal cavity and paranasal sinuses. Archives of Otolaryngology 97: 322–325
183. Holdcraft J, Gallagher J C 1969 Malignant melanomas of the nasal and paranasal sinus mucosae. Annals of Otology, Rhinology and Laryngology 78: 1–20
184. Snow G B, Van der Esch E P, Van Slooten E A 1978 Mucosal melanoma of the head and neck. Head and Neck Surgery 1: 24–30
185. Trodahl J N, Sprague W G 1970 Benign and malignant melanocytic lesions of the oral mucosa. Cancer 25: 812–823
186. Eneroth C M, Lundberg C 1975 Mucosal malignant melanomas of the head and neck. Acta Otolaryngologica 80: 452–458
187. Lund V J 1982 Malignant melanoma of the nasal cavity and paranasal sinuses. Journal of Laryngology and Otology 96: 347–355
188. Soman C S, Sirsat M V 1974 Primary malignant melanoma of the oral cavity in Indians. Oral Surgery 38: 426–434
189. Crone R P 1966 Malignant amelanotic melanomas of the nasal septum and maxillary sinus. Laryngoscope 76: 1826–1833
190. Gallagher J C 1970 Upper respiratory melanoma: pathology and growth rate. Annals of Otology, Rhinology and Laryngology 79: 551–556
191. Williams R A, Rode J, Milroy C M, Charton G, Drewe R H, Lund V J 1991 Ploidy analysis and proliferative activity in nasal melanoma. Presented XIII European Congress of Pathology
192. Clark W H, From L, Bernadino E A, Mihm M C 1969 The histogenesis and histologic behaviour of primary human melanoma of the skin. Cancer Research 29: 707–720
193. Harrison D F N 1976 Malignant melanomata arising in the nasal mucous membrane. Journal of Otolaryngology 90: 993–1005
194. Conley J 1990 Melanoma of the head and neck. Georg Thieme Verlag, Stuttgart, pp 37–44
195. Rhomberg W 1991 Radiotherapie beim malignen Melanom. In: Waclawiczek H W, Gebhart W, Manfreda D, Schlag P (eds) Das Maligne Melanom. Springer-Verlag, Berlin, pp. 229–237
196. Kokoschka E-M 1991 Chemotherapie des malignen Melanoms. In: Waclawiczek H W, Gebhart W, Manfreda D, Schlag P (eds) Das Maligne Melanom. Springer Verlag, Berlin, pp. 222–228
197. Balch C M, Hersey P 1985 Current status of adjuvant therapy. In: Balch C M, Milton G W, Shaw H M, Soong S (eds) Cutaneous melanoma. Clinical management and treatment results worldwide. Lippincott, Philadelphia, pp. 197–218
198. Bystryn J C 1985 Immunology and immunotherapy of human malignant melanoma. Dermatology Clinics 3: 327–334
199. Ho V C, Sober A J 1990 Therapy for cutaneous melanoma: an update. Journal of the American Academy of Dermatology 22: 159–176
200. Batsakis J G, Regezi J A, Solomon A R, Rice D H 1982 The pathology of head and neck tumours: mucosal melanomas, Part 13. Head and Neck Surgery 4: 404–418
201. Ravid J M, Esteves J A 1960 Malignant melanoma of nose and paranasal sinuses and juvenile melanoma of the nose. Archives of Otolaryngology 72: 431–444
202. Mundth E D, Guralnick E A, Raker J W 1965 Malignant melanoma: a clinical study. Annals of Surgery 162: 15–28
203. Panje W R, Moran W J 1986 Melanoma of the upper aerodigestive tract: a review of 21 cases. Head and Neck Surgery 8: 309–312
204. Trapp T K, Fu Y-S, Calcaterra T C 1987 Melanoma of the nasal and paranasal sinus mucosa. Archives of Otolaryngology, Head and Neck Surgery 113: 1086–1089
205. Batsakis J J 1987 Melanotic neuroectodermal tumour of infancy. Annals of Otology, Rhinology and Laryngology 96: 128–129
206. Johnson R E, Scheithaver B W, Dahlin D C 1983 Melanotic neuroectodermal tumour of infancy. Cancer 52: 661–666
207. Hupp J R, Topazian R G, Krutchkoff D J 1981 The melanotic neuroectodermal tumour of infancy, report of two cases and review of the literature. International Journal of Oral Surgery 10: 432–446
208. Cutler L S, Chaudry A P, Topazian R G 1981 Melanotic neuroectodermal tumour of infancy: an ultrastructural study. Cancer 48: 257–262
209. Williams A F 1967 Melanotic neuroectodermal tumour of infancy. Journal of Pathology and Bacteriology 93: 545–548
210. Brekke J H, Gorlin R J 1975 Melanotic neuroectodermal tumour of infancy. Journal of Oral Surgery 33: 858–865
211. Slootweg P J, Straks W, van der Dussen M 1983 Primitive neuroectodermal tumour of the maxilla. Journal of Maxillofacial Surgery 11: 54–57

212. Misugi K, Okajima H, Newton W 1965 Mediastinal origin of a melanotic prognoma or retinal anlage tumour. Cancer 18: 477–484
213. Dehner L P, Sibley R K, Sauk J J 1979 Malignant melanotic neuroectodermal tumour of infancy: a clinical, pathological, ultrastructural and tissue culture study. Cancer 43: 1389–1410
214. Nikai H, Ijuhin N, Yamajaki A 1977 Ultrastructural evidence for a neural crest origin of the melanotic neuroectodermal tumour of infancy. Journal of Oral Pathology 6: 221–230
215. Stowens D, Lin T H 1974 Melanotic prognoma of the brain. Human Pathology 5: 105–108
216. McCormick M V, Hogg D S, Chrystal V 1983 Melanotic neuroectodermal tumour of infancy. Journal of Laryngology and Otology 97: 755–757

20. Surgical options in the management of nose and sinus neoplasia

D. J. Howard and V. J. Lund

The biological nature of sinonasal tumours necessitates surgery in the management of the majority of cases. A considerable spectrum of surgical procedures is now available ranging from endoscopic techniques to base of skull resection. Accurate determination of extent and histological diagnosis has refined our choice but in selecting the appropriate procedure, the surgeon attempts to combine cure with quality of life in respect to function and cosmesis. This requires a diversity of skills but above all depends upon an understanding of the natural history of the disease. It is this which should ultimately dictate our radicality. Cure is always at a price to the patient and as is apparent from the foregoing chapters in this book, a frequently unattained goal. However, that cost is minimized by procedures such as midfacial degloving and craniofacial resection and in this area genuine palliation can be an achievable surgical aim.

It is not within the remit of this book to offer a manual of operative techniques but rather to assess the respective roles and limitations of the surgical options.

The immensely improved optics afforded by rigid and flexible endoscopes has greatly facilitated our examination technique and might ultimately lead to earlier diagnosis of disease. Sadly this will probably continue to be confounded by the late clinical presentation of patients who have ignored the early innocuous symptoms of sinonasal malignancy. Certainly the use of such instruments greatly enhances the accuracy of biopsy and has largely superseded conventional assaults via an inferior meatal antrostomy or Caldwell–Luc approach. Indeed it is difficult on oncologic grounds to support the breaching of an intact anterior maxillary wall in such a pursuit. The endoscopes also offer an invaluable adjunct to postoperative follow-up and can readily be utilized, with biopsy, on an out-patient basis in addition to repeated imaging.

Caution should, however be exercised when considering the use of endoscopic techniques for resection. Demonstrably limited benign disease as can occasionally occur in inverted papilloma may be suitable and certainly an important role exists in the management of many of the conditions simulating neoplasia (see Ch. 4) but it would be inappropriate as the primary surgical approach in malignancy.

External fronto-ethmoidectomy and the osteoplastic flap have been mentioned in relation to some benign tumours such as osteomas and conditions such as mucocoeles but the paucity of benign lesions confined to the frontal sinus significantly limits the role of these procedures and they have no place in oncologic resection.

The lateral rhinotomy approach, attributed to Moure in 1902[1] but described as early as 1848,[2] was originally intended for removal of fronto-ethmoidal tumours combined with radiotherapy if disease had comprised the cribriform plate or roof of the ethmoids. Limiting the superior extent of the incision to the medial canthus and careful repair of the alar margin diminishes the cosmetic problems which originally limited its popularity (Fig. 20.1).[3] It affords excellent access to the nasal cavity for tumours such as malignant melanoma and benign neoplasms arising within the nasal cavity, medial maxilla, pterygomaxillary region and nasopharynx, e.g. angiofibroma, inverted papilloma, osteoma, ossifying fibroma and neurofibroma.[4-6] Haemostasis can be effected in the more vascular lesions by ligation of the sphenopalatine artery in the lateral nasal wall or of the internal maxillary artery via the antrum.

However, the majority of such cases can be better managed via a midfacial degloving approach which offers even greater bilateral access and avoids all external scars (Fig. 20.2).[7-9] Its only limitations are the extra time taken in closure to avoid vestibular stenosis and oro-antral fistula and less satisfactory access to the frontal sinus. For younger patients and those with extensive benign disease of the upper jaw it is the procedure of choice and is particularly suitable for angiofibroma, inverted papilloma and fibro-osseous disease. The combination of oncologic resection and rhinoplasty technique is especially appealing.

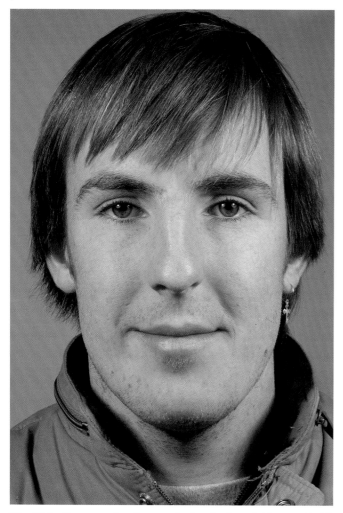

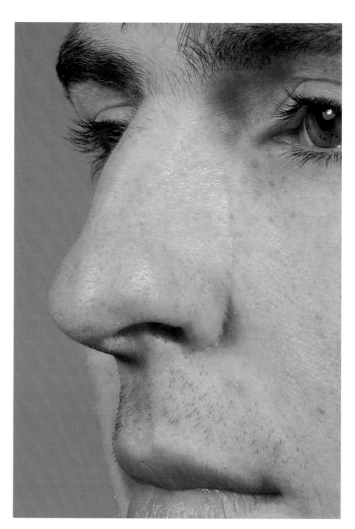

Fig. 20.1   Post-operative photographs showing lateral rhinotomy incision.

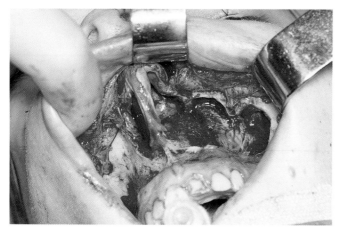

Fig. 20.2   Intraoperative photograph showing access via midfacial degloving approach (courtesy of D. J. Howard).

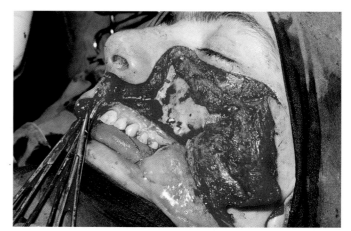

Fig. 20.3   Intraoperative photograph showing Weber-Fergusson approach to maxilla.

Thus the Weber–Fergusson incision is confined to those older patients with malignancy of the upper jaw, requiring conventional radical maxillectomy with or without orbital clearance and for procedures such as the maxillary swing[10] designed for access to the nasopharynx (Fig. 20.3). Many patients who would in the past have undergone total maxillectomy and orbital clearance are now managed by a craniofacial approach and this change is reflected in the frequency with which maxillectomies have been performed each year on the Professorial Unit. Between 1970 and 1980, 47% of cases of sinonasal malignancy underwent total maxillectomy with or without orbital clearance, between 1981 and 1991 this had fallen to 26%.

Distinction should be made between orbital clearance and orbital exenteration in which the eyelids are also removed. For the pathology encountered in the sinonasal region which may compromise the orbit there is rarely any oncologic advantage to the sacrifice of the lids. Preservation of the skin and orbicularis muscle results in a skin-lined socket which is cosmetically more acceptable and in which the prosthetic eye can comfortably be fitted (p. 337).

Rhinectomy is fortunately rarely indicated except for extensive nasal tumours and heroic and lengthy attempts at soft tissue reconstruction of the nose are usually inappropriate.[11] The patient's rehabilitation and palliation is better served in most instances by a skilled prosthedontist.

It is well recognized that the poor prognosis associated with malignant tumours of the nose and paranasal sinuses is a consequence of local recurrence engendered by inadequate resection. Realization that every tumour affecting the inferior surface of the cribriform plate and roof of ethmoid theoretically had spread intracranially, led to the development of the craniofacial approach which offered access and a more rational resection dependent on anatomical considerations. Thus the combined approach craniofacial procedure has become well established.[12–15]

The craniofacial operation was originally described in 1954[16] and was subsequently developed by Ketcham et al[13] and by Terz et al[15]. Clifford[17] promoted the concept of a single team approach which has been extended by Cheesman and others[18–21] for use in extensive benign and malignant disease.

Previously total maxillectomy with orbital clearance or lateral rhinotomy allowed wide resection of such anteriorly placed tumours but could not encompass safe resection of the cribriform plate and entire ethmoid block leading to inevitable local recurrence. Present experience indicates that a combination of radiotherapy and radical surgery offers the best prognosis for radiosensitive tumours, with radical resection optimally performed 6 weeks following radiotherapy irrespective of response. The procedure is also eminently suitable for the safe excision of large benign lesions.

The majority of patients undergo radiology, contrast-enhanced (direct coronal and axial) CT and MRI (axial, coronal and sagittal planes). Previous studies on craniofacial patients have shown a correlation of 85% between CT and histology. MRI improves this correlation to 94% and the addition of the paramagnetic agent, gadolinium DTPA, improves the accuracy of tumour delineation to 98%, distinguishing it from inflamed mucosa, retained secretions and normal mucosa.[22] The imaging is repeated postoperatively, at 6 months and on an annual basis where appropriate in combination with examination of the cavity under general anaesthetic (Figs 20.4 and 20.5).

The craniofacial operation uses an extended lateral rhinotomy incision with access to the anterior cranial fossa effected via a 'shield-shaped window' craniotomy which can be rewired in place at the end of the procedure (Figs 20.6 and 20.7). Through the craniotomy, the frontal lobes and overlying dura are retracted as dissection of the dura is carried out on a wide front, progressing posteriorly onto the smooth bone of the jugum sphenoidale and exposing crista galli, cribriform plate, ethmoid and orbital roofs (Figs 20.8 and 20.9). Thus an en bloc removal of both ethmoidal complexes, cribriform plate and posterior end of septum can now be performed with additional resection of surrounding structures dependent upon the extent of the disease (Fig. 20.10). In particular, accurate evaluation of orbital involvement is possible as the procedure gives excellent visualization of the posterior portion of the medial orbital wall. In cases where the medial bony wall of the orbit has been breached but the periosteum is intact, the compromised area of periosteum can often be resected and grafted with a split skin graft with preservation of the globe and its musculature. Any significant dural defect can be repaired with fascia lata to which a thin fenestrated split skin graft is applied. As for lateral rhinotomy and maxillectomy, the surgical cavity is packed with ribbon gauze soaked in Whitehead's varnish (compound iodoform paint: iodoform, benzoin, prepared storax, tolu balsam and solvent ether) which decreases bleeding and

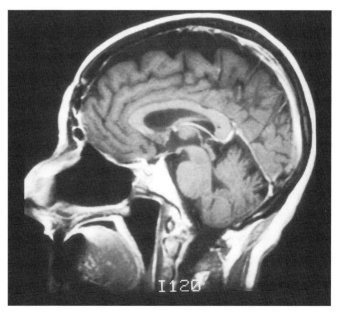

Fig. 20.4 Sagittal MR scan, T1 weighted with gadolinium. Postoperative follow-up to craniofacial resection.

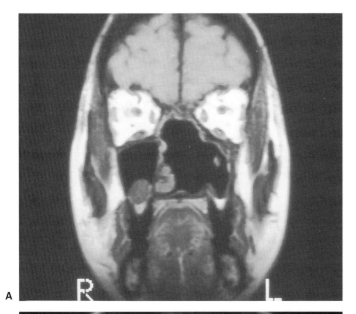

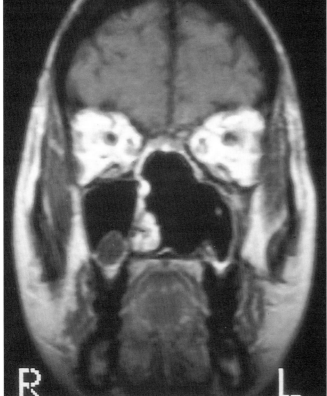

Fig. 20.5 **A**, coronal MR scan, T2 weighted sequence and **B**, T1 weighted sequence with gadolinium in patient who has previously undergone craniofacial resection for olfactory neuroblastoma. A small area of high signal from recurrence is shown in the middle of the roof of the nasal cavity.

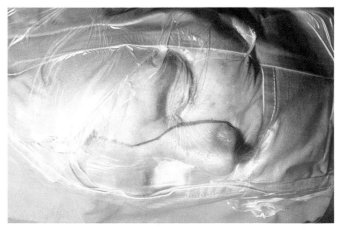

Fig. 20.6 Intraoperative photograph showing position of incision for craniofacial resection (courtesy of A. D. Cheesman).

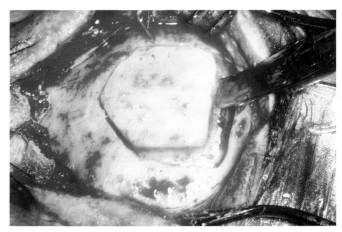

Fig. 20.7 Intraoperative photograph showing removal of shield-shaped frontal osteotomy.

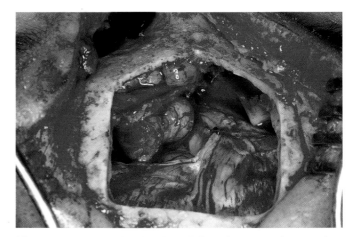

Fig. 20.8 Intraoperative view through frontal osteotomy into anterior cranial fossa.

is removed under a short general anaesthetic at 10 days. The standard closure can be modified using local flaps and bone grafts if required following excision of extensive anteriorly placed disease.

160 patients have had craniofacial resections performed between 1978 and 1992. Their ages ranged from 9–74 years, with an average of 49 years, the majority

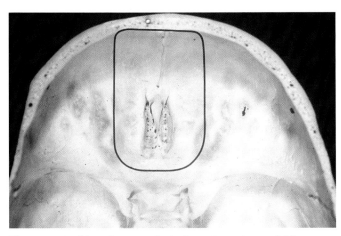

Fig. 20.9 Position of osteotomies in floor of anterior cranial fossa shown on skull (courtesy of A. D. Cheesman).

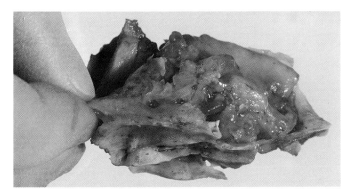

Fig. 20.10 Surgical specimen removed via craniofacial approach (Courtesy of A.D. Cheesman).

Table 20.1 Range of malignant histology in patients undergoing craniofacial resection

Histology	No. of patients
Adenocarcinoma	34
Olfactory neuroblastoma	19
Chondrosarcoma	13
Adenoid cystic carcinoma	13
Squamous cell carcinoma	13
Anaplastic carcinoma	11
Malignant melanoma	7
Transitional cell carcinoma	4
Rhabdomyosarcoma	3
Malignant fibrous histiocytoma	2
Primitive neuroblastoma	2
Cylindric cell carcinoma	2
Carcinosarcoma	1
Osteogenic sarcoma	1
Angiosarcoma	1
Spindle cell carcinoma	1
Haemangiopericytoma	1
Alveolar soft part sarcoma	1
Total	129

Table 20.2 Range of benign histology in patients undergoing craniofacial resection

Histology	No. of patients
Meningioma	7
Osteoma	6
Meningoencephalocoele	3
Reparative granuloma	2
Osteoblastoma	2
Phycomycete granuloma	2
Leiomyoblastoma	2
Angioma	1
Neurofibroma	1
Cholesterol granuloma	1
Cementifying fibroma	1
Dermoid	1
Pseudotumour	1
Osteomyelitis	1
Total	31

(63%) being between 40–70. There were 104 (65%) men and 56 (35%) women. The range of histopathology was extremely wide (Tables 20.1 and 20.2). The commonest type of tumour was adenocarcinoma (21%) (8 of whom were wood-workers) followed by olfactory neuroblastoma (12%) though virtually all other types of histopathology affecting this area were represented.

In the majority of patients (52%), disease arose in the ethmoid region, though tumours primarily affecting the nasal cavity, septum, maxilla, orbit and frontal sinus also necessitated this approach. 56% had undergone previous surgery, 31% had received radiotherapy and 5% had been given chemotherapy in the past. Of those recurrences which had undergone previous surgery, adenocarcinoma again predominated and as a consequence the ethmoids were the commonest site of recurrent disease but all other areas were represented. Previous surgery ranged from lateral rhinotomy, internal and external ethmoidectomy, maxillectomy and orbital clearance.

Complications following this procedure have been few with an average postoperative stay of 16 days (Table 20.3). Prophylactic broad-spectrum antibiotics and anticonvulsants have minimized infection and epileptiform attacks. The majority of the serious sequelae resulted in the early part of the series from precipitate mobilization (two cerebrovascular accidents) or radiotherapy given shortly after surgery (two frontal lobe abscesses). 5 days

Table 20.3 Complications in series of 160 patients undergoing craniofacial resection

Complication	No.	Result
Immediate/peroperative		
Convulsions	1	Recovery
Haemorrhage	2	1, embolization
		1, death
Air embolism	1	Recovery
Pneumoencephalocoele	1	Recovery
Intermediate		
CVA	2	1, partial recovery
		1, death
Long-term		
Haemorrhage	1	Death
Frontal lobe abscess	2	Death
Bone necrosis	2	Recovery after debridement
Convulsions	3	Control with phenytoin
CSF leak	7	4, surgical repair
		3, spontaneous recovery
Epiphora	3	Dacrocystorhinotomy
Serous otitis media	8	Myringotomy & grommet
Pituitary insufficiency	1	Steroid replacement

CSF, cerebrospinal fluid; CVA, cerebrovascular accident

bed-rest and postponement of radiotherapy for 2 months if not given preoperatively have avoided further problems.

The excellent cosmetic results are unquestionable in both adults and children (Figs 20.11–20.13). Sequential standardized radiologic and photographic follow-up has not demonstrated any distortion of mid-facial growth in over 20 children and adolescents. This approach can readily be repeated (10%), up to six times in one individual with chondrosarcoma.

The orbit may be cleared at the time of the initial surgery (27%) but the exposure offered by this approach may allow preservation of the eye if disease abuts but has not breached the orbital periosteum. In these cases (10%), resection of the affected periosteum can be performed, under frozen section control, without adverse effect on survival and only three individuals have required subsequent clearance. This approach to the orbital periosteum has been used with similar success by Perry et al.[23]

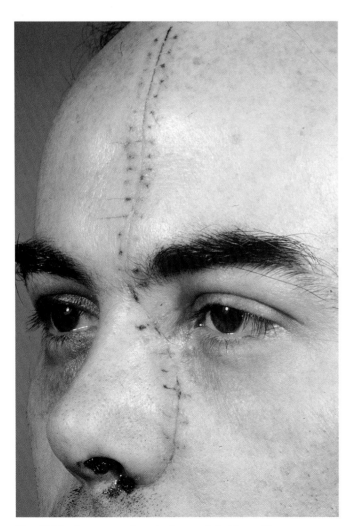

Fig. 20.11 Appearance 1 week after craniofacial resection.

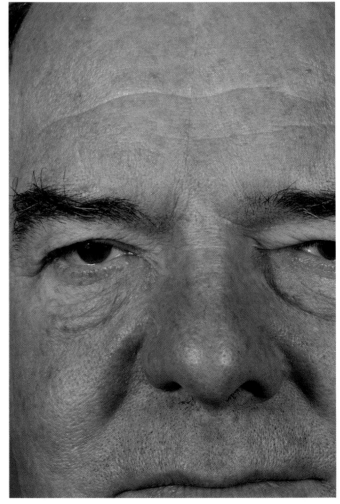

Fig. 20.12 Cosmetic appearance some months following craniofacial resection.

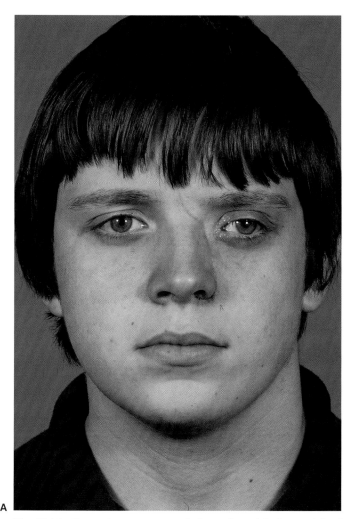 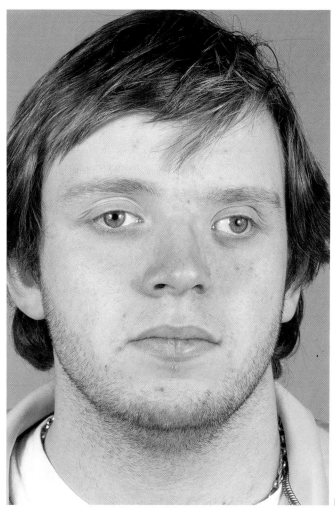

A   B

Fig. 20.13   Cosmetic appearance at **A**, 3 months and **B**, 7 years following craniofacial resection. Patient was 14 years old at time of craniofacial resection for a reparative granuloma.

Assessing the results of this series is, nevertheless, compromised by the diversity of pathologies, the lack of large numbers with long-term follow-up and the range of disease extent, factors which have bedevilled evaluation of all results in this area. Over half the patients have already failed previous treatment and 5-year follow-up is relatively meaningless for many of the malignancies.

Complete excision of many benign pathologies can be effected via this approach but the 'benign' nature of tumours such as meningioma as defined by their inability to metastasize, can be seriously questioned in a site where they frequently lead to blindness and death. Involvement of the middle cranial fossa and pterygopalatine fossa, irrespective of the pathology compromises cure but the minimal morbidity and mortality of this procedure offers meaningful palliation. Survival in this particular group is necessarily poor and when the brain is involved few survive beyond a year.

Thus with these considerations in mind, of 100 patients with malignant disease and follow-up in excess of 5 years, actuarial survival is 38%. When patients with 'incurable' or extensive disease and those with curable benign conditions are excluded, a group of patients emerge by whom the efficacy of the procedure must be judged. 50 patients are in this category, 27 with 5–14 years' follow-up, of whom 17 are alive and well, one with evidence of recurrent disease, seven have died (three of postoperative complications or intercurrent disease) and two have been lost. This suggests a crude survival rate of 67%.

56 patients (36%) have died following surgery, 84% due to local and/or metastatic disease. This occurred on average 18 months following surgery. The incidence of metastatic disease (54%) may reflect improved local control, unmasking systemic spread previously obscured by the rapid demise of the patient.

Notwithstanding this possible change in the natural history of sinonasal malignancy, the oncologic advantages of the approach over previous techniques are clear. Craniofacial resection allows access, accurate staging and monoblock resection. It is not the ultimate panacea as it cannot cure the incurable, but it does offer palliation with minimal morbidity and represents one of the major surgical advances in this region.

Endnote

The craniofacial patients presented represent a combined series operated on at the Royal National Throat, Nose and Ear Hospital by ourselves and Mr A. D. Cheesman. We would like to take this opportunity to gratefully acknowledge the unique contribution made by Tony Cheesman in the development of this procedure.

REFERENCES

1. Moure E J (1902) Traitement des tumeurs malignes primitives de l'ethmoide. Revue Hebdomadaire de Laryngologie 2: 401–412
2. Mertz J S, Pearson B W, Kern E B 1983 Lateral rhinotomy: indications, technique and review of 226 patients. Archives of Otolaryngology 109: 235–239
3. Bernard P J, Lawson W, Biller H F, Lebenger J 1989 Complications following rhinotomy: review of 148 patients. Annals of Otology, Rhinology and Laryngology 98: 684–692
4. Harrison D F N 1977 Lateral rhinotomy: a neglected operation. Annals of Otology, Rhinology and Laryngology 86: 756–759
5. Lund V J 1992 Lateral rhinotomy. In: McGregor I A, Howard D J (eds) Head and neck surgery, Part 2, 4th edn. Butterworth-Heinemann, London, pp 551–554
6. Schramm V L, Myers E N 1978 Lateral rhinotomy. Laryngoscope 88: 1042–1045
7. Howard D J 1992 Midfacial degloving. In: McGregor I A, Howard D J (eds) Head and neck surgery, Part 2, 4th edn. Butterworth-Heinemann, London, pp 571–575
8. Price J C, Holliday M J, Johns M E 1988 The versatile midface degloving approach. Laryngoscope 98: 291–295
9. Sacks M E, Conley J, Rabuzzi D D 1984 Degloving approach for total excision of inverted papillomas. Laryngoscope 94: 1595–1598
10. Wei W I, Lam K H, Sham J S T 1991 New approach to the nasopharynx: the maxillary swing approach. Head and Neck Surgery 13: 200–207
11. Harrison D F N 1982 Total rhinectomy – a worthwhile operation? Journal of Laryngology and Otology 96: 1113–1123
12. Ketcham A S, Wilkins R H, Van Buren J M, Smith R R 1963 A combined intracranial approach to the paranasal sinuses. American Journal of Surgery 106: 698–703
13. Ketcham A S, Chretien P B, Van Buren J M, Hoye R C, Beazley R M, Herdt J R 1973 The ethmoid sinuses: a re-evaluation of surgical excision. American Journal of Surgery 126: 469–476
14. Lund V J, Howard D J, Lloyd G A S 1983 CT evaluation of paranasal sinus tumours for craniofacial resection. British Journal of Radiology 56: 439–446
15. Terz J J, Young H F, Lawrence W 1980 Combined craniofacial resection for locally advanced carcinoma of the head and neck. American Journal of Surgery 140: 613–624
16. Smith R R, Klopp C T, Williams J M 1954 Surgical treatment of cancer of the frontal sinus and adjacent areas. Cancer 7: 991–994
17. Clifford P 1977 Transcranial approach for cancer of the antroethmoidal area. Clinical Otolaryngology 2: 115–130
18. Cheesman A D, Lund V J, Howard D J 1986 Craniofacial resection for tumors of the nasal cavity and paranasal sinuses. Head and Neck Surgery 8: 429–435
19. Jackson I T, Laws E R Jr, Martin R D 1983 A craniofacial approach to advanced recurrent cancer of the central face. Head and Neck Surgery 5: 474–488
20. Jackson I T, Munro I R, Hide T A H 1984 Treatment of tumours involving the anterior cranial fossa. Head and Neck Surgery 6: 901–913
21. Schramm V L Jr, Myers E N, Maroon J C 1979 Anterior skull base surgery for benign and malignant disease. Laryngoscope 89: 1077–1091
22. Lund V J, Howard D J, Lloyd G A S, Cheesman A D 1989 Magnetic resonance imaging of paranasal sinus tumors for craniofacial resection. Head and Neck Surgery 11: 279–283
23. Perry C, Levine P A, Williamson B R, Cantrell R W 1988 Preservation of the eye in paranasal sinus cancer surgery. Archives of Otolaryngology, Head and Neck Surgery 114: 632–634

21. Disability and rehabilitation following surgery for sinonasal malignancy

The oncologic surgeon is faced with the unhappy task of reconciling complete excision of disease with maximal preservation of appearance and function. Whilst the first criterion must take precedence, the emotional impact of postoperative disfigurement and dysfunction is becoming increasingly recognized as a critical factor in physical and psychological rehabilitation of patients. Considerable emotional upheaval is inevitable since acquired facial deformity and dysfunction constitute an enormous threat to self-perception.[1] Whilst the degree and duration of distress will vary from individual to individual, the patient faces the dual burden of coping with the diagnosis of cancer and the physical changes engendered by treatment. Patients are particularly vulnerable as social interaction and emotional expression depend to a great extent upon the structural and functional integrity of the head and neck region and these individuals cannot hide their disfigurement which is constantly on show.

Psychiatric morbidity has been estimated to affect between 20% and 35% of all cancer patients.[2] However, it is often ignored as the distress is judged to be an inevitable and understandable consequence.[3] It is estimated that approximately 25% of cancer patients suffer from depression[4,5] and patients with head and neck malignancy are at an even greater risk due to the mutilating surgery.[6] It has been suggested that psychosocial problems in addition to adversely affecting patients' quality of life also interfere with treatment and rehabilitation of head and neck cancer patients.[7] Herzon & Boshier[8] have observed that patients' fears about their altered facial appearance and dysfunction, as well as the prospect of re-entering society, outweighed their fears of recurrent disease.

In addition the functional impact of such surgery on speech and eating and on the senses of sight, smell, taste and even hearing can be profound, with far-reaching consequences on social activities and occupation. Quality of life is a difficult concept to define.[9] However, there appears to be agreement in the literature with regard to its multidimensional nature.[9–13] Nevertheless, despite the critical importance of the attendant problems, reliable measurement has remained elusive. In a study designed to assess perception of relative severity of 11 common facial disfigurements resulting from surgery, orbital exenteration and radical maxillectomy scored highest with rhinectomy only outweighed by mandibulectomy.[14]

Sinonasal malignancy can affect both the young and the old. In a study of 116 patients with head and neck cancer, aged 16–35 years, 32 (28%) had sinonasal disease, representing the largest group by site.[15] At the other end of the age spectrum, in 100 patients over 70 years undergoing head and neck surgery, 14% had sinonasal malignancy.[16]

In order to assess quality of life, it needs to be broken down into its component parts and at least the following four aspects should be considered: physical complaints (somatic sensations, disease symptoms and treatment side effects), social functioning, psychological distress and functional status.[17] A modified EORTC core questionnaire was used to examine these aspects in 49 patients who had undergone ablative surgery for head and neck malignancy during the preceding 2 years.[18] This included 11 craniofacial patients who reported significant problems with vision (blurring), smell, taste and headaches. High levels of fatigue were reported by this group. This has also been described in other studies[19] and could represent a somatic manifestation of psychological distress. However, by contrast with patients undergoing laryngectomy, pull-up, glossectomy and other buccal resections, they scored well functionally with only moderate feelings of self-consciousness, minimal impairment of sexual activity and reasonable social and occupational rehabilitation. These sort of problems may in part be alleviated by careful pre- and postoperative counselling, the help of individuals who have similarly suffered and support groups (p. 339).

In those patients undergoing radical maxillectomy, more tangible physical rehabilitation is required and the surgeon must work closely with a maxillo-facial prosthedontist. The patient must be assessed preoperatively to obtain dental impressions, modify existing dentures and the likely extent of excision discussed. The surgical cavity may be modified to facilitate the design and construction of the most appropriate prosthesis thus allowing the immediate placement of a temporary obturator at the end of the procedure. This can be done using gutta percha moulded to the self-retaining pre-prepared denture base.[20] Thus on waking, normal speech and feeding will considerably bolster the patient's morale. The technical 'tips' that make this branch of reconstructive medicine such an art are to be found in the maxillo-dental literature and are beyond the scope of this book. Suffice to say that once the surgical cavity is healed, a permanent hard acrylic or soft polymer obturator can be fashioned and the use of sectional, sprung and swivel-retained obturators can be used if needed in 'difficult' cases (Figs 21.1 and 21.2).[20,21] Every case requires frequent visits and sympathetic care to obtain the optimum tailor-made fit.

The advent of the osseo-integration techniques has greatly improved the retention of prostheses, both intra-oral and facial. This is particularly relevant to the nose and eye following excision. In the past these prostheses required attachment on spectacles or with tissue glues which were often unsatisfactory (Fig. 21.3). The Brane-mark system of osseo-integrated implants works by the use of titanium screws which become an integral part of the skeleton and to which the prosthesis can be firmly attached (Fig. 21.4).[22] The life of the prosthesis can be extended when it is not being continually manipulated.

The screws can be implanted at the time of the resection or as a secondary procedure. The bone must be at least 3–4 mm in depth, limiting the sites available and radiotherapy can adversely affect integration. In the orbit it is advisable to wait at least 6 months or even up to 1 year if radiotherapy has been given, before exposing the fitments and attaching the prosthesis as integration is less successful in this region for reasons which are not entirely

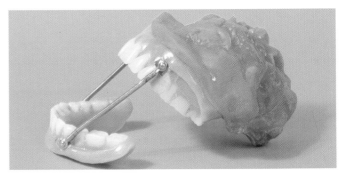

Fig. 21.2 Spring-loaded obturator for patient who had undergone bilateral maxillectomies.

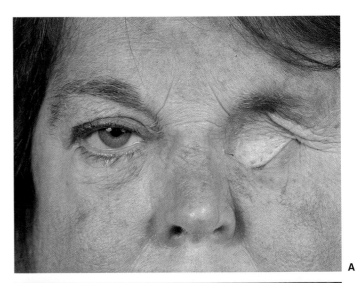

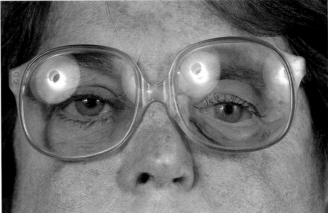

Fig. 21.3 **A**, socket following orbital clearance lined by skin of eyelids. **B**, same patient with orbital prosthesis attached to spectacles.

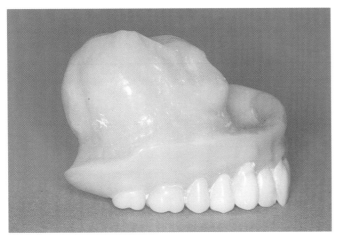

Fig. 21.1 Permanent acrylic obturator for use following radical maxillectomy.

understood. A temporary prosthesis should be offered during the interim.

The availability of these specialized techniques have dramatically improved the postoperative rehabilitation of our patients although in pursuit of that ultimate but often

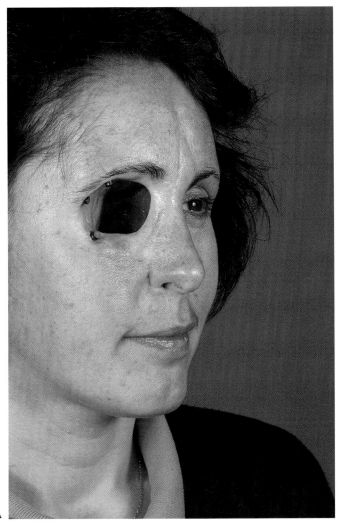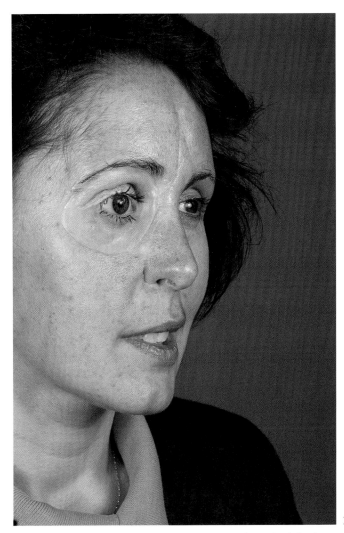

Fig. 21.4 The Branemark system. **A**, socket with three Branemark screws exposed in lateral margin. **B**, same patient with orbital prosthesis in place.

elusive goal, we as surgeons can never fully comprehend the impact of our best efforts to cure.

LIVING WITH A CHANGED FACE

Christine Piff

What many professionals and the public do not realize, is that it isn't necessarily the visible and measurable physical extent of damage that is of major importance to the patient. It is the damage done by the surgeon in saving a life that has to a degree 'spoiled' the image that the patient has of themself; causing grief, humiliation, embarrassment and an immeasurable degree of deep psychological suffering. Patients themselves cannot explain or even begin to understand these strange emotions that are overtaking them. The feeling of isolation and rejection causes withdrawal, an inability to share these feelings and an inability to identify with this new face. Some do eventually, after years of bereavement for their old face, recover enough to undertake a fairly normal life style but still hiding their pain and fears about the way they look. Avoiding crowds, public transport and areas where people may look and stare. Unfortunately, there are many who never can accept their new faces and can never live a normal life again. They shut themselves away, protecting themselves from inquisitive remarks and stares which cause so much pain and grief.

No matter how hard we try to help, it is only the patients themselves who can fight to try and gain some degree of normality. But if you are in pain and discomfort and trying to come to terms with a poorly fitting obturator that is making it difficult to eat or drink, life becomes impossible. Reliance on others who cannot understand these privations, once you have left the protection of the hospital, accentuates these stresses. I write as one who has 'been there', having lived for over 14 years following total maxillectomy and orbital loss.

Living through the terrifying experiences of fittings for obturators and facial prostheses with the nightmare of facing family and friends with a 'changed' face. The pain never goes away!

Surprisingly, some people have an inner strength to cope with stress and since starting the Support Network for the Facially Disfigured, I have found that patients with families and friends who give wonderful support suffer less although still having withdrawal from their loved ones. However, there are many who are sent home to cope alone and still make a dramatic recovery in facing the world determined to get on with their lives – come what may. No individual patient is the same as another and we cope in our own way and in our own time, or perhaps not at all.

The great fear is of rejection, of not being loved anymore, of being worthless, a burden to family and friends and this is quickly felt on returning home and seeing our changed faces in familiar surroundings, where we have previously felt most secure. How we come to terms with this depends again on the individual. Some of us cannot cry in company, cannot discuss fears with our loved ones or closest friends. Losing one's face means losing one's identity, for our faces are our lives and mark in the world. We have grown accustomed to this all our lives and suddenly it is changed although we know we are the same people. Alas, so many professional carers fail to understand this or its importance to the patient. It is now that we desperately need support from somebody who has themselves 'been there'. A voice who can share the tears of regret and suffering, who's mouth was ulcerated during radiotherapy and who couldn't eat without dribbling. Reassurance that it would improve in time helps to make the waiting time shorter.

The need to talk with someone who has a facial prosthesis is of the utmost importance as there are so many questions we never seem to be able to ask the experts. A patient who is now living a normal existence with such a prosthesis is so great an encouragement, for failure to eat or drink properly or even talk is shattering. This experience encouraged me to talk on television about this need for help and this led to the launching of 'LET'S FACE IT', a support network which now extends throughout the United Kingdom and in many countries elsewhere. My life and that of the supporters of the network, is dedicated to improving the lives of all facially disfigured people for I know from experience that in a society that values physical beauty it is hard to understand the feelings of isolation and rejection that comes with facial abnormality. Do please look us in the eye, accept our anxieties, acknowledge anger, fear and bewilderment for at heart we still are the same people, grateful to be alive.

Christine Piff, at the age of 36 years and in September 1977 had a total maxillectomy with orbital clearance for a radiation-failed squamous carcinoma. As a result of this experience she wrote a book entitled 'Let's Face It'. This was a moving account of the effect of this traumatic time and the support she received from a loving and caring family. She remains free from disease 14 years later, and has used her talents to promote her highly successful Support Network to assist those who have also suffered some form of facial disfigurement. A truly remarkable woman!

REFERENCES

1. Dropkin M J 1980 Changes in body image associated with head and neck cancer. In Marino L (ed) Cancer Nursing. Mosby, St Louis, pp 379–384
2. Feinnmann C, Hapwood P 1990 Emotional disturbance of patients with functional symptoms. Journal of Royal Society of Medicine 83: 596–597
3. Massie M J, Holland J C 1984 Diagnosis and treatment of depression in cancer patients. Journal of Clinical Psychology 45: 25–28
4. Bukberg J, Penman D, Holland J 1984 Depression in hospitalized cancer patients. Psychosomatic Medicine 46: 199–212
5. Derogatis L R, Morrow G R, Fetting J 1983 The prevalence of psychiatric disorders among cancer patients. Journal of American Medical Association 249: 715–757
6. Breitbart W, Holland J 1988 Psychological aspects of head and neck cancer. Seminars in Oncology 15: 61–69
7. Mathog R H 1991 Rehabilitation of head and neck cancer patients: Consensus on recommendations from the International Conference on Rehabilitation of the Head and Neck Cancer Patient. Head and Neck Surgery: 1–14
8. Herzon F, Boshier M 1979 Head and neck cancer – emotional management. Head and Neck Surgery 2: 112–118
9. Calman K C 1984 Quality of life in cancer patients – an hypothesis. Journal of Medical Ethics 10: 124–127
10. Ferrell B R, Wisdom C, Wenzl C 1989 Quality of life as an outcome variable in the management of cancer pain. Cancer 63: 2321–2327
11. Flanagan J C 1982 Measures of quality of life. Current state of the art. Archives of Physical Medicine and Rehabilitation 63: 56–59
12. Schipper H, Clinch J, McMurray A, Levitt M 1984 Measuring the quality of life of cancer patients. The Functional Living Index for Cancer. Journal of Clinical Oncology 2: 472–483
13. Smart C R, Yates J W 1987 Quality of life. Cancer 60: 620–622
14. Dropkin M J, Malgady R G, Scott D W, Oberst M T, Strong E W 1983 Scaling of disfigurement and dysfunction in postoperative head and neck patients. Head and Neck Surgery 6: 559–570
15. Lund V J, Howard D J 1990 Head and neck cancer in the young: a prognostic conundrum? Journal of Laryngology and Otology 104: 544–548
16. Harries M, Lund V J 1989 Head and neck surgery in the elderly: a maturing problem. Journal of Laryngology and Otology 103: 306–309
17. Aaronson N K, Bullinger M, Ahmedzai S 1988 A modular approach to quality of life assessment in cancer clinical trials. Recent Results in Cancer Research 111: 231–249
18. Jones E, Lund V J, Howard D J, Greenberg M P, McCarthy M 1992 Quality of life of patients treated surgically for head and neck cancer. Journal of Laryngology and Otology 106: 238–242
19. Krouse J H, Krouse H J, Fabian R L 1989 Adaptation to surgery for head and neck cancer. Laryngoscope 99: 789–794

20. Manderson R D 1992 Prosthetics in head and neck surgery. In: McGregor I A, Howard D J (eds) Head and neck surgery, Part 2, 4th edn. Butterworth-Heinemann Ltd, London, pp 576–592

21. Harrison R E 1979 Prosthetic management of the maxillectomy patient. Head and Neck Surgery 1:366–369

22. Tjellstrom A 1989 Osseointegrated systems and their application in the head and neck. Archives of Otolaryngology, Head and Neck Surgery 3: 39–70.

Index

Cysts (*contd.*)
  calcifying odontogenic, 215–17
  dermoid, 261, 262–3
  epidermoid, 261
  odontogenic, 215–17
  primordial, 217–19
  teratoid, 261
Cytosine, 258
Cytotoxic drugs *see* Chemotherapy

Dacarbazine
  juvenile angiofibroma, 174
  malignant fibrous histiocytoma, 148
  rhabdomyosarcoma, 194
Dactinomycin
  Ewing's sarcoma, 151
  juvenile angiofibroma, 174
Deafness, 287–8
Denker, A., 10
Dermoid cysts, 261, 262–3
Dermoplasty, intranasal, 163
Desmoid tumours, 135
Diagnosis, pathological *see* Histopathology
Diagnostic imaging *see* Radiology
Diathermy, 5
Dickson, D., 2
Dieffenbach, Johann Friedrich, 6, 8
Diethylenetriamine penta-acetic acid (DTPA), 47–50
Diethylnitrosamine
  adenocarcinoma, 117
  olfactory neuroblastoma, 312
Diethylstilboestrol, 172–3
Dimethyltriazenoimidazole carboxamide (DTIC) *see* Dacarbazine
Diplopia
  mucocoeles, 57
  post-mucocoele surgery, 60–61
Disability, postoperative, 337–41
Disfigurement, 339–40
Doxorubicin
  juvenile angiofibroma, 174
  non-Hodgkin's lymphoma, 271
Dupuytren, Guillaume, 1

Ear
  chordoma, 255
  Wegener's granulomatosis, 287–8
Earle (19th century surgeon), 2, 8
Ecchondroma, 199–200
Ectoturbinals, 35–6
Embolization techniques, 49–52
  adenoid cystic carcinoma, 112–13
  epistaxis, 163–4
  juvenile angiofibroma, 171–2
  traumatic epistaxis, 163–4
Encephalocoeles, nasal, 295–9
Endoscopic techniques, 329
Endoturbinals, 35–6
Endoxan *see* Cyclophosphamide
Entomophthora coronatus, 68
Eosinophilic granulomas, 257–9
Epidermoid cyst, 261
Epiphora, 33
  mucocoeles, 57
Epithelium
  olfactory, 23
  respiratory, 22–3
Epstein–Barr virus, 265, 267
Epulis of pregnancy, 158
ESR (erythrocyte sedimentation rate)
  midline destructive granuloma, 278
  Wegener's granulomatosis, 285, 290, 291

Ethinyloestradiol, 164, 173
Ethmoid bone
  blood and nerve supply, 27–8
  foramen, 31
  histology, 27
  infundibulum, 22
  lymphatic drainage, 28
  ossification, 19
  osteology, 26
  uncinate process, 22
Ethmoid sinuses, 26
  comparative anatomy, 40
  development, 19
  osteology, 26
Ethmoidectomy
  nasal polyps, 65–6
  sinonasal papillomas, 78
Ethmoido-maxillo-orbito-malar complex, historical resections, 8–9
Ethmoturbinals, 35–6
Etoposide, 258
External fronto-ethmoidectomy, 329
Ewing's papilloma, 73
Ewing's sarcoma, 148–51
Eye
  maxillary sinus carcinoma, 98–100
  Wegener's granulomatosis, 288
  see also Orbit

Falx cerebri, 35
Familial haemorrhagic telangiectases (Osler-Rendu-Weber disease), 159–64
Farabeuf, 10
Fat suppression studies, 48–9
Fergusson, Sir William, 1, 4
  lion forceps, 5
  maxillectomy incision, 8
Fibro-osseus lesions, 223–4
Fibroblasts, 57
Fibromas, 135–6
  ameloblastic, 214
  historical, 3–4
  ossifying, 224–8
Fibromatosis, 135–6
  peripheral (schwannoma), 299–302
Fibromyxomas, 143
Fibrosarcoma, 136–9
Fibrous dysplasia, 228–32
  secondary osteogenic sarcoma, 246
Fistulas
  arteriovenous *see* Arteriovenous fistulas
  mucocoeles, 57
  oro-antral, 247
Fluorouracil
  maxillary sinus carcinoma, 100
  olfactory neuroblastoma, 316
Fontanelles, 22
Forceps, Fergusson's lion-jawed, 5
Formaldehyde
  malignant melanoma, 317
  nasal carcinoma, 88–9
Frontal bone, 29–30
Frontal sinus, 29–30
  development, 20
Fronto-ethmoidal mucocoeles, 55, 56–7, 60–62
Frontonasal processes, 17
Fungal infections, 66–9

Gadolinium DTPA, 47–50
Gadolinium-enhanced magnetic resonance, 43, 46–50
Gardner's syndrome, 239
Gensoul, P.J., 1